Low Back Pain: A Scientific and Clinical Overview

American Academy of Orthopaedic Surgeons

Based on a workshop

Supported by the
American Academy of Orthopaedic Surgeons

and the
North American Spine Society

and the
National Institute of Arthritis and Musculoskeletal and Skin Diseases

and the
Orthopaedic Research and Education Foundation

This workshop was also supported in part by educational grants from
Sofamor Danek Group
Synthes Spine
Electrobiology, Inc.
DePuy, Inc.
Smith & Nephew Richards, Inc.

Workshop Discussion Leaders and Section Editors
Gunnar B.J. Andersson, MD, PhD
Joseph A. Buckwalter, MS, MD
Richard A. Deyo, MD, MPH
Steven R. Garfin, MD
Edward N. Hanley, Jr, MD
Jeffrey N. Katz, MD, MS
Björn L. Rydevik, MD, PhD

Workshop
San Diego, California
November 1995

Low Back Pain: A Scientific and Clinical Overview

Edited by
James N. Weinstein, DO, MS
Professor of Surgery and Community and Family Medicine
Center for the Evaluative Clinical Sciences
Dartmouth Medical School
Hanover, New Hampshire

Stephen L. Gordon, PhD
Vice President
Advanced Technology Development
Osiris Therapeutics, Inc.
Baltimore, Maryland

American Academy of Orthopaedic Surgeons
6300 North River Road
Rosemont, IL 60018

American Academy of Orthopaedic Surgeons

Low Back Pain: A Scientific and Clinical Overview

The material presented in *Low Back Pain: A Scientific and Clinical Overview* has been made available by the American Academy of Orthopaedic Surgeons for educational purposes only. This material is not intended to present the only, or necessarily best, methods or procedures for the medical situations discussed, but rather is intended to represent an approach, view, statement, or opinion of the author(s) or producer(s), which may be helpful to others who face similar situations.

Some drugs and medical devices demonstrated in Academy courses or described in Academy print or electronic publications have Food and Drug Administration (FDA) clearance for use for specific purposes or for use only in restricted settings. The FDA has stated that it is the responsibility of the physician to determine the FDA status of each drug or device he or she wishes to use in clinical practice, and to use the products with appropriate patient consent and in compliance with applicable law.

At the time of this writing, bone screws placed posteriorly into vertebral elements have not been cleared for use in this specific manner by the Food and Drug Administration (FDA). These are Class III devices. This category includes screws placed transfacetally, within pedicles, or in articular, lateral masses. Some bone screws for use within the sacrum have been approved as Class II devices. Some companies have received Class II clearance for use of screws in lumbar pedicles specifically to supplement fusions in the treatment of grade III and IV spondylolisthesis with the proviso that these devices are removed after the arthrodesis has healed. Anterior vertebral body screws (cervical, thoracic, and lumbar) are Class II devices and can be used as labeled in vertebral bodies. Many of the posterior screw-based devices have been shown in laboratory and clinical testing to be useful and may be used in an off-label manner if the physician feels this is appropriate and important for the treatment of the patient. As with all surgeries, informed consent should explain the procedure and why a particular technique has been chosen, as well as its risks and benefits. The question of whether informed consent regarding pedicle screws must include a discussion of the device's FDA clearance status is currently being litigated in several jurisdictions. In cases that have been included in the multidistrict litigation in the Eastern District of Pennsylvania, this additional requirement has not been imposed.

Furthermore, any statements about commercial products are solely the opinion(s) of the author(s) and do not represent an Academy endorsement or evaluation of these products. These statements may not be used in advertising or for any commercial purpose.

The material contained in this volume was submitted as previously unpublished material, except in the instances in which credit has been given to the source from which some of the illustrative material was derived.

Materials appearing in this book prepared by individuals as part of their official duties as U.S. Government employees are not covered by the above-mentioned copyright.

First Edition
Copyright © 1996 by the American Academy of Orthopaedic Surgeons

ISBN: 0-89203-160-3

Library of Congress Cataloging-in-Publication Data

Low back pain : a scientific and clinical overview / edited by James
   N. Weinstein, Stephen L. Gordon ; workshop discussion leaders and
   section editors, Joseph A. Buckwalter . . . [et al.]. — 1st ed.
      p.   cm.
   "Workshop, San Diego, California, November 1995."
   Includes bibliographical references and index.
   ISBN 0-89203-160-3
   1. Backache—Congresses.   2. Backache—Pathophysiology—
Congresses.   I. Weinstein, James N.   II. Gordon, Stephen L.
III. Buckwalter, Joseph A.
   [DNLM: 1. Low Back Pain—etiology—congresses.   2. Spinal
Diseases—complications—congresses.   WE 755 L9124 1996]
RD771.B217L68   1996
617.5'64—dc21
DNLM/DLC
for Library of Congress   96-44528
                                                            CIP

American Academy of Orthopaedic Surgeons

Contributors and Participants

Howard An, MD†
  Associate Professor
  The Medical College of Wisconsin
  Milwaukee, Wisconsin

Gunnar B.J. Andersson, MD, PhD*†
  Professor and Chairman
  Department of Orthopaedic Surgery
  Rush-Presbyterian-St. Luke's Medical
    Center
  Chicago, Illinois

Shirley Ayad, BSc, PhD†
  School of Biological Sciences
  University of Manchester
  Manchester, England

Federico Balagué, MD†
  Médecin-Chief Adjoint
  Rheumatology, Physical Medicine and
    Rehabilitation Department
  Cantonal Hospital
  Fribourg, Switzerland

Michele Crites Battié, PhD*†
  Professor and Chairman
  Department of Physical Therapy
  Faculty of Rehabilitation Medicine
  University of Alberta
  Edmonton, Alberta, Canada

Michael T. Bayliss, PhD†
  Head, Division of Biochemistry
  Kennedy Institute of Rheumatology
  London, England

Gordon R. Bell, MD*†
  Head, Section of Spinal Surgery
  Department of Orthopaedic Surgery
  Cleveland Clinic Foundation
  Cleveland, Ohio

Edward C. Benzel, MD, FACS*†
  Division of Neurosurgery
  University of New Mexico School of
    Medicine
  Albuquerque, New Mexico

Scott D. Boden, MD*†
  Associate Professor of Orthopaedics
  Emory University School of Medicine
  Director, The Emory Spine Center
  Atlanta, Georgia

Nikolai Bogduk, MD, PhD, BSc*†
  Professor, Faculty of Medicine and Health
    Sciences
  University of Newcastle
  Newcastle, New South Wales, Australia

Joseph A. Buckwalter, MS, MD*†
  Professor of Orthopaedic Surgery
  University of Iowa
  Iowa City, Iowa

John M. Cavanaugh, MS, MD*†
  Wayne State University
  Bioengineering Center
  Detroit, Michigan

Ken-ichi Chatani, MD, PhD†
  Director, Department of Orthopaedic
    Surgery
  Kyoto Prefectural Yosanoumi Hospital
  Kyoto, Japan

Raymond W. Colburn, BS†
  Department of Pharmacology
  Dartmouth-Hitchcock Medical Center
  Lebanon, New Hampshire

Douglas A. Conrad, PhD*†
  Professor, Department of Health Services
  School of Public Health and Community
    Medicine
  University of Washington
  Seattle, Washington

Joyce A. DeLeo, PhD*†
  Assistant Professor of Anesthesiology and
    Pharmacology
  Dartmouth-Hitchcock Medical Center
  Lebanon, New Hampshire

Marshall Devor, PhD*†
  Department of Cell and Animal Biology
  Life Sciences Institute
  Hebrew University of Jerusalem
  Jerusalem, Israel

Richard A. Deyo, MD, MPH*†
  Professor of Medicine and Health Services
  University of Washington
  Seattle, Washington

Christopher H. Evans, PhD†
  Professor, Department of Orthopaedic
    Surgery
  Molecular Genetics and Biochemistry
  University of Pittsburgh School of
    Medicine
  Pittsburgh, Pennsylvania

Kenneth A. Follett, MD, PhD*†
  Associate Professor of Neurosurgery
  University of Iowa Hospitals and Clinics
  Iowa City, Iowa

Robert J. Foster, ScD†
  Associate Research Scientist
  Department of Orthopaedic Surgery
  Columbia University
  New York, New York

Steven R. Garfin, MD*†
  Professor of Orthopaedic Surgery
  University of California, San Diego
    Medical Center
  San Diego, California

Gerald F. Gebhart, PhD*†
  Professor of Pharmacology
  University of Iowa
  Iowa City, Iowa

Vijay K. Goel, PhD*†
  Professor and Chairman
  Department of Biomedical Engineering
  University of Iowa
  Iowa City, Iowa

Stephen L. Gordon, PhD*†
  Vice President
  Advanced Technology Development
  Osiris Therapeutics, Inc.
  Baltimore, Maryland

Scott Haldeman, MD, PhD*
  Department of Neurology
  University of California, Irvine
  Irvine, California

Edward N. Hanley, Jr, MD*†
  Chairman, Department of Orthopaedic
    Surgery
  Carolinas Medical Center
  Charlotte, North Carolina

Hiroshi Hashizume, MD†
  Clinical Physician
  Department of Orthopedic Surgery
  Wakayama Medical College
  Wakayama City, Wakayama, Japan

Victor M. Haughton, MD*†
  Professor of Radiology and Biophysics
  Medical College of Wisconsin
  Milwaukee, Wisconsin

Harry N. Herkowitz, MD*†
  Chairman, Department of Orthopaedic
    Surgery
  William Beaumont Hospital
  Royal Oak, Michigan

Richard J. Herzog, MD*†
  Associate Professor
  Department of Radiology
  University of Pennsylvania Medical
    Center
  Philadelphia, Pennsylvania

John P. Holland, MD, MPH†
  Clinical Assistant Professor
  Department of Orthopedics and
    Environmental Health
  University of Washington
  Seattle, Washington

James C. Iatridis, PhD†
  Postdoctoral Associate
  Department of Orthopaedics and
    Rehabilitation
  McClure Musculoskeletal Research Center
  University of Vermont
  Burlington, Vermont

Brian Johnstone, PhD*†
  Assistant Professor
  Department of Orthopaedics
  Case Western Reserve University
  Cleveland, Ohio

Parviz Kambin, MD*†
  Clinical Associate Professor of
    Orthopaedic Surgery
  University of Pennsylvania Medical
    School
  Philadelphia, Pennsylvania

James D. Kang, MD*†
  Assistant Professor, Orthopaedic Surgery
  Division of Spinal Surgery
  University of Pittsburgh School of
    Medicine
  Pittsburgh, Pennsylvania

Jaakko Kaprio, MD, PhD†
  Academy of Finland Senior Research
    Fellow
  Department of Public Health
  University of Helsinki
  Helsinki, Finland

Jeffrey N. Katz, MD, MS*†
  Assistant Professor of Medicine
  Harvard Medical School
  Division of Rheumatology
  Brigham & Women's Hospital
  Boston, Massachusetts

Mamoru Kawakami, MD, PhD*†
  Assistant, Department of Orthopaedic
    Surgery
  Wakayama Medical College
  Wakayama City, Wakayama, Japan

Shigeru Kobayashi, MD, PhD†
  Assistant Professor
  Department of Orthopaedic Surgery
  Fujita Health University
  Toyoake-City, Aichi, Japan

Martin Krag, MD*†
  Department of Orthopaedics and
    Rehabilitation
  McClure Musculoskeletal Research Center
    and Vermont Rehabilitation Engineering
    Center for Low Back Pain
  University of Vermont
  Burlington, Vermont

Richard L. Lieber, PhD*†
  Professor of Orthopaedics and
    Bioengineering
  University of California, San Diego and
    VA Medical Centers
  San Diego, California

Tae-Hong Lim, PhD†
  Assistant Professor
  Department of Orthopaedic Surgery
  Medical College of Wisconsin
  Milwaukee, Wisconsin

Jilan Liu, MD, MHA†
  J.R. & Associates, Inc.
  Seattle, Washington

Donlin M. Long, MD, PhD*
  Director, Department of Neurosurgery
  Johns Hopkins University Medical Center
  Baltimore, Maryland

James Martin, PhD†
  Research Scientist
  Department of Orthopaedic Surgery
  University of Iowa
  Iowa City, Iowa

Robert F. McLain, MD*†
  Associate Professor
  Department of Orthopaedic Surgery
  Director of Spine Research
  University of California, Davis
  Sacramento, California

Steven Demetrios Meletiou, MD*†
  Resident, Department of Orthopaedic
    Surgery
  University of Iowa Hospitals and Clinics
  Iowa City, Iowa

Tomofumi Morita, MD, PhD†
  Department of Orthopaedic Surgery
  Fujita Health University
  Toyoake-City, Aichi, Japan

Van C. Mow, PhD†
  Professor of Mechanical Engineering and
    Orthopaedic Bioengineering
  Departments of Mechanical Engineering
    and Orthopaedic Surgery
  Columbia University
  New York, New York

Robert R. Myers, PhD*†
  Professor
  VA Medical Center and the University of
    California, San Diego
  Departments of Anesthesiology and
    Pathology (Neuropathology)
  La Jolla, California

Sadaaki Nakai, MD, PhD†
  Assistant Professor
  Department of Orthopaedic Surgery
  Fujita Health University
  Toyoake-City, Aichi, Japan

Margareta Nordin, Dr Sci*†
  Director, Occupational Industrial
    Orthopaedic Center
  Hospital for Joint Diseases Orthopaedic
    Institute
  New York University Medical Center
  New York, New York

Bruce H. Nowicki, BS†
  Manager, Spine Research
  Medical College of Wisconsin
  Department of Radiology
  Milwaukee, Wisconsin

Theodore R. Oegema, Jr, PhD*†
  Professor, Departments of Orthopaedic
    Surgery and Biochemistry
  University of Minnesota
  Minneapolis, Minnesota

Kjell Olmarker, MD, PhD*†
  Lundberg Laboratory of Orthopaedics
  Department of Orthopaedics
  Gothenburg University
  Sahlgren Hospital
  Gothenburg, Sweden

James S. Panagis, MD, MPH*
  Program Director, Section on
    Orthopaedics, Musculoskeletal Disease
    Branch, Extramural Program
  National Institute of Arthritis and
    Musculoskeletal and Skin Diseases
  National Institutes of Health
  Bethesda, Maryland

Manohar M. Panjabi, PhD*†
  Professor and Director, Biomechanics
    Laboratory
  Yale University School of Medicine
  Department of Orthopaedics
  New Haven, Connecticut

Malcolm H. Pope, Dr Med Sci, PhD*†
  Professor and Director
  Iowa Spine Research Center
  University of Iowa
  Iowa City, Iowa

Jan K. Richardson, PT, PhD, OCS*†
  Director, Professor
  Graduate School of Physical Therapy
  Slippery Rock University
  Slippery Rock, Pennsylvania

Björn L. Rydevik, MD, PhD*†
  Associate Professor, Department of
    Orthopaedics
  Sahlgren Hospital
  Gothenburg University
  Gothenburg, Sweden

Jeffrey A. Saal, MD*
  Clinical Associate Professor
  Stanford University
  Stanford, California

Linda J. Sandell, PhD*†
  Professor
  Seattle Veterans Affairs Medical Center
  Seattle, Washington

Lori A. Setton, PhD†
  Assistant Professor
  Department of Biomedical Engineering
  Duke University
  Durham, North Carolina

Paul G. Shekelle, MD, PhD*†
  Assistant Professor of Medicine
  University of California, Los Angeles and
    West Los Angeles
  Veterans Administration Medical College
  Los Angeles, California

Naoyuki Shizu, MD†
  Department of Orthopaedic Surgery
  Fujita Health University
  Toyoake-City, Aichi, Japan

Kanwaldeep S. Sidhu, MD†
  Spine Surgery Fellow
  Department of Orthopaedic Surgery
  William Beaumont Hospital
  Royal Oak, Michigan

Kevin F. Spratt, PhD*
  Research Scientist
  Spine Diagnostic and Treatment Center
  University of Iowa Hospitals and Clinics
  Iowa City, Iowa

Keisuke Takahashi, MD, PhD*†
  Department of Orthopaedic Surgery
  Ishikawa Prefectural Central Hospital
  Kanazawa, Ishikawa, Japan

Tetsuya Tamaki, MD, PhD†
  Chairman, Professor
  Department of Orthopaedic Surgery
  Wakayama Medical College
  Wakayama City, Wakayama, Japan

Alexander R. Vaccaro, MD†
  Assistant Professor
  Department of Orthopaedics
  Thomas Jefferson University
  Philadelphia, Pennsylvania

Tapio Videman, MD, Dr Med Sci*†
  Professor in Sports Medicine
  Department of Health Sciences
  University of Jyväskylä
  Jyväskylä, Finland

Mark Weidenbaum, MD*†
  Associate Professor
  Department of Orthopaedic Surgery
  College of Physicians and Surgeons
  Columbia University
  New York, New York

James N. Weinstein, DO, MS*†
  Professor of Surgery and Community and
    Family Medicine
  Center for the Evaluative Clinical
    Sciences
  Dartmouth Medical School
  Hanover, New Hampshire

Hidezo Yoshizawa, MD, PhD*†
  Professor and Chairman
  Department of Orthopaedic Surgery
  Fujita Health University
  Toyoake-City, Aichi, Japan

Hansen A. Yuan, MD*
  Professor, State University of New York
  Health Science Center at Syracuse
  Syracuse, New York

* Workshop Participant
† Contributor to Volume

Preface

This book is based on a workshop entitled "New Horizons in Low Back Pain" that was held in November 1995 in San Diego, California. This was the third in a series of three workshops on low back pain spanning the past 15 years. Each workshop has been sponsored by the American Academy of Orthopaedic Surgeons and the National Institute of Arthritis and Musculoskeletal and Skin Diseases (NIAMS), National Institutes of Health. This workshop had significant support from the North American Spine Society (NASS) and the Orthopaedic Research and Education Foundation (OREF). The workshop was also supported in part by educational grants from Sofamor Danek Group, Synthes Spine, Electrobiology, Inc., DePuy, Inc., and Smith & Nephew Richards, Inc. There was a large and valuable effort put forth by the book editors and the section leaders, the contributors and workshop participants, and the publishing staff. We would like to thank Marilyn Fox, PhD, Director of the Department of Publications; Lisa Moore, associate senior editor who was responsible for organizing and managing this project; Bruce Davis, senior editor, and Joan Abern, associate senior editor, who assisted in editing the manuscripts; Loraine Edwalds, production manager, and Sophie Tosta, production coordinator, who oversaw the smooth flow of manuscripts through the production process. We would also like to acknowledge the efforts of Jana Ronayne, production assistant, and Geraldine Dubberke and Thomas Pender, publications secretaries.

The first workshop, entitled "Idiopathic Low Back Pain" was held in December 1980 in Miami, Florida. The subsequent book was published in 1982. Co-chairpersons were Augustus A. White III and Stephen L. Gordon. The effort was organized along classic scientific disciplines: epidemiology, anatomy, biomechanics, biochemistry, and neurology. There was a broad understanding of the tissue properties and possible mechanisms to explain low back pain. A clear pathophysiology was not known in most patients. Therefore, more research was needed.

The second workshop, "New Directions in Low Back Pain Research", was held in May 1988 in Airlie, Virginia. The resulting book, *New Perspectives in Low Back Pain,* was published in 1989. This project was designed to consider clinical and basic science issues of four anatomic components of the lumbar spine—nerves, intervertebral disks, posterior support structures, and muscles. Many advances had been achieved since the first workshop, yet there were still many unanswered questions.

The format of the 1995 symposium was that of a case study model. On each day, clinical issues were discussed in the morning, with afternoon sessions devoted to the basic science related to the clinical problem. A summary of the chapters in each section was presented by the section leader. This overview served as a nidus for a 2-hour discussion, represented by the overview and future directions as presented at the beginning and end of each section in this book.

Finally, the group addressed clinical questions that are often asked by the lay public or journalists who seek more information about this very common and costly condition. The topics were based on issues and questions often noted in public inquiries to the NIAMS. The summary of these discussions is presented at the end of this book.

Overall, there is a tremendous need for expanded research. Low back pain is the second most common cause for seeing a doctor, at a cost of $30 billion a year. Interdisciplinary treatment and research efforts appear to be the most rewarding. Studies of biomechanics, muscle, neurophysiology, pathology, anatomy, epidemiology, and biostatistics, as well as clinical and diagnostic medicine, are needed in order to find solutions to a problem for which there are currently few answers. The efforts of all contributors and workshop participants are greatly appreciated. This book by leading academic clinicians and scientists is a thorough compendium of current knowledge, but also details gaps in knowledge. The new findings and new models presented throughout this book provide strong encouragement for the next period of research.

JAMES N. WEINSTEIN, DO, MS
STEPHEN L. GORDON, PHD

Table of Contents

Section One

Epidemiologic and Clinical Issues of Lumbar Radiculopathy

Section Editors:
Richard A. Deyo, MD, MPH
Gunnar B.J. Andersson, MD, PhD

Federico Balagué, MD
Michele Crites Battié, PhD
Scott D. Boden, MD
Douglas A. Conrad, PhD
Edward N. Hanley, Jr, MD
John P. Holland, MD, MPH
Parviz Kambin, MD

Jaakko Kaprio, MD, PhD
Jilan Liu, MD, MHA
Robert F. McLain, MD
Margareta Nordin, PT, Dr Sci
Tapio Videman, MD, Dr Med
  Sci

Overview

Epidemiology and Natural History of Herniated Disks

Disk herniation with sciatica is certainly less common than simple low back pain, although studies of prevalence are plagued by methodologic problems. Epidemiologic studies, which are often vague and based on reports of hospitalization for sciatica or on symptom reports that have not been confirmed, provide varying results. Thus, the reported prevalence of sciatica ranges from 1% to 24%, although studies reporting a lifetime prevalence of 1% to 3% in the general population may be more accurate. The reliability of epidemiologic studies is also compromised by a dissociation between the anatomic finding and the clinical syndrome, because imaging studies show evidence of herniated disks in over 20% of normal, asymptomatic persons.

Wide variations in medical care, and especially in surgical rates (numbers of procedures), are observed geographically, and cannot be explained by differences in the prevalence of back problems. A number of risk factors have been identified for sciatica, including personal characteristics such as age, height, and obesity, but also occupational factors such as heavy lifting and vibration. Familial aggregation is striking, although the relative contribution of genetics and environment remains unclear. Spinal morphology plays a role in the likelihood of symptomatic disk herniations, because conditions such as a narrow canal can lead to back problems. Disk herniations in the cervical spine are less common than in the lumbar spine, but some of the risk factors are similar.

The natural history of disk herniations is quite favorable, with symptomatic improvement in nearly half of afflicted persons within 2 weeks and approximately 70% recovery after 6 weeks. Clinical studies also show good resolution of at least minor neurologic deficits even in the absence of surgery.

Exercise in the Prevention and Treatment of Herniated Disks

Exercise might be a valuable physiologic factor in preventing intervertebral disk herniations. Exercise improves circulation and disk metabolism, mechanical loading in childhood development, and the role of motion and activity in the healing process. Epidemiologic studies suggest that leisure time activity does not predict the likelihood of a herniated disk or of sciatica. An increased incidence of herniated disks is identified in athletes in some sports, but this incidence varies with the sport. Studies of the association between exercise and sciatica are also affected by the unreliability of past exercise reports. Overall, there is little evidence of either a preventive or a causal effect of exercise in annular degeneration, nerve root entrapment, or healing rate. There may be metabolic benefits of exercise on the disk, although any possible preventive or therapeutic mechanisms remain speculative.

Diagnostic Considerations

The history and physical examination usually suggest the possibility of radiculopathy in a patient complaining of back or leg pain. Although a history of sciatica is usually the first indication of radiculopathy, the definition of sciatica is not well standardized and there is no consistent operational definition in research studies. Straight leg raising signs are useful in the diagnosis of radiculopathy, although the ipsilateral straight leg raise is sensitive, though not specific, while the crossed straight leg raise is specific but not sensitive. Isolated neurologic findings are of limited value in distinguishing patients with and without radiculopathy, but combinations of findings may be substantially more valuable.

Because of the high prevalence of abnormal anatomic findings in asymptomatic persons, imaging results must always be closely correlated with clinical findings. Symptoms of disk herniation often resolve during the first 8 to 12 weeks of care; therefore, advanced imaging tests are generally unnecessary until surgery is being considered. Other important issues in imaging include the timing of studies, the choice of an optimal study, and the need for invasive investigations.

Therapeutic Interventions

Epidural steroids have become a popular treatment for disk herniations, acting to impede a number of inflammatory mediators in and around the affected nerve root. Unfortunately, there is enormous variability in the techniques reported, a wide variety of indications, and few controlled trials. Available studies have conflicting results, but overall suggest a small clinical effect of epidural steroid injections. Intrathecal injections should be avoided because of the risk of arachnoiditis. The need for rigorous randomized trials of epidural injections is still apparent.

It seems clear that surgical diskectomy can accelerate relief of symptoms for carefully selected patients with disk herniations who have symptoms persisting beyond 6 weeks. However, there is little evidence to demonstrate which diskectomy technique is optimal, and a number of techniques are now available. There is little evidence to suggest that spinal fusion is indicated for patients who undergo a primary diskectomy. The value of fusion in patients undergoing repeat diskectomy is less clear, although rigorous studies to support its use are lacking. Arthroscopic disk surgery is growing in popularity, and allows a direct visualization of the disks, nerve roots, and dural sac. Arthroscopic techniques are now also being studied for certain patients with lateral recess stenosis and for some patients undergoing spinal fusion. The technique is also useful for obtaining material for culture and debridement when disk space infection is suspected. However, arthroscopic techniques have not yet been rigorously compared to those of standard diskectomy clinical trials.

Costs of Care for Patients With Herniated Disks

The Agency for Health Care Policy and Research (AHCPR) has provided general strategies for the early identification of patients with radicular symptoms and their evaluation and treatment. This guideline also deals with isolated low back pain and the problem of identifying patients with underlying systemic diseases. In an analysis of a hypothetical strategy based on the guideline, it has been found that compared with current practice (based on insurance claims), the AHCPR guideline might reduce by 38% the overall costs of care for back pain. However, this result is sensitive to the assumptions as to how frequently magnetic resonance imaging (MRI) is performed to rule out underlying infection or cancer; what proportion of patients will experience persistent neurologic symptoms and functional limitation beyond 4 weeks of care; and the proportion of such patients who chose surgical over nonsurgical care. Very recent studies suggest that the cost effectiveness of lumbar diskectomy in carefully selected patients, as measured by cost per quality-adjusted life year, may be comparable to many widely accepted medical treatments, such as treatment of moderate hypertension.

Summary

There is general agreement that the data on which many clinical decisions regarding prevention, diagnosis, and treatment of disk herniations are based is inadequate. More randomized, controlled trials of treatment methods (surgical and nonsurgical) are needed. These studies should use strict inclusion and exclusion criteria. For some strategies, the timing of intervention may be an important study variable. Outcome measures must be further developed, and outcomes assessed by blinded observers. We also need to further assess the value of our diagnostic methods: history and physical examination, imaging, and neurophysiologic tests. Many of these methods have poorly defined reproducibility, and the validity, sensitivity, and predictive value of each remains unclear. Preventing herniated disks is problematic because risk factors remain uncertain, with a few exceptions. Preventing disability as a result of the herniated disk may be a more fruitful approach, as would preventing recurrences.

Patients with classic symptoms and signs of disk herniation and confirmatory imaging studies in whom conservative treatment has failed respond well to surgical intervention. Spontaneous recovery is slow after 3 months. For patients without the classic symptoms and signs and whose imaging studies are suggestive but not conclusive, the results of surgery are poor.

Because of the high prevalence of herniation in asymptomatic populations, surgery based on imaging alone might be considered an illogical treatment choice.

Chapter 1

Intervertebral Disk Herniation: Epidemiology and Natural History

Gunnar B.J. Andersson, MD, PhD

Epidemiologic research on disk herniations is limited because of disagreement on definition and classification of cases. Further, because all disk herniations are not symptom-producing, and cross-sectional and longitudinal studies of asymptomatic patients using modern imaging techniques are impractical, most data are based on either symptom reports or insurance and hospital data. Acknowledging the difficulties in defining cases, symptomatic disk herniations are better researched than back pain in general from an epidemiologic perspective. In this review, I will discuss the incidence and prevalence of "sciatic and/or rhizopathic symptoms," hospital and surgical data, risk factor data, imaging information, and limited information about the natural history of disk herniations. Most literature is concerned with the lumbar spine, and some with the cervical spine, while very little is known about the epidemiology of thoracic disk herniations. This chapter is, in part, based on a previous review.[1]

Incidence and Prevalence of Sciatic and/or Rhizopathic Symptoms

Early studies typically defined sciatica as pain radiating from the back down one or both legs. Using such a definition, the Arthritis and Rheumatism Council of the United Kingdom surveyed a large cross section of the population in the 1950s. Sciatica, suggestive of a herniated disk, was found in 3.1% of all men and 1.3% of women.[2] The highest prevalence, 9.6%, was in 55- to 64-year-old men, while for women the peak prevalence was 5% occurring after the age of 64. Much higher numbers were reported in a cross-sectional study of 15- to 71-year-old women that was performed in Gothenburg, Sweden.[3] Almost 14% of all women had "referred leg pain of the sciatica type." The highest prevalence was 22.4% among women aged 45 to 54 years. A contemporary Copenhagen survey of 4,753, 50- to 59-year-old men reports a 1-year prevalence of 11%.[4]

More recent studies report very high prevalence rates of sciatica. In a sample of 295 male, 15- to 64-year-old, Finnish concrete reinforcement workers, 42% of the men and as many as 60% of those aged 45 years or older reported a lifetime history of sciatica.[5] Five years later, the lifetime prevalence of all men had increased to 59%.[6-8] At that time, a reference group of house painters had a lifetime prevalence of 42%. The 5-year incidence of sciatica was 34% among the concrete workers, compared to 23% among the house painters. In these studies, predictors of sciatica were occupation (risk ratio (RR) 1.5), history of back accidents (RR 2.0), and previous low back pain (RR 3.9). Body height and stress were weakly associated with sciatic pain, whereas abdominal and back muscle strength, body mass index, and smoking were not. The studies performed on the concrete reinforcement workers[5-8] suggest that the risk of sciatica is increased in workers performing heavy physical work. Other studies support this.[9-11] Confounding factors may exist, however, and the level at which physical workload becomes dangerous is not determined.

Other Finnish studies of female health care workers confirm the high prevalence of sciatica. Random samples of 764 Finnish female nurses and 453 nursing aides were studied.[12] Thirty-eight percent of the nurses and 43% of the nursing aides had experienced pain of sciatic distribution at least once previously. Reports of six or more previous episodes were given by 18% of the nurses and 23% of the nursing aides. Among 370 Finnish nursing school applicants (average age 22.1 years), 5% reported a previous history of sciatic pain.[13]

United States cross-sectional studies report similar prevalence rates. Hrubec and Nashold[9] studied 1,095 army hospital admissions for herniated nucleus pulposus (HNP), and compared those to age and service period matched holders of Army National Service life insurance policies. Factors associated with hospital admission were occupation of craftsman or foreman, marital status, rural residence, above average height, obesity, large frame, good posture, ground combat military occupation, and rank of sergeant or staff sergeant. A negative association was found with clerical occupation, earned battle stars, and officer rank. Essentially the same relationships were found among a subgroup who had surgically confirmed HNP.

Kelsey[14-19] studied women and men aged 20 to 64 years residing in the New Haven, Connecticut area who had lumbar radiographs taken over a 2-year period for suspected HNP. The sample was divided into two groups: those with surgically confirmed herniated disks, and those who had probable or possible herniated disks based on clinical signs and symptoms. A case-control design was used, and two control groups were employed. One control group was patients admitted to emergency rooms for reasons other than back pain and matched for sex and age; the second group was patients who had radiographs of their spines, but who did not have symptoms and signs of a disk herniation. Associations were found between disk herniations and sedentary occupations; driving of motor vehicles; chronic cough and chronic bronchitis; lack of physical exercise; participation in baseball, golf, and bowling; suburban residence; and pregnancy. Jobs involving lifting, pushing, and pulling were not found to be associated with increased risk of HNP.[14-16,19-21]

Kelsey and associates[10,22,23] later performed another case-control study in Connecticut with minor methodologic modifications. The study population was 20- to 64-year-old women and men who had had radiographs and myelograms. A control group of nonback patients admitted for in-hospital services was matched for sex and age. In contrast to Kelsey's earlier studies, frequent lifting of heavy objects and twisting were both identified as significant risk factors (Table 1).[10,22,23] The odds ratio for HNP in subjects performing frequent lift-

Table 1 Odds ratios for association between a prolapsed lumbar disk and lifting of 11.3 kg[10,22,47]

Variable	Frequency	Odds Ratio
No lifting	—	1.10
Lifting	< 5	0.8
	5-25	0.9
	> 25	3.8
Lifting and twisting*	< 5	3.0
	5-25	1.9
	> 25	3.4

*Twisting refers to a situation where a twist occurs half or more of the time when lifting

ing of heavy weights while twisting was 3.4. The number of hours spent in a motor vehicle and smoking were also associated with an increased risk, whereas pregnancy, height, weight, and participation in sports were not.[10] The risk of HNP was also found to be related to the type of vehicle used.[22]

Data from the United States National Health Interview Surveys (1985-1988)[24] reveal that 4.1 million persons annually report "intervertebral disk disorders." Men are more likely to report these disorders than women (2% compared to 1.5%). The highest prevalence rate was found in the 45- to 64-year-old age group (23.7/100 persons).

Heliövaara and associates[25-28] surveyed a sample of 8,000 persons representative of the Finnish population aged 30 years or older. They carefully defined a diagnosis "lumbar disk syndrome (LDS)" based on medical history, symptom history, and a standardized physical examination. Lumbar disk syndrome was found in 5.3% of men and 3.7% of women. In both sexes the prevalence rates were highest in the 45- to 64-year age group. The prevalences for definite herniated disks were 1.9% for men and 1.3% for women, while 0.2% of both sexes had a probable HNP (Table 2). Disability as a result of LDS was estimated at 3.5% in men and 4.5% in women. At clinical examination, 56% of the patients were at least slightly limited in their performance of daily activities, while 5% were severely limited.

Table 2 Prevalence (%) of lumbar disk syndrome and other low back syndromes by sex (age adjusted)[27]

Diagnosis	Men	Women
Lumbar disk syndrome	5.3	3.8
Herniated nucleus pulposus (HNP)		
Definite	1.9	1.3
Probable	0.2	0.2
Sciatica		
Definite	1.9	1.3
Probable	1.3	1.0
Other low back pain (LBP)	12.5	13.2

Hospitalizations and Operations

Generalizations from studies based on surgical samples are difficult, because multiple factors other than disease severity influence the decision to perform surgery. Further, the benign clinical history of a herniation means many will recover spontaneously or at least without surgery. The diagnosis in patients who have had surgery is more definite, however.

In a review of 15,235 operations, Spangfort[29] found that 46.9% involved the L5-S1 level and 49.8% the L4-5 level, whereas 3.3% were performed at higher levels. In his own case material, which included 2,504 operations, the distribution was 50.5% L5-S1, 47.4% L4-5, and 2.1% at higher lumbar levels. While the peak incidence of operations was around age 40, the proportions of herniations occurring at different levels were age dependent. At a younger age most herniations were at L5-51, while from age 40 or older, L4/L5 herniations were the most common. The proportions of herniations at higher levels increased with advancing age (Fig. 1).

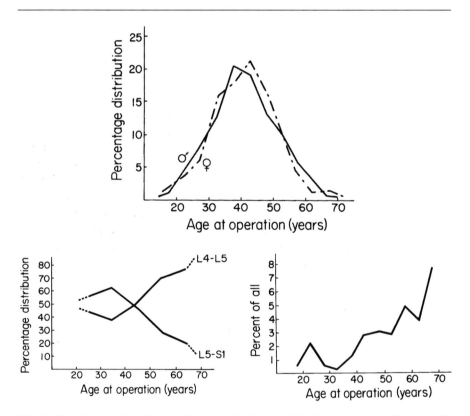

Fig. 1 **Top,** *Percent distribution of surgery for lumbar disks by age and sex.* **Bottom left,** *Percent distribution of operations for herniated lumbar disks by age and level.* **Bottom right,** *Incidence of high lumbar herniations (above L4) by age at operation. (Reproduced with permission from Spangfort EV: The lumbar disc herniation: A computer-aided analysis of 2,504 operations.* Acta Orthop Scand *1972;142(suppl):1–95.)*

Heliövaara and associates[29] studied hospital admission records for HNP and sciatica in a group of 57,000 Finnish women and men who had participated in screening examinations over a period of 11 years (1966 to 1977). Using various social and health registers they attempted to identify factors predicting back diseases. For each case accepted into the study, four control subjects matched for sex, age, and place of residence were selected. A total of 1,537 subjects were hospitalized because of back disease during the 558,074 person-years of follow-up. The discharge diagnosis was HNP, 30%; sciatica, 24%; and other back disease, 46%. Men had a 1.6-fold increased risk of HNP compared to women, and a 1.3-fold increased risk of sciatica (Table 3). The risk of HNP was higher in tall people of both sexes; in obese men but not obese women; in men who were industrial workers and motor vehicle drivers (Fig. 2); in women who did "strenuous work," were smokers, or had multiple pregnancies; and in subjects with symptoms indicating physical distress.[25-28] Marital status and leisure time physical activities were not risk factors. The relative risk of HNP and sciatica was lower in rural than in urban areas. The main influences on risk were sex, occupation, workload, and body height; the other factors were of lesser predictive importance.

In the United States, 125 persons per 100,000 population were discharged from acute care hospitals with a first-listed diagnosis of herniated lumbar intervertebral disk in 1983.[30] Men were hospitalized more often than women; 151.7 per 100,000 for men and 99.9 per 100,000 for women. The rate of hospitalization increased with patient age. The rate for persons aged 15 to 44 years was 157.2, whereas it was 213.4 per 100,000 in the 45- to 64-year age group.

Table 3 Multivariate relative risk (RR) of herniated intervertebral disk (herniated nucleus pulposus; HNP) or sciatica: Case-control studies[25-28]

Factors	RR HNP	RR sciatica (including HNP)
Sex		
Women	1.0	1.0
Men	1.6	0.3
Occupation		
White collar	1.0	1.0
Men		
Motor vehicle drivers	2.9	4.6
Metal workers	3.0	4.2
Construction	2.4	3.1
Women		
Nurses	2.2	1.5
Housewives	0.4	0.8
Height		
Men (180 cm or taller)	2.3	
Women (170 cm or taller)	3.7	

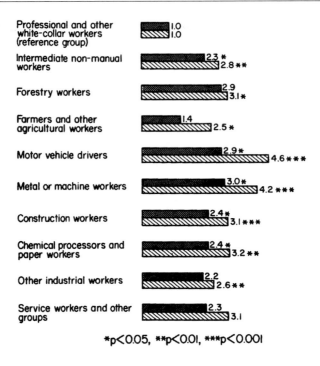

*p<0.05, **p<0.01, ***p<0.001

Fig. 2   *Relative risk of herniated lumbar intervertebral disk (dotted columns) and of herniated disk or sciatica combined (lined columns) in men. (Reproduced with permission from Heliövaara M:* Epidemiology of Sciatica and Herniated Lumbar Intervertebral Disc. *Helsinki, Finland, Social Insurance Institution, 1988.)*

Volinn and associates[31] examined the National Hospital Discharge Survey from 1979 though 1987. The rate of low back surgery in the United States increased 49% over that time period, while the rate of nonsurgical low back pain hospitalization decreased by 33% (Fig. 3). The average length of stay decreased for both surgical and nonsurgical admissions. Table 4 from Deyo and associates[32] further illustrates the dramatic increase in back operations in the United States. The number of fusions increased more than laminectomies or diskectomies. Volinn and associates[31] also reported that in 1987 the rate of surgery ranged regionally from 77 per 100,000 adults in the northeastern region to 146 per 100,000 in the southern region. Apparently, cultural differences and prac-

Table 4   Rates of selected back operations in the United States per 100,000 of general population[32]

Procedure	1979	1981	1983	1985	1987	% Increase
Laminectomy	31	36	41	41	38	23
Diskectomy	59	57	81	96	103	75
Lumbar fusion	5	9	10	18	15	200

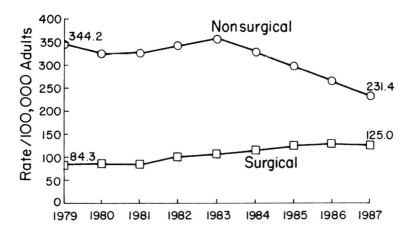

Fig. 3 *Low back hospitalization in the U.S. per 100,000 adults. (Reproduced with permission from Volinn E, Turczyn KM, Loeser JD: Patterns in low back pain hospitalizations: Implications for the treatment of low back pain in an era of health care reform.* Clin J Pain *1994;10:64–70.)*

tice patterns have a major influence on hospitalizations and procedures. Taylor and associates[33] extended the analysis of the National Hospital Survey Data through 1990. Their data indicate a further increase in the number of surgical procedures from 1987 to 1990. Over the 11-year time period, adult low back operations increased by 55% from 147,500 (1979) to 279,000 (1990); an increase from 102 to 158 per 100,000 adults. Fusions increased by 100% from 13 to 26 per 100,000, but the more common nonfusion operations increased as well by 47% from 89 to 131 per 100,000. In 1990 there were 46,500 lumbar fusions and 232,500 low back operations without fusion in the United States. Increases in the number of operations were particularly great for patients aged 60 years and older (Fig. 4). Nonsurgical hospitalizations decreased from 402 per 100,000 in 1979 to 150 per 100,000 in 1990. The average back surgery rates for 1988 to 1990 were lowest in the West (113 per 100,000 adults) and highest in the South (171 per 100,000 adults) (Fig. 5). The same regional differences were found for nonsurgical hospitalizations as well.

Available data suggest marked intercountry variations in rates of back surgery.[32,34] The number of surgical procedures for HNP in Sweden has remained stable at 20 per 100,000 inhabitants per year from the mid-1950s through 1980s.[35] The corresponding number in Finland (1967-1977) was 35,[28] and in Great Britain, 10.[36,37] The number of people operated on for HNP per 100,000 per year in the U.S. has been variable, assessed in the past as ranging between 45 to 90.[21,38,39] The data by Taylor and associates[33] reveal that in 1990 the rate was 131 per 100,000 per year. A recent international comparison of the rates of back surgery from 13 countries reveals the rate in the United States is at least 40% higher than in any other country, and more than five times that of Scotland and England[34] (Fig. 6). Differences in the underlying prevalence of back pain were not believed to explain the differences in surgical rates. Cultural differences and practice patterns are more likely explanations.

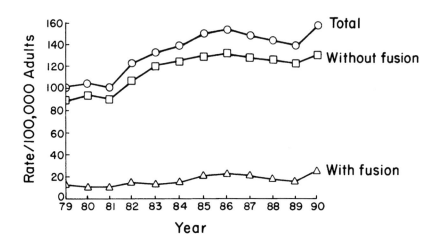

Fig. 4 *Low back surgery rates per 100,000 adults, by age, 1979-1990. (Reproduced with permission from Taylor VM, Deyo RA, Cherkin DC, et al: Low back pain hospitalization: Recent United States trends and regional variations. Spine 1994;19:1207–1213.)*

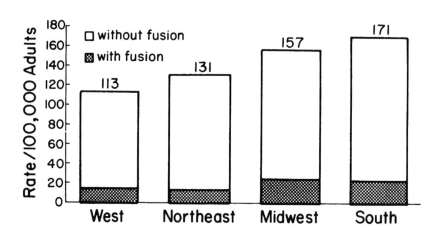

Fig. 5 *Annual low back surgery rates per 100,000 adults divided by region (averages 1988-1990). (Reproduced with permission from Taylor VM, Deyo RA, Cherkin DC, et al: Low back pain hospitalization: Recent United States trends and regional variations. Spine 1994;19:1207–1213.)*

Individual Factors and Herniated Nucleus Pulposus

The relative role of genetic and environmental factors in sciatica was studied in a nationwide Finnish twin cohort. Environmental factors explained more than 80% of the etiology of sciatica[40] and low back pain.[12] Thus, the common low back syndromes seem to be mainly caused by environmental factors,

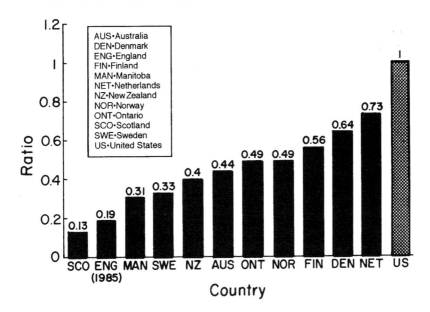

Fig. 6 *Ratios of back surgery rates in 11 countries and Canadian states compared to the back surgery rate in the U.S. (1988-89). (Reproduced with permission from Cherkin DC, Deyo RA, Loeser JD, et al: An international comparison of back surgery rates.* Spine *1994;19:1201–1206.)*

although a familial predisposition to lumbar herniated disks has been reported.[41-44]

As discussed, age is a major factor influencing the prevalence of sciatica, rhizopathy, and herniated disk operations. Although older individuals have more symptoms,[2,24-28] the majority of operations are in patients 35 to 50 years old[28,29] (Fig. 1). Operations for lumbar disk herniations are performed 1.5 to 3 times as often in men as in women.[19,28,29,45,46] Cervical herniations are most frequent in the fourth decade of life, and both symptoms and surgical procedures are more frequent in men than women.[47,48]

Height and weight have been studied as possible risk factors for sciatica and disk herniation. Hrubec and Nashold[9] found that body height was a predictor of herniated lumbar disks among army recruits. Heliövaara[25,28] found body height to be a significant predictor of HNP in both women and men. In tall men (taller than 179 cm) the relative risk (RR) was 2.3, and in tall women (taller than 169 cm) 3.7 in relation to subjects who were at least 10 cm shorter (RR 1.0). Riihimaki and associates[8] found a weak correlation between tallness (taller than 180 cm versus shorter than 169 cm) and the lifetime prevalence of sciatica (RR 1.7), but not with the 5-year incidence. A case control study of 15-year-old children using magnetic resonance imaging identified more disk protrusions among taller children.[49] Although in summary, tallness appears to be a risk factor for sciatica and herniated disks, all studies do not agree. Kelsey[14] did not observe differences in height between disk patients and controls. The significance of obesity to the occurrence of HNP is even more complex. Heliövaara[25,28] found that a moderately increased body mass index predicted the development of HNP in men but not in women, whereas severe obesity appeared to carry less than moderate risk. Body mass index was not a predictor of risk of sciatica in the study by Riihimaki and associates.[8] Hrubec and Nashold,[9] on the other hand, report that above average patient weight at enrollment into military service predicted a higher risk of developing a lumbar disk herniation.

Patients with sciatica or prolapsed disks have been found to have more narrow canals than control groups.[50,51] It is possible that smaller canal diameters make smaller disk herniations more clinically important.

The role of physical exercises is another uncertain area. Kelsey[14,15] found "insufficient physical exercise," as well as baseball, golf, and bowling, to be associated with the occurrence of prolapsed lumbar disks. But Weber[46] reported an unexpectedly low percentage of physically active men in his study of patients with herniated disks, and Hurme and associates[52] found no difference in recreational physical leisure activities between patients operated on for HNP and the general population.

Smoking has been found to be associated with HNP.[14] Whether smoking is in fact a risk factor or only a confounding factor remains unclear. Kelsey and associates[23] reported an increased risk of developing a herniated disk of 20% with ten cigarettes smoked per day in the previous year (odds ratio, 1.2).

Cervical Herniated Disks

Kondo and associates[48] determined the incidence of cervical disk herniations in Rochester, Minnesota, from 1950 through 1974, based on medical records from medical facilities. Residence in Rochester for at least 1 year was required of subjects studied. Both protrusions and herniations were accepted as long as they caused radicular symptoms. A total of 56 cases met the criteria. The annual incidence rates by sex were 6.5 and 4.6 per 100,000 for men and women, respectively, for a combined incidence of 5.5 per 100,000. The incidence for both sexes was highest between 45 and 54 years of age and slightly lower between the ages of 35 and 44 years. C5-6 was the disk most frequently affected, followed by C4-5 and C6-7.

Kelsey and associates[47] surveyed people aged 20 to 64 years in New Haven and Hartford, Connecticut, who were identified as having a prolapsed cervical disk as determined by radiographs and myelograms performed between 1979 and 1981. Patients were divided into three groups: a surgical group, a probable group, and a possible group. People in the fourth decade of life were affected somewhat more often than individuals in other age groups. Men were more frequently affected than women with a ratio of 1.4. C5-6 and C6-7 were the affected disks in 75% of patients. Twenty-three percent of disks were believed to be related to a car accident. The odds ratio was calculated for a number of factors, and comparatively high ratios were found for frequent lifting, cigarette smoking, and frequent diving from a board (Table 5). Operating of vibrating equipment and driving or time spent in motor vehicles were weak positive associations. Factors not associated with increased risk were participation in sports other than diving, number of pregnancies and live births, frequent twisting of the neck at work, prolonged sitting, wearing high heels, and smoking of cigars and pipes.

Table 5 Adjusted odds ratio for association between several factors and a prolapsed cervical disk[10]

Factor	Odds Ratio
Lifting	
0 times	1.0
< 5	1.6
5-25	2.7
> 25	4.9
Smoking	1.7
Diving	
< 10 times	1.0
10-25	2.3
> 25	4.9
Golfing	2.0
Operating vibrating equipment	2.0

Herniations on Imaging

A few studies exist in which imaging has been performed in healthy individuals to determine the prevalence of pathologic changes, including disk herniations. For the lumbar spine, myelography, diskography, and computed tomography have all shown prevalences of herniated disks ranging from 19% to 27%[53-55] in spite of absence of symptoms. More recently, magnetic resonance imaging has permitted larger patient samples and better definitions of herniations. Boden and associates[56] performed imaging in 67 individuals who had never had symptoms. These scans were independently reviewed by three "blinded" neuroradiologists. Of subjects younger than 60 years of age, 20% had a herniated disk, while 36% of those 60 years and older had herniations. Most (84%) of the herniated disks were at L4-5 or L5-S1. A subsequent study by Jensen and associates[57] included 98 asymptomatic patients. Careful definition of what constituted a herniation and division of findings into bulges, protrusions, and extrusions provided additional information. Twenty-seven percent of the subjects had a protrusion, one an extrusion. The findings were similar in men and women. Age did not influence the prevalence up to 60 years. The L4-5 and L5-S1 disks were again those most frequently herniated (75%).

Boden and associates[58] obtained images of the cervical spine in asymptomatic individuals as well. Sixty-three volunteers participated. In 10% of 40 individuals younger than 40 years of age, a herniated disk was identified, while in the older than 40 years population (n = 23), the corresponding percentage was 5. For the whole group, this means a prevalence of 8%.

Although the imaging information is helpful to determine prevalences, it should be remembered that all symptomatic individuals were excluded, making the data an underestimate. Further, the populations are not cross-sectional. Even so, the high prevalence indicates that herniations are more common than suspected from clinical and surgical reports.

Natural History of Disk Herniation

The natural history of sciatica and disk herniation is not quite as favorable as for simple low back pain, yet is still excellent. About 50% of patients recover in the first 2 weeks, 70% in 6 weeks.[59] Hakelius[60] treated patients with sciatica with a corset and rest. Thirty-eight percent improved in the first month, 52% in the second, and 73% by 3 months. Weber[46] reported that 25% of patients admitted with a documented disk herniation improved after a 2-week hospital stay. However, 25% remained significantly symptomatic and were operated on. The remaining 126 patients were randomized to nonsurgical and surgical treatment. At 1 year, good results were found in 90% of surgically treated patients compared to 60% in the conservative group. Seventeen patients in that group had been operated on because of intolerable pain. At 4 and 10 years, the results were similar in the two groups. Return of muscle function was the same irrespective of treatment at 10 years, as was sensory function, which remained abnormal in 35%. These neurologic findings were confirmed by Saal and Saal,[61] who followed 58 patients with herniated disks, 52 of whom were treated without surgery. After 31 months, 93% had returned to work, and 96% reported "good" or "excellent" outcome. Only three of 15 patients with extruded fragments required surgery.

Only a small percentage of individuals with sciatica require surgery. One cross-sectional study reported a lifetime incidence of sciatica of 40%, but a lifetime incidence of disk surgery of 1% to 2%.[62] In patients with documented lumbar disk herniations, surgery has a favorable influence on the natural history measured by symptom reduction and return to work.[46] Yet, long-term pain and function were minimally influenced in this study. Hurme and Alaranta[63] reported better results in patients operated on during the first 2 months than later. Initially, treating patients without surgery takes advantage of the favorable natural history. The optimal time for surgery remains unclear. The risk of developing chronic pain increases after the third month. Recurrences of sciatica are common, but the incidence is less well reported than that for acute low back pain. Hakelius[60] found increased prevalences of back pain and residual and recurrent sciatica in patients treated nonsurgically who were followed up after 7 years compared to those treated surgically. Weber,[46] on the other hand, reported almost identical recurrence rates in nonsurgically and surgically treated patients after 10 years.

Summary and Recommendation

The epidemiologic literature on herniated disks leaves much to be desired. Better case definitions would be an excellent start. Still it is obvious that the incidence of HNP in the general population is high. All patients with sciatica do not have herniated disks, and all herniated disks do not produce symptoms. Also, the effect of treatment on the natural history of herniated disks—which is good—is unclear. The opportunity for research is clearly at hand.

References

1. Andersson GBJ: The epidemiology of spinal disorders, in Frymoyer JW (ed): *The Adult Spine, Principles and Practice*, ed 2. Philadelphia, PA, JB Lippincott, 1996.
2. Lawrence JS (ed): *Rheumatism in Populations*. London, England, Heinemann Medical, 1977.
3. Hirsch C, Jonsson B, Lewin T: Low-back symptoms in a Swedish female population. *Clin Orthop* 1969;63:171–176.
4. Gyntelberg F: One year incidence of low back pain among male residents of Copenhagen aged 40-59. *Dan Med Bull* 1974;21:30–36.
5. Wickstrom G, Hanninen K, Lehtinen M, et al: Previous back syndromes and present back symptoms in concrete reinforcement workers. *Scand J Work Environ Health* 1978;4(suppl 1):20–29.
6. Riihimaki H: Back pain and heavy physical work: A comparative study of concrete reinforcement workers and maintenance house painters. *Br J Ind Med* 1985;42:226–232.
7. Riihimaki H: *Back Disorders in Relation to Heavy Physical Work.* Helsinki, Finland, Institute of Occupational Health, pp 1–72. Thesis.
8. Riihimaki H, Wickstrom G, Hanninen K, et al: Predictors of sciatic pain among concrete reinforcement workers and house painters: A five-year follow-up. *Scand J Work Environ Health* 1989;15:415–423.
9. Hrubec Z, Nashold BS Jr: Epidemiology of lumbar disc lesions in the military in World War II. *Am J Epidemiol* 1975;102:367–376.
10. Kelsey JL, Githens PB, White AA III, et al: An epidemiologic study of lifting and twisting on the job and risk for acute prolapsed lumbar intervertebral disc. *J Orthop Res* 1984;2:61–66.
11. Videman T, Nurminen T, Tola S, et al: Low-back pain in nurses and some loading factors of work. *Spine* 1984;9:400–404.
12. Videman T, Heikkilä JK, Koskenvuo M, et al: The role of environmental factors in the development of back pain and sciatica: An epidemiological study with adult twin pairs. *Orthop Trans* 1990;14:6.
13. Cedercreutz G, Videman T, Tola S, et al: Individual risk factors of the back among applicants to a nursing school. *Ergonomics* 1987;30:269–272.
14. Kelsey JL: An epidemiological study of acute herniated lumbar intervertebral discs. *Rheumatol Rehabil* 1975;14:144–159.
15. Kelsey JL: An epidemiological study of the relationship between occupations and acute herniated lumbar intervertebral discs. *Int J Epidemiol* 1975;4:197–205.
16. Kelsey JL: Epidemiology of radiculopathies. *Adv Neurol* 1978;19:385–398.
17. Kelsey JL: Idiopathic low back pain: Magnitude of the problem, in White AA III, Gordon SL (eds): American Academy of Orthopaedic Surgeons *Symposium on Idiopathic Low Back Pain*. St. Louis, MO, CV Mosby, 1982, pp 5–8.
18. Kelsey JL, Hardy RJ: Driving motor vehicles as a risk factor for acute herniated lumbar intervertebral disc. *Am J Epidemiol* 1975;102:63–73.
19. Kelsey JL, Ostfeld AM: Demographic characteristics of persons with acute herniated lumbar intervertebral disc. *J Chronic Dis* 1975;28:37–50.
20. Kelsey JL, Pastides H, Bisbee GE (eds): *Musculo-skeletal Disorders: Their Frequency of Occurrence and Their Impact on the Population of the United States.* New York, NY, Prodist, 1978.
21. Kelsey JL, White AA III: Epidemiology and impact on low-back pain. *Spine* 1980;5:133–142.
22. Kelsey JL, Githens PB, O'Conner T, et al: Acute prolapsed lumbar intervertebral disc: An epidemiologic study with special reference to driving automobiles and cigarette smoking. *Spine* 1984;9:608–613.
23. Kelsey JL, Golden AL: Occupational and workplace factors associated with low-back pain. *Occup Med* 1988;3:7–16.
24. Praemer A, Furner S, Rice DP (eds): *Musculoskeletal Conditions in the United States.* Park Ridge, IL, American Academy of Orthopaedic Surgeons, 1992.
25. Heliövaara M: Body height, obesity, and risk of herniated lumbar intervertebral disc. *Spine* 1987;12:469–472.

19

26. Heliövaara M: Occupation and risk of herniated lumbar intervertebral disc or sciatica leading to hospitalization. *J Chronic Dis* 1987;40:259–264.

27. Heliövaara M, Knekt P, Aromaa A: Incidence and risk factors of herniated lumbar intervertebral disc or sciatica leading to hospitalization. *J Chronic Dis* 1987;40:251–285.

28. Heliövaara M: *Epidemiology of Sciatica and Herniated Lumbar Intervertebral Disc.* Helsinki, Finland, Social Insurance Institution, 1988.

29. Spangfort EV: The lumbar disc herniation: A computer-aided analysis of 2,504 operations. *Acta Orthop Scand* 1972;142(suppl):1–95.

30. Kozak LJ, Moien M: *Detailed Diagnoses and Surgical Procedures for Patients Discharged From Short-Stay Hospitals. United States, 1983.* Washington, DC, National Center for Health Statistics, US Department of Health and Human Services, Vital Health Statistics Series 13, No 82. DHHS Publication No (PHS) 85-1743, 1985.

31. Volinn E, Turczyn KM, Loeser JD: Patterns in low back pain hospitalizations: Implications for the treatment of low back pain in an era of health care reform. *Clin J Pain* 1994;10:64–70.

32. Deyo RA, Cherkin D, Conrad D, et al: Cost, controversy, crisis: Low back pain and the health of the public. *Annu Rev Public Health* 1991;12:141–156.

33. Taylor VM, Deyo RA, Cherkin DC, et al: Low back pain hospitalization: Recent United States trends and regional variations. *Spine* 1994;19:1207–1213.

34. Cherkin DC, Deyo RA, Loeser JD, et al: An international comparison of back surgery rates. *Spine* 1994;19:1201–1206.

35. Nachemson AL: *Report to the Swedish Department of Economy.* Stockholm, Sweden, Civil Tryck, 1989.

36. Benn RT, Wood PH: Pain in the back: An attempt to estimate the size of the problem. *Rheumatol Rehabil* 1975;14:121–128.

37. Wood PHN, Badley EM: Musculoskeletal system, in Holland WW, Detels R, Knox G, et al (eds): *Oxford Textbook of Public Health: Specific Applications.* Oxford, England, Oxford University Press, 1985, vol 4, pp 279–297.

38. Frymoyer JW: Back pain and sciatica. *N Engl J Med* 1988;318:291–300.

39. Kane WJ: Worldwide incidence rates of laminectomy for lumbar disc herniations. Proceedings of the Annual Meeting of the International Society for the Study of the Lumbar Spine, Toronto, Canada. New Orleans, LA, International Society for the Study of the Lumbar Spine, 1980.

40. Heikkilä JK, Koskenvuo M, Heliövaara M, et al: Genetic and environmental factors in sciatica: Evidence from a nationwide panel of 9,365 adult twin pairs. *Ann Med* 1989;21:393–398.

41. Matsui H, Tsuji H, Terahata N: Juvenile lumbar herniated nucleus pulposus in monozygotic twins. *Spine* 1990;15:1228–1230.

42. Porter RW, Thorp L: Familial aspects of disc protrusion. *Orthop Trans* 1986;10:524.

43. Postacchini F, Lami R, Pugliese O: Familial predisposition to discogenic low-back pain: An epidemiologic and immunogenetic study. *Spine* 1988;13:1403–1406.

44. Varlotta GP, Brown MD, Kelsey JL, et al: Familial predisposition for herniation of a lumbar disc in patients who are less than twenty-one years old. *J Bone Joint Surg* 1991;73A:124–128.

45. Braun W: *Ursachen des lumbalen Bandscheiberverfalls: Die Wirbelsaule in Forschung und Praxis 43.* Stuttgardt, Germany, Hippocrates, 1969.

46. Weber H: Lumbar disc herniation: A controlled, prospective study with ten years of observation. *Spine* 1983;8:131–140.

47. Kelsey JL, Githens PB, Walter SD, et al: An epidemiological study of acute prolapsed cervical intervertebral disc. *J Bone Joint Surg* 1984;66A:907–914.

48. Kondo K, Molgaard CA, Kurland LT, et al: Protruded intervertebral cervical disk: Incidence and affected cervical level in Rochester, Minnesota, 1950-1974. *Minn Med* 1981;64:751–753.

49. Salminen JJ, Erkintalo-Tertti MO, Paajanen HE: Magnetic resonance imaging findings of lumbar spine in the young: Correlation with leisure-time physical

activity, spinal mobility, and trunk muscle strength in 15-year-old pupils with or without low-back pain. *J Spinal Disord* 1993;6:386–391.

50. Ramani PS: Variations in size of the bony lumbar canal in patients with prolapse of lumbar intervertebral discs. *Clin Radiol* 1976;27:301–307.

51. Winston K, Rumbaugh C, Colucci V: The vertebral canals in lumbar disc disease. *Spine* 1984;9:414–417.

52. Hurme M, Alaranta H, Torma T, et al: Operated lumbar disc herniation: Epidemiological aspects. *Ann Chir Gynaecol* 1983;72:33–36.

53. Hitselberger WE, Witten RM: Abnormal myelograms in asymptomatic patients. *J Neurosurg* 1968;28:204–206.

54. Holt EP Jr: The question of lumbar discography. *J Bone Joint Surg* 1968;50A:720–726.

55. Wiesel SW, Tsourmas N, Feffer HL, et al: A study of computer-assisted tomography: I. The incidence of positive CAT scans in an asymptomatic group of patients. *Spine* 1984;9:549–551.

56. Boden SD, Davis DO, Dina TS, et al: Abnormal magnetic-resonance scans of the lumbar spine in asymptomatic subjects: A prospective investigation. *J Bone Joint Surg* 1990;72A:403–408.

57. Jensen MC, Brant-Zawadzki MN, Obuchowski N, et al: Magnetic resonance imaging of the lumbar spine in people without back pain. *N Engl J Med* 1994;331:69–73.

58. Boden SD, McCowin PR, Davis DO, et al: Abnormal magnetic-resonance scans of the cervical spine in asymptomatic subjects: A prospective investigation. *J Bone Joint Surg* 1990;72A:1178–1184.

59. Andersson GB, Svensson HO, Odén A: The intensity of work recovery in low back pain. *Spine* 1983;8:880–884.

60. Hakelius A: Prognosis in sciatica: A clinical follow-up of surgical and non-surgical treatment. *Acta Orthop Scand* 1970;129(suppl):1–76.

61. Saal JA, Saal JS: Nonoperative treatment of herniated lumbar intervertebral disc with radiculopathy: An outcome study. *Spine* 1989;14:431–437.

62. Frymoyer JW, Pope MH, Clements JH, et al: Risk factors in low-back pain: An epidemiological survey. *J Bone Joint Surg* 1983;65A:213–218.

63. Hurme M, Alaranta H: Factors predicting the result of surgery for lumbar intervertebral disc herniation. *Spine* 1987;12:933–938.

Chapter 2

Biomechanics and Ergonomics in Disk Herniation Accompanied by Sciatica

Margareta Nordin, PT, Dr Sci
Federico Balagué, MD

Introduction

In 1987, Spitzer and associates[1] suggested a classification of activity related to spinal disorders (Table 1). The classification considered symptoms such as duration of symptoms and signs from onset, and working status at the time of evaluation. The classification acknowledges that back pain with or without leg pain is a symptomatology rather than a diagnosis. The bibliography of the Quebec Task Force report[1] was the starting point in the expanded literature search for the Agency for Health Care Policy and Research Guideline on Acute Low Back Problems in Adults.[2] The guideline suggests a classification into three descriptive clinical categories—potentially serious condition, sciatica (Fig. 1), and nonspecific low back symptoms—based on medical history and physical examination findings. This chapter will focus on the patient who has sciatica as a result of a disk herniation.

We do not understand the exact pathophysiologic mechanism of sciatica. Several authors[3,4] point to a multifactorial genesis consisting of mechanical deformation and chemical irritation in the acute stage. The mechanism of chronic sciatica may even be more complicated; impairment of axonal transport and intraneural microcirculation may have occurred. This chapter will focus on the mechanical aspects of disk herniation and sciatica and on possible ergonomic intervention to reduce these factors.

How Big is the Problem?

The epidemiologic data on disk herniation with accompanying sciatica symptoms is the focus of chapter 1. Nevertheless, some key figures are helpful as background for a discussion of prevention. An overall lifetime prevalence of 1% to 3% in the general population has been reported in industrial countries.[5-7] Men have almost twice the prevalence of women, 4.8% and 2.5%, respectively. Most prolapsed disks occur between the ages of 20 and 64 years, and the highest frequency occurs at 35 to 45 years of age.[8,9] Individuals in this age group are active, usually working, and at the peak of their active lifestyle. The type of work influences the incidence of disk herniation; the prevalence in individuals who

Table 1 Classification of activity-related spinal disorders

Classification*	Symptoms	Duration of Symptoms From Onset
1	Pain without radiation	
2	Pain + radiation to extremity, proximally	a (< 7 days)
3	Pain + radiation to extremity, distally[†]	b (7 days to 7 weeks)
4	Pain + radiation to upper/lower limb neurologic signs	c (> 7 weeks)
5	Presumptive compression of a spinal nerve root on a simple radiograph (ie, spinal instability or fracture)	
6	Compression of a spinal nerve root confirmed by specific imaging techniques (ie, computed tomography, myelography, or magnetic resonance imaging)	
7	Spinal stenosis	
8	Postsurgical status, 1 to 6 months after intervention	
9	Postsurgical status, 1 to 6 months after intervention	
10	Chronic pain syndrome	
11	Other diagnoses	

*Working status at time of evaluation can be either working or idle. Idle is defined as absent from work, unemployed, or inactive

[†]Not applicable to the thoracic segment

(Adapted with permission from Spitzer WO, Dupuis M, Leblanc FE, et al: Scientific approach to the assessment and management of activity-related spinal disorders: A monograph for clinicians. Report of the Quebec Task Force on Spinal Disorders. *Spine* 1987;12(suppl 1):S17.)

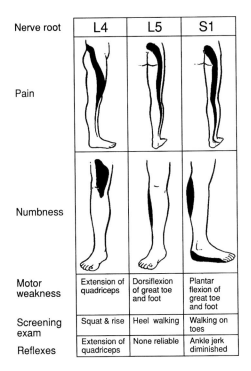

Nerve root	L4	L5	S1
Pain			
Numbness			
Motor weakness	Extension of quadriceps	Dorsiflexion of great toe and foot	Plantar flexion of great toe and foot
Screening exam	Squat & rise	Heel walking	Walking on toes
Reflexes	Extension of quadriceps	None reliable	Ankle jerk diminished

Fig. 1 *Sciatica clinical representation from nerve root compromise in the lumbar spine. (Adapted with permission from Bigos S, Bowyer O, Braen G, et al: Acute low back problems in adults, in* Clinical Practice Guideline No 14. *Rockville, MD, US Department of Health and Human Services (AHCPR Publication No. 95-0642), 1994.*

do heavy work leads to more patients reporting symptoms of sciatica. Wickström and Hänninen[10] studied reinforcement workers and painters in Finland and found 51% and 15%, respectively, of workers reporting sciatica symptoms. Abenhaim and associates[11] studied a cohort of 1,848 Canadian workers who represented all sectors of industry. Sciatica was found in 3.4% and disk herniations in an additional 2.1% of the cohort. Kelsey and Hardy[8] reported a 4.5 times higher risk for truck drivers and a 2.5 times higher risk for sedentary work in subjects older than 35 years of age. In summary, the reported prevalence rate for sciatica varies from 1% to 50%, and it is reported more often in heavy work and in work in which there is long-lasting exposure to whole body vibration.

Risk factors associated with sciatica have been studied by Heliövaara,[12] Wickström and Hänninen,[10] Kelsey and associates,[13] and Riihimäki and associates.[14] Factors significantly associated with reporting sciatica were multifactorial. One study related the highest association (relative risk) of prior episodes of sciatica to the number of reported back accidents, when compared with an individual with no history of sciatica or back accidents.[14] Kelsey and associates[13] found a significant increase in reported sciatica associated with frequent lifting. When the authors combined lifting with twisting or holding a load far away from the body, the relative risk increased 12 times for reporting low back pain and four times for reporting sciatica. Exposure from operation of vehicles on the job also was associated significantly with a higher risk for reporting sciatica.[8,15] Kelsey and Hardy[8] found a relative risk of sciatica to be 2.75 for car drivers and 4.67 for truck drivers compared to nondriving subjects. Load exposure is also significant in elite sports. Swärd and associates[16] and Afshani and Kuhn[17] studied elite gymnasts and found an increased prevalence of disk herniation, but Tertti and associates[18] refuted these findings. Finally, microgravity induces back pain;[19] but there is a lack of data about whether back pain induced by microgravity is accompanied by sciatica.

Weber[9,20] reports that long-term outcome of sciatica is favorable. Fifty percent of the patients reporting sciatica recover within 6 weeks.[11] Other authors[21,22] recognize sciatica, whether or not it is related to disk diseases, to be a predictor of poor outcomes for return to work. Compared to nonspecific low back pain, sciatica symptoms are associated with longer duration of painful episodes, more severe episode, significantly reduced return to work, increased disability, and pension.[22-25] The recurrence rate for sciatica after follow-up to 10 years has been reported to be about 12% for disk herniations at L4 to S1 levels.[9,26]

Load Imposition on the Disk

The theoretical rationale that a disk herniation results in sciatica needs discussion. Load imposition in moderate daily activities provides the disk with nutrition; inadequate nutrition may lead to hastened disk degeneration.[27] During flexion of the trunk, when the posterior portion of the anulus fibrosus is under tension, it becomes thinner. This enhances the transport of metabolites from the periphery of the disk into the posterior part of the anulus.[28] The type of motion affects the fluid transport differently. A fast motion, which results in rapid fluid transport, will affect the periphery of the anulus; slow motion, such as changes in posture, will have a larger effect.[29] No motion has a detrimental effect because the metabolic rates are decreased and the disk loses matrix.[30] Excessive and/or repeated loading of the lumbar spine may lead to fatigue of the disk structures and, ultimately, to disk bulging and/or herniation with accompanying symptoms of sciatica. The most harmful exposure for the disk structures is forward flexion in combination with side bending and rotation of the trunk and/or whole body vibration.

Theoretical Courses of Events in Disk Herniation

The mechanical theory behind nontraumatic disk herniation is based on diskography and cadaver studies.[5,31] Peripheral annular tears occur at the anulus–bone junction. These junctions serve as stress concentration sites and are biomechanically weak links. Patient studies have shown, however, that annular tears can occur first centrally. Once the annular "cage" is disrupted, the nucleus pulposus migrates peripherally because the disk is under prestressed load. The migration causes a bulge that may produce irritation in the well-innervated posterior ligament. If the nuclear tissue migrates completely into the spinal canal, the disk has herniated, mechanical compression of the nerve root occurs gradually, irritates the nerve, and an inflammatory reaction develops and leads to symptomatic sciatica. A pathoanatomic reason is found.

Basic Biomechanics of the Disk

We believe that there is a mechanical component to disk herniation. This statement is made with some caution because genetic and immunologic factors may be found to play a larger role as research progresses.[32,33] The influence of loads on the disk structures is complex and not completely understood. The disk is subjected in vivo to large mechanical loads that represent several times body weight.

The functional unit of the spine is the motion segment, which consists of two vertebrae and their intervening soft tissues (Fig. 2). The vertebral bodies are designed mainly to bear compressive loads. The intervertebral disk bears and distributes loads imposed on the lumbar spine and restrains excessive motion. Disks are subjected to a combination of compression, tension, shear, bending, and torsion loads. The nucleus pulposus and the anulus fibrosus compose the disk. In the lumbar spine, the nucleus pulposus, a gelatinous mass that is rich in hydrophilic glycoaminoglycans that are water binding, is located posterior in the mo-

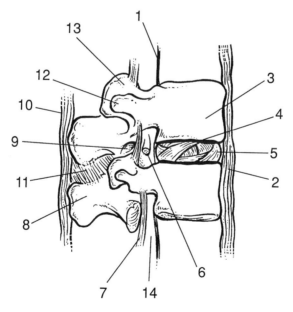

Fig. 2 *Schematic representation of a motion segment in the lumbar spine (sagittal view).* **Anterior portion:** *1, posterior longitudinal ligament; 2, anterior longitudinal ligament; 3, vertebral body; 4, cartilaginous end plate; 5, intervertebral disk; 6, intervertebral foramen with nerve root.* **Posterior portion:** *7, ligamentum flavum; 8, spinous process; 9, intervertebral joint formed by the superior and inferior facets (the capsular ligament is not shown); 10, supraspinous ligament; 11, interspinous ligament; 12, transverse process (the intertransverse ligament not shown); 13, arch; and 14, vertebral canal (the spinal cord is not depicted).*

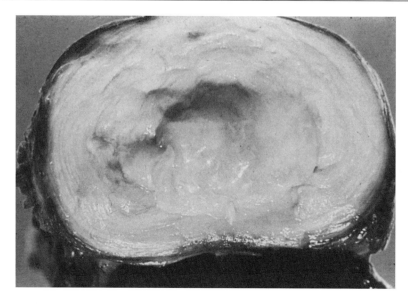

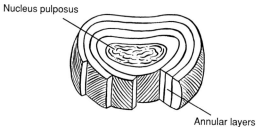

Nucleus pulposus

Annular layers

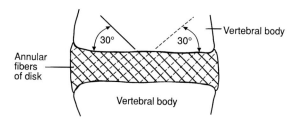

Vertebral body

30°   30°

Annular fibers of disk

Vertebral body

Fig. 3 **Top,** *Photograph of a transverse section of the disk including the anulus fibrosus and the nucleus pulposus.* **Bottom,** *Schematic representation of the layers of the anulus fibrosus. (Adapted with permission from White AA, Panjabi MM:* The Clinical Biomechanics of the Spine. *Philadelphia, PA, JB Lippincott, 1978.)*

tion segment. The glycoaminoglycan content diminishes with age, and the disk is progressively less hydrated.[34] The anulus fibrosus is a tough outer covering composed of collagen fibers arranged in a series of sheets, each of which is at a 30° angle about the next sheet. This covering allows the disk to withstand high bending and torsional loads (Fig. 3).

Vertical transection of a cadaveric lumbar motion segment resulted in a protrusion of the nucleus pulposus, which shows that the lumbar disk is under pressure. Nachemson[35] showed that the intrinsic pressure in unloaded nuclei pulposi is about 10 N cm^2 in normal lumbar spines. The longitudinal ligaments and the ligamenta flava cause the intrinsic pressure in the disk. During loading of the spine, the nucleus pulposus acts hydrostatically and uniformly distributes the load throughout the disk.[36] The disk acts as a "cushion" between the vertebral bodies to store energy. Nachemson[37] has studied the distribution of stress in a cross-section of a lumbar disk under loading. During compressive loading, the compressive stress was highest in the nucleus pulposus; it was approximately 1.5 times the externally applied load per unit area. As the disk bulges during compressive loads, the tensile stresses per unit area on the posterior annular fibers are about four to five times greater than the externally applied load (Fig. 4). These findings have been the key argument in many discussions concerning a mechanical cause for a bulging or prolapsed disk. In several cadaver studies, the nuclear material shifted posteriorly under different loading conditions.[28,38,39] Brinckmann[40] simulated a disk bulging in vitro under physiologic loading (1,000 N). When he made a 1-mm thick radial cut within the anulus fibrosus peripheral layer in lumbar disk motion segments, the disk bulged 0.5 mm posteriorly. The bulge increased when a compression fracture of the vertebral

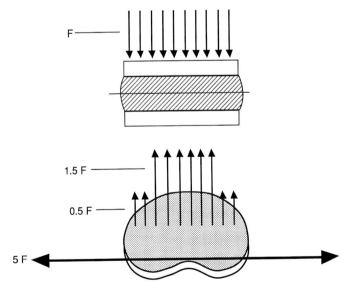

Fig. 4 *Distribution of stress in a cross section of a lumbar disk under compressive loading in vitro. The compressive stress is highest in the nucleus pulposus, 1.5 times the externally applied load (F) per unit area. By contrast, the compressive stress on the anulus fibrosus is only about 0.5 times the externally applied load. This part of the disk bears predominantly tensile stress, which is four to five times greater than the externally applied load per unit area. (Adapted with permission from Nachemson A: Lumbar mechanics as revealed by lumbar intradiscal pressure measurements, in Jayson M (ed): The Lumbar Spine and Back Pain. London, England, Churchill Livingstone, 1992, pp 157–171.)*

body was simulated. These findings support the theory that mechanical tears can produce bulges.

Direction of Loading

The disk is most vulnerable in loading conditions including a combination of compression, forward bending, and lateral bending. Adding axial torsion may increase the risk for herniation.[28,41] This combined motion places high tensile stresses on the posterior part of the anulus, increases the intradiskal pressure, and stretches the interspinous ligament.[40,42] When the motion segment was loaded in flexion, disk prolapse occurred at a range of 2,800 to 13,000 N of compressive force in experimental in vitro studies.[41,43] These loads are within the physiologic ranges computed by biomechanical models.[44-46]

Creep Behavior and Cyclic Loading of the Disk

The spine is inherently unstable. Lucas and Bresler[47] showed that buckling in thoracolumbar spine segments devoid of muscles occurs at 20 N when they are loaded axially. When the disk is subjected to a constant load, it exhibits creep, that is, it continuously deforms. This time-dependent behavior comes from the fluid flow of the disk under applied load and the inherent viscoelastic behavior of the collagen and proteoglycan matrix. Kazarian[48] has shown time-dependent behavior in autopsy specimens; he found that disks with degenerative changes had a higher rate of deformation. Keller and associates[49] showed creep response in vivo in porcine intervertebral disks. Wilder and associates[50] focused on the behavior of the motion segment in a simulated sitting environment. During testing, a motion segment could suddenly buckle and produce high tensile stresses on the posterolateral region of the disk (Fig. 5). Combined cyclic loading caused tracking tears throughout the disk—from the nucleus pulposus through the anulus fibrosus. This loading may be a mechanism for disk herniation in vivo where exposure to whole body vibration, repeated trauma, or repetitive motion causes muscle fatigue and indirect loss of protection from mechanical perturbation.

Cyclic loading of the lumbar motion segments has been performed in several studies.[41,50-52] In summary, these authors suggest that cyclic loading leads to changes in the mechanical properties of the disk that could explain the mechanism of disk herniation. The most important changes are (1) distortions of the lamellae, (2) increase of axial rotation in the motion segment, and (3) sudden buckling creating large forces. Using a mathematical model, Shirazi-Adl[53] simulated strain in fibers of the lumbar anulus fibrosus. He showed that very small changes in axial rotation (< 1 °) produced large increases in strain (up to six times). The direct relationship between in vivo load exposure and in vitro laboratory testing is still unclear and needs further discussion.[54]

Spine creep has been indirectly measured in humans by measuring the change in overall height over time.[55-57] The diurnal loss was about 17 mm.[58] It is not known how this loss in height is distributed over each motion segment in the spine; nevertheless, the disks have exhibited creep. McGill and Brown[56] found

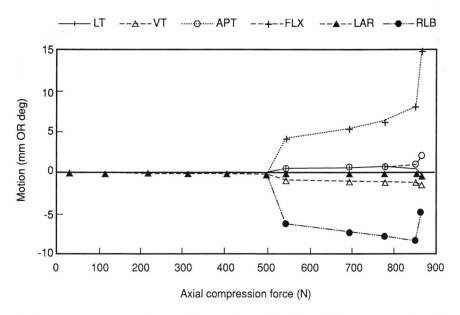

Fig. 5 *Plots of typical stable (0 to 500 N) and unstable (500 to 870 N) responses of an L4 motion segment tested using a 10-s load ramp. The individual responses are noted as LT, left lateral translation; VT, vertical translation; APT, anterior translation; FLX, flexion rotation; LAR, left axial rotation; RLB, right lateral bend. This segment was exposed to an hour of vibration and a subsequent overload event. (Adapted with permission from Pope MH, Wilder DG, Krag MH: Biomechanics of the lumbar spine: Basic principles, in Frymoyer JW (ed): The Adult Spine: Principles and Practice. New York, NY, Raven Press, 1991, pp 1487–1501.)*

a similar response when the spine was loaded in prolonged full flexion. Hedman and Fernie[57] used magnetic resonance imaging (MRI) to study lumbar spine creep in a healthy 31-year-old man in two seated positions: one with the trunk extended and the other with the trunk flexed. A gravity inversion posture resembling autotraction maintained for 10 minutes was compared to the trunk flexed versus the trunk extended with a load of 50% of body weight maintained for 30 minutes. Imaging and measurements were performed immediately before and after each loading situation at the L2-S1 level. Lumbosacral creep was larger in the extended than in the flexed position, 9% (3.58 mm) and 7% (2.92 mm), respectively. System resolution was 0.78 mm. This study has limitations, but it merits attention because it uses a more direct measurement of creep in vivo and demonstrates a rather significant creep response to loading.

Whole body vibration exposure is most common in sitting, where it adds a load component to the sitting posture. The effects of whole body vibration on the spine are not completely understood.[58] The mechanical pathway for exposure is the sitting posture and the dynamic response of the trunk to vibration. The natural frequency of the seated human being is 4 to 6 Hz,[59,60] which coincides with the vibration produced by many vehicles. Whole body vibration simulation studies in vivo have indicated (1) an increased strain in the lumbar region, (2) an increased rate of development of muscle fatigue in the erector spinae muscles, (3) an increased response of creep behavior of the spine, and (4) a significant increase in energy expenditure.[58] Animal studies have shown that disk pressure peaks at 5 Hz exposure exponentially, which could be a partial explanation for the increased rate of reported disk herniations in drivers.[13,61] Bongers and Boshuizen[62] propose a four pathways mechanism for structural damage to the motion segment. The pathways are (1) direct structural damage to the end plate and subchondral bone, anulus fibrosus, and facet joints and/or pars articularis; (2) direct interference with supply of nutrient to the intervertebral disk and/or indirect tampering with the supply as a result of microfractures of the end plate; (3) loss of intervertebral disk height, which causes increased load on the facet joints and increased stiffness of the intervertebral disk; and (4) increased trunk muscular fatigue, which leads to destabilization of the spine and eventual buckling.

The biochemical reaction to whole body vibration exposure may be damage to the dorsal root ganglion neuropeptides. Recently, McLain and Weinstein[63,64] exposed adult rabbits to whole body vibration 3 hours per day over a period of 2 weeks. The study used immobilized rabbits and nonimmobilized rabbits as controls. The authors found a marked increase in pain-related neuropeptide concentration, increased nuclear clefting, increased density of nuclear pores, and aggregation of metabolic clefts. The ultrastructural changes generated by a physiologically valid vibration provides an anatomic link between the clinical observation of increased back pain and biochemical changes involving the pain-related neuropeptides. Further studies are needed to show if this is a dose-response reaction. In prolonged exposure to whole body vibration, we can postulate a mechanism of loss of energy absorbing capacity in vivo, that is, the disk becomes more vulnerable to mechanical perturbations. We can also postulate a mechanically induced damaging effect to the ganglion tissues that leads to a neurochemical reaction. It is not well understood if the two mechanisms occur simultaneously or in an orderly fashion.

Biomechanical Characteristics of the Degenerated and Denucleated Disk

Substantial changes have been reported in the mechanical behavior in motion segments with degenerative or denucleated disks. A number of studies have provided compiled data from experimental testing of the motion segment[65-78] with (1) degenerated disks, (2) mechanically denucleated disks, and (3) disks that have undergone chemonucleolysis before regeneration. The changed mechanical characteristics are compared to normal disk mechanics and related to possible clinical relevance. The most relevant findings for this review are the increased lateral bulge formation[65-68] and the increased mobility[73-75] in degenerated and denucleated disks. The degenerative changes imply a decreased ability to absorb shocks in normal life; the degenerated disk is less viscoelastic in its behavior. In summary, the disk with pathophysiology exhibits (1) an increased amount of creep response, particularly in flexion; (2) a decreased range of motion, and (3) a longer recovery time. These findings suggest that prolonged sitting or forward bending of the trunk followed by immediate strenuous activity should be avoided. This situation may lead to abnormally high stressors, resulting in injury.[38]

Disk Bulging and Clinical Relevance to Sciatica

The clinical relevance of a bulging disk is still unclear. Data from early experimental studies have shown that mild compression on the normal dorsal root ganglion generates bursts of nerve impulses, that is, repetitive firing of sensory axons that produces radicular pain.[79,80] This result was refuted by Kuslich and associates,[81] who found that only a stretched, compressed, and swollen nerve root reproduced sciatica in patients when stimulated. The closer the stimulation to the site of the compression, the greater the pain response. No other tissue in the spine was capable of reproducing leg pain. Computed tomography (CT) and MRI have been used to evaluate the association between a disk bulge and back and/or sciatica symptoms. Site and size are poorly correlated in asymptomatic individuals and in patients.[82-85] Montaldi and associates[86] and Tullberg[87] showed that a residual herniation does not necessarily result in sciatica.

Thelander and associates[88] studied patients with sciatica caused by a disk herniation. The patients were treated nonsurgically, and CT scans were performed at 3 and 24 months after the first diagnostic CT scan. Three indices were used to determine the size of the herniation in relation to the size of the spinal canal. The results showed that the index was correlated significantly to the degree of decrease in reported sciatica. The area of the herniations decreases markedly over time. The authors claim that there seems to be an individual threshold in the ratio of relative hernia size to spinal canal size under which sciatica disappears. If the ratio is above this level, the mechanical contribution stimulus persists by triggering a painful local inflammatory reaction in the nerve root. This ratio can be a useful tool in better understanding the eventual mechanical stimulus of sciatica. It may also describe the large individual variations in pain reporting in response to bulging/herniation and mechanical stimuli. The biomechanical or ergonomic posture or position interventions would have the best effect if the posture relieved the pressure on the inflamed nerve tissue.

The Influence of Spine Muscle Activity and Load on the Disk

We discuss the influence of trunk muscle in relation to disk herniation from two points of view: muscle recruitment and muscle fatigue that can influence the injury mechanism of the disk. Cumulative evidence in the literature leads to the hypothesis that motion is beneficial for the musculoskeletal structures.[89] The question is how much and how long should we expose the system.

Parnianpour and associates[90] showed that motion of the trunk until exhaustion decreased motor control. The subjects exposed to controlled dynamic submaximal trunk flexion and extension exhibited increased coupled motion of the trunk. In this study, about one third of the subjects tested reported muscle soreness in the lumbar spine. That none reported sciatica may be due to the limited range of motion that was exerted. Marras and associates[91] studied trunk mobility in five asymmetric positions using a triaxial goniometer. More than 500 subjects participated (339 subjects without and 171 subjects with low back pain). The patients with pain were classified according to the Quebec categories.[1] Marras and associates[91] used an eight variables model that included velocity and range of motion and derivatives thereof. Patients diagnosed with herniated disk had a significantly changed motion pattern. Specificity for these patients' motion patterns was 99% and sensitivity ranged from 16% to 42%, depending on the pain intensity. Velocity and acceleration were the best discriminators; range of motion performed poorly. The authors concluded that trunk motion reflects the biomechanical limitations of the diseased spine as well as the guarding process learned by the patient.[91] These measurements can be used in rehabilitation to indicate the effect of treatment, normalization of trunk motion, and the need for ergonomic intervention.

Muscle fatigue theory implies a loss of motor control,[92-94] which can yield very high loads on the lumbar spine. During increased coupled motion, the spine is subjected to asymmetric loads. Gallagher and associates[95] investigated dynamic biomechanical stresses associated with lifting in stooping and kneeling postures. Eight trunk muscles were recorded with electromyography (EMG). The analysis of muscle recruitment indicated that during asymmetric lifting, recruitment was shifted to ancillary muscles that had a smaller cross-sectional area and less fatigue resistance. This shift may, in turn, lead to increased shear forces on the lumbar spine and the anulus fibrosus.

The current research on improving mathematical optimization models is promising in attempting a better understanding of the load estimates on the lumbar spine. Previous models were adequate for estimating load distribution on the spine structures in symmetrical postures.[44,45] The newer models take into account individual anthropometric data, such as muscle cross-sectional size determined using MRI, larger number of trunk muscles, and EMG of each muscle (wire and surface). The literature suggests that optimization-based biomechanical models are not adequate for the study of asymmetric tasks. In these tasks, the internal loads increase as a result of high coactivation of trunk muscles rather than of changes in force prediction.[96,97] The EMG-driven models compared to mathematical models are better load predictors of asymmetric postures; however, their reliability and validity need further improvement. The researcher using anthropometric data must base muscle parameters of individual subjects on an accurate imaging system and base the EMG-derived force on individual characteristics.[96] Biomechanical compression load models have been shown to create errors up to 40% in the prediction of spinal loads.[97,98] There is a lack of understanding of the load on the lumbar disk in asymmetric posture and dynamic tasks and its contribution to eventual injury.

Muscle pattern recruitment activity in patients with a disk herniation is disturbed. Pope and associates[99] report marked changes in the "flexion-relaxation" response of the erector spinae of a patient before and following a disk herniation. Figure 6, *top*, shows the normal burst pattern of the erector spinae muscles during a forward maximal flexion of the trunk. Floyd and Silver[100] reported this muscle recruitment pattern earlier. The first burst activity occurs at the initial flexion of the trunk, and after that there is a relaxation of the activity. A second burst occurs when the trunk is erected. In the patient with a disk herniation, the erector spinae muscles activity remains constant over the whole motion (Fig. 6,

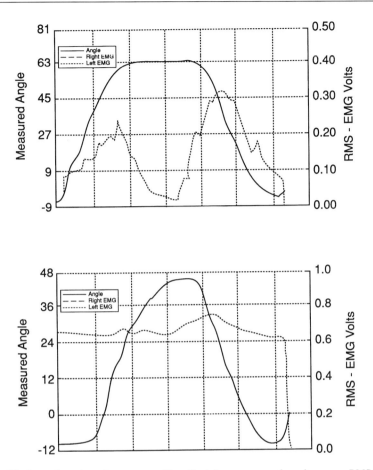

Fig. 6 *Flexion-relaxation phenomenon.* **Top**, *Preinjury measured angle versus RMS-EMG.* **Bottom**, *Postinjury measured angle versus RMS-EMG. (Adapted with permission from Pope MH, Wilder DG, Krag MH: Biomechanics of the lumbar spine: Basic principles, in Frymoyer JW (ed): The Adult Spine: Principles and Practice. New York, NY, Raven Press, 1991, pp 1487–1501.)*

bottom). This finding would infer that the disk is under constant pressure. The lack of intermittent burst activity may lead to decreased disk nutrition, which eventually may be detrimental for the disk tissues. We could find no study of the normalization of muscle recruitment patterns in patients with disk herniation. Trunk muscle recruitment studies are expensive and difficult; however, they are essential to the increased understanding of intrinsic and extrinsic asymmetric load patterns of the spine.

In Vivo Measurement of Disk Pressure

Nachemson[37] performed disk pressure measurements by introducing a needle directly into the nucleus pulposus in vivo. The needle was connected to a pressure gauge, and the change in intradiskal pressure in healthy, young individuals was registered during slow motion and static loads. The pressure changes are usually presented in reference to the upright relaxed standing position (Fig. 7). The studies have had an enormous impact on the discussion of load contribution to the lumbar spine, workplace design, lifting, exercises and training, and conservative treatment. The measurements showed that the load on the third intervertebral disk in standing is approximately body weight; any deviations from the upright standing posture increase the relative pressure, and any extrinsic added load further increases the relative pressure. The highest increase in pressure is in the sitting position with the trunk forward flexed and rotated, with an external load in the hands far away from the body. Coughing and laughing increase the upright standing pressure about 20% as does sitting. Use of a lumbar backrest support or an increase in the backrest inclination decreases the load in the sitting position; thoracic support increases the load. Lying down reduces the load by approximately 50%. The limitations of these studies are that they were performed in a semistatic fashion, that is, the acceleration forces were virtually absent.

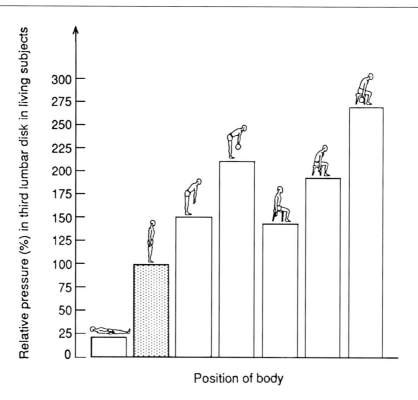

Fig. 7 *Relative increase and decrease in intradiskal pressure in different spine standing and sitting postures compared to the reference pressure in upright standing (100%). (Adapted with permission from Lindh M: Biomechanics of the lumbar spine, in Nordin M, Frankel VH (eds):* Basic Biomechanics of the Musculoskeletal System. *Philadelphia, PA, Lea & Febiger, 1989, pp 183–208.)*

Lelong and associates[101] and Drevet and associates[102] studied 42 subjects using intradiskal pressure measurements. In the study, 17 subjects had healthy disks and 25 slightly degenerated disks. By means of a piezoresistive device that allowed static and dynamic measurements of intradiskal pressure in vivo, the authors found that there are large differences in pressure in healthy disks among subjects with the same age and morphology. Further, they found that hyperlordosis immediately increases intradiskal pressure (30% to 100% according to the values of lordosis). The same phenomenon occurs with kyphosis greater than 30°. Drevet and associates[102] found that posterior tilting of the pelvis did not significantly modify intradiskal pressure, passive stretching of the paraspinal muscles by autotraction reduced the intradiskal pressure by 30% to 50%, and contraction of the back muscles raised the intradiskal pressure by 100% to 400%.

The long-term effect of high-pressure posture could outwear the slow healing mechanism of the disk by continuously disturbing the formation of new collagen and/or rupturing the newly formed collagen of less tension capacity.[45,103] If the anulus fibrosus is considered to be a soft collagenous tissue, there is a convincing body of literature to promote early controlled motion, even for a painful disk herniation. This motion would enhance healing by stimulating collagen synthesis, increasing tension strength, and aligning the repaired cells and collagen fibers.[104] Premature or excessive motion, on the other hand, can mechanically increase the damage and the inflammatory reaction.[89,104] We return to the initial question of how much exposure is a risk factor. Do excessive mechanical loads exacerbate the risk of disk herniation and accompanying sciatica? If the answer is a cautious yes, how can we reduce these loads to avoid disk reinjury and to enhance healing of an injured disk treated conservatively or surgically that has residual symptoms of sciatica? Longitudinal prospective epidemiologic studies answer the first item. Outcome and intervention studies will shed light on the two following questions.

Prevention Interventions

In-depth epidemiologic knowledge is necessary when designing prevention intervention strategies. We can divide prevention into primary, secondary, and tertiary interventions. Primary prevention aims at reducing the occurrence before it happens. Secondary prevention aims to reduce the severity and/or the recurrence of sciatica. Tertiary prevention involves the reduction of disability and restoration of function in patients with chronic sciatica. This chapter focuses on primary and secondary prevention. The first question is, can we prevent disk herniation and sciatica from occurring? The second question is, if a patient has a disk herniation and sciatica, can we reduce the symptoms and/or prevent recurrences?

Primary Prevention of Disk Herniation and Sciatica

Primary prevention programs for the population at large are uncommon for several reasons.[105] Accurate identification of the individual at risk is difficult; primary prevention programs have to address a substantial segment of the population. Given the size of this task, the lack of epidemiologic data, and the cost, such a study currently is difficult to justify. Nevertheless, primary prevention strategies for nonspecific low back pain will probably reduce the occurrence of sciatica because many of these strategies involve reduction in the imposition of excessive load on the lumbar spine. This would be the ergonomic and/or risk reduction approach. The National Institute for Occupational Safety and Health (NIOSH)[106] recommends four strategies for work-related musculoskeletal disorders: identifying the biomechanical hazards, developing effective health-control interventions, changing management concepts and operational policies with respect to work performance, and devising strategies for disseminating knowledge on control.

The biomechanical hazards, the focus of this paper, point to reported and perceived accidents (slip, falls, unspecific trauma, lift, strenuous posture), poor design or poor work technique (lift with twist and object held far away, posture), and exposure to whole body vibration. These items would be the targets for primary prevention.

Biomechanical Hazards

Accidents including slips, falls, unspecific trauma, lifts, and strenuous postures are related to workplace design, work technique, and hazard control. We could make an argument here that if we eliminate all lifts by increasing the load so much that no human being could lift it, injuries due to overexertion would disappear. This solution is impractical and hypothetical. Therefore, we have to take a more realistic approach, that is, hazard control and redesign of job tasks and environments that necessitate excessive forward bending and rotation of the trunk. Hazard control involves a proactive surveillance system in industry, but it may not necessarily account for leisure activities. A low-cost strategy may be to relate the number of reported incidences to the task performed instead of the individual. The more accidents reported related to the task itself, the more the reason to change the task. For each incident reported, a detailed analysis is performed of the workplace and work technique. Table 2 shows examples of the parameters that are included in an ergonomic evaluation of load exposure, that is, loads, object design, lifting technique, workplace layout, task design, psychology, environment, and work organization. It is a diagnosis of the physical task and its modifier. This report forms a database for decision making about future intervention. If such a system is implemented, accident-promoting tasks can be eliminated or reduced.

One study used an ergonomic intervention program that involved workers in a large automobile plant in the United States. The load imposed on the lumbar spine was reduced by 40% according to the NIOSH guidelines. Redesign of large machinery was costly. A follow-up period of 1 year was not sufficient to show an impact on the reported injury data.[107] In a similar intervention in a car assembly plant, Lifshitz and associates[108] reported a reduction of 50% (from 6.5% to 3.2%) of reported back and upper extremity injuries and disorders. The greatest reduction of injuries took place in the jobs that require heavy lifting. Some tasks are more difficult to eliminate because of the type of work involved, for example, concrete work, railway spiking, and manhole-cover pulling. In such a case, work technique training may be implemented. Work technique training re-

Table 2 Examples of parameters of interest for physical load exposure measurements and possible confounders

Parameter*	Example(s) of Exposure and Modifier
Load (E)	The weight of the object handled
Object design (E)	The size of the object handled, the shape, location, and size of the handles
Lifting technique (E)	The lever arm of the object, posture, twisting of the trunk, feet placement
Workplace layout (E)	The spatial features of the task, such as carrying distance, range of motion of the trunk and arms, obstacles such as stairs
Task design (E)	Frequency and duration of task, muscle fatigue
Psychology (C)	Job satisfaction, autonomy and control, expectations
Environment (E,C)	Whole body vibration, temperature, humidity, noise
Work organization (E,C)	Team work, incentives, shifts, job rotation, machine pacing, job security

*E denotes mainly physical exposure and C denotes possible modifier to physical exposure (Adapted with permission from Halpern M: Prevention of low back pain: Basic ergonomics in the workplace and the clinic, in Nordin M, Vischer TL (eds): *Common Low Back Pain: Prevention of Chronicity*. London, England, Baillière Tindall, 1992, p 716.)

lated to nonspecific low back pain has had little impact. We could not find any study related to workplace intervention and disk herniation with or without sciatica.

Field intervention studies on whole body vibration are sparse. Özkaya and associates[109-111] reported the results of a comprehensive field study conducted on train operators for a large metropolitan subway system. The study was undertaken to measure mechanical vibrations transmitted to the train operators, to calculate daily whole-body vibration exposure levels, and to compare these levels with maximum acceptable exposure levels according to the international standard on whole-body vibration (ISO 2631, 1985).[112] The investigators also sought to identify factors that might influence mechanical vibrations transmitted to the operators. As a result of the study, six out of 20 subway lines were determined to have vibration levels higher than daily exposure limits provided in the ISO 2631 standard. Train speed was the most significant factor influencing the vibration exposure levels. Moreover, there were varying degrees of vibration transmissibility between different car types used in the subway system. Different cars of a single car type could transmit vibrations differently as well. This finding suggested that car maintenance was another factor that influenced the vibration levels. The continuous or welded rail contributed less to the vibration levels than the bolted rail. Operator experience in terms of the number of years on the job was observed to have some effect on the vibration levels: the more experienced the operator, the lower the measured vibration levels.

In a follow-up study, the same research group carried out a project to determine the vibration characteristics of two "new" operator seats and two "new-technology" trains that the authority in charge of the subway system was testing and planning to acquire.[113] The new seats with technologically more advanced appearance exhibited worse vibration characteristics than relatively simple old seats; the reasons for the difference could be explained through simple structural and kinematic analysis. Although it is very important to consider operator comfort and ergonomically correct posture, the vibration transmissibility must also be addressed in the design of new seats. The new seats tested could be satisfactory for use in a static (nonvibrating) environment, but would not protect the operator from the long-term effects of vibration exposure. As far as mechanical vibrations transmitted to the train operators were concerned, the two new-technology trains tested were superior to the trains currently operated on the subway system and also were in compliance with the limits provided in the ISO 2631 standard. Vibration should be reduced at the source. If this is not possible, other interventions could be used, such as seat redesign, cushion selection, or isolating the vibration at its source. Large field studies on whole body vibration are costly and difficult to perform. Nevertheless, they are important and challenge current design to protect the individual. Recent designs, including an active suspension system, are being tested that may reduce the long exposure levels.[114,115]

Ergonomic and Biomechanically-Based Advice to Patients With Sciatica

The patient with sciatica symptoms also commonly complains of low back pain. About two thirds of the patients reporting symptoms will have back pain as their chief symptom, and one third will have leg pain as their chief symptom. Numbness and muscle weakness can accompany these symptoms. Several authors report that patients with sciatica have a loss of sensation.[9,116,117] The prevalence of muscle weakness varies from 87% to 45%.[116-118] Pain usually develops first, and muscle weakness follows. The extensor hallucis longus is most affected, and the results are similar to those for patients operated on for a disk herniation.[119,120] We believe that the real prevalence of muscle weakness is underestimated because of the clinical method of muscle testing and the presence of compensatory mechanisms, as suggested by Bohannon and Gajdosik.[121] The recovery of muscle function is not well understood whether or not the patient has undergone surgery. However, such information is essential to the decision to return to work, particularly for individuals in safety-sensitive positions. For example, can a bus driver resume work with reduced pain but residual fatigue in the right foot? Can a utility employee climb a ladder safely several times a day with residual numbness, or is restricted duty indicated? If the pain is intolerable, must we recommend change of duty; and if the answer is yes, what kind of duty? Should an ergonomic workplace evaluation be recommended? There is no immediate answer to these questions, but they are important to the patient and to the treating physician.

The following suggested advice to be given to the patient with sciatica for personal prevention is based on biomechanical, epidemiologic, and outcome studies. We found no study related to the prevention of recurrence of sciatica. The long-term outcome for sciatica is relatively good if the condition is related to a disk herniation.[20,116,122,123] It is unclear if active[116] versus passive[124] treatment has a better outcome in the acute stage. This may reflect the natural history of sciatica.[125] No study has demonstrated the benefit of rest for sciatica. The support for bed rest would come from the biomechanical literature. Lying down exerts the lowest disk pressure, and the inflamed nerve root may be less mechanically irritated. Clinical observations support this theory.[9]

In the early stage, the patient should avoid heavy lifting and lifting in combination with twisting and lateral bending. The patient also should reduce driving time in the acute stage to a minimum and should adapt sitting posture in such a way as to maintain a neutral posture or to support the lumbar area.[101,102,126] Walking impact on the spine can be reduced by 40% with viscoelastic shoe inserts.[127] If morning stiffness is increased, the patient should avoid heavy physical loading for a couple of hours until the morning ''swelling'' of the disk is stabilized.[128] There is no evidence that immobilizing the spine with a corset would hasten recovery. There is some evidence that a program of weight control, regular exercise, and posture correction may reduce the frequency and severity of recurrent disk herniation and reported pain,[129] but the program needs further validation.

Johannsen and associates[130] compared supervised endurance training to a home program for patients with lumbar diskectomy. They state that ''It is not worthwhile to implement 3 months of supervised endurance training rather than home training on all first lumbar diskectomized patients.'' This study did not look at recurrence. Further studies are needed to understand the effect of exercise in relation to the natural history of sciatica, accompanying low back pain, and protection mechanisms for disk herniation. Fathallah and associates[131] showed diurnal variations in trunk flexibility and challenge the concept that injuries ocurring in the early morning hours may be a result of insufficient trunk mobility. A stretching program before starting work may be beneficial. Maigne and associates[132] and Matsubara and associates[133] showed that progression to painless working and leisure activities can vary from less than 1 month to 12 months. These two studies relate the time to recovery to the large individual differences in the reduction of size of the disk herniation. Surin[134] stated that ''the patient himself controls the duration of disability after surgery for lumbar disk prolapse.'' Finally, we could not find any ergonomic intervention studies related to sciatica.

Conclusion

Experimental studies show biomechanical evidence that disk herniation occurs after excessive load. Flexion of the motion segment in combination with lateral bending and axial torsion is damaging to the disk structure. In continuous repetitive motion or exposure to vibration, the motion segment exhibits creep and sudden buckling that can lead to disk herniation. Load to failure point for the disk structure corresponds to load calculated by mathematical models. The translation of these findings in vivo are still unclear. Studies in vivo indicate that the spine exhibits creep, muscle fatigue, loss of motor control, and thereby, increased load on the disk during exposure to repetitive motion, peak loads, and whole body vibration. Some epidemiologic data supports these findings. Existing available data indicate that disk herniation is a continuum of chronic, repetitive low grade trauma.

The situation for sciatica is more confusing. Experimental studies reveal that mechanical pressure and vibration on the nerve root ganglion are detrimental to the nerve tissue. The clinical findings of sciatica bear some correlation with the size and site of the herniated disk in nonsurgically treated patients over time. In patients who underwent surgery, no correlation was found between the size of the herniated disk and the reported pain. Sciatica pain only can be reproduced by compression or stretching if the nerve root itself is inflamed. Biomechanical or ergonomic principles, therefore, only can have an effect if relief of pressure on the inflamed nerve is obtained.

We could not find any primary prevention intervention studies specifically related to disk herniation and sciatica, nor could we find any outcome studies related to ergonomic intervention or reduction of mechanical load exposure related to this diagnosis and symptomatology. Strategies of prevention are based on the cumulative evidence from experimental studies, sparse epidemiology, and clinical studies and observations. Two strategies are presented for primary and secondary prevention. Primary prevention interventions should focus on eliminating excessive peak loads and reducing whole body vibration exposure. This type of intervention may affect the incidence of disk herniation. It may affect the incidence of reported sciatica differently. Secondary prevention is focused on advice to the patient with sciatica. The strategy here is to relieve the perceived pain by simple biomechanical and ergonomic concepts at home and in the workplace.

Acknowledgments

We would like to thank Dr. Nihat Özkaya for valuable advice, Ben Willems for compiling searches, Judy Trucios for manuscript preparation, and Dr. Dawn Leger for final editing. This paper was supported by The Reicher Foundation, Hospital for Joint Diseases Orthopaedic Institute, New York University Medical Center, New York, New York.

References

1. Spitzer WO, LeBlanc FE, Dupuis M, et al: Scientific approach to the assessment and management of activity-related spinal disorders: A monograph for clinicians. Report of the Quebec Task Force on Spinal Disorders. *Spine* 1987;12:S1–S59.
2. Bigos SJ, Bowyer O, Braen G, et al: Acute Low Back Problems in Adults, in *Clinical Practice Guideline No 14*. Rockville, MD, US Department of Health and Human Services, (AHCPR Publication No 95-0642), 1994.
3. Hasue M: Pain and the nerve root: An interdisciplinary approach. *Spine* 1995;18:2053–2058.
4. Kitano T, Zerwekh JE, Usui Y, et al: Biochemical changes associated with the symptomatic human intervertebral disk. *Clin Orthop* 1993;293:372–377.
5. Frymoyer JW: Back pain and sciatica. *N Engl J Med* 1988;318:291–300.
6. Bell GR, Rothman RH: The conservative treatment of sciatica. *Spine* 1984;9:54–56.
7. Nachemson AL: The natural course of low back pain, in White AA III, Gordon SL (eds): *Symposium on Idiopathic Low Back Pain*. St. Louis, MO, CV Mosby, 1982, pp 46–51.
8. Kelsey JL, Hardy RJ: Driving of motor vehicles as a risk factor for acute herniated lumbar intervertebral disc. *Am J Epidemiol* 1975;102:63–73.
9. Weber H: The natural history of disc herniation and the influence of intervention. *Spine* 1994;19:2234–2238.
10. Wickström G, Hänninen K: Determination of sciatica in epidemiologic research. *Spine* 1987;12:692–698.

11. Abenhaim L, Rossignol M, Gobeille D, et al: The prognostic consequences in the making of the initial medical diagnosis of work-related back injuries. *Spine* 1995;20:791–795.
12. Heliövaara M: Body weight, obesity and risk of herniated lumbar intervertebral disk. *Spine* 1987;12:469–472.
13. Kelsey JL, Golden AL, Mundt DJ: Low back pain/prolapsed lumbar intervertebral disc. *Rheum Dis Clin North Am* 1990;16:699–716.
14. Riihimäki H, Wickström G, Hanninen K, et al: Predictors of sciatic pain among concrete reenforcement workers and house painters: A five-year follow-up. *Scand J Work Environ Health* 1989;15:415–423.
15. Heliövaara M: Occupation and risk of herniated lumbar intervertebral disk or sciatica leading to hospitalization. *J Chron Dis* 1987;40:250–264.
16. Swärd L, Hellström M, Jacobsson B, et al: Disc degeneration and associated abnormalities of the spine in elite gymnasts: A magnetic resonance imaging study. *Spine* 1991;16:437–443.
17. Afshani E, Kuhn JP: Common causes of low back pain in children. *Radiographics* 1991;11:269–291.
18. Tertti M, Paajanen H, Kujala UM, et al: Disc degeneration in young gymnasts: A magnetic resonance imaging study. *Am J Sports Med* 1990;18:206–208.
19. Wing PC, Tsang IK, Susak L, et al: Back pain and spinal changes in microgravity. *Orthop Clin North Am* 1991;22:255–262.
20. Weber H: Lumbar disc herniation: A controlled, prospective study with ten years of observation. *Spine* 1983;8:131–140.
21. Biering-Sorensen F: Physical measurements as risk indicators for low-back trouble over a one-year period. *Spine* 1984;9:106–119.
22. Nykvist F, Hurme M, Alaranta H, et al: Severe sciatica: Troubles after years may still exist. A 13 year follow-up of 342 patients. *Eur Spine J*, in press.
23. Wood PHN, Baddeley EM: Epidemiology of back pain, in Jayson M IV (ed): *The Lumbar Spine and Low Back Pain,* ed 2. London, England, Pitman, 1980, pp 29–55.
24. Damkot DK, Pope MH, Lord J, et al: The relationship between work history, work environment and low-back pain in men. *Spine* 1984;9:395–399.
25. Moeri R, Balagué F, Carron R, et al: Chronic backache and occupational rehabilitation: Prognostic factors. *Schweiz Med Wochenschr* 1991;121:1897–1899.
26. Hakelius A: Prognosis in sciatica: A clinical follow up of surgical and nonsurgical treatment. *Acta Orthop Scand* 1970;129(suppl):1–76.
27. Nachemson A, Lewin T, Maroudas A, et al: In-vitro diffusion of dye through the end-plates and the annulus fibrosus of human lumbar intervertebral discs. *Acta Orthop Scand* 1970;41:589–607.
28. Adams MA, Hutton WC: Gradual disc prolapse. *Spine* 1985;10:524–531.
29. Holm S, Maroudas A, Urban JP, et al: Nutrition of the intervertebral disc: Solute transport and metabolism. *Connect Tissue Res* 1981;8:101–119.
30. Holm S, Nachemson A: Nutritional changes in the canine intervertebral disc after spinal fusion. *Clin Orthop* 1982;169:243–258.
31. Mooney V, Brown M, Modic M: Clinical perspectives, in Frymoyer JW, Gordon SL (eds): *New Perspectives on Low Back Pain.* Park Ridge, IL, American Academy of Orthopaedic Surgeons, 1989, pp 133–146.
32. Postacchini F, Lami R, Pugliese O: Familial predisposition to discogenic low-back pain: An epidemiologic and immunogenetic study. *Spine* 1988;13:1403–1406.
33. Varlotta GP, Brown MD, Kelsey JL, et al: Familial predisposition for herniation of a lumbar disc in patients who are less than twenty-one years old. *J Bone Joint Surg* 1991;73A:124–128.
34. Urban JP, McMullin JF: Swelling pressure of the inervertebral disc: Influence of proteoglycan and collagen contents. *Biorheology* 1985;22:145–157.
35. Nachemson A: Lumbar intradiscal pressure: Experimental studies on post-mortem material. *Acta Orthop Scand* 1960;43(suppl):1–104.
36. Virgin WJ: Experimental investigations into the physical properties of the intervertebral disc. *J Bone Joint Surg* 1951;33B:607–611.

37. Nachemson A: Lumbar mechanics as revealed by lumbar intradiscal pressure measurements, in Jayson M (ed): *The Lumbar Spine and Back Pain*. London, England, Churchill Livingstone, 1992, pp 157–171.
38. Goel VK, Weinstein JN (eds): *Biomechanics of the Spine: Clinical and Surgical Perspective*. Boca Raton, FL, CRC Press, 1990, pp 157–179.
39. Krag MH, Seroussi RE, Wilder DG, et al: Internal displacement distribution from in vitro loading of human thoracic and lumbar spinal motion segments: Experimental results and theoretical predictions. *Spine* 1987;12:1001–1007.
40. Brinckmann P: Injury of the annulus fibrosus and disc protrusions: An in vitro investigation on human lumbar discs. *Spine* 1986;11:149–153.
41. Adams MA, Hutton WC: Prolapse intervertebral disc: A hyperflexion injury. *Spine* 1982;7:184–191.
42. Panjabi MM, Goel VK, Takata K: Physiologic strains in the lumbar spinal ligaments: An in vitro biomechanical study. *Spine* 1982;7:192–203.
43. Adams MA, Dolan P: Recent advances in lumbar spinal mechanics and their clinical significance. *Clin Biomech* 1995;10:3–19.
44. Chaffin DB: A computerized biomechanical model: Development of and use in studying gross body actions. *J Biomech* 1969;2:429–441.
45. Schultz A, Andersson GB, Örtengren R, et al: Analysis and quantitative myoelectric measurements of loads on the lumbar spine when holding weights in standing postures. *Spine* 1982;7:390–397.
46. McGill SM, Norman RW: Dynamically and statically determined low back moments during lifting. *J Biomech* 1985;18:877–885.
47. Lucas DB, Bresler B (eds): *Stability of the Ligamentous Spine*. San Francisco, CA, University of California, 1961.
48. Kazarian L: Dynamic response characteristics of the human vertebral column: An experimental study on human autopsy specimens. *Acta Orthop Scand* 1972;146(suppl):1–186.
49. Keller TS, Hansson TH, Holm SH, et al: In vivo creep behavior of the normal and degenerated porcine intervertebral disk: A preliminary report. *J Spinal Disord* 1988;1:267–278.
50. Wilder DG, Pope MH, Seroussi RE, et al: The balance point of the intervertebral motion segment: An experimental study. *Bull Hosp Joint Dis Orthop Inst* 1989;49:155–169.
51. Goel VK, Nishiyama K, Weinstein JN, et al: Mechanical properties of lumbar spinal motion segments as affected by partial disc removal. *Spine* 1986;11:1008–1012.
52. Liu YK, Goel VK, De Jong A, et al: Torsional fatigue of the lumbar intervertebral joints. *Spine* 1985;10:894–900.
53. Shirazi-Adl A: Strain in fibers of a lumbar disc: Analysis of the role of lifting in producing disc prolapse. *Spine* 1989;14:96–103.
54. Brinckmann P, Wilder DG, Pope MH: Effects of repeated loads and vibration, in Wiesel SW, Weinstein JN, Herkowitz H, et al (eds): *The Lumbar Spine*. Philadelphia, PA, WB Saunders, 1996, pp 181–202.
55. Eklund JA, Corlett EN: Shrinkage as a measure of the effect of load on the spine. *Spine* 1984;9:189–194.
56. McGill SM, Brown S: Creep response of the lumbar spine to prolonged full flexion. *Clin Biomech* 1992;7:43–46.
57. Hedman TP, Fernie GR: In vivo measurement of lumbar spinal creep in two seated postures using magnetic resonance imaging. *Spine* 1995;20:178–183.
58. Magnusson ML: *Effects of Seated Whole Body Vibrations on the Spine: An Experimental Study in Man*. Gothenburg, Sweden, University of Gothenburg, 1991. Thesis.
59. Panjabi MM, Andersson GB, Jorneus L, et al: In vivo measurements of spinal column vibrations. *J Bone Joint Surg* 1986;68A:695–702.
60. Pope MH, Wilder DG, Jorneus L, et al: The response of the seated human to sinusoidal vibration and impact. *J Biomech Eng* 1987;109:279–284.

61. Hansson TH, Keller TS, Spengler DM: The effect of static and dynamic load on disc pressure in the human lumbar spine. *Trans Orthop Res Soc* 1984;9:255.

62. Bongers HC, Boshuizen PM: *Back Disorders and Whole Body Vibration at Work.* Amsterdam, The Netherlands, University of Amsterdam, 1990. Thesis.

63. McLain RF, Weinstein JN: Ultrastructural changes in the dorsal root ganglion associated with whole body vibration. *J Spinal Disord* 1991;4:142–148.

64. McLain RF, Weinstein JN: Effects of whole body vibration on dorsal root ganglion neurons: Changes in neuronal nuclei. *Spine* 1994;19:1455–1461.

65. Hirsch C, Nachemson A: New observations on the mechanical behavior of lumbar discs. *Acta Orthop Scand* 1954;23:254–283.

66. Lin HS, Liu YK, Adams KH: Mechanical response of the lumbar intervertebral joint under physiological (complex) loading. *J Bone Joint Surg* 1978;60A:41–55.

67. Reuber M, Schultz A, Denis F, et al: Bulging of lumbar intervertebral disks. *J Biomech Eng* 1982;104:187–192.

68. Brinckmann P, Horst M: The influence of vertebral body fracture, intradiscal injection, and partial discectomy on the radial bulge and height of human lumbar discs. *Spine* 1985;10:138–145.

69. Ritchie JH, Fahrni WH: Age changes in lumbar intervertebral discs. *Can J Surg* 1970;13:65–71.

70. Krag MH, Seroussi RE, Wilder DG, et al: Internal displacement distribution from in vitro of the human lumbar spinal motion segments: Experimental results and theoretical predictions. *Spine* 1987;12:1001–1007.

71. Erlacher PR: Nucleography. *J Bone Joint Surg* 1952;34B:204–210.

72. Andersson GB, Schultz AB: Effects of fluid injection on mechanical properties of intervertebral discs. *J Biomech* 1979;12:453–458.

73. Knutsson F: The instability associated with disk degeneration in the lumbar spine. *Acta Radiol* 1944;25:593–609.

74. van Akkerveeken PF, O'Brien JP, Park WM: Experimentally induced hypermobility in the lumbar spine: A pathologic and radiologic study of the posterior ligament and annulus fibrosus. *Spine* 1979;4:236–241.

75. Harris RI, Macnab I: Structural changes in the lumbar intervertebral discs: Their relationship to low back pain and sciatica. *J Bone Joint Surg* 1954;36B:304–322.

76. Bradford DS, Swedenburg SM, Carpenter RJ, et al: Facet joint changes after surgical excision of the nucleus pulposus of mature dogs. *Trans Orthop Res Soc* 1987;12:324.

77. Takahashi K, Inoue S, Takada S, et al: Experimental study of chemonucleolysis: With special reference to the change of intradiscal pressure. *Spine* 1986;11:617–620.

78. Tsuchida T, Suguro T, Inoue S, et al: Regeneration of the nucleus pulposus after experimental chemonucleolysis: Collagenase. *Trans Orthop Res Soc* 1987;12:325.

79. Howe JF, Loeser JD, Calvin WH: Mechanosensivity of dorsal root ganglia and chronically injured axons: A physiological basis for the radicular pain of nerve root compression. *Pain* 1977;3:25–41.

80. Wall PD, Devor M: Sensory afferent impulses originate from dorsal root ganglia as well as from the periphery in normal and nerve injured rats. *Pain* 1983;17:321–339.

81. Kuslich SD, Ulstrom CL, Michael CJ: The tissue origin of low back pain and sciatica: A report of pain response to tissue stimulation during operations on the lumbar spine using local anesthesia. *Orthop Clin North Am* 1991;22:181–187.

82. Boden SD, Davis DO, Dina TS, et al: Abnormal magnetic-resonance scans of the lumbar spine in asymptomatic subjects: A prospective investigation. *J Bone Joint Surg* 1990;72A:403–408.

83. Wiesel SW, Tsourmas N, Feffer HL, et al: A study of computer-assisted tomography: I. The incidence of positive CAT scans in an asymptomatic group of patients. *Spine* 1984;9:549–551.

84. Weinreb JC, Wolbarsht LB, Cohen JM, et al: Prevalence of lumbosacral intervertebral disk abnormalities on MR images in pregnant and asymptomatic nonpregnant women. *Radiology* 1989;170:125–128.

45

85. Jensen MC, Brant-Zawadzki MN, Obuchowski N, et al: Magnetic resonance imaging of the lumbar spine in people without back pain. *N Engl J Med* 1994;331:69–73.

86. Montaldi S, Fankhauser H, Schnyder P, et al: Computed tomography of the postoperative intervertebral disc and lumbar spinal canal: Investigation of twenty-five patients after successful operation for lumbar disc herniation. *Neurosurgery* 1988;22:1014–1022.

87. Tullberg T: *Lumbar Disc Herniation Results of Micro and Standard Surgical Treatment Evaluated by Clinical, Radiological and Neurophysiological Methods.* Stockholm, Sweden, St. Göran Hospital and Karolinska Hospital, 1993. Thesis.

88. Thelander U, Fagerlund M, Friberg S, et al: Describing the size of lumbar disc herniations using computed tomography: A comparison of different size index calculations and their relation to sciatica. *Spine* 1994;19:1979–1984.

89. Buckwalter JA: Editorial: Should bone, soft-tissue, and joint injuries be treated with rest or activity? *J Orthop Res* 1995;13:155–156.

90. Parnianpour M, Nordin M, Kahanovitz N, et al: The triaxial coupling of torque generation of trunk muscles during isometric exertions and the effect of fatiguing isoinertial movements on the motor output and movement patterns. *Spine* 1988;13:982–992.

91. Marras WS, Parnianpour M, Ferguson SA, et al: Classification of anatomic- and symptom-based low back disorders using motion measure models. *Spine* 1995;20:2531–2546.

92. Chaffin DB: Localized muscle fatigue: Definition of and measurement. *J Occup Med* 1973;15:346–354.

93. Bates BT, Osternig LR, James SL: Fatigue effects in running. *J Motor Behav* 1977;9:203–207.

94. Bigland-Ritchie B, Woods JJ: Changes in muscle contractile properties and neural control during human muscular fatigue. *Muscle Nerve* 1984;7:691–699.

95. Gallagher S, Hamrick CA, Love AC, et al: Dynamic modelling of symmetric and asymmetric lifting tasks in restricted postures. *Ergonomics* 1994;37:1289–1310.

96. Hakkinen K, Keskinen KL: Muscle cross-sectional area and voluntary force production characteristics in elite strength- and endurance-trained athletes and sprinters. *Eur J Appl Physiol* 1989;59:215–220.

97. McGill SM, Norman RW: Effects of an anatomically detailed erector spinae model on L4/L5 disc compression and shear. *J Biomech* 1987;20:591–600.

98. Genaldy A, Houshyar H: Optimization techniques in occupational biomechanics, in *Proceedings of the Human Factors Society, 33rd Annual Meeting.* Santa Monica, CA, Human Factors Society, 1989, pp 672–676.

99. Pope MH, Wilder DG, Krag MH: Biomechanics of the lumbar spine, in Frymoyer JW, Ducker TB, Hadler NM, et al (eds): *The Adult Spine: Principles and Practice.* Raven Press, New York, NY, 1991, vol 2, pp 1487–1501.

100. Floyd WF, Silver PHS: The function of erectores spinae muscles in certain movements and postures in man. *J Physiol* 1955;129:184–203.

101. Lelong C, Drevet JG, Chevallier R, et al: Spinal biomechanics and the sitting position. *Rev Rhum Mal Ostéoartic* 1988;55:375–380.

102. Drevet JG, Lelong C, Plas F, et al: Les pressions intra-discales lombaires in vivo: application aux techniques de rééducation des lombo-radiculalgies. *Rev de Méd Orthopédique* 1991;23:9–12.

103. Belytschko T, Kulak RF, Schultz AB, et al: Finite element stress analysis of an intervertebral disc. *J Biomech* 1974;7:277–285.

104. Buckwalter JA, Goldberg VM, Woo SL-Y (eds): *Musculoskeletal Soft-Tissue Aging: Impact on Mobility.* Rosemont, IL, American Academy of Orthopaedic Surgeons, 1993.

105. Nordin M, Weiser S, Halpern N: Education: The prevention and treatment of low back disorders, in Frymoyer JW, Ducker TB, Hadler NM, et al (eds): *The Adult Spine: Principles and Practice.* New York, NY, Raven Press, 1991, vol 2, pp 1641–1651.

106. National Institute for Occupational Safety and Health: *Proposed National Strategy for the Prevention of Musculoskeletal Injuries.* Cincinnati, Ohio, US Department of Health and Human Services, DHHS (NIOSH) Publication No 89-129, 1986.

107. Joseph BS: Ergonomic considerations and job design in upper extremity disorders. *Occup Med* 1989;4:547–557.

108. Lifshitz YR, Armstrong TJ, Seagull FBJ, et al: The effectiveness of an ergonomics program in controlling work-related disorders in an automotive plant: A case study, in Queinnec Y, Daniellou F (eds): *Designing for Everyone.* London, England, Taylor & Francis, 1991, pp 323–325.

109. Özkaya N, Willems B, Goldsheyder D: Vibration exposure study conducted on train operators part I: Exposure levels. *BED* 1992;22:565–566.

110. Özkaya N, Willems B, Goldsheyder D, et al: Whole-body vibration exposure experienced by subway train operators. *J Low Frequency Noise Vibration* 1994;13:13–18.

111. Özkaya N, Willems B, Goldsheyder D: Whole-body vibration exposure: A comprehensive field study. *Am Ind Hyg Assoc J* 1994;55:1164–1171.

112. International Standard Organization: *Evaluation of Human Exposure to Whole-Body Vibration: Part I. General Requirements.* Geneva, Switzerland, International Organisation for Standardization, ISO 2631/1, 1985, pp 1–17.

113. Özkaya N, Goldsheyder D, Willems B: Effect of subway car design on vibration exposure. *Int J Indust Ergo,* in press.

114. Koizumi S, Hirata T, Ishihara K, et al: Active suspension system for railway vehicles. *Sumito Search* 1994;56:55–61.

115. Nagai M, Mori H, Nakadai S: Active vibration control of electrodynamic suspension system. *JSME Int J* 1995;38:48–54.

116. Saal JA, Saal JS: Nonoperative treatment of herniated lumbar intervertebral disc with radiculopathy: An outcome study. *Spine* 1989;14:431–437.

117. Saal JA, Saal JS, Herzog RJ: The natural history of lumbar intervertebral disc extrusions treated nonoperatively. *Spine* 1990;15:683–686.

118. Garfin SR, Rydevik B, Lind B, et al: Spinal nerve root compression. *Spine* 1995;20:1810–1820.

119. Kortelainen P, Puranen J, Koivisto E, et al: Symptoms and signs of sciatica and their relation to the localization of the lumbar disc herniation. *Spine* 1985;10:88–92.

120. Jönsson B, Strömqvist B: Symptoms and signs in degeneration of the lumbar spine: A prospective, consecutive study of 300 operated patients. *J Bone Joint Surg* 1993;75B:381–385.

121. Bohannon RW, Gajdosik RL: Spinal nerve root compression: Some clinical implications. A review of the literature. *Phys Ther* 1987;67:376–382.

122. Bush K, Cowan N, Katz DE, et al: The natural history of sciatica associated with disc pathology: A prospective study with clinical and independent radiologic follow-up. *Spine* 1992;17:1205–1212.

123. Sany J, Kalfa G, Bataille R, et al: La sciatique paralysante en milieu rhumatologique, in Simon L (ed): *La sciatique et le nerf sciatique.* Paris, France, Masson, 1980, pp 202–210.

124. Delauche-Cavallier MC, Budet C, Laredo JD, et al: Lumbar disc herniation: Computed tomography scan changes after conservative treatment of nerve root compression. *Spine* 1992;17:927–933.

125. Ellenberg MR, Ross ML, Honet JC, et al: Prospective evaluation of the course of disc herniations in patients with proven radiculopathy. *Arch Phys Med Rehabil* 1993;74:3–8.

126. Andersson GBJ, Örtengren R, Herberts P: Quantitative electromyographic studies of back muscle activity related to posture and loading. *Orthop Clin North Am* 1977;8:85–96.

127. Wosk J, Voloshin AS: Low back pain: Conservative treatment with artificial shock absorbers. *Arch Phys Med Rehabil* 1985;66:145–148.

128. Porter RW, Trailescu IF: Diurnal changes in straight leg raising. *Spine* 1990;15:103–106.

47

129. Gilmer HS, Papadopoulos SM, Tuite GF: Lumbar disk disease: Pathophysiology, management and prevention. *Am Fam Physician* 1993;47:1141–1152.
130. Johannsen F, Remvig L, Kryger P, et al: Supervised endurance exercise training compared to home training after first lumbar diskectomy: A clinical trial. *Clin Exp Rheumatol* 1994;12:609–614.
131. Fathallah FA, Marras WS, Wright PL: Diurnal variation in trunk kinematics during a typical work shift. *J Spinal Disord* 1995;8:20–25.
132. Maigne JY, Rime B, Deligne B: Computed tomographic follow-up study of forty-eight cases of nonoperatively treated lumbar intervertebral disc herniation. *Spine* 1992;17:1071–1074.
133. Matsubara Y, Kato F, Mimatsu K, et al: Serial changes on MRI in lumbar disc herniations treated conservatively. *Neuroradiology* 1995;37:378–383.
134. Surin VV: Duration of disability following lumbar disc surgery. *Acta Orthop Scand* 1977;48:466–471.

Chapter 3

Exercise in the Prevention and Treatment of Herniated Nucleus Pulposus

Tapio Videman, MD, Dr Med Sci

Introduction

The early explanation for sciatic pain was purely "mechanical," entrapment of a nerve root by a herniated nucleus pulposus (HNP), and the prevention strategies and treatment principles were thought to be relatively clear. More recent demonstrations of biochemical and immunologic mechanisms of sciatic nerve inflammation suggest the pathogenesis is more complicated than once thought.

Defining Intervertebral Disk Herniation and Sciatica

Although HNP is one of the best understood severe back-related symptom disorders, its definition is not clear. The clinical diagnosis of HNP has included, in addition to herniation of material from the nucleus pulposus and anulus fibrosus, back pain radiating to the extremity (sciatic pain distribution). Recent studies, which show that inflammation of neural elements caused by biochemical factors alone can cause sciatic pain,[1-3] have called into question the earlier "clear" clinical principles and further confused the issue about the clinical relevance of herniation (Fig. 1).

No generally accepted terminology or classification of herniations exists.[4] Only a portion of disk herniations cause sciatica; in one study, 37% of asymptomatic subjects had abnormalities of the intervertebral space as assessed from myelograms.[5] In two other studies, about 20% of subjects had disk herniations identified on imaging studies, but no recollection of ever having had back or sciatic pain.[6,7] HNP and sciatica are not synonyms; HNP does not always produce sciatic pain, nor do all patients with sciatica have a herniated disk or all annular ruptures lead to inflammation of the sciatic nerve. Most epidemiologic studies of sciatica are based purely on questionnaire data of "back pain radiating to the extremity" because usually it is not possible to obtain data from clinical examinations, such as myelograms, computed tomography (CT), or magnetic resonance imaging (MRI), which include risks for subjects or are expensive.

The Role of Biomechanics

Annular ruptures occur when the anulus is exposed to mechanical forces of either peak loads or repeated loading that exceed its strength. The individual

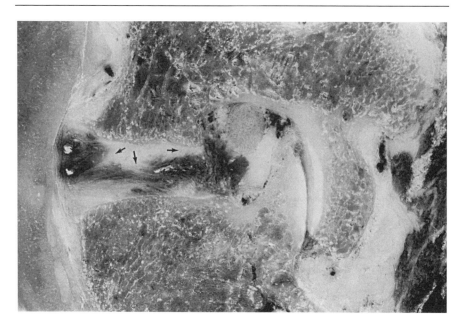

Fig. 1 *A cryomicrotomic section (made by Dr. W. Rauschning) through the edge of the disk and intervertebral foramina. Methylene blue (arrows) was injected into the nucleus pulposus and the dye leaked through tears in the anulus and is communicating with the nerve root. (It is not known whether this situation causes back or sciatic pain.)*

variation in the strength of the anulus may be due mainly to the stage of degeneration. A common explanation for the development of HNP is that the anulus fibrosus degenerates to such an extent that during normal daily activity parts of the nucleus pulposus can herniate through it. The extruded disk material also swells by more than twice its original size in the surrounding fluid during the first 4 hours; this swelling can worsen the entrapment of the nerve root[8] and cause inflammation from mechanical irritation. Spinal canal dimensions are associated with pain, but it is not clear how these dimensions affect symptoms from herniation.

The training effect responsible for increased strength of muscles, tendons, ligaments, and bone that is clearly demonstrated in athletes may influence the anulus as well. Data from a few studies have indicated that loading strengthens the connective tissues of the disk,[9] but data from other studies have not revealed this association[10,11] (Table 1). A complicated relationship may exist between

Table 1 Disk bulging and herniations among former elite athletes[11]

MRI Finding*	Runners	Soccer Players	Weight Lifters	Shooters
Disk bulging	1.1	1.3	1.4	1
Disk herniation	1.2	1.7	1.6	1

*MRI, magnetic resonance imaging

structural failure, current mechanical loading, and adaptive remodeling due to past loading.[12]

Major methodologic problems limit the evaluation of the strength and thickness of the anulus fibrosus in living persons. As an example, a thin anulus fibrosus is usually classified as ''degenerated'' in diskographic evaluations, but in theory, the thinning could be due partly to atrophy from a lifelong activity (the absence of a training effect). Biomechanical experiments using cadaveric material have shown that compressive loading alone usually cannot produce disk damage before damage to the adjacent vertebral body.[13,14] Adams and Dolan[12] wrote, ''The only loading condition known to cause posterior disk prolapse involves a combination of compression, lateral bending, and forward bending.'' Repeated compressions in a flexed spine can cause posterolateral annular fissures and gradual disk herniation in nondegenerated disks.[15]

Normal-looking lumbar disks from cadavers of individuals younger than 50 years of age prolapse the most readily, while severely degenerated disks could not be made to prolapse.[15] One explanation for the peak in lumbar disk prolapses in middle-aged adults has been that the risk for prolapse decreases in later years due to depletion of hydrophilic glycosaminoglycans and increased fibrosis in the nucleus as part of disk degeneration. When disk degeneration starts is a matter of controversy. Osti and associates[16] found that around the age of 20 years, the outer anulus commonly shows rim lesions, the first macroscopic degenerative changes of the anulus. In a review article, Buckwalter[17] underlined that age-related degeneration of the human disk, including declining nutrition and loss of viable cells, begins in the nucleus. The possible role of vertebral end plate defects in disk degeneration has been described as a consequence of decreased intradiskal pressure, which leads to less stimuli of disk cells and, further, to decreased synthesis of collagen and glycosaminoglycans.[12]

Although degeneration related to biologic aging cannot be prevented, some factors accelerate it, and some may have beneficial effects in slowing it. Increased physical activity improves blood circulation around the intervertebral disk, diffusion between the disk and surrounding tissues, and accelerates metabolism in general. All these phenomena have been considered beneficial for the disk. This conclusion is based on experimental studies, which show that spinal movements give rise to positive nutritional variations.[18] Another theory also suggests that free radical formation in connection with strenuous exercise could accelerate degeneration.[19] In general, exercise improves metabolism; however, accelerated metabolism during physical activity reflects the body's response to increased needs, and the final gain from accelerated metabolism and further exercise is unclear. Hereditary factors are likely to exert a major role both in the structure of intervertebral disks and their degeneration; the ability to identify those at highest risk could increase markedly the chances for prevention.

Exercise Considerations

The physical loading patterns vary in different exercise modes and sport events. In respect to the back, leisure time physical activities can be grossly grouped. Endurance activities, for example, swimming, jogging, and cross-country skiing, are believed to have mainly beneficial effects on the back. Power sports, which increase axial loading across the entire thoracolumbar spine with high peak loads and increased loading in flexion and extension, and sometimes also in twisted positions, show an increased risk for spine degeneration. Sports with variable loading, which include occasional contact, forceful twisting, and falling (gymnastics, boxing, wrestling, game sports, and downhill and water skiing), include increased risk for injuries and also for degeneration, especially of the two lowest lumbar disk levels. In addition to the different types of exercises, the content of sessions of the same event can vary in duration, intensity, and frequency. The number of years of the activity is crucial in studying the long-term effects of exercise. The leisure time activities have shorter duration, but often higher intensity, than does occupational physical loading, and the chances to rest after physical activity sessions usually can be individually decided.

The physical demands of the job represent an important confounder for recreational physical activities: those with physically light work seem to participate in more leisure time physical activities than do those with heavier jobs.[20] Because the time spent in exercise is a small portion of that spent in work, accurate lifetime information about both work and exercise and sport participation is important when studying the effects of either.

Exercise as a Risk/Preventive Factor for Herniated Nucleus Pulposus

The Epidemiologic Evidence

It has been estimated that the incidence of a new prolapsed lumbar intervertebral disk is between 0.1% to 0.5% of the population per year in the age range of 20 to 64 years.[21,22] A history or sign of nerve root involvement was found in 10% of those with moderate or severe lumbar disk degeneration.[23] Among 2,504 consecutive lumbar disk operations performed in Sweden, the proportion of men to women was seven to three, and the mean age increased from 38 to 44 years from 1951 to 1962.[24] A prospective study of sciatica among concrete reinforcement workers and house painters showed that during a 5-year follow-up period, 60% of the concrete reinforcement workers and 42% of the house painters had experienced sciatica. These high percentages may reflect different underlying diagnostic criteria than were used in some earlier studies.[25] However, the apparently high incidence of sciatica reported by concrete reinforcement workers and house painters was supported by another study, in which it was found that sciatica had been diagnosed in approximately 25% of a general population sample of working age Finnish men.[26] In a prospective study of World War II United States military recruits, military rank and occupations of craftsman or foreman were factors associated with higher occurrence rates of hospitalizations, whereas rates were lower among recruits with clerical occupations.[27] Men who were taller and heavier at the time of their recruitment also had a higher incidence of hospitalizations.

In a Finnish population-based study of 57,000 men and women followed over an 11-year period, men were 1.6 times more likely than women to be hospitalized for disk herniation.[28] Taller men and women also were more likely to be hospitalized; an association with weight was less clear. Kelsey and Hardy[29] reported that the risk of being hospitalized due to a herniated lumbar disk or sciatica was lowest in professional occupations and highest among blue-collar workers and motor vehicle drivers. A multivariate model of the predictors of sciatic pain in concrete reinforcement workers and painters[25] included a history of prior sciatica and back "accidents." The relative risk for a person with a history of previous sciatica was 3.4 times that of someone without such a history, and the relative risk for someone with a previous back "accident" was 1.2 times higher. Stress also was associated with a higher incidence of sciatica during follow-up. A separate analysis of the subset of workers without a history of sciatica prior to the 5-year follow-up showed that concrete reinforcement workers (with physically heavier jobs) had a relative risk of 1.5 times that of house painters. A history of prior back "accidents" was associated with a relative risk of 1.4.[25]

For sciatica, as for all multifactorial diseases, it is very difficult to separate a true causal risk factor from a risk indicator; for example, heavy physical work and smoking are likely to be causal factors for many health problems, but they are also indicators for many other risk factors. Heliövaara and associates[28] wrote, "Although none of the suspected risk factors can be described as having been conclusively investigated epidemiologically, the results of published studies show that there are modifiable factors contributing to low back pain." In an autopsy study, the probability for at least one annular rupture, identified by diskography, increased with age. By age 64 years, almost all patients had had at least one annular rupture, but the lifetime incidence of sciatic pain was 15%. Although the validity of a pain history obtained from close family members can be questioned, it would appear that only a small portion of annular ruptures lead to severe back pain, even if annular leaking at the time of diskography has been shown to be highly associated with pain reproduction in surgery candidates.[30]

In summary, the main suspected risk factors for HNP are manual handling of materials, twisting, bending, and driving;[29] however, less than 20% of the cases could be attributed to such activities.[31] Although smoking, obesity, and parity in women have been associated with sciatica, their causal relation is questionable.[32,33] Body height may be the only sciatica-specific risk factor; taller persons have increased incidence of surgically treated sciatica.[28] Leisure time physical activity did not predict HNP or sciatica in a population sample,[28] nor in former top athletes[11] (Table 2). Overall, the suspected physical risk factors for HNP are similar to those for low back pain and disk degeneration; psychologic distress, self-assessed strenuousness of work, and social class also are associated with sciatica (Table 3).

The Effect of Exercise on Herniated Nucleus Pulposus

It is obvious that exercise will avoid the side effects of inactivity and that the musculoskeletal system needs some use to function optimally. Experimental and clinical studies have demonstrated that immobilization causes disorganization, weakening, and shortening of connective tissues. The common experience is, however, that physical activities exacerbate sciatic pain, which restricts and limits most physical activities. There are a few studies demonstrating that repeated end-range lumbar flexion and extension movements ("McKenzie-method") performed by the patients can affect back pain intensity and location in a beneficial way, that is, they decrease the distribution of the radiating pain. This is called

Table 2 Odds ratio for sciatica and for hospitalization due to sciatica among former athletes and referents[11]

Sport	Adjusted for Age and Occupational Loading*	
	Sciatica	Hospitalization
Endurance	1.5	0.8
Sprint	1.0	1.1
Jumping	0.8	0.5
Throwing	1.2	2.4
Games	1.1	1.2
Contact	0.7	1.9
Weightlifting	1.5	1.8
Shooting	1.2	3.0
Referents	1.00	1.00

*None of the odds ratios were statistically significant

Table 3 Age-adjusted odds ratios of some covariates for sciatica, hospitalization due to sciatica, and back pain[11]

Covariate	Sciatica	Hospitalization	Back Pain
Education (low)	1.2	1.5	1.3
Divorced/widowed	1.1	0.8	0.9
Heavy occupational load	1.6	2.0	3.1§
Forced work pace	1.3	0.3	1.8*
Monotonic work	2.2	1.1	1.8†
Not working	1.2	3.2†	1.3
Smoking	0.9	1.3	1.3*
Alcohol (much)	0.9	0.8	1.0
Strenuous exercise	1.4*	1.4	0.7*
Body mass index (kg/m²) > 30	1.4*	1.0	1.3
Height	1.0	1.0	1.0
Poor sleep quality	1.5*	0.5	3.1§
Life dissatisfaction	1.6	1.3	2.6§
Extroversion	1.2	0.8	1.3*
Neuroticism	1.6*	0.5	2.5§
Hostility	1.9*	1.6	1.8*

* $p < 0.05$
† $p < 0.01$
§ $p < 0.001$

the "centralization phenomenon," and is a predictor of a more rapid recovery without surgery.[34,35] The common explanation of this phenomenon is a "mechanical effect" on the nucleus pulposus. In theory, increased metabolism could accelerate resorption of herniated material, but this has not been clearly documented.

Animal experiments show that increased motion and associated loading can increase scar tissue formation. In a rabbit experiment, the anterior anulus of two

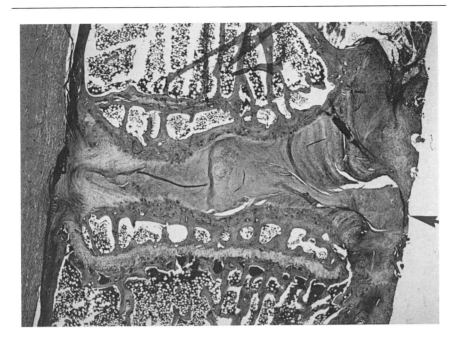

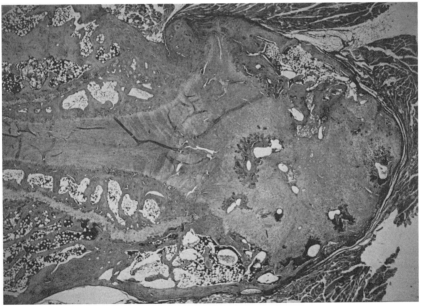

Fig. 2   *Histologic sections from an intervertebral disk operated on 12 weeks earlier show the effect of increased motion and loading on healing. The upper section is from a rabbit living in a standard cage, which allows limited movement, and shows a partly herniated nucleus pulposus with some healing of the anulus (arrow). The lower picture is from a rabbit that was allowed to move freely in a large cage with other rabbits; the section shows a large fibrocartilaginous proliferation at the site of incision. (Reproduced with permission from Gill K, Videman T, Shimizu T, et al: Experimental intervertebral disc degeneration: Studies on the pathogenesis and therapy.* Orthop Trans *1988;12:96–97.)*

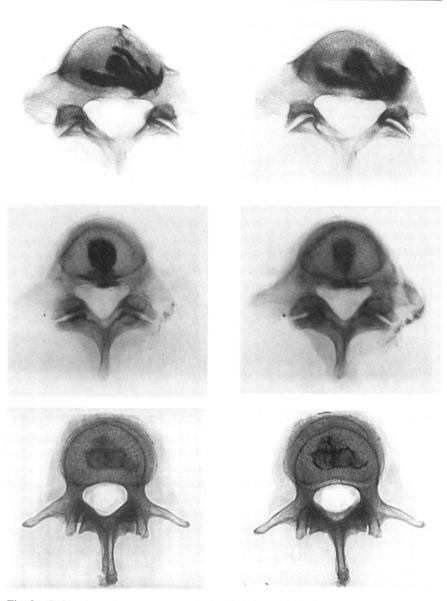

Fig. 3 *Cadaveric motion segments studied with diskography before and after repeated extensions.* **Top left** *(axial view), There is a posterolateral leaking of contrast media.* **Top right**, *Further dye extravasation has occurred, with increased bulging and narrowing of the canal.* **Middle left**, *There is a central fissure and bulge.* **Middle right**, *After 270 repeated extensions the dye is extravasated into the spinal canal with changes in the diskogram pattern.* **Bottom left** *and* **right**, *Diskograms without leaking and no significant changes after repeated extensions. (Reproduced with permission from Gill K, Videman T, Shimizu T, et al: The effect of repeated extensions on the discographic dye patterns in cadaveric lumbar motion segments. Clin Biomech 1987;2:205–210).*

lumbar disks was first cut using the technique described by Lipson and Muir.[36] One group of animals was put together in a cage built by combining three dog cages. The rabbits from the other group were separated and kept in individual small cages. When the groups were compared after 12 weeks, the cut disks from the group that was free to move showed marked proliferative reaction in histologic examination and more severe osteophyte formation and disk space narrowing than did the cut disks from rabbits kept separately in standard cages (Fig. 2). It could be concluded that deconditioning can be avoided by exercise, but the type of exercise may be important because some activities may have deleterious effects.

There are many anecdotal reports of beneficial outcomes and sudden recovery from manipulative and traction therapies. However, there are no adequate clinical studies demonstrating these effects. The mechanisms for possible beneficial effects are also unclear. Most of these treatment methods are based on biomechanical theories, but there is no clear experimental evidence that nerve entrapment can be resolved by mechanical forces applied through exercise and activity. Fifty-four cadaveric motion segments were studied using diskography and tested thereafter with repeated extension/compression moments. Analysis of changes in diskogram dye patterns showed increased dye leaking in 43%, while the observed bulging increased in 31% and decreased in 2%.[37] The major effect of repeated extension moments appears to lie in forcing dye from the nucleus pulposus into the spinal epidural space, or some peridiskal space in disks with a degenerated anulus. If the anulus was intact, no major changes occurred in the dye patterns (Fig. 3). These results did not explain how extension treatment methods may have favorable clinical results, but it is possible that some beneficial biochemical changes may be involved. There is a dearth of scientific evidence supporting a beneficial biomechanical effect of physical activity on nerve entrapment or the healing process of disk ruptures. Exercise could have beneficial metabolic effects on the mechanism underlying the sciatic pain, but this association has not been demonstrated.

References

1. Cavanaugh JM: Neural mechanisms of lumbar pain. *Spine* 1995;20:1804–1809.
2. Saal JS: The role of inflammation in lumbar pain. *Spine* 1995;20:1821–1827.
3. Weinstein J, Claverie W, Gibson S: The pain of discography. *Spine* 1988;13:1344–1348.
4. Garfin SR, Rydevik B, Lind B, et al: Spinal nerve root compression. *Spine* 1995;20:1810–1820.
5. Hitselberger WE, Witten RM: Abnormal myelograms in asymptomatic patients. *J Neurosurg* 1968;28:204–206.
6. Boden SD, Davis DO, Dina TS, et al: Abnormal magnetic-resonance scans of the lumbar spine in asymptomatic subjects: A prospective investigation. *J Bone Joint Surg* 1990;72A:403–408.
7. Wiesel SW, Tsourmas N, Feffer HL, et al: A study of computer-assisted tomography: I. The incidence of positive CAT scans in an asymptomatic group of patients. *Spine* 1984;9:549–551.
8. Dolan P, Adams MA, Hutton WC: The short-term effects of chymopapain on intervertebral discs. *J Bone Joint Surg* 1987;69B:422–428.
9. Porter RW: Does hard work prevent disc protrusion? *Clin Biomech* 1987;2:196–198.

10. Videman T, Nurminen M, Troup JD: Lumbar spinal pathology in cadaveric material in relation to history of back pain, occupation, and physical loading. *Spine* 1990;15:728–740.
11. Videman T, Sarna S, Battié MC, et al: The long-term effects of physical loading and exercise lifestyles on back-related symptoms, disability, and spinal pathology among men. *Spine* 1995;20:699–709.
12. Adams MA, Dolan P: Recent advances in lumbar spinal mechanics and their clinical significance. *Clin Biomech* 1995;10:3–19.
13. Brickmann P, Biggemann M, Hilweg D: Fatigue fracture of human lumbar vertebrae. *Clin Biomech* 1988;3(suppl 1):1–23.
14. Hutton WC, Adams MA: Can the lumbar spine be crushed in heavy lifting? *Spine* 1982;7:586–590.
15. Adams MA, Hutton WC: Gradual disc prolapse. *Spine* 1985;10:524–531.
16. Osti OL, Vernon-Roberts B, Fraser RD: Anulus tears and intervertebral disc degeneration: An experimental study using an animal model. *Spine* 1990;15:762–767.
17. Buckwalter JA: Aging and degeneration of the human intervertebral disc. *Spine* 1995;20:1307–1314.
18. Holm S, Nachemson A: Variations in the nutrition of the canine intervertebral disc induced by motion. *Spine* 1983;8:866–874.
19. Jenkins RR, Goldfarb A: Introduction: Oxidant stress, aging, and exercise. *Med Sci Sports Exerc* 1993;25:210–212.
20. Ilmarinen J, Louhevaara V, Korhonen O, et al: Changes in maximal cardiorespiratory capacity among aging municipal employees. *Scand J Work Environ Health* 1991;17(suppl 1):99–109.
21. Glower JR: Occupational health research and the problem of back pain. *Trans Soc Occup Med* 1970;21:2–8.
22. Gyntelberg F: One year incidence of low back pain among male residents of Copenhagen aged 40–59. *Dan Med Bull* 1974;21:30–36.
23. Lawrence JS: Disc degeneration: Its frequency and relationship to symptoms. *Ann Rheum Dis* 1969;28:121–138.
24. Spangfort EV: The lumbar disc herniation: A computer-aided analysis of 2,504 operations. *Acta Orthop Scand* 1972;142(suppl):1–95.
25. Riihimäki H, Wickström G, Hänninen K, et al: Predictors of sciatic pain among concrete reinforcement workers and house painters: A five-year follow-up. *Scand J Work Environ Health* 1989;15:415–423.
26. Battié MC, Videman T, Sarna S: A comparison of risk indicators of osteoarthritis and back-related symptom complaints, hospitalizations, and pensions. *Orthop Trans* 1994;18:868.
27. Hrubec Z, Nashold BS Jr: Epidemiology of lumbar disc lesions in the military in World War II. *Am J Epidemiol* 1975;102:367–376.
28. Heliövaara M, Knekt P, Aromaa A: Incidence and risk factors of herniated lumbar intervertebral disc or sciatica leading to hospitalization. *J Chronic Dis* 1987;40:251–258.
29. Kelsey JL, Hardy RJ: Driving of motor vehicles as a risk factor for acute herniated lumbar intervertebral disc. *Am J Epidemiol* 1975;102:63–73.
30. Moneta GB, Videman T, Kaivanto K, et al: Reported pain during lumbar discography as a function of anular ruptures and disc degeneration: A re-analysis of 833 discograms. *Spine* 1994;19:1968–1974.
31. Walsh K, Varnes N, Osmond C, et al: Occupational causes of low-back pain. *Scand J Work Environ Health* 1989;15:54–59.
32. Heliövaara M: Occupation and risk of herniated lumbar intervertebral disc or sciatica leading to hospitalization. *J Chron Dis* 1987;40:259–264.
33. Heliövaara M: Risk factors for low back pain and sciatica. *Ann Med* 1989;21:257–264.
34. Donelson R, Grant W, Kamps C, et al: Pain response to sagittal end-range spinal motion: A prospective, randomized, multicentered trial. *Spine* 1991;16(suppl 6):S206–S212.

35. Donelson R, Silva G, Murphy K. Centralization phenomenon: Its usefulness in evaluating and treating referred pain. *Spine* 1990;15:211–213.
36. Lipson SJ, Muir H: Proteoglycans in experimental intervertebral disc degeneration. *Spine* 1981;6:194–210.
37. Gill K, Videman T, Shimizu T, et al: The effect of repeated extensions on the discographic dye patterns in cadaveric lumbar motion segments. *Clin Biomech* 1987;2:205–210.

Chapter 4

Accuracy of the History and Physical Examination for Detecting Clinically Important Lumbar Disk Herniations

Richard A. Deyo, MD, MPH

Back pain is a common problem that will affect approximately two thirds of the adult population. Only a small percentage of these adults will exhibit symptoms of radiculopathy beyond 2 weeks. A majority of those with persistent radiculopathy will prove to have herniated disks, and lumbar diskectomy is the most common type of back surgery in the United States. Because there is strong evidence that invasive procedures can accelerate pain relief from disk herniations, it is important to consider the accuracy of the history and physical examination in detecting patients with this condition. The ability to make an accurate diagnosis from the history and physical examination will help in providing the patient with prognostic information, making treatment decisions, and choosing diagnostic imaging tests and specialists.

The mere presence of severe back or leg pain does not automatically indicate the presence of a herniated disk. Many observers believe that the diagnosis of herniated disk has been overused, especially when referring to patients with severe functional impairments resulting from their back pain. The term "herniated disk" is sometimes applied in the absence of confirmatory clinical or imaging evidence, resulting in a "nominal" diagnosis, which should be avoided.[1] The term can be frightening to the layperson, because it can imply disability, leading to suggestions of blame and compensability for the condition.

Even the finding of a herniated disk on imaging tests such as computed tomography (CT) or magnetic resonance imaging (MRI) does not prove that this is the cause of a patient's pain and other symptoms. This is because lumbar disks may herniate without causing symptoms, creating a dilemma for both physicians and patients when imaging is performed in the absence of clinical findings of radiculopathy. Thus, myelography, CT, and MRI studies all demonstrate that 20% to 30% of normal asymptomatic adults have herniated disks, with the prevalence increasing with age.[2,3] These herniations apparently do not result in nerve root irritation, radicular symptoms, or back pain. In contrast to the high prevalence of imaging abnormalities, only about 2% of all persons with back pain undergo surgery for a disk herniation,[4] suggesting that a majority of disk herniations seen on imaging tests may be unrelated to symptoms (Table 1). Thus, a strong association between imaging results and clinical findings of radicul-

Table 1 Prevalence of back pain and sciatica in the entire adult population

Characteristic	Prevalence (%)
Any low back pain	60 to 80
Ever had low back pain persisting at least 2 weeks	14
Low back pain persisting at least 2 weeks at a given time (point prevalence)	7
Back pain with features of sciatica lasting at least 2 weeks	1.6
Lumbar spine surgery	1 to 2

(Reproduced with permission from Deyo RA, Loeser JD, Bigos SJ: Herniated lumbar intervertebral disk. *Ann Intern Med* 1990;12:598–603.)

opathy is essential in selecting candidates for surgery, further emphasizing the importance of an accurate history and physical examination.

Differential Diagnosis

Current evidence suggests that a clinically important disk herniation is one that is associated with radiculopathy. The differential diagnosis of a herniated disk, therefore, includes other conditions that may cause radiculopathy or mimic its symptoms. Perhaps the most common cause of radiculopathy aside from herniated disks is spinal stenosis: narrowing of the central spinal canal or its lateral recesses, usually resulting from hypertrophic degenerative changes in the facet joints, disks, and ligamentum flavum.

Other less common conditions that may cause sciatica are synovial cysts, congenital anomalies at the lumbar nerve roots, primary neural or bone tumors, metastatic cancer, and epidural abscesses. Transient sciatic nerve irritation may occur with local external pressure such as that caused by a wallet in the back pocket. Also, pain from other sources in the lumbar spine, such as the facet joints, may radiate into the upper leg in patterns that mimic sciatica. Finally, in the setting of chronic pain complaints, clinicians must often distinguish vague complaints of radiating pain from a syndrome of clear-cut neurologic impairment.

Once a consistent history and physical findings suggestive of true radiculopathy (often including pain, reflex loss, sensory changes, and weakness) have been identified, imaging tests are usually necessary to determine the precise cause and location of any pathoanatomic changes. Thus, a major goal of the physical examination is simply to identify patients who have true radiculopathy.

The Quality of Research Evidence for the Accuracy of the History and Physical Examination

Gold Standard for Diagnosis

In order to assess the accuracy of the history and physical examination, these findings must be compared with some reasonable ''gold standard'' of diagnosis for a herniated disk. As the previous discussion implies, anatomic criteria based on imaging tests are not sufficient for determining whether a herniated disk actually constitutes a clinical problem. Indeed, it is a pervasive problem in the study of low back pain that a precise anatomic diagnosis is often impossible, because of the weak associations among symptoms, pathoanatomic changes, and imaging results.

For many studies of diagnostic accuracy, the gold standard has been surgical findings. This is a good indicator, though not a perfect one, because limited surgical exposure, destruction of anatomic structures in establishing exposure, limited visibility, or exposure at the wrong level may all cause diagnostic errors.[5] Even the surgical finding of a herniated disk may not establish that this was the cause of a patient's symptoms because, as previousy noted, many asymptomatic persons have such findings. Finally, surgery cannot be used to establish the absence of a herniated disk in patients for whom a diagnostic test (such as the history and physical examination) is normal, to establish that the test is a true negative. An alternative for studying herniated disks may be some combination of imaging findings and electrophysiologic results, although the imaging results suffer from limited specificity, and the operating characteristics of electrophysiologic tests are poorly characterized. In some studies of imaging tests, the gold standard has been the consensus of a multidisciplinary expert panel after reviewing the clinical course of patients over time, the evolution of clinical findings, all test results, and the outcomes of treatments that were administered. If this procedure is consistently applied, such an expert consensus may be a perfectly reasonable gold standard.

Criteria for Research Quality

Aside from the choice of a gold standard, other criteria for evaluating studies of diagnostic test accuracy have been proposed, and a typical list is presented in Outline 1.

Quality of Existing Studies

In the overview by van den Hoogen and associates,[6] methodologic shortcomings in the existing literature were common. On a quality rating scale from 0 to 100, studies on the history and physical examination for herniated disks had a median score of 55, with a maximum of 70. The most common methodologic shortcomings in the literature on back pain history and physical examination were in technical quality of the maneuver being performed and of the gold standard comparison, blinded interpretations, clinical description of patients, and appropriate assembly of the study population. The problems of variability in interpretation of both the physical examination maneuvers and the gold standard tests were rarely addressed.

Of the 19 studies on radiculopathy that were included, all were potentially biased because they were based on case series of patients who underwent surgery, therefore representing only the most severe part of the range of clinical severity. The process of selecting patients for surgery generally omits patients with both false and true negative clinical findings, leading to an overestimation of sensitivity and an underestimation of specificity for the physical examination maneuvers.

Outline 1 Criteria for diagnostic research methods

Technical quality of performing the history and physical examination. This would include a standardized method for performing the tests, explicit criteria for positive and negative test results, and consideration of interobserver variability.

Technical quality of the "gold standard": anatomic findings at surgery or overall clinical impression as previously described would be regarded as high quality gold standards for evaluating radiculopathy.

Application of the same gold standard test for every case evaluated.

The items of history and physical examination and the gold standard test would each be interpreted independently (blindly) of the other.

Adequate clinical description of subjects, including duration of symptoms, percentage of patients with sciatica, age, and sex.

Appropriate assembly of the study population. This includes explicit description of inclusion and exclusion criteria, and an adequate spectrum of disease severity to challenge a test's diagnostic accuracy.

Inclusion of subjects both with and without the disease, in order to assess both test sensitivity and specificity.

Sufficient sample size for the confidence intervals around estimates of sensitivity and specificity to be appropriately narrow. In previous studies of imaging tests, it has been suggested that at least 35 subjects with and 35 subjects without the disease would be most appropriate (this number is sufficient so that if true sensitivity or specificity were 1.0, the lower bound of the 95% confidence interval would be 0.9).[7]

Presentation of sufficient data to calculate both sensitivity and specificity, and information concerning missing values.

Medical History

The typical history for a middle-aged patient with a herniated disk is the onset of leg or foot pain accompanied by numbness and tingling. In many cases, back pain precedes leg pain by months or even years, but when leg pain develops it often overshadows the back pain. Deviations from this typical history are common, however, and can confound even experienced physicians.

The first clue to a herniated disk is usually a history suggestive of sciatica. The onset of leg pain may be gradual or sudden, and frequently there is no identifiable precipitating event.[7] It has been observed that attribution of symptoms to a specific incident (often lifting) is more common among patients with workers' compensation claims than among those with noncompensable incidents. Recent studies suggest that among all patients with back pain, those who were not involved in compensation claims or litigation can identify a triggering event about one third of the time.[8]

Unfortunately, there is not a standardized or consistent definition of sciatica. Some define sciatica as any leg pain associated with back pain, while others describe sciatica as pain that radiates distally below the knee, is distributed in a radicular fashion, and is associated with abnormal straight leg raising or neurologic deficits. Typical sciatica radiates down the posterior or lateral aspect of the leg, and is often associated with numbness or paresthesia. Symptoms are usually aggravated by coughing, sneezing, or the Valsalva maneuver. Many patients find sitting painful, and experience at least partial pain relief while supine. This may be because of the minimization of intradiskal pressure, and also the reduction in spine motion, when supine. Unfortunately, very little investigation has been conducted into which of these symptoms is most strongly associated with actual electrophysiologic or anatomic evidence of radiculopathy. Thus, the sensitivity and specificity of any of these symptoms for true radiculopathy remains unknown. It is generally agreed that the presence of sciatica is a sensitive test for herniated disks (80% to 95%),[6,9] but estimates of specificity are lower.

Table 2 Estimated accuracy of physical examination for lumbar disk herniation among patients with sciatica

Test	Source	Sensitivity*	Specificity*	Comments
Ipsilateral straight leg raising	Kosteljanetz et al[13]; Hakelius and Hindmarsh[14]	0.80	0.40	Positive test result: leg pain at < 60°
Crossed straight leg raising	Spangfort[12]; Hakelius and Hindmarsh[14,15]	0.25	0.90	Positive test result: reproduction of contralateral pain
Ankle dorsiflexion weakness	Spangfort[12]; Hakelius and Hindmarsh[14]	0.35	0.70	HNP† usually at L4-5 (80%)
Great toe extensor weakness	Hakelius and Hindmarsh[14]; Kortelainen et al[11]	0.50	0.70	HNP usually at L5-S1 (60%) or L4-5 (30%)
Impaired ankle reflex	Spangfort[11]; Hakelius and Hindmarsh[14]	0.50	0.60	HNP usually at L5-S1; absent reflex increases specificity
Sensory loss	Kosteljanetz et al[13]; Kortelainen et al[11]	0.50	0.50	Area of loss poor predictor of HNP level
Patella reflex	Aronson and Dunsmore[16]	0.50	—	For upper lumbar HNP only
Ankle plantar flexion weakness	Hakelius and Hindmarsh[14]	0.06	0.95	
Quadriceps weakness	Hakelius and Hindmarsh[14]	< 0.01	0.99	

*Sensitivity and specificity were calculated by the authors of the present report; values represent rounded averages where multiple references were available; all results are from surgical case series
† HNP, herniated nucleus pulposus
(Reproduced with permission from Deyo RA, Rainville J, Kent DL: What can the history and physical examination tell us about low back pain? *JAMA* 1992;268:760–765.)

Table 3 Accuracy of history and physical examination for detecting radiculopathy

Test	Sensitivity	Specificity
Sciatica	0.79 - 0.91	0.14
Paresthesia	0.30 - 0.74	0.18 - 0.58
SLR*	0.88 - 1.00	0.11 - 0.44
SLR < 30°	0.12 - 0.27	0.94
Crossed SLR	0.23 - 0.44	0.86 - 0.95
Impaired ankle reflex	0.31 - 0.56	0.57 - 0.89
Impaired patellar reflex	0.04 - 0.15	0.67 - 0.96
Great toe extensor weakness	0.30 - 0.82	0.52 - 0.89

* SLR, straight leg raising
(Adapted with permission from van den Hoogen HMM, Koes BW, van Eijk JTM, et al: On the accuracy of history, physical examination, and erythrocyte sedimentation rate in diagnosing low back pain in general practice. *Spine* 1995;20:318–327.)

Physical Examination

In addition to pain, radiculopathy is often associated with motor, reflex, or sensory dysfunction in the lower extremities, and (rarely) bowel or bladder dysfunction. Furthermore, patients with nerve root irritation experience pain when the sciatic nerve is stretched by straight leg raising from the supine position.

Straight Leg Raising

A positive straight leg raising test generally reproduces sciatica when the leg is raised between 30° and 60° of elevation. As shown in Tables 2 and 3, this test is moderately sensitive, but nonspecific, for herniated disks because limitations in straight leg raising occur often in the absence of herniated disks.[9] The crossed straight leg raising sign refers to reproduction of sciatica when the opposite leg is raised. This test is less sensitive than ipsilateral straight leg raising, but much more specific (Table 2). In this circumstance, a positive test greatly enhances the likelihood of a disk herniation, but a negative test does not rule out the condition.

Although straight leg raising is usually regarded as positive or negative, depending on whether it is limited to 60° or less, the actual angle of a positive straight leg raise has diagnostic value. The lower the angle that reproduces pain, the more specific the test is, and the larger the herniated disk that is found at surgery.[10,11] The straight leg raising test is most appropriate for evaluating the two lowest lumbar nerve roots, where the vast majority of herniated disks occur. Radiculopathy of the higher lumbar nerve roots must be tested with a femoral nerve stretch test, for which data on sensitivity and specificity have not been identified. Various enhancements of the straight leg raising test, such as forced foot dorsiflexion when the leg is fully raised, have not been evaluated for their diagnostic accuracy.

Neurologic Abnormalities

Over 95% of clinically important lumbar disk herniations occur at the two lowest intervertebral levels, L4-5 and L5-S1. Thus, impairments of the L5 and S1 nerve roots are by far the most common. Accordingly, the most frequent neurologic deficits are weakness of ankle dorsiflexion, great toe dorsiflexion, ankle reflexes, and sensation of the feet. Tables 2 and 3 provide estimates of the sensitivity and specificity of these aspects of the physical examination.[6,9,11-16]

Higher lumbar nerve roots account for only a small percentage of all disk herniations. Thus, there is far less information on the accuracy of physical maneuvers for the evaluation of upper lumbar nerve roots. Testing for higher levels of impairment includes evaluation of patellar reflexes, quadriceps strength, and psoas strength. The low sensitivity of quadriceps weakness for detecting herniated disks (Table 2) is a reflection of the infrequency of upper lumbar disk herniations.

Reproducibility of Findings

The techniques used to elicit physical signs may be important in their reproducibility and therefore in their accuracy. In most instances, studies of test accuracy have not specified the exact techniques used for eliciting the physical findings. For example, visual estimation in assessing straight leg raising is moderately accurate, but the use of goniometers or inclinometers improves the reproducibility of the results. Similarly, it appears that manual methods for testing ankle dorsiflexion and plantar flexion weakness may be more reproducible than the patient's ability to heel stand or toe walk.[9] Positioning for eliciting ankle reflexes is important, and some believe that side-lying, prone, or kneeling are positions preferable to sitting. Sensory impairments may be more accurately detected by pin prick than light touch or temperature assessment. Because these details of test performance are likely to be important, they should be specified in studies of test accuracy. Table 4 indicates the reproducibility of several physical findings, based on a small number of studies.[17-21] Most of the tabled values are kappa statistics, which measure agreement above and beyond that expected by chance alone, and for practical purposes, range from zero (no better than chance agreement) to 1 (perfect agreement).

Combinations of Findings

As suggested by Table 2, the accuracy of any individual neurologic finding for detecting herniated disks is quite limited. However, the complete clinical picture, with the full combination of history and physical findings, provides the most useful diagnostic impression. Further studies of the accuracy of various combinations of findings would be a substantial contribution to the existing literature. The limited data available suggest the power of combinations of findings. For example, the finding of either impaired ankle reflexes or weak foot dorsiflexion has a sensitivity of almost 90% for patients with surgically proven disk herniations, compared to a sensitivity of 0.50 or less for each finding alone.[10] It has also been shown that multiple findings related to straight leg raising or neurologic examination increase the probability of finding a herniated disk at surgery.[22]

Table 4 Reproducibility of physical examination findings

Category	Test	Unit of Measurement†	Interobserver Agreement (Statistic)	Source
Tenderness	Bone tenderness	Yes/no	0.40 (k)	McCombe et al[17]
	Soft-tissue tenderness	Yes/no	0.24(k)	McCombe et al[17]
	Muscle spasm	Yes/no	"Discarded—too unreliable"	Waddell et al[18]
SLR*	Ipsilateral SLR, inclinometer	Degrees	0.78 to 0.97 (r)	Hoehler and Tobis[19]; Hsieh et al[20]
	Ipsilateral SLR, goniometer	Degrees	0.69 (r)	McCombe et al[17]
	SLR causes leg pain	Yes/no	0.66 (k)	McCombe et al[17]
	Ipsilateral SLR < 75° by visual estimation	Yes/no	0.56 (k)	Waddell et al[18]
	Crossed SLR, causes pain	Yes/no	0.74(k)	McCombe et al[17]
Neurologic examination	Ankle dorsiflexion weak	Yes/no	1.00 (k)	McCombe et al[17]
	Great toe extensors weak	Yes/no	0.65(k)	McCombe et al[17]
	Ankle reflexes normal	Yes/no	0.39-0.50 (k)	McCombe et al[17]; Schwartz et al[21]
	Any sensory deficit	Yes/no	0.68 (k)	McCombe et al[17]
	Calf wasting	Yes/no	0.80 (k)	McCombe et al[17]
Inappropriate signs	Superficial tenderness	Yes/no	0.29 (k)	McCombe et al[17]
	Simulated rotation or axial loading causes pain	Yes/no	0.25 (k)	McCombe et al[17]
	SLR with distraction causes pain	Yes/no	0.40 (k)	McCombe et al[17]
	Inexplicable pattern, neurologic examination	Yes/no	0.03 (k)	McCombe et al[17]
	Overreaction	Yes/no	0.29 (k)	McCombe et al[17]

*SLR, straight leg raising
†Yes/no indicates measurement of whether or not finding was present
(Reproduced with permission from Deyo RA, Rainville J, Kent DL: What can the history and physical examination tell us about low back pain? *JAMA* 1992;268:760–765.)

Other Causes of Radiculopathy

Spinal stenosis is one of the most common conditions in the differential diagnosis of radiculopathy. Factors that distinguish patients with spinal stenosis from those with herniated disks include age, which is typically higher for those with stenosis (a mean of 55 years in one overview)[23] and a history of neurogenic claudication rather than sciatica. Neurogenic claudication is pain that occurs in the legs after walking and is sometimes associated with neurologic deficits. This syndrome may mimic intermittent ischemic claudication, but is associated with neurologic symptoms and normal arterial pulses.[24]

Little is known about features of the physical examination that would distinguish spinal stenosis from herniated disks. However, it appears that pain on spine extension is typical of spinal stenosis, whereas pain with spinal flexion is more common in patients with herniated disks. Unfortunately, actual data on the sensitivity and specificity of these findings is unavailable. It appears that abnormal straight leg raising and neurologic deficits may be less frequent in patients with spinal stenosis,[23] but again few data are available on the accuracy of these physical findings. Involvement of multiple nerve root levels, and bilateral signs and symptoms may be more common in spinal stenosis than with herniated disks, but the accuracy of such findings has not been quantified.

van den Hoogen and associates[6] have highlighted the importance of sciatica and neurologic abnormalities among patients with vertebral cancer. Sciatica is reported in 58% to 93% of patients hospitalized with vertebral cancer. Although the neurologic findings can be similar to those of other causes of radiculopathy, they are typically late findings in patients with spinal malignancies.

Cauda Equina Syndrome

The cauda equina syndrome is a rare complication of lumbar disk herniations, occurring in only 1% to 2% of all surgical cases.[12] In part because the syndrome is so rare, data on the accuracy of physical findings for this syndrome are particularly scarce. Table 5 presents representative estimates of sensitivity of various clinical findings, but data on their specificity are unavailable.[25-27]

Evidence of Social or Psychologic Distress

An important aspect of patient evaluation for a possible herniated disk is the examination of factors that may predict a poor surgical outcome. Such factors,

Table 5 Approximate sensitivity of findings for cauda equina syndrome

Finding	Sensitivity
Urinary retention	0.90
Sciatica	0.80
Abnormal SLR	0.80
"Saddle anesthesia"	0.75
Decreased anal sphincter tone	0.70

(Adaped with permission from Deyo RA, Rainville J, Kent DL: What can the history and physical examination tell us about low back pain? *JAMA* 1992;268:760–765.)

independent of pathoanatomic changes, are often social, economic, or psychologic. Thus, for example, depression, alcohol or drug abuse, and disability and litigation claims all may affect patient prognosis in response to therapy.

There is evidence that patients with psychologic distress may amplify their pain, and may present with findings that mimic radiculopathy. Waddell[28] has proposed several features of the medical history that suggest abnormal illness behavior and would influence diagnostic impressions. For example, complaints of whole leg pain, tailbone pain, whole leg numbness, the whole leg giving way, intolerance of previous treatments, emergency admissions to the hospital, or a complaint of persistent pain are all suggestive of abnormal illness behavior despite some superficial resemblance to symptoms of radiculopathy. Unfortunately, these findings have not been evaluated for their accuracy in detecting psychologic distress or in ruling out true radiculopathy.

Similarly, Waddell and associates[29] have also proposed five categories of so-called "nonorganic" physical signs as markers of abnormal illness behavior. These include inappropriate tenderness that is superficial or widespread; pain on simulated loading produced by pressing on the top of the head or simulated spine rotation; distraction signs such as inconsistency between straight leg raising in the supine position and straight leg raising in the seated position; regional disturbances in sensation and strength in nonradicular patterns; and overreaction during the physical examination. As in the case of other physical findings, the presence of any one sign was of limited value, but positive findings in three of these five categories were found to be strongly associated with psychologic distress.[29] Subsequent studies have found limited reproducibility for some of these findings (Table 3), but fair reproducibility for others.[17] Again, data on the sensitivity or specificity of these signs for either psychologic distress or for ruling out true radiculopathy are unavailable.

Acknowledgments

Thanks to Sandra Coke for assistance in preparing this manuscript.

References

1. Waddell G: A new clinical model for the treatment of low-back pain. *Spine* 1987;12:632–644.
2. Wiesel SW, Tsourmas N, Feffer HL, et al: A study of computer-assisted tomography: I. The incidence of positive CAT scans in an asymptomatic group of patients. *Spine* 1984;9:549–551.
3. Boden SD, Davis DO, Dina TS, et al: Abnormal magnetic-resonance scans of the lumbar spine in asymptomatic subjects: A prospective investigation. *J Bone Joint Surg* 1990;72A:403–408.
4. Deyo RA, Loeser JD, Bigos SJ: Herniated lumbar intervertebral disk. *Ann Intern Med* 1990;112:598–603.
5. Deyo RA, Haselkorn J, Hoffman R, et al: Designing studies of diagnostic tests for low back pain or radiculopathy. *Spine* 1994;19(suppl 18):2057S–2065S.
6. van den Hoogen HM, Koes BW, van Eijk JT, et al: On the accuracy of history, physical examination, and erythrocyte sedimentation rate in diagnosing low back pain in general practice: A criteria-based review of the literature. *Spine* 1995;20:318–327.
7. White AA III, Gordon SL: Synopsis: Workshop on idiopathic low-back pain. *Spine* 1982;7:141–149.

8. Hall H: The back page. *Back Let* 1995;10:73–82.
9. Deyo RA, Rainville J, Kent DL: What can the history and physical examination tell us about low back pain? *JAMA* 1992;268:760–765.
10. Xin SQ, Zhang QZ, Fan DH: Significance of the straight-leg raising test in the diagnosis and clinical evaluation of lower lumbar intervertebral-disc protrusion. *J Bone Joint Surg* 1987;69A:517–522.
11. Kortelainen P, Puranen J, Koivisto E, et al: Symptoms and signs of sciatica and their relation to the localization of the lumbar disc herniation. *Spine* 1985;10:88–92.
12. Spangfort EV: The lumbar disc herniation: A computer-aided analysis of 2,504 operations. *Acta Orthop Scand* 1972;142(suppl):1–95.
13. Kosteljanetz M, Espersen JO, Halaburt H, et al: Predictive value of clinical and surgical findings in patients with lumbago-sciatica: A prospective study (Part 1). *Acta Neurochir* 1984;73:67–76.
14. Hakelius A, Hindmarsh J: The comparative reliability of preoperative diagnostic methods in lumbar disc surgery. *Acta Orthop Scand* 1972;43:234–238.
15. Hakelius A, Hindmarsh J: The significance of neurological signs and myelographic findings in the diagnosis of lumbar root compression. *Acta Orthop Scand* 1972;43:239–246.
16. Aronson HA, Dunsmore RH: Herniated upper lumbar discs. *J Bone Joint Surg* 1963;45A:311–317.
17. McCombe PF, Fairbank JC, Cockersole BC, et al: Reproducibility of physical signs in low-back pain. *Spine* 1989;14:908–918.
18. Waddell G, Main CJ, Morris EW, et al: Normality and reliability in the clinical assessment of backache. *Br Med J* 1982;284:1519–1523.
19. Hoehler FK, Tobis JS: Low back pain and its treatment by spinal manipulation: Measures of flexibility and asymmetry. *Rheumatol Rehabil* 1982;21:21–26.
20. Hsieh CY, Walker JM, Gillis K: Straight-leg-raising test: Comparison of three instruments. *Phys Ther* 1983;63:1429–1433.
21. Schwartz RS, Morris JG, Crimmins D, et al: A comparison of two methods of eliciting the ankle jerk. *Aust N Z J Med* 1990;20:116–119.
22. Morris EW, Di Paola M, Vallance R, et al: Diagnosis and decision making in lumbar disc prolapse and nerve entrapment. *Spine* 1986;11:436–439.
23. Turner JA, Ersek M, Herron L, et al: Surgery for lumbar spinal stenosis: Attempted meta-analysis of the literature. *Spine* 1992;17:1–8.
24. Hawkes CH, Roberts GM: Neurogenic and vascular claudication. *J Neurol Sci* 1978;38:337–345.
25. Kostuik JP, Harrington I, Alexander D, et al: Cauda equina syndrome and lumbar disc herniation. *J Bone Joint Surg* 1986;68A:386–391.
26. O'Laoire SA, Crockard HA, Thomas DG: Prognosis for sphincter recovery after operation for cauda equina compression owing to lumbar disc prolapse. *Br Med J* 1981;282:1852–1854.
27. Tay EC, Chacha PB: Midline prolapse of a lumbar intervertebral disc with compression of the cauda equina. *J Bone Joint Surg* 1979;61B:43–46.
28. Waddell G: Biopsychosocial analysis for low back pain. *Ballieres Clin Rheumatol* 1992;6:523–557.
29. Waddell G, McCulloch JA, Kummel E, et al: Nonorganic physical signs in low-back pain. *Spine* 1980;5:117–125.

Chapter 5

Imaging of the Patient With Lumbar Radiculopathy

Scott D. Boden, MD

Introduction

The past 20 years have resulted in a technologic revolution in the area of neuroradiologic imaging. Existing modalities have been refined and new noninvasive imaging modalities have been developed as well, thus rendering "exploratory" spine surgery obsolete. The ready availability of detailed anatomic visualization of the spine can be a mixed blessing when dealing with lumbar degenerative disorders, which may affect 60% to 80% of the population. The primary issues involved with decision-making for imaging of the patient with lumbar radiculopathy include: (1) the timing of the study during the patient's clinical course; (2) matching the clinical indications to the choice of the optimal imaging study; and (3) precise correlation of imaging abnormalities with clinical symptoms. The goals of this chapter are to review the general principles of spinal imaging and then discuss each of these three issues in the context of the most common clinical presentations of radiculopathy with and without previous spine surgery.

General Imaging Considerations

Timing for Advanced Diagnostic Imaging

As with any diagnostic test, the ideal time to obtain a lumbar spine imaging study in the patient with radiculopathy is when study results will affect the treatment plan. The appropriate timing may vary based on the working diagnosis and other patient factors. Imaging studies should not be obtained prematurely because of changes that can occur in the patient's anatomy. For example, in the case of a herniated lumbar disk, significant resorption of the disk can occur in just a few months, rendering the prematurely obtained imaging scan outdated as a guide for surgical planning.[1,2]

Role of Diagnostic Imaging in the Lumbar Spine

Diagnostic imaging should be used to confirm information obtained from a thorough patient history and physical examination. In general, advanced neurodiagnostic imaging studies should not be used for general screening in the absence of a working clinical diagnosis, nor should they ever be used in place of a careful physical examination. Most imaging modalities are highly sensitive and relatively unselective. "Let's get a magnetic resonance imaging scan to see if there is anything wrong with the spine" is the beginning of a dangerous thought process. This danger arises from the high prevalence of abnormal imaging findings in asymptomatic individuals.[3] Excessive reliance on diagnostic studies without precise clinical correlation can lead to suboptimal treatment of lumbar radiculopathies.

Markers of Imaging Test Performance

To evaluate the clinical performance of any diagnostic study, the physician must know its sensitivity, which is a reflection of the false negative results, or the ability of the test to detect the presence of disease. More relevant to avoiding overtreatment is the specificity, which is a reflection of the false positive results, or the ability of the test to remain negative in the absence of disease. Most often the false positive rate of spine diagnostic imaging tests has been measured in a population of symptomatic patients who have undergone surgery to confirm the imaging findings. However, this design can underestimate the actual rate of false positive results because it does not assess the frequency of abnormal findings in asymptomatic individuals. To best interpret abnormal imaging findings in symptomatic patients with degenerative spinal disorders, it is important to know the spectrum and frequency of abnormalities that can be present without causing symptoms (Table 1).

Lumbar Radiculopathy

Patients with or without low back pain who have a significant amount of leg pain or sciatica in the absence of trauma, tumor, or infection warrant a conservative approach to diagnostic imaging. Emergent neurodiagnostic imaging is only indicated in the face of trauma, suspected tumor or infection, cauda equina syndrome with loss of bowel or bladder control, progressive neurologic loss, or a pattern inconsistent with a monoradiculopathy. Thus, most patients with radicular leg pain, including those with intermittent neurogenic claudication, should be managed nonsurgically for at least 6 to 8 weeks. The most common causes of leg pain are herniated nucleus pulposus and lumbar spinal stenosis. The ideal choice and sequence of imaging studies will depend on which diagnosis is most likely as well as the quality and availability of magnetic resonance imaging (MRI).

Table 1 Prevalence of disk herniations in studies of asymptomatic individuals

Modality	Prevalence (%)	No. of Subjects	Mean Age (years)
Diskography	37	30	26
Myelography	24	300	51
Computed tomography	20	52	40
Magnetic resonance	28	67	42
imaging	28	98	42

In patients with leg pain, plain radiographs are generally not useful. Identification of spondylolisthesis, congenital stenosis, tumor, or infection may be possible, but these diagnoses are easily made from other tests that provide additional information about the presence and location of neural compression.[4] Computed tomography (CT) replaced myelography in the 1980s as the study of choice to confirm a herniated lumbar disk.[5] One report of 461 patients compared myelography to CT for sensitivity (82% versus 73%), specificity (67% versus 77%), and positive predictive value (93% versus 94%).[6] Another study has shown the accuracy of myelography to be comparable at 77%.[7] CT improved detection of far lateral disk herniations[8,9] and eliminated the complications associated with myelography.[10-12] However, a study of 52 asymptomatic patients revealed the presence of a herniated disk or spinal stenosis in 24% of the subjects.[13] While CT alone was once the study of choice to confirm the diagnosis of disk herniation, this modality does not provide adequate information regarding neural compression, unless combined with myelography. This combination increases diagnostic accuracy when compared to that of either study alone.[7,14,15]

In patients with radiculopathy who are older than 55 years, the possibility of isolated foraminal stenosis with or without a disk herniation is increased. In patients with leg pain and a history suggestive of neurogenic claudication, many clinicians prefer to use myelography followed by postmyelographic CT. The rationale for postmyelographic CT over MRI in patients with suspected spinal stenosis is the improved visualization of bone and hypertrophic spurs. In addition, CT offers the improved delineation of pedicle size and anatomy, which may be useful information for planning surgical reconstruction. To some extent, the optimal choice of imaging also depends on its quality. There is less of a tendency to overestimate neural compression, which can be a problem with MRI, particularly T2-weighted sequences. Finally, the myelogram provides the added benefit of demonstrating thecal sac compression that is severe enough to result in a functional block of dye (or cerebrospinal fluid) through the stenotic area. In patients with far lateral disk herniations, MRI is generally thought to be more accurate, although no prospective study has formally compared its accuracy with that of CT. For this cause of lumbar radiculopathy, MRI has the advantage of demonstrating readily obtainable parasagittal reconstructions that show the relationship of the disk herniation and exiting nerve root in the foramen (Fig. 1).

In patients with a history and physical findings consistent with a herniated disk, MRI has proved to be the most accurate study for demonstration of the anatomy of the cauda equina and confirmation of the presence of a disk herniation.[16-18] As with all spinal imaging studies, MRI scans should be used to confirm the clinical diagnosis only in those patients who do not respond to nonsurgical management and should ideally be obtained just prior to surgical intervention. The justification for this delayed imaging rationale is twofold: (1) herniated disks tend to diminish in size over time, so a scan obtained too early may no longer be accurate;[19-22] and (2) there is a 28% prevalence of herniated disks in asymptomatic individuals, so a disk herniation visualized may or may not be the source of a patient's pain.[3,23] The prevalence of abnormal findings in asymptomatic volunteers increases with age (Table 2). This problem of abnormal scans in asymptomatic individuals highlights the limitations of using lumbar MRI scans as a screening tool, as well as the importance of precise cor-

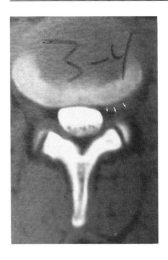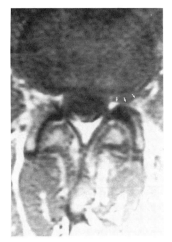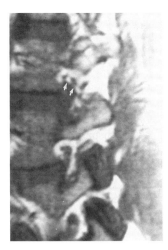

Fig. 1 *Imaging studies from a patient with left anterior thigh pain and a positive femoral nerve stretch test.* **Left,** *Myelogram/CT scan demonstrates a soft tissue shadow suggestive of a far lateral disk herniation at L3-4 on the left side.* **Center,** *Axial MRI scan demonstrates the lateral disk herniation on the left side.* **Right,** *Parasagittal MRI scan demonstrates the foraminal component of the disk herniation at L3-4 migrating upward in the foramen and obliterating the signal from the exiting nerve root.*

Table 2 Correlation of age with abnormal magnetic resonance images of the lumbar spine in 67 asymptomatic subjects*

	Age in years (no. of patients)		
Finding	20 to 39 (35)	40 to 59 (18)	60 to 80 (14)
Herniated disk	21	22	36
Spinal stenosis	1	0	21
Bulging disk	56	50	79
Degenerative disk	34	59	93

* Data represent the percentage of subjects in each age group who had the indicated finding in at least one lumbar level

relation of imaging findings with clinical signs and symptoms prior to invasive treatment (Fig. 2).

In an effort to distinguish symptomatic from asymptomatic disk herniations on MRI scans, nerve root enhancement after gadolinium contrast administration has been observed. A strong correlation between intrathecal root enhancement and radicular symptoms from herniated lumbar disks has been reported by some.[24-26] One animal study has suggested that root enhancement is associated with inflammation and disruption of capillary endothelium.[27] A series of 115 patients treated with surgical diskectomy for disk herniation demonstrated root enhancement in 39% preoperatively and 59% postoperatively, with no correlation to postoperative radicular pain.[28] In a report describing MRI scans in 30 asymptomatic volunteers, 18 had root enhancement thought to be related to

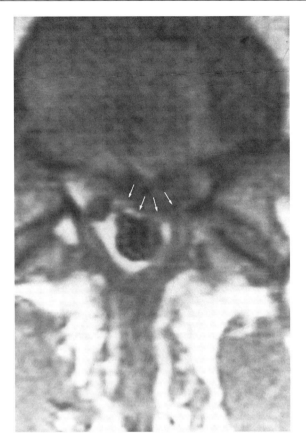

Fig. 2 *Axial MRI scan from a patient with left leg radiculopathy demonstrates a large posterolateral disk herniation at L5-S1 on the left side. The herniated disk obliterates the signal from the S1 nerve root on the left side.*

prominent radicular veins.[29] Thus, at present, nerve root enhancement is a potentially interesting phenomenon with unknown clinical relevance.

Other attempts at distinguishing symptomatic from asymptomatic disk herniations have examined factors including the size and position of disk herniation, and the size and morphology of the spinal canal. At present there is no method to reliably determine which disk herniations on MRI images are symptomatic. It is also not possible to determine which disk herniations are least likely to respond to nonsurgical management; this information would be useful to enable earlier surgical intervention in appropriate cases to afford quicker return to normal function.

The development of minimally invasive treatments, such as intradiskal enzyme therapy, percutaneous nucleotomy, arthroscopic diskectomy, and endoscopically assisted transforaminal disk excision, has increased the need to distinguish sequestered disk herniations from contained or subligamentous disk herniations. MRI is the only imaging modality that can reliably make this distinction. The accuracy of MRI for distinguishing between these types of disk herniation is thought to be 85%, although one report was as low as 52%.[30-32] With gadolinium contrast, a sequestered fragment will often display a peripheral ring of enhancement which is caused by surrounding inflammatory and scar tissue.[33,34]

In patients with lumbar radiculopathy, MRI may also demonstrate two less common pathologic problems: synovial facet joint cysts and isthmic spondylolisthesis. Cysts of the facet joints occur most commonly at the junction of the fourth and fifth lumbar vertebrae and appear as a dorsal epidural mass of variable signal intensity.[35-37] In 17 patients with isthmic spondylolisthesis, the shape of the neural foramen on sagittal MRI scans was abnormal in all cases.[38] In the 33 foramina examined, appearance of the exiting nerve correlated with the side of symptoms; eight had a normal appearing nerve root, 16 a compressed nerve, and nine showed disappearance of the fat signal precluding identification of the nerve. This observation supports my clinical impression that sagittal MRI scans provide superior visualization of foraminal stenosis as compared with axial CT or myelography.

Diskography is most commonly performed as a provocative test to reproduce axial diskogenic low back pain. While the literature does not support the use of diskography in patients with predominant leg pain, there is one potential application. In a patient with leg pain but no significant disk herniation causing nerve root impingement or displacement, it has been postulated that a chemical radiculitis may result from leakage of irritants from the nucleus pulposus out through an annular tear. In such a case, diskography may demonstrate dye extravasation at the correct level and side of the affected nerve root.[39] Results from surgical treatment of this problem, however, are unpredictable.

Leg Pain in Patients With Previous Lumbar Surgery

Because the occurrence of a herniated disk increases the likelihood of a recurrent disk at the same or a different lumbar level, this discussion would be incomplete without recognition of the unique issues involved with imaging in patients who have had previous surgery. It is estimated that 300,000 de novo laminectomies are performed annually in the United States and that up to 15% of these patients may experience continued or recurrent pain and disability.[40] Interpretation of lumbar spinal imaging in patients who have had previous surgery is more complex because of the superimposition of normal postsurgical imaging changes with normal age-related degenerative changes. The primary objective in such patients is to distinguish mechanical and nonmechanical causes of pain. The most common mechanical sources of pain include recurrent or residual herniated disk material, spinal instability (including pseudarthrosis after unsuccessful arthrodesis), spinal stenosis, and intervertebral diskitis, which can all produce symptoms by placing direct pressure on neural elements, or indirect pressure as a result of excessive motion. All of these conditions are amenable to surgical intervention. In contrast, the nonmechanical entities include scar tissue, either intrathecal (arachnoiditis) or extradural (epidural fibrosis), psychosocial problems, or systemic medical disease, and surgical intervention has no effect on these conditions.[41]

The most critical challenge of postoperative imaging in the patient with leg pain following previous surgery is to distinguish scar from treatable conditions such as a residual or recurrent herniated disk or spinal stenosis. When unenhanced CT is used in this assessment, scar can be separated from disk in 43% to 60% of cases.[42,43] Use of CT with intravenous contrast increases the likelihood of an overall correct diagnosis to 70% to 83%.[42-47] Unenhanced MRI is reported to have an accuracy comparable to that of contrast-enhanced CT, 76% to 89%.[44,45,48-50] The diagnostic accuracy of contrast-enhanced MRI approaches 96% to 100%.[49,51] Digital subtraction may further enhance the diagnostic confidence in more difficult cases.[52] Thus, when obtaining an MRI scan in a patient who has had lumbar surgery, intravenous paramagnetic contrast material should always be used. For patients in whom MRI is contraindicated (for example, those with ferromagnetic implants or pacemakers) myelography with postmyelographic CT would be the modality of choice.

It is important to be able to distinguish normal postsurgical changes on MRI scans from findings that can result in symptoms. Postoperative studies using CT have shown that approximately 40% of asymptomatic patients show persistent herniated disks or other findings that are indistinguishable from those of symptomatic patients.[51,53,54] Postoperative studies show that 69% of diskectomy patients had an epidural mass effect resembling the preoperative disk herniation in a study with unenhanced MRI scans.[55] The timing and sequence of changes observed on MRI scans following uncomplicated diskectomy have also been documented.[56] The consensus from these reports is that mass effect on the thecal sac observed with MRI scans obtained in the early (first 3 months) postoperative period can be misleading because of the presence of immature hematoma/scar that can mimic residual herniated disk material.[57-59] It is thought that these early postoperative changes consistent with disk material result from avascular hematoma and scar, which becomes increasingly vascular and shrinks during the first 3 to 6 months following diskectomy.[60-62]

In patients who have had lumbar surgery, nerve root enhancement has been observed on MRI scans, but this finding is presently of unknown clinical significance. The involved nerve root may demonstrate increased signal intensity on gadolinium T1-weighted sequences tracking proximally to the conus medullaris. Although this finding has been seen in some patients with radiculopathy preoperatively and may be seen quite frequently following surgical diskectomy, it does not seem to correlate with residual symptoms postoperatively.[28,63] The prevalence of this finding decreases dramatically during the first 6 months following surgery.[57]

Arachnoiditis may be the cause of postoperative leg pain and may be seen on MRI scans. It may appear as one of three distinct patterns: central clumping, peripheral clumping, or empty sac.[64] Arachnoiditis is seen postoperatively in less than 5% of patients with persistent symptoms, far less than was once thought.[65,66] When arachnoiditis is present, chances for surgical reduction in postoperative pain are diminished unless a clear mechanical lesion is also identified.

Summary

Patients with radiculopathy are fortunate in that noninvasive examination of the anatomy of the lumbar spine with superb resolution is possible. However, a high frequency and broad spectrum of abnormal findings can exist as part of the normal aging process without generating clinical symptoms. In addition, mechanical causes of nerve root compression that may result in radicular symptoms can be distinguished. Despite the extraordinary progress in the diagnostic imaging of entities that result in leg pain or other radicular symptoms, the ability to determine which herniated disks are clinically symptomatic and which disk herniations are asymptomatic is limited. Physicians cannot predict, on the basis of morphology or location, whether or not the herniation is likely to be one of the few that will not respond to nonsurgical treatment, thereby allowing earlier intervention and faster return to function. Finally, the decisions and interventions based on improved anatomic visualization of lumbar disk herniations with MRI must result in improved clinical outcomes for all patients.

References

1. Ellenberg MR, Ross ML, Honet JC, et al: Prospective evaluation of the course of disc herniations in patients with proven radiculopathy. *Arch Phys Med Rehabil* 1993;74:3–8.
2. Bozzao A, Gallucci M, Masciocchi C, et al: Lumbar disk herniation: MR imaging assessment of natural history in patients treated without surgery. *Radiology* 1992;185:135–141.
3. Boden SD, Davis DO, Dina TS, et al: Abnormal magnetic-resonance scans of the lumbar spine in asymptomatic subjects: A prospective investigation. *J Bone Joint Surg* 1990;72A:403–408.
4. Dailey EJ, Buehler MT: Plain film assessment of spinal stenosis: Method comparison with lumbar CT. *J Manipulative Physiol Ther* 1989;12:192–199.
5. Hashimoto K, Akahori O, Kitano K, et al: Magnetic resonance imaging of lumbar disc herniation: Comparison with myelography. *Spine* 1990;15:1166–1169.
6. Schipper J, Kardaun JW, Braakman R, et al: Lumbar disk herniation: Diagnosis with CT or myelography. *Radiology* 1987;165:227–231.
7. Voelker JL, Mealey J Jr, Eskridge JM, et al: Metrizamide-enhanced computed tomography as an adjunct to metrizamide myelography in the evaluation of lumbar disc herniation and spondylosis. *Neurosurgery* 1987;20:379–384.
8. Godersky JC, Erickson DL, Seljeskog EL: Extreme lateral disk herniation: Diagnosis by computed tomographic scanning. *Neurosurgery* 1984;14:549–552.
9. Spanu G, Rodriguez y Baena R, Rainoldi F: Reliability of clinical examination and computed tomography in the diagnosis of extreme lateral disc herniation. *Neurochirurgia (Stuttg)* 1987;30:112–114.
10. Gabrielsen TO, Gebarski SS, Knake JE, et al: Iohexol versus metrizamide for lumbar myelography: Double-blind trial. *Am J Roentgenol* 1984;142:1047–1049.
11. Postacchini F, Massobrio M: Outpatient lumbar myelography: Analysis of complications after myelography comparing outpatients with inpatients. *Spine* 1985;10:567–570.
12. Tate CF III, Wilkov HR, Lestrange NR, et al: Outpatient lumbar myelography: Initial results in 79 examinations using a low-dose metrizamide technique. *Radiology* 1985;157:391–393.
13. Wiesel SW, Tsourmas N, Feffer HL, et al: A study of computer-assisted tomography: I. The incidence of positive CAT scans in an asymptomatic group of patients. *Spine* 1984;9:549–551.
14. Goldberg AL, Soo MS, Deeb ZL, et al: Degenerative disease of the lumbar spine: Role of CT-myelography in the MR era. *Clin Imaging* 1991;15:47–55.
15. Herkowitz HN, Garfin SR, Bell GR, et al: The use of computerized tomography in evaluating non-visualized vertebral levels caudad to a complete block on a lumbar myelogram: A review of thirty-two cases. *J Bone Joint Surg* 1987;69A:218–224.
16. Cohen MS, Wall EJ, Kerber CW, et al: The anatomy of the cauda equina on CT scans and MRI. *J Bone Joint Surg* 1991;73B:381–384.

17. Weisz GM, Lamond TS, Kitchener PN: Spinal imaging: Will MRI replace myelography? *Spine* 1988;13:65–68.
18. Albeck MJ, Hilden J, Kjaer L, et al: A controlled comparison of myelography, computed tomography, and magnetic resonance imaging in clinically suspected lumbar disc herniation. *Spine* 1995;20:443–448.
19. Fagerlund MK, Thelander U, Friberg S: Size of lumbar disc hernias measured using computed tomography and related to sciatic symptoms. *Acta Radiol* 1990;31:555–558.
20. Delauche-Cavallier MC, Budet C, Laredo JD, et al: Lumbar disc herniation: Computed tomography scan changes after conservative treatment of nerve root compression. *Spine* 1992;17:927–933.
21. Cowan NC, Bush K, Katz DE, et al: The natural history of sciatica: A prospective radiological study. *Clin Radiol* 1992;46:7–12.
22. Dullerud R, Nakstad PH: CT changes after conservative treatment for lumbar disk herniation. *Acta Radiol* 1994;35:415–419.
23. Jensen MC, Brant-Zawadzki MN, Obuchowski N, et al: Magnetic resonance imaging of the lumbar spine in people without back pain. *N Engl J Med* 1994;331:69–73.
24. Jinkins JR: MR of enhancing nerve roots in the unoperated lumbosacral spine. *Am J Neuroradiol* 1993;14:193–202.
25. Toyone T, Takahashi K, Kitahara H, et al: Visualisation of symptomatic nerve roots: Prospective study of contrast-enhanced MRI in patients with lumbar disk herniation. *J Bone Joint Surg* 1993;75B:529–533.
26. Crisi G, Carpeggiani P, Trevisan C: Gadolinium-enhanced nerve roots in lumbar disk herniation. *Am J Neuroradiol* 1993;14:1379–1392.
27. Nguyen C, Haughton VM, Ho KC, et al: Contrast enhancement in spinal nerve roots: An experimental study. *Am J Neuroradiol* 1995;16:265–268.
28. Taneichi H, Abumi K, Kaneda K, et al: Significance of Gd-DTPA-enhanced magnetic resonance imaging for lumbar disk herniation: The relationship between nerve root enhancement and clinical manifestations. *J Spinal Disord* 1994;7:153–160.
29. Lane JI, Koeller KK, Atkinson JL: Contrast-enhanced radicular veins on MR of the lumbar spine in an asymptomatic study group. *Am J Neuroradiol* 1995;16:269–273.
30. Masaryk TJ, Ross JS, Modic MT, et al: High-resolution MR imaging of sequestered lumbar intervertebral disks. *Am J Roentgenol* 1988;150:1155–1162.
31. Kim KY, Kim YT, Lee CS, et al: Magnetic resonance imaging in the evaluation of the lumbar herniated intervertebral disc. *Int Orthop* 1993;17:241–244.
32. Silverman CS, Lenchik L, Shimkin PM, et al: The value of MR in differentiating subligamentous from supraligamentous lumbar disk herniations. *Am J Neuroradiol* 1995;16:571–579.
33. Wasserstrom R, Mamourian AC, Black JF, et al: Intradural lumbar disk fragment with ring enhancement on MR. *Am J Neuroradiol* 1993;14:401–404.
34. Yamashita K, Hiroshima K, Kurata A: Gadolinium-DTPA: Enhanced magnetic resonance imaging of a sequestered lumbar intervertebral disk and its correlation with pathologic findings. *Spine* 1994;19:479–482.
35. Jackson DE Jr, Atlas SW, Mani JR, et al: Intraspinal synovial cysts: MR imaging. *Radiology* 1989;170:527–530.
36. Liu SS, Williams KD, Drayer BP, et al: Synovial cysts of the lumbosacral spine: Diagnosis by MR imaging. *Am J Roentgenol* 1990;154:163–166.
37. Xu GL, Haughton VM, Carrera GF: Lumbar facet joint capsule: Appearance at MR imaging and CT. *Radiology* 1990;177:415–420.
38. Annertz M, Holtas S, Cronqvist S, et al: Isthmic lumbar spondylolisthesis with sciatica: MR imaging vs myelography. *Acta Radiol* 1990;31:449–453.
39. McCutcheon ME, Thompson WC III: CT scanning of lumbar discography: A useful diagnostic adjunct. *Spine* 1986;11:257–259.
40. Waddell G: Failures of disc surgery and repeat surgery. *Acta Orthop Belg* 1987;53:300–302.

81

41. Finnegan WJ, Fenlin JM, Marvel JP, et al: Results of surgical intervention in the symptomatic multiply-operated back patient: Analysis of sixty-seven cases followed for three to seven years. *J Bone Joint Surg* 1979;61A:1077–1082.

42. Braun IF, Hoffman JC Jr, Davis PC, et al: Contrast enhancement in CT differentiation between recurrent disk herniation and postoperative scar: Prospective study. *Am J Neuroradiol* 1985;6:607–612.

43. Firooznia H, Kricheff II, Rafii M, et al: Lumbar spine after surgery: Examination with intravenous contrast-enhanced CT. *Radiology* 1987;163:221–226.

44. Bundschuh CV, Modic MT, Ross JS, et al: Epidural fibrosis and recurrent disk herniation in the lumbar spine: MR imaging assessment. *Am J Roentgenol* 1988;150:923–932.

45. Sotiropoulos S, Chafetz NI, Lang P, et al: Differentiation between postoperative scar and recurrent disk herniation: Prospective comparison of MR, CT, and contrast-enhanced CT. *Am J Neuroradiol* 1989;10:639–643.

46. Tullberg T, Grane P, Rydberg J, et al: Comparison of contrast-enhanced computed tomography and gadolinium-enhanced magnetic resonance imaging one year after lumbar diskectomy. *Spine* 1994;19:183–188.

47. Kieffer SA, Witwer GA, Cacayorin ED, et al: Recurrent post-discectomy pain: CT-surgical correlation. *Acta Radiol* 1986;369(suppl):719–722.

48. Bundschuh CV, Stein L, Slusser JH, et al: Distinguishing between scar and recurrent herniated disk in postoperative patients: Value of contrast-enhanced CT and MR imaging. *Am J Neuroradiol* 1990;11:949–958.

49. Hueftle MG, Modic MT, Ross JS, et al: Lumbar spine: Postoperative MR imaging with Gd-DTPA. *Radiology* 1988;167:817–824.

50. Hochhauser L, Kieffer SA, Cacayorin ED, et al: Recurrent postdiskectomy low back pain: MR-surgical correlation. *Am J Roentgenol* 1988;151:755–760.

51. Cervellini P, Curri D, Bernardi L, et al: Computed tomography after lumbar disc surgery: A comparison between symptomatic and asymptomatic patients. *Acta Neurochir Suppl (Wien)* 1988;43:44–47.

52. Murray JG, Stack JP, Ennis JT, et al: Digital subtraction in contrast-enhanced MR imaging of the postoperative lumbar spine. *Am J Roentgenol* 1994;162:893–898.

53. Montaldi S, Fankhauser H, Schnyder P, et al: Computed tomography of the postvertebral intervertebral disk and lumbar spinal canal: Investigation of twenty-five patients after successful operation for lumbar disk herniation. *Neurosurgery* 1988;22:1014–1022.

54. Ilkko E, Lahde S, Koivukangas J, et al: Computed tomography after lumbar disc surgery. *Acta Radiol* 1988;29:179–182.

55. Ross JS, Masaryk TJ, Modic MT, et al: Lumbar spine: Postoperative assessment with surface-coil MR imaging. *Radiology* 1987;164:851–860.

56. Dina TS, Boden SD, Davis DO: Lumbar spine after surgery for herniated disk: Imaging findings in the early postoperative period. *Am J Roentgenol* 1995;164:665–671.

57. Boden SD, Davis DO, Dina TS, et al: Contrast-enhanced MR imaging performed after successful lumbar disk surgery: Prospective study. *Radiology* 1992;182:59–64.

58. Balagura S, Neumann JF: Magnetic resonance imaging of the postoperative intervertebral disk: The first eight months. Clinical and legal implications. *J Spinal Disord* 1993;6:212–217.

59. Tullberg T, Grane P, Isacson J: Gadolinium-enhanced magnetic resonance imaging of 36 patients one year after lumbar disc resection. *Spine* 1994;19:176–182.

60. Ross JS, Delamarter R, Hueftle MG, et al: Gadolinium-DTPA-enhanced MR imaging of the postoperative lumbar spine: Time course and mechanism of enhancement. *Am J Roentgenol* 1989;152:825–834.

61. Nguyen CM, Ho KC, Yu SW, et al: An experimental model to study contrast enhancement in MR imaging of the intervertebral disk. *Am J Neuroradiol* 1989;10:811–814.

62. An HS, Nguyen C, Haughton VM, et al: Gadolinium-enhancement characteristics of magnetic resonance imaging in distinguishing herniated intervertebral disc versus scar in dogs. *Spine* 1994;19:2089–2095.

63. Jinkins JR, Osborn AG, Garrett D Jr, et al: Spinal nerve enhancement with Gd-DTPA: MR correlation with the postoperative lumbosacral spine. *Am J Neuroradiol* 1993;14:383–394.
64. Delamarter RB, Ross JS, Masaryk TJ, et al: Diagnosis of lumbar arachnoiditis by magnetic resonance imaging. *Spine* 1990;15:304–310.
65. Cavanagh S, Stevens J, Johnson JR: High-resolution MRI in the investigation of recurrent pain after lumbar discectomy. *J Bone Joint Surg* 1993;75B:524–528.
66. Fitt GJ, Stevens JM: Postoperative arachnoiditis diagnosed by high resolution fast spin-echo MRI of the lumbar spine. *Neuroradiology* 1995;37:139–145.

Chapter 6

The Role of Genetic Influences in Disk Degeneration and Herniation

Michele Crites Battié, PhD
Jaakko Kaprio, MD, PhD

The etiology of intervertebral disk degeneration and herniation remains speculative. Yet, the conditions commonly have been attributed to the accumulation of environmental effects, primarily mechanical insults and injuries, imposed on ''normal'' aging changes. Environmental factors have received much attention as possible risk factors,[1] but until recently, detailed studies focusing on hereditary aspects of disk degeneration and failure have been lacking.[2]

There is little surprise that, in humans, the size and shape of the spinal structures are more similar in family members than in unrelated individuals. The case reports and reports on series of twin pairs that demonstrate similarities in spinal and other skeletal morphology simply provide confirmatory evidence.[3-7] Such similarities have been amply demonstrated for other anthropometrics, such as height and dental structure.[8,9] In a review of the scientific literature on the heritability of traits in a wide variety of other species, Mousseau and Roff[10] found that the heritability of morphologic traits is larger on average than that of behavioral and life history traits (for example, fecundity and developmental rate), and such is the case in humans as well. Of greater interest are the ideas that degenerative changes commonly attributed primarily to environmental factors may be, in part, a function of genetic predisposition, and that, in some cases, this contributory role may be substantial.

Several mechanisms have been suggested through which hereditary factors could influence disk degeneration and herniation. Genetic effects on the size and shape of spinal structures could affect the spine's mechanical properties, and thus its vulnerability to external forces.[11] Biologic processes associated with the synthesis and breakdown of the disk's structural and biochemical constituents could be genetically predetermined, in part, leading to accelerated degenerative changes in some persons relative to others.[12-16] We could speculate, for example, that specific genes, which code for a structural protein contained in the disk, and which are defective in some proportion of the population, may lead to accelerated disk degeneration. Other defective genes may guide the development of the disk during embryogenesis, leading to larger or smaller disks than normal. These disks would be functionally normal, but more liable in the presence of unfavorable environmental agents to result in disk degeneration.

Recent studies undertaken to explore possible genetic influences primarily have investigated the presence of familial aggregation. These studies have been focused on juvenile lumbar disk herniation, sciatica, and disk degeneration and herniation among adults, as well as on back pain interfering with work.

Juvenile Lumbar Disk Herniation

The occurrence of juvenile disk herniation typically has been reported as a percentage of the total number of operations for lumbar disk herniation.[17-25] These figures, in part, reflect the standards of practice of the surgeons from various geographical regions, and the era of the reports. What is clear from these reports, however, is that surgery for disk herniation in children and adolescents is far less common than for these problems in adults. Reports of studies from North America and Europe indicate that less than 1% to as high as 6.6% of patients in these surgical cases are younger than 20 years of age.[17-21,23-25] Reports from Japan, however, have noted a higher percentage of juvenile disk herniations. Kurihara and Kataoka[22] found that 70 of 456 patients (15.4%) who underwent surgery for lumbar disk herniation between 1951 and 1977 at Kobe University Hospital were younger than 20 years of age. They also noted several other studies published in Japanese that reported that childhood and adolescent cases constituted between 7.8% and 22.3% of all surgically treated cases.

Population-based studies revealing the incidence of surgeries for juvenile disk herniation are rare. One such study was reported by Matsui and associates[26] who determined the incidence rate among more than 75,000 Japanese elementary, junior high, and high school students. The incidence rates of surgically treated lumbar disk herniations were calculated at 1.69 per 100,000 person-years for 10- to 12-year-olds, 3.15 for 13- to 15-year olds, and 9.36 for 16- to 18-year olds. The mean incidence rate for all the school children was 5.42 per 100,000 person-years. In comparison, the overall incidence of surgically treated herniated disks among adults in a population-based study in Minnesota was approximately ten times greater.[27]

Injury or trauma have commonly been presented as important antecedents to juvenile disk herniation,[19,24,25] including that arising from sport participation.[22,28] However, others have noted that although trauma may influence disk herniation, the percentage of juvenile cases for which such precipitating factors have been reported is similar to that for adults.[17,29] Degeneration of the disk has been suggested as the primary cause, with trauma acting as a precipitating factor.[17] An interaction between gender and age also has been suspected of influencing risk, with the ratio of females to males being greater in childhood and younger adolescent years than in later adolescence and into adulthood.[17] Yet, this finding has not been supported by all studies.[29,30] DeOrio and Bianco[18] found that, in a large series of patients from the Mayo Clinic, the children who underwent disk removal surgery were much taller than their peers. It has been postulated that this might be due to stresses associated with rapid periods of growth.[31] Nelson and associates[30] compared three age groups of young patients who had undergone diskectomy, those 9 through 15, 16 through 19, and 20 through 25 years of age, and found that younger patients were significantly more likely to have a family history of back disorders. Such a finding would be consistent with genetic epidemiologic literature, which indicates that stronger genetic effects are associated with earlier onset. It was not until more recent years, however, that familial aggregation and indications of possible genetic influences on juvenile disk herniation were pursued.[2,7,32]

Several investigators have reported on observations of familial aggregation. Matsui and associates[7] documented a case of a 16-year-old female identical twin who was admitted to a hospital for low back and left leg pain of approximately 1 year duration. Myelography and subsequent laminotomy revealed a protruded mass at the L4-5 level with left L5 root compression. Two years later, the patient's twin was admitted complaining of back pain of 2 years duration and right leg symptoms of approximately 8 months. Results from myelography and diskography prompted the surgeon to perform laminotomy and diskectomy at the L4-5 and L5-S1 levels, which immediately relieved the pain. The observation that herniated lumbar disks in young patients are relatively rare,[7,25,29,33] and the absence of a history of trauma, suggested that the similarity of the local disk pathology in the twins was not a chance occurrence. Matsui and associates[7] thus concluded that their findings suggest that genetic factors are involved in the development of juvenile herniated nucleus pulposus.

During the same year, Gunzburg and associates[2] documented a case of female identical twins who experienced radicular pain within 1 year of one another when they were approximately 13 years of age. Computed tomography (CT) scans revealed posterior bulging at the L4-5 level and herniation at the L5-S1 level in both. As in the case presented by Matsui and associates,[7] the onset of symptoms was similar and neither twin cited an injury or trauma. The twins experienced progressive symptoms that led to surgery in one case and chemonucleolysis in the other, with subsequent pain relief and return to normal activities.

These case reports demonstrate that familial aggregation occurs; whether it occurs more often than would be expected through random occurrence is not clear without comparison to controls or referents. However, the generally low incidence of juvenile disk herniation would suggest that such aggregation would be an extremely unlikely chance event.[26] The relative contribution of genetic and environmental factors also is not available from such data.

Two subsequent papers reported on the degree of familial aggregation in cases versus control groups. Varlotta and associates[32] investigated the incidence of severe low back pain, sciatica, and surgically treated herniated disks among the parents of 63 patients under 21 years of age who had herniated lumbar disks and the parents of a control group of nonback patients. They also tried to eliminate reporting bias by family members by requiring confirmation from medical records. The estimated risk of developing a herniated disk before the age of 21 was four to five times greater for patients who had a positive family history, as compared to those who did not. Of the patients, 73% had a single precipitating traumatic event.

A year later, a report was published on the occurrence of lumbar disk herniation in the siblings and parents of 40 patients who had undergone surgery for lumbar disk herniation and a referent group composed of the families of 120 controls (patients treated in the same department who had "normal spines").[26] The odds ratio for a family member of a patient with juvenile disk herniation to have had surgery for lumbar disk herniation was greater than 5.61 times that of a family member of a patient without disk herniation. The authors conclude that their results "strongly suggest that lumbar disk herniation in patients aged 18 years or younger shows familial predisposition and clustering."

These two papers are similar in using a control series to test for the degree of familial aggregation. Because family members can become affected even though the disease is not familially transmitted, the risk in family members needs to be compared with the population risk. Matsui and associates[26] found that six of 40 consecutive patients had a positive family history, which yielded an odds ratio of 5.61 (p risk estimate is, of course, directly useful clinical information when combined with the baseline incidence of five per 100,000 revealed from more than 75,000 children and adolescents.[26] Varlotta and associates[32] used matched patient-control pairs in their series of 63 disk herniations under 21 years of age. The age-adjusted relative risk of herniation in family members of patients compared to family members of controls was 4.5, which was quite similar to that found by Matsui and associates,[26] despite differences in methods and sample populations.

Collectively, these investigations make a fairly convincing case that juvenile intervertebral disk herniations are indeed influenced by genetic factors. The studies do not, however, provide data on the relative contributions and complex interactions of genetic and environmental factors.

Lumbar Disk Herniation in Adults

Bruske-Hohlfeld and associates[27] found first-time operations for suspected disk prolapse in residents of a county in Minnesota from 1950 through 1979 to be 46.3 per 100,000 person years (36.0 for women, 57.4 for men), and the overall incidence to be 52.3 per 100,000 person years. They made a distinction between surgically proven and unproven cases of disk prolapse and found the cumulative risk of having a second disk prolapse to be 8% in the following 20 years (a risk ten times that of the general population in the first 10 years and five times that of the population in the next 10 years). The surgery rates are likely to vary, however, from those of other geographic areas. Although diskectomy may appear to be a clear indication of the presence of symptomatic disk herniation, the significant regional variations in rates of spine surgery demonstrate that this outcome is likely to be significantly influenced by other factors as well. Thus, some degree of classification error is involved when equating the presence or absence of diskectomy with the presence or absence of a severe symptomatic herniated disk.

Among the most commonly suspected risk factors are occupations involving manual labor versus clerical or white-collar jobs,[34-36] vehicular vibration,[34,36] and being of greater height.[34,35] It also has been observed that men are at greater risk of being hospitalized for disk herniation than are women.[27,34]

Several reported observations of familial aggregation have raised the possibility of a genetic component.[37-40] Perhaps the most striking is the report of a family history of a 44-year-old patient who had surgery for lumbosacral disk herniation.[38] Of the patient's 14 siblings (eight men, six women), six (five men, one woman) had undergone surgery for lumbar disk herniation. Two other siblings, one man and one woman, had been diagnosed as having lumbar disk herniation on the basis of physical and electromyographic findings and were treated conservatively. The authors noted an early onset of symptoms, usually in the third decade, that was not precipitated by trauma. They also noted unusually large volumes of herniated disk material. They concluded that the high proportion of members of this generation affected could be due to transmission by both branches of the family of a genetic predisposition to premature degeneration or soft-tissue weakness. Alternatively, they postulated that a defective autosomal dominant major gene with low penetrance may be responsible for increasing risk among some persons.

Similarly, Varughese and Quartey[39] reported on the case histories of four brothers who had severe leg pain associated with disk herniation and concomitant spinal stenosis, which led to spinal surgery between 27 and 39 years of age. Both parents reported similar histories of symptoms and spine surgery. The authors concluded that the familial aggregation, along with the relatively young ages of the brothers at the time of their acute radicular symptoms, suggest that developmental or hereditary factors may have been responsible for the pathogenesis of spinal problems in this family.

Heikkilä and associates[41] investigated the role of genetic factors in sciatica and hospitalization for disk herniation by comparing pairwise concordance of monozygotic versus dizygotic twins. The Finnish data are valuable in that both self-report and hospital data are available and cover mild cases, which are less reliably reported, and generally more severe cases, which are more reliably categorized but more selected. In addition, the series was large (more than 9,000 same-sex twin pairs) and representative. The estimated heritability was approximately 21% for sciatica and 11% for associated hospitalizations. Perhaps most informative are the analyses of monozygotic to dizygotic ratios. The fact that reported sciatica had a lesser monozygotic to dizygotic ratio than did hospitalized cases suggests a greater genetic component in more severe cases. Also, the difference in the observed versus expected incidence of sciatica between monozygotic and dizygotic pairs decreased with increasing age. Thus, genetic influences were more significant in persons under 40 years of age. These findings are consistent with the literature, which indicates that stronger genetic effects are associated with an earlier onset of disease.[42] However, the apparently greater genetic influence in younger subjects may be due, in part, to the progressively higher rate of misclassifications caused by forgetfulness that occurred with increasing age.

Lumbar Disk Degeneration

Because disk degeneration is believed to be an important factor in the pathogenesis of disk herniation, it is also of interest to explore possible genetic influences on this process. Our research group[12,43] recently reported two studies related to this topic. The first study[12,43] dealt with similarities in degenerative findings in the lumbar disks of 20 pairs of monozygotic twins from 36 to 60 years of age, and we investigated whether the frequency of similar findings at the same spinal level between twins could be explained by chance based on the prevalence of the findings by level among all 40 subjects. The magnetic resonance imaging (MRI) assessments of disk bulging/herniation were done blinded to twinship and revealed a higher degree of twin similarities than would be expected by chance (Fig. 1). The percentage of variability in disk bulging/herniation explained by familial aggregation rose to 54% in the L1-L4 disks from

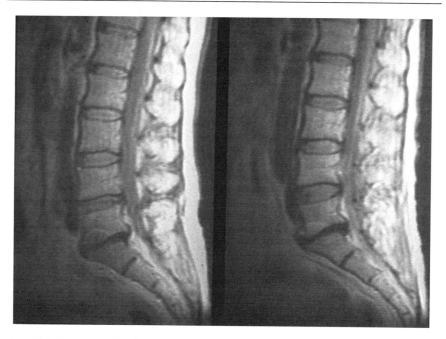

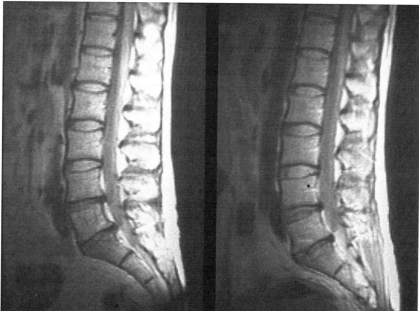

Fig. 1 **Top**, *Spine-density weighted sagittal lumbar magnetic resonance imaging of a pair of 60-year-old male identical twins reveals more advanced changes at the L4–5 disk in the twin on the left, but changes at the L5–S1 disk are strikingly similar.* **Bottom**, *Note the similarities in osteophyte formation, disk height, and posterior disk protrusions at L4–5 and L5–S1. (Reproduced with permission from Battié MC, Haynor DR, Fisher LD, et al: Similarities in degenerative findings on MRI of the lumbar spine of identical twins.* J Bone Joint Surg *1995;77A:1662–1670.)*

the 15% explained by age and smoking. Approximately 26% of the variability in such findings was explained in the L4-5 and L5-S1 levels by familial aggregation. These results were compatible with a significant genetic influence on lumbar degenerative disk changes and warranted further investigation.

In a later study,[12] we used spine MRIs from 115 pairs of identical twins to estimate the effects of commonly suspected risk factors on disk degeneration, as determined from signal intensity, bulging, and height narrowing, relative to the effects of age and familial aggregation. In the multivariate analysis of the T12-L4 region, occupational physical loading conditions explained 7% of the variability in disk degeneration scores among the 230 subjects; this rose to 16% with the addition of age and to 77% with the addition of a variable representing familial aggregation. In the L4-5 and L5-S1 region, leisure-time physical loading was the only behavioral or environmental factor investigated to enter the multivariate model and explained only 2% of the variability in disk degeneration summary scores. The amount of variability of lower lumbar disk degeneration scores explained rose to 9% with the addition of age and to 43% with the addition of familial aggregation. Significantly more of the variability in degeneration remained unexplained in the lower lumbar region. This discrepancy could be due to environmental conditions, which are likely mechanical in nature, that interact with spinal anthropometrics in such a way as to have a disproportional effect on the lower lumbar levels. However, the factors involved may be largely unpredictable and, for example, may result from a complex interaction and occasional convergence of conditions leading to degenerative changes. These study findings suggest that disk degeneration may be explained primarily by genetic influences and as yet unidentified factors, which may include complex, unpredictable interactions.

This study[12] provides a first estimate of the relative importance of specific environmental agents and overall genetic factors, which may be confounded with early childhood environmental factors because only monozygotic twins were studied (Fig. 2). The remaining variance that is unaccounted for by these two sources of variation (specific environmental and overall genetic) is due to measurement error and as yet unknown environmental effects. What is not known is whether specific gene effects of relatively large magnitude exist or if the genetic contribution is due to small effects of many genes. For example, about 50% of the population variability in cholesterol levels is due to genetic effects and 50% is due to environmental, mainly dietary effects. Of the genetic variability, more than half is attributed to specific genes in lipid metabolism, in particular apolipoprotein genes, and the remainder is presumed polygenic.[44]

Back Pain

Bengtsson and Thorson[45] investigated possible genetic influences on back pain that interfered with work by studying concordance of symptoms in twin pairs. The subjects were from a cohort of 5,029 monozygotic and 7,876 dizygotic Swedish twin pairs. Back pain was identified by an affirmative answer to the questionnaire item, ''Have you had so much back pain during the last few years that you found it difficult to work?'' Such pain was reported by about 17% of the males and 13% of the females in this fairly young cohort of twins ranging from 15 to 47 years of age. Pain concordance among twins with similar physi-

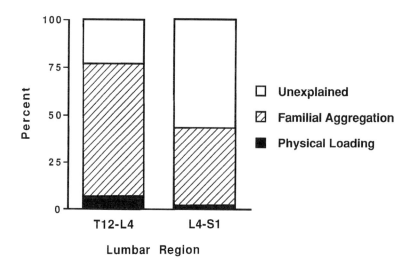

Fig. 2 *The graph displays the percentage of variability in disk degeneration in the T12–L4 and L4–S1 spinal regions explained by specific occupational and leisure physical loading variables relative to that explained by familial aggregation. Significantly more variability remains unexplained in the lower lumbar region. (Reproduced with permission from Battié MC, Videman T, Gibbons LE, et al: Determinants of lumbar disc degeneration. Spine 1995;20:2601–2612.)*

cal work demands was statistically significantly greater in monozygotic than in dizygotic pairs, with the exception of men engaged in light work, where the difference was not significant. Concordance with respect to pain, however, within monozygotic or dizygotic pairs was not enormous. For example, in all pairs where at least one member reported back pain interfering with heavy work activities, 25.3% of monozygotic twins reported similar problems versus 14.8% of dizygotic twins. The authors viewed these findings as supportive of a relationship between genetic factors and the occurrence of pain. The Swedish data are reported by gender, workload, and zygosity, but not by age, which is unfortunate given the findings of Heikkilä and associates[41] of a differential effect of heredity by age on sciatica and associated hospitalizations.

Identifying and Confirming Genetic Influences

Studies of the genetic epidemiology of back pain and spinal pathology start with determining whether familial aggregation of the disease or disorder being studied can be detected. In general terms, this is done by examining the frequency of disease in relatives compared to the frequency of disease in the general population. If relatives are at increased risk, the pattern of familial aggregation can be further defined through studies of different types of families, such as twin pairs, nuclear families, large pedigrees, or adoptee.[42] Most of the studies on disk herniation and degeneration fall into this category. Once evidence for familial aggregation has been obtained, there is a need to distinguish be-

tween biologic (genetic) and social (cultural inheritance) sources of familial similarity.[46] This would be the next logical step, for example, in the study of juvenile disk herniation and disk degenerative changes in adults.

Normal traits and common diseases generally have a genetic contribution from
more than one gene locus. The genetic architecture of a trait includes information on how many gene loci are involved and at which of these loci there are at
least two common forms of the genes or alleles, ie, are polymorphic. If the locus is not polymorphic, there will be no associated genetic variation. For each
gene locus, we ask how many alleles exist, and what the allele frequencies are.
Allele frequencies and average effects associated with the alleles determine the
contribution of allelic variation (which can be further partitioned into additive
genetic variance, due to gene ''dosage,'' and variance due to dominance) to the
overall genetic variation.[47]

A growing number of monogenic diseases have been successfully analyzed
down to the molecular level. Thus, monogenic diseases have shown how a biochemical defect evolves from a single mutation, which parts of a gene are indispensable for normal function, and how phenotypes develop from different mu-
tations. Based on these insights, molecular genetics can yield information on
normal traits and common disease.

Biochemical and molecular genetics of coronary heart disease can serve as a
useful example. The genetic architecture of traits involved in coronary artery
disease is being studied in increasing detail.[47] Genes possibly involved in the
etiology of disease are called candidate genes. Candidate genes may be used as
targets, with potential genetic variation leading to differences in the proteins encoded by these genes. These proteins are part of the physiologic system that,
when disturbed, gives rise to the disease being studied. For example, genetic
variation in only a few specific genes (apolipoprotein E, apolipoprotein B, and
the low density lipoprotein-receptor gene) accounts for about one half of the
total genetic variation (estimated by twin and family studies) in plasma cholesterol levels in the population.[47]

A prerequisite for these measured genotype approaches is more knowledge
of the intermediate physiologic levels linking genes, gene products, and intermediate metabolites to biochemical and behavioral outcomes. In orthopaedics,
knowledge both of the responsible genes and of the intervening variables and
relevant physiologic systems is poor compared to knowledge of lipid metabolism. The candidate gene approach is promising for the analysis of common diseases, which are complex in their etiology and development. Further, for specific genes and some environmental factors (diet, medications, and smoking),
gene-gene interactions, gene-environment interactions, and genotype-dependent
relationships of concomitants with serum lipid levels in lipid metabolism have
been demonstrated. Thus, simple linear models fail to grasp the complexity of
the real world, thereby indicating the difficulty of unraveling the contribution of
genes and environment in the etiology of a disease.[48] Molecular methods will
need to be further integrated with family and twin studies in the near future. For
example, dizygotic pairs either concordant for disease or extremely discordant
are highly informative genetically[49] and can serve as age-matched sib pairs,
whereas stratifying monozygotic pairs by genotype can illustrate the genotype-
specific variability of the trait.

Summary

The investigation of possible genetic influences on disk degeneration and herniation is in its infancy. An initial step along this line of inquiry has been to identify cases of familial aggregation, which indicate that shared genes and/or shared environments influence the likelihood of disease or the outcome of interest. Familial aggregation has been found for outcomes, such as hospitalizations for disk herniation in juveniles and adults, sciatica, back pain, and disk degeneration (encompassing changes in disk signal intensity, height, and bulging). It has been found that the degree of aggregation in family members is well beyond what would be expected by chance occurrence. Familial aggregation also has been found to be greater in younger than older subjects in the case of hospitalizations for disk herniation and in more severe cases when comparing having experienced sciatica to having had an associated hospitalization. These findings provide additional support for a possible genetic component to these conditions. Although these findings are congruent with a genetic influence, little has been done to differentiate the effects of shared genes from shared environments. Thus, the complex contributions of genetic and environmental factors, including possible interactions, is unknown.

A substantial genetic influence is sometimes interpreted as meaning that outcomes are predetermined and interventions are useless. However, finding a genetic effect does not preclude meaningful intervention or a role for environmental factors. By changing the environment, the role of genetic effects can be decreased or in some cases eliminated. In any event, genetic effects, given their basic role in determining cell structure and function, and hence tissue and organ structure and function, can provide key insights into the mechanisms underlying back disorders.

References

1. Riihimäki H: Low-back pain, its origin and risk indicators. *Scand J Work Environ Health* 1991;17:81–90.
2. Gunzburg R, Fraser RD, Fraser GA: Lumbar intervertebral disc prolapse in teenage twins: A case report and review of the literature. *J Bone Joint Surg* 1990;72B:914–916.
3. Bull J, el Gammal T, Popham M: A possible genetic factor in cervical spondylosis. *Br J Radiol* 1969;42:9–16.
4. King JB: A radiographic survey of nine pairs of elderly identical twins. *Clin Radiol* 1971;22:375–378.
5. King JB: A second radiographic skeletal survey of identical twins. *Clin Radiol* 1968;19:315–317.
6. Hurxthal LM: Schmorl's nodes in identical twins: Their probable genetic origin. *Lahey Clinic Foundation Bull* 1966;15:89–92.
7. Matsui H, Tsuji H, Terahata N: Juvenile lumbar herniated nucleus pulposus in monozygotic twins. *Spine* 1990;15:1228–1230.
8. Langinvainio H, Koskenvuo M, Kaprio J, et al: Finnish twins reared apart: II. Validation of zygosity, environmental dissimilarity, and weight and height. *Acta Genet Med Gemmellol* 1984;33:251–258.
9. Potter RH, Nance WE, Yu P-L: Genetic determinants of dental dimension: A twin study. *Prog Clin Biol Res* 1978;24:235–240.
10. Mousseau TA, Roff DA: Natural selection and the heritability of fitness components. *Heredity* 1987;59:181–197.
11. Palmer PE, Stadalnick R, Arnon S: The genetic factor in cervical spondylosis. *Skeletal Radiol* 1984;11:178–182.

12. Battié MC, Videman T, Gibbons LE, et al: Determinants of lumbar disc degeneration: A study relating lifetime exposures and magnetic resonance imaging findings in identical twins. *Spine* 1995;20:2601–2612.
13. Taylor TKF: Abstract: Lumbar intervertebral disc prolapse in children and adolescents. *J Bone Joint Surg* 1982;64B:135–136.
14. Rowe ML: Disc surgery and chronic low back pain. *J Occup Med* 1965;7:196–202.
15. Szypryt EP, Twining P, Wilde GP, et al: Diagnosis of lumbar disc protrusion: A comparison between magnetic resonance imaging and radiculography. *J Bone Joint Surg* 1988;70B:717–722.
16. Gibson MJ, Szypryt EP, Buckley JH, et al: Magnetic resonance imaging of adolescent disc herniation. *J Bone Joint Surg* 1987;69B:699–703.
17. Borgensen SE, Vang PS: Herniation of the lumbar intervertebral disk in children and adolescents. *Acta Orthop Scand* 1974;45:540–549.
18. DeOrio JK, Bianco AJ Jr: Lumbar disc excision in children and adolescents. *J Bone Joint Surg* 1982;64A:991–996.
19. Epstein JA, Epstein NE, Marc J, et al: Lumbar intervertebral disc herniation in teenage children: Recognition and management of associated anomalies. *Spine* 1984;9:427–432.
20. Fernström U: Protruded lumbar intervertebral disc in children: Report of a case and review of the literature. *Acta Chir Scand* 1956;111:71–79.
21. Raaf J: Some observations regarding 905 patients operated upon for protruded lumbar intervertebral disc. *Am J Surg* 1959;97:388–399.
22. Kurihara A, Kataoka O: Lumbar disc herniation in children and adolescents: A review of 70 operated cases and their minimum 5-year follow-up studies. *Spine* 1980;5:443–451.
23. Webb JH, Svien HJ, Kennedy RLJ: Protruded lumbar intervertebral disks in children. *JAMA* 1954;154:1153–1154.
24. Beks JW, ter Weeme CA: Herniated lumbar discs in teenagers. *Acta Neurochir* 1975;31:195–199.
25. Bulos S: Herniated intervertebral lumbar disc in the teenager. *J Bone Joint Surg* 1973;55B:273–278.
26. Matsui H, Terahata N, Tsuji H, et al: Familial predisposition and clustering for juvenile lumbar disc herniation. *Spine* 1992;17:1323–1328.
27. Bruske-Hohlfeld I, Merritt JL, Onofrio BM, et al: Incidence of lumbar disc surgery: A population-based study in Olmsted County, Minnesota, 1950–1979. *Spine* 1990;15:31–35.
28. Grobler LJ, Simmons EH, Barrington TW: Intervertebral disc herniation in the adolescent. *Spine* 1979;4:267–278.
29. Bradford DS, Garcia A: Lumbar intervertebral disc herniations in children and adolescents. *Orthop Clin North Am* 1971;2:583–592.
30. Nelson CL, Janecki CJ, Gildenberg PL, et al: Disk protrusions in the young. *Clin Orthop* 1972;88:142–150.
31. O'Connell JE: Intervertebral disk protrusions in childhood and adolescence. *Br J Surg* 1960;47:611–616.
32. Varlotta GP, Brown MD, Kelsey JL, et al: Familial predisposition for herniation of a lumbar disc in patients who are less than twenty-one years old. *J Bone Joint Surg* 1991;73A:124–128.
33. Rugtveit A: Juvenile lumbar disc herniations. *Acta Orthop Scand* 1966;37:348–356.
34. Heliövaara M, Knekt P, Aromaa A: Incidence and risk factors of herniated lumbar intervertebral disc or sciatica leading to hospitalization. *J Chron Dis* 1987;40:251–258.
35. Hrubec Z, Nashold BS Jr: Epidemiology of lumbar disc lesions in the military in World War II. *Am J Epidemiol* 1975;102:367–376.
36. Kelsey JL, Githens PB, O'Conner T, et al: Acute prolapsed intervertebral disc: An epidemiologic study with special reference to driving automobiles and cigarette smoking. *Spine* 1984;9:608–613.
37. Porter RW, Thorp L: Familial aspects of disc protrusion. *Orthop Trans* 1986;10:524.

38. Scapinelli R: Lumbar disc herniation in eight siblings with a positive family history for disc disease. *Acta Orthop Belgica* 1993;59:371–376.
39. Varughese G, Quartey GR: Familial lumbar spinal stenosis with acute disc herniations: Case reports of four brothers. *J Neurosurg* 1979;51:234–236.
40. Wilde GP, Narth AD, Kerslake R, et al: The familial incidence of disc degeneration. Proceedings of the Society for Back Pain Research, Oswestry, England. Hastings, England, Society for Back Pain Research, 1990, pp 51–52.
41. Heikkilä JK, Koskenvuo M, Heliövaara M, et al: Genetic and environmental factors in sciatica: Evidence from a nationwide panel of 9365 adult twin pairs. *Ann Med* 1989;21:393–398.
42. Khoury MJ, Beaty TH, Cohen BH (eds): *Fundamentals of Genetic Epidemiology.* New York, NY, Oxford University Press, 1993.
43. Battié MC, Haynor DR, Fisher LD, et al: Similarities in degenerative findings on magnetic resonance images of the lumbar spines of identical twins. *J Bone Joint Surg* 1995;77A:1660–1670.
44. Sing CF, Boerwinkle EA: Genetic architecture of inter-individual variability in apolipoprotein, lipoprotein and lipid phenotypes. *Ciba Found Symp* 1987;130:99–127.
45. Bengtsson B, Thorson J: Back pain: A study of twins. *Acta Genet Med Gemellol* 1991;40:83–90.
46. Cavalli-Sforza LL, Feldman MW (eds): *Cultural Transmission and Evolution: A Quantitative Approach.* Princeton, NJ, Princeton University Press, 1981.
47. Sing CF, Moll PP: Genetics of atherosclerosis. *Annu Rev Genet* 1990;24:171–187.
48. Zerba KE, Sing CF: The role of genome type-environment interaction and time in understanding the impact of genetic polymorphisms on lipid metabolism. *Curr Opin Lipidol* 1993;4:152–162.
49. Risch N, Zhang H: Extreme discordant sib pairs for mapping quantitative trait loci in humans. *Science* 1995;268:1584–1589.

Chapter 7

Epidural Corticosteroid Therapy for Acute Disk Herniations

Robert F. McLain, MD

Introduction

Although mechanical compression is thought to be the primary cause of sciatic pain in patients with lumbar disk herniation, it is unlikely that pressure on the nerve root is the only cause. First, several studies have demonstrated that not all disk herniations are symptomatic. Although Lindblom and Rexed,[1] in their histologic analysis of cadaver specimens, studied pathologic changes in nerve roots exposed to prolonged compression, other investigators have demonstrated that roughly 40% of postmortem examinations will reveal disk herniation in patients with no history of sciatic pain.[2] Similarly, myelographic abnormalities can be found in as many as 35% of normal individuals,[3] and magnetic resonance imaging (MRI) abnormalities in as many as 60% of asymptomatic subjects.[4]

Second, sciatic symptoms typically resolve over a course of 2 to 6 weeks, occurring more quickly than resorption of the extruded disk. Patients treated surgically may experience slightly improved results compared to those treated nonsurgically, but this difference is apparent only during the initial postoperative period.[5] On the other hand, some patients with complete surgical decompression, and others, with no radiographic evidence of frank nerve root compression, will have persistent sciatic pain.

In addition, findings by Howe and associates[6,7] indicate that the nerve root (as opposed to ganglion) must be sensitized before it can become an ectopic pain generator.[6,7] While acute compression of the nerve will produce weakness and anesthesia, it is not until an inflammatory process has been generated that the nerve begins to transmit pain signals. Once inflammation is present, however, the nerve becomes exquisitely sensitive to pressure, giving rise to prolonged, pain-producing discharges with even gentle manipulation or pressure.[8]

Hence, the current theories of sciatic pain related to disk herniation must consider inflammatory and neurochemical mediators as principal modulators, if not precipitators of, radicular symptoms. It is this aspect of the pain problem that physicians are trying to address when steroid and local anesthetic medicines are injected into the facet joints, disk, or epidural space.

History of Epidural Steroid Therapy

Viner[9] introduced the procedure of injecting large volumes of saline and procaine into the lumbar epidural space to treat back pain and lumbar radiculopathy in the 1920s. Evans[10] reported his results with a similar procedure in 1930, claiming a 14% success rate in 40 patients. Corticosteroids were added to the epidural injection in 1953.[11] In the United States, the effects of epidural steroid injection were first reported by Brown and by Goebert and associates in 1960.[12,13] Brown injected 80 mg methylprednisolone in 40 to 100 ml of saline into four patients with long-term (6 to 24 months' duration) sciatica. He reported complete transient relief in all four. Goebert and associates administered three injections of 1% procaine and 125 mg hydrocortisone to 239 patients with sciatica. Injections were given on consecutive or alternating days. Results were good (greater than 60% relief of symptoms) in 58% of patients. Since these reports were published, the technique and indications of epidural steroid injection have been constantly changing.

Epidural injections have been attempted with saline alone, anesthetic alone, steroid alone, and with combinations of each. A variety of anesthetics have been used (procaine, lidocaine, bupivacaine) as well as a number of corticosteroid agents (hydrocortisone, methylprednisolone, triamcinolone). Dosages of each medication, and number and timing of injections have varied widely as well. Both caudal and lumbar approaches have been used to reach the epidural space,[14,15] and injections may be carried out with or without fluoroscopic confirmation of needle position. Intrathecal injections were popular for a time, but the significant incidence of steroid-induced arachnoiditis by either the steroid or its vehicle, as well as the less common occurrence of meningitis (aseptic, septic, cryptococcal, and tuberculous), has made this an uncommon approach to pain management.[15-17]

The indications for epidural steroids have included acute and chronic pain, back or leg pain, and diagnoses ranging from acute herniated nucleus pulposus to end-stage degenerative disk disease and spinal stenosis. Likewise, the myriad associated modalities usually referred to as ''conservative therapy'' range from prolonged bed rest to lumbar traction to any of a variety of antiinflammatory medications, and have rarely been uniform within any one treatment group. The end result of this wide variety of approaches and indications for epidural steroid use is the difficulty in finding studies that can be compared along any level, irrespective of the presence or absence of controls. The fact that very few studies have been carried out prospectively, and that even fewer have included controls, makes it very difficult to find a firm footing in the existing clinical literature.

Scientific Basis for Steroid's Postulated Effect

Inflammation has been implicated as a cause of radicular pain in nerve root compression by studies that have demonstrated inflammatory changes in patients with pain and that have shown improvement in symptoms when patients were treated to relieve inflammation.

In 1950, Lindahl and Rexed[18] took biopsy samples from posterior nerve roots of patients undergoing laminectomy for lumbar disk degeneration. Inflammation, edema, and proliferative or degenerative changes were noted in seven of ten patients. Berg[19] used myelography to follow patients with sciatica and noted a consistent reduction in the size of the swollen nerve root coincident to the patient's improvement in symptoms. Green[20] reported a similar experience with one patient treated with intramuscular dexamethasone. He also reported on results of 100 patients treated with this protocol, and found that 67% had mild residual pain and 15% had no recurrent pain 1 year after treatment, numbers comparable to a surgical cohort. Systemic anti-inflammatory medication appeared to be just as effective as mechanical decompression, suggesting that the inflammatory component of sciatica might be just as important as the compressive one. This hypothesis is supported by the finding that the nucleus pulposus contains histamine, and that extracts of glycoprotein from the nucleus cause release of histamine, interstitial fluid, and protein from perfused tissues.[21] Saal and associates[22] recently demonstrated an immunocompetent cellular reaction present at the site of acute human disk herniations.[22] They identified macrophage and T lymphocyte aggregates at the interface of herniated nuclear material and the epidural space, and they noted that this reaction decreased in patients with a longer interval from symptom onset to surgery.

Corticosteroids act either locally or systemically to inhibit the inflammatory response produced by mechanical, chemical, infectious, or immunologic agents. The anti-inflammatory and immunosuppressive effects produced by corticosteroids both stem from glucocorticoid's ability to inhibit specific functions of leukocytes, ameliorating both the early phenomena of inflammation (edema, fibrin deposition, capillary dilatation, leukocyte aggregation, and phagocytosis) and late effects (capillary and fibroblast proliferation, collagen deposition, and cicatrization).

Corticosteroids combat inflammation by inhibiting the synthesis or release of a number of proinflammatory substances. They inhibit production of arachidonic acid and its metabolites (prostaglandins and leukotrienes) through glucocorticoid-induced synthesis of proteins (lipocortin and macrocortin), which inhibit the activity of phospholipase A_2.[23] Lipocortin also appears to inhibit the release of platelet-activating factor (PAF).[24] Corticosteroids inhibit activity of a number of lymphokines, including tumor necrosis factor-alpha (TNF-α), normally released from phagocytic cells in response to exposure to bacterial endotoxins. TNF-α is an endogenous pyrogen capable of inducing interleukin-1 (IL-1) production and stimulating synovial cell production of prostaglandin E_2 (PGE$_2$).[25-27] As a modulator of acute phase inflammatory responses, IL-1 plays a key role in the inflammatory process. It stimulates production of PGE$_2$ and collagenase, activates T lymphocytes, induces fibroblast proliferation, and acts as a chemo-attractant for leukocytes. In addition to the indirect anti-IL-1 effect they generate through TNF-α inhibition, corticosteroids also directly inhibit IL-1 production through their influence over monocyte and macrophage function.[28]

The nature of glucocorticoid activity is still not well defined. Recent studies have suggested that at least one mechanism of action is by decreasing endothelial adhesiveness for resting polymorphonuclear leukocytes (PMNs). By inhibiting the display of chemotactic molecules on the surface of endothelial cells, glucocorticoids prevent leukocyte aggregation and prevent endothelial injury due to diapodesis.[29] This inhibition may occur when glucocorticoid molecules, acting through specific cytoplasmic receptors within the endothelial cell, interrupt the transcription and expression of proinflammatory molecules responsible for endothelial-leukocyte adhesion. Leukocytes damage and disrupt endothelial membranes as they adhere and then transmigrate across the vascular wall. The damage to endothelial integrity, and to the cells themselves, results in an increase in capillary permeability and leads to subsequent tissue edema.[30] Ito[31] performed clearance studies that suggested an increase in vascular perfusion and clearance in the epidural space of patients with sciatica. Compared with patients with mild symptoms and those controls with no symptoms, patients with severe sciatica were believed to have increased circulatory clearance of the epidural space because of increased capillary permeability, increased capillary numbers, or dilatation of capillaries and other vessels.

Endothelial cells may also release a variety of cytokines, some of which act as chemo-attractants to monocytes and activated macrophages.[32,33] Once engaged in the local inflammatory process, these mononuclear phagocytes may elaborate a wide variety of secretory products into the surrounding milieu, including substance P (SP), IL-1, IL-6, TNF, PGE_2, leukotrienes, and PAF (Fig. 1).[34] Once released, these substances are capable of propagating both the early and late effects of the inflammation process, and of directly stimulating local and regional nociceptive nerve endings.

It should be noted, however, that while the glucocorticoid effect on endothelial adhesiveness is prominent for some inflammatory triggers, it is not effective for others. Cells exposed to lipopolysaccharide endotoxin are protected by glucocorticoids from developing an increased adhesiveness for leukocytes. Cells

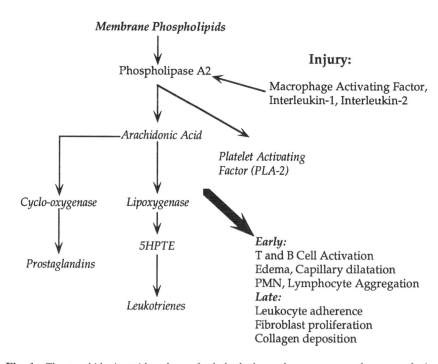

Fig. 1 *The arachidonic acid pathway feeds both the cyclooxygenase pathway, producing prostaglandins, and the lipoxygenase pathway, producing leukotrienes.*

exposed to TNF or IL-1 are not protected, however, suggesting that the inflammatory responses generated by endotoxin, TNF, and IL-1 must occur by different mechanisms, only some of which are sensitive to corticosteroid inhibition.[35]

Phospholipase A_2 (PLA$_2$) is a known agent in the process of inflammation, playing a crucial role in the regulation of free arachidonate and eicosanoid production.[36] Its action as a mediator in inflammatory conditions of the musculoskeletal system has been supported by a number of animal and human studies, and elevated PLA$_2$ levels have been demonstrated in serum and synovium of patients with rheumatoid arthritis.[37,38] High levels of PLA$_2$ have also been found in the human intervertebral disk, suggesting both a role for inflammation as a part of painful disk pathology, and as a humeral process that might have topical and diffuse local effects on adjacent neural tissues.[39,40]

Pain generated by nerve fibers in the outer layers of the anulus fibrosis is thought to affect the back but not to manifest as radicular symptoms. Recent studies have demonstrated the ramification of fine nerve endings over the anulus itself and throughout the posterior longitudinal ligament, and have suggested a reason why diskographic injection may produce pain.[41-44] Neurohistochemical studies have shown that pain-related neuropeptides (calcitonin gene-related peptide [CGRP], vasoactive intestinal peptide [VIP], and SP) are resident within the neural investments of the anulus, supporting the conclusion that these fine endings are nociceptive fibers.[45,46] An inflammatory process that stimulates these fibers directly may produce back pain, while release of neuropeptides from these fibers into the local milieu of the dorsal root ganglion could generate leg pain. Hence, an anti-inflammatory modality might be effective against back pain or leg pain in different patients.

In addition to a direct role as mediators of nociceptive transmission, these neurotransmitters may also impact spinal health through the paracrine effects of their release into surrounding connective tissues. CGRP and VIP may have an indirect effect on skeletal mechanics; VIP stimulates bone resorption while CGRP inhibits it.[47,48] At the same time, SP stimulates synovial proliferation and the release of prostaglandins, collagenase, IL-1, and TNF.[49] These peripheral effects may be important in the evolution of spinal instability, degeneration, and nerve root irritation.

One important question (and a prominent confounder of previous clinical studies) is the failure to define what pain investigators have been treating—back pain or leg pain? It is possible that appropriately administered epidural corticosteroids may ameliorate either back *or* leg pain in specific patients, assuming that an inflammatory mechanism is responsible for that patient's symptoms.

Clinical Studies of Efficacy: Effectiveness of Epidural Corticosteroid Injections

Clinical studies of epidural steroid therapy are, by and large, flawed. Studies have typically contained one or more of the following flaws: (1) Most studies have had no control group with which to compare treatment. (2) Many studies have included patients who have undergone a variety of other therapies concurrent with their treatment with epidural steroids. (3) In some studies the steroid treatment has not been standardized, varying with respect to steroid type, dose, delivery method, and the inclusion of local anesthetics. (4) None of the studies has been randomized, prospective, or blinded in such a way as to provide really valuable data. (5) Criteria for determining outcome have not been standardized.[50]

Swerdlow and Sayle-Creer[51] retrospectively reviewed 325 patients undergoing epidural injection for lumbosciatic syndrome. This study included no controls, and patients were not described. Similarly, the patients' symptoms were not described in detail. Patients in this study were roughly grouped according to symptoms: acute pain, chronic pain, and recurrent pain. Outcomes for these patients were roughly described as relieved, assisted, or valueless. There was no difference in results with epidural injections of local anesthetic versus saline alone, or between either of these modalities and corticosteroids in the acute pain group. However, the addition of methylprednisolone did provide more good results in chronic pain patients, and fewer "valueless" results in the recurrent pain group.

Bush and associates[52] described their results with conservatively treated patients receiving triamcinolone and procaine epidural injections, noting that 14% of patients got no relief and required surgical decompression. With no control group or objective measures of outcome, it is impossible to draw firm conclusions from this study. Nonetheless, the authors were able to correlate objective evidence of disk resorption with a subjective measure of clinical improvement, and to demonstrate the key feature of most studies: that the majority of patients improve with conservative therapy.

In the few well-controlled studies of epidural steroid use, results have been variable (Table 1). Dilke and associates[53] found steroids effective in their controlled, randomized, double-blind trial of 100 consecutive patients treated for unilateral sciatica. Patients in the treatment group were given 80 mg of methylprednisolone via the lumbar epidural route, while controls received an injection of saline into the interspinous ligament. If no clinical progress was observed, the patient would then be given a second injection of the same substance. The two groups were comparable with respect to age, sex, neurologic deficit, symptom complex, duration of symptoms, and occupational demands. Treated patients showed a significantly decreased need for analgesics during admission, a higher rate of return to work, a lower rate of surgery, and greater subjective pain relief both initially and at 3 months. Unfortunately, the authors truncated follow-up at 3 months, so long-term benefit is unknown. They also did not discuss the 30% dropout from both groups during the study.

In contrast, Snoek and associates[54] found no difference between epidural steroid and placebo in their double-blind study of 51 patients treated for lumbar root compression of variable duration. In this study, patients received either 2 ml (80 mg) methylprednisolone or 2 ml normal saline. Again, the two groups were comparable, the approach was lumbar epidural, and compression was confirmed by myelography prior to treatment. Outcome criteria in this series included physical findings (improvement of straight-leg raise, assessments of muscle and reflex function) and analgesic use, as well as subjective impressions of pain relief. Early outcome assessment was carried out 24 to 48 hours after injection (steroid response may not be seen for up to 6 days). Although the treated group experienced greater early improvement in sagittal motion, sciatic stretch, motor weakness, back, radicular, and impulse pain, and analgesic con-

Table 1 Epidural steroid injections: Outcomes in controlled series

Author	Patients (No.)	Patient Diagnosis*	Study Design[†]	Outcome Measures[§]	Treatment	Controls/Other Groups	Efficacy[¶]
Beliveau (1971)[55]	24	Mixed: Acute and chronic sciatic pain	Prosp; Rand; Tr Cont	Sub pain rel	Procaine w/ methylprednisolone	Procaine alone	(+/-)
Breivik (1976)[56]	35	Mixed: Acute HNP and chronic arachnoiditis	Prosp; Rand; Tr Cont	Sub pain rel	Bupivacaine w/ methylprednisolone	Bupivacaine w/ saline	(+)
Snoek (1977)[54]	51	Uniform: Unilateral sciatica	Prosp; Dble Bld; Plac Cont	Sub pain rel Physical signs Analg use Surg rate	2 ml methyl-prednisolone	2 ml saline	(-)
Yates (1978)[57]	20	Mixed: Acute and subacute sciatica	Prosp; Rand; Tr Cont	Sub pain rel Physical signs	Lidocaine w/ triamcinolone	Saline; lidocaine; saline and triamcinolone	(+)
Klenerman (1984)[60]	63	Uniform: Unilateral sciatica	Prosp; Rand; Plac Cont	Sub pain rel Physical signs	Methylprednisolone	Needle placement w/o injection	(-)
Cuckler (1985)[59]	73	Mixed: Acute HNP or spinal stenosis	Prosp; Rand; Dble Bld; Tr Cont	Sub pain rel Physical signs	Procaine w/ methylprednisolone	Procaine w/saline	(-)
Ridley (1988)[58]	39	Uniform: Unilateral sciatica	Prosp; Rand; Dble Bld; Plac Cont	Sub pain rel	Methylprednisolone, 80 mg	Injection of saline into interspinous ligament	(+/-)
Bush (1991)[61]	23	Uniform: Unilateral sciatica	Prosp; Rand; Dble Bld; Plac Cont	Sub pain rel Physical signs	Procaine w/ triamcinolone	Saline	(+/-)

* Uniform = all patients fit the same diagnostic criteria prior to enrollment; Mixed = multiple diagnostic groups were combined under each treatment arm
[†] Prosp = Prospective; Rand = Randomized; Dble Bld = Double blind; Plac Cont = Placebo controlled; Tr Cont = Treatment controlled
[§] Sub Pain Rel = Subjective pain relief; Analg use = Analgesic use; Surg Rate = Rate of treatment failure requiring surgery
[¶] (+) = Authors demonstrated a significant benefit of epidural steroids relative to treatment or placebo controls; (-) = Authors demonstrated no significant benefit of epidural steroids relative to treatment or placebo controls; (+/-) = Only some criteria showed steroid benefit, or benefit was not maintained over time

103

sumption, these were not statistically significant. Likewise, though more of the treated patients experienced improved physical findings (67% versus 42%) and the physiotherapists assessed more of the treated patients as improved (70% versus 43%), these differences did not reach statistical significance. Long-term follow-up in this study consisted of a late chart review to see which patients had required surgery in the interval since treatment. Fourteen patients in each group had undergone diskectomy; hence, the authors concluded no long-term benefit for the use of corticosteroids. Benzon[50] has also pointed out that Snoek used no diluent in his injections, and gave only one injection, limiting the likelihood of effective therapy.

Beliveau[55] compared caudal epidural injections of procaine with and without methylprednisolone in patients with acute and chronic sciatic pain. He found no difference in overall efficacy; 75% of patients in either group experienced subjective improvement after injection. Patients with acute symptoms apparently benefited from either type of injection, while those with severe, chronic pain got relief only when steroid was included. The numbers of acute and chronic patients were not discussed, however, and physical findings were not assessed in any detail. This study was prospective and randomized, but there was no untreated control for comparison.

Breivik and associates[56] specifically studied patients with chronic back pain, and included 11 previously operated patients in their 35-patient study group. Their prospective, randomized study included patients with diagnoses ranging from acute disk herniation to arachnoiditis. Patients received one to three injections of bupivacaine with either methylprednisolone or saline. If no clinical benefit was seen, patients then crossed over into the other treatment group for three more injections. During initial therapy, nine of 16 patients (56%) receiving steroid experienced significant relief, compared to five of 19 patients (26%) receiving bupivacaine with saline. In the crossover only one of seven patients (14%) who had failed steroid therapy got any relief from the subsequent bupivacaine and saline injections. Eight of the 11 (73%) who failed the bupivacaine and saline injections reported satisfactory relief after receiving the second series of injections containing methylprednisolone.

In 1978, Yates[57] reported a series of 20 patients randomized to a series of four different epidural caudal injections. Patients were injected with either saline, lidocaine, saline and triamcinolone, or lidocaine and triamcinolone. Physical findings of decreased straight leg raise and limited sagittal range of motion most improved with the use of injections containing steroid. However, follow-up was brief, and patients who improved before completing the series of injections were removed from the study.

Most recent studies that have been controlled and randomized have, at best, attributed a rather marginal benefit to corticosteroid therapy. Ridley and associates[58] found a significant initial difference between treated patients and controls in their randomized trial of 39 patients treated with epidural steroids. While treated patients noted a significant decrease in pain at 2 weeks, there was no residual benefit to the treatment; treated and untreated patients were indistinguishable at 6 months. Cuckler and associates[59] found no benefit with steroid injection in their prospective, double-blind, randomized study of 73 patients with lumbar pain. Methylprednisolone and procaine were compared to physiologic saline with procaine in treating patients with documented nerve root compression caused by acute disk herniation or spinal stenosis. There was no significant difference in outcomes for either group, either initially or at long-term (20-month) follow-up. Klenerman and associates[60] found that 75% of their patients with acute sciatica had satisfactory improvement regardless of whether they had injections of saline, methylprednisolone, or bupivacaine. In this prospective, randomized, and controlled study, the only group that did not improve was that in which needle placement was not associated with any injection. It was concluded that the benefit of epidural steroid injection might be attributed partly to placebo effect and partly to the natural history of sciatica.

Bush and Hillier,[61] on the other hand, found triamcinolone with procaine hydrochloride significantly superior to placebo in a double-blind, controlled study of caudal epidurals. At 4 weeks follow-up the actively treated group exhibited significantly greater pain relief and mobility relative to placebo. Patients had a significantly improved quality of life following triamcinolone injection. At 1 year follow-up both treatment and placebo groups showed subjective and objective improvement. The treated patients showed greater improvement than placebo patients, but only the improvement in straight leg raise was significant.

Uncontrolled studies abound.[14,62-66] Power and associates[67] declared epidural steroids an unmitigated failure and concluded that it would be unethical to continue their study after all of their 16 patients failed to benefit from injections of bupivacaine and methylprednisolone. Although 10 patients were believed to have some initial relief (24 hours to 3 months), none avoided surgery. All patients were shown to have large disk protrusions or sequestrations on CT or myelogram. Six patients were subjected to surgery when injection failed to produce relief in the first 24 hours. This time frame is inadequate to realistically assess the benefit of the steroid medication. Nonetheless, epidural steroids failed to alter the treatment course for any of these patients with large disk herniations. No explanation was given as to why this population had a much poorer outcome than would have been expected from natural history had no treatment been given at all. Ito[31] reported that 12% of 161 patients with disk protrusion had excellent results and 46% had fair results when injected with 20 mg prednisolone; 40 patients subsequently underwent surgery. In this study, patients with spondylosis or degenerative spondylolisthesis had better results from epidural steroids than did those with acute disk herniation (84% and 83% fair to excellent results, respectively, versus 58%).

Anderson and Mosdal[68] reported on a mixed group of seven women and nine men treated with methylprednisolone and lidocaine, with outcome determined by visual analog pain scale. They found that 10 of 17 patients felt significant improvement initially, but that only one patient experienced substantial long-term benefit.

Berman and associates[69] reported on 367 patients with leg pain treated with epidural steroids in a multidisciplinary pain management program. All patients had failed a 2-week program of conservative management prior to injection with either methylprednisolone or hydrocortisone. They found best results for steroids in patients with subacute or chronic radicular pain who had not had any previous surgery. In this uncontrolled, retrospective study, 70% of patients with this profile experienced good to excellent results from their injections. Outcomes were determined based on the subjective relief of pain, return to work, and need for further treatment. Outcomes deteriorated over time, but 60% good to excellent results were reported 1 year after treatment.

Reasons for Treatment Failure

Surprisingly little has been said about factors predisposing patients to success or failure with epidural steroid therapy. Although the influence of psychosocial factors has long been recognized with respect to surgical and overall outcomes, only a few studies have specifically addressed these confounders with respect to epidural injections.

Hopwood and Abram[70] analyzed 33 factors relative to treatment outcome in 209 patients treated for low back pain. An increased risk of treatment failure was associated with a prolonged duration of symptoms, nonradicular symptomatology, lack of employment at the start of treatment, and smoking. Ferrante and associates,[71] in their study of cervical epidurals, also found that axial (neck) pain carried a poorer prognosis than radicular pain. Jamison and associates[72] identified four factors predictive of poor outcome in their prospective analysis of 249 patients with chronic low back pain: (1) greater number of previous treatments for pain; (2) greater dependence on medications; (3) pain not necessarily increased by activity; and (4) pain increased by cough. Lack of employment was again predictive of a poor long-term result.

From a technical point of view, failure to apply the steroid medication to the appropriate area could be a cause of treatment failure. Renfrew and associates[73] noted that, even in experienced hands, blind placement of the injection needle was optimal in only 60% of cases. They recommended fluoroscopic control and contrast administration to eliminate incorrect needle placement and inadvertent venous injections.

Current Usage: What Constitutes an Adequate Epidural Injection?

Current treatment regimens vary, but some basic principles can be presented.

Steroids should be introduced into the epidural space, with care taken to avoid unintentional intrathecal injection. Either a caudal or interspinal lumbar approach may be used, depending on the practitioner's preference and experience.[66,74]

Blind needle placement is effective in the hands of some practitioners, but can lead to significant complications including meningitis or chemical arachnoiditis from accidental intradural injection.[75] Brown[76] described the technique for interspinous injection, placing the needle in the upper lumbar region in the seated patient. He reported excellent results, with no complications, in a small series of selected patients.

As previously noted, some physicians advocate needle placement under fluoroscopic control, using contrast instillation to document an epidural, extravascular placement before injection of medications.[73] Epidural injections are performed on an outpatient basis.

Corticosteroids may be injected alone[77] or with a local anesthetic or saline diluent.[53,62] The local anesthetic, procaine, lidocaine, or bupivacaine, may serve to acutely relieve pain and muscle spasm, and can, through the extent of neural blockade, indicate whether needle placement was correct. Large volume injections of saline are not indicated and may result in complications.[78] Harley[63] demonstrated that a 6.0-ml injection was sufficient to disperse radio-opaque contrast from the level of the sacrum up to L1. A 10.0-ml infiltration of steroid and saline, or steroid with 0.25% bupivacaine or 0.5% lidocaine should be sufficient for any application.

There are no data to suggest that any one corticosteroid medication performs better than others. Usual dosages include methylprednisolone 80 mg or triamcinolone 80 mg. Although most patients benefit from a single injection, administration of a series of three injections is recommended before assuming failure.

Gaps in Current Knowledge

A better understanding of the cause of radicular pain is needed in order to establish the role of epidural steroids, or any injectable or topical medicine for that matter, in treating acute disk herniation with nerve root pain. The questionable benefit of steroids brought out by the studies reviewed herein may relate either to the inability to administer an effective medication to the focus of pain generation, or to the inherent inability of corticosteroids to impact this pain-producing pathway. Recent studies have demonstrated that human PLA_2 is not sensitive to nonsteroidal medications acting through inhibition of cyclooxygenase, and that dexamethasone, naproxen, ibuprofen, ketoprofen, and piroxicam are completely inactive as PLA_2 inhibitors in vitro.[79,80]

Additionally, the safety of epidural steroid therapy is in question. Nelson points out an apparent incongruency between scientific understanding of steroid effects and the reported clinical experience. While intrathecal steroid injections are known to produce a high rate of adhesive arachnoiditis,[81] and inadvertent intrathecal puncture is not uncommon during epidural injection,[53] the reported incidence of clinical arachnoiditis following injection is far lower than would be expected.[82] Although it is possible that the steroid medication is inhibiting the inflammatory response to the polyethylene glycol vehicle, it is also possible that subacute and mild to moderate cases of clinical arachnoiditis are not being recognized in those patients with persistent pain, and failed back syndrome.

Summary

Epidural steroids may or may not be beneficial to some patients with back and/or leg pain; it depends somewhat on the patient: if all patients have acute sciatica, a 90% or higher success rate is expected, to be comparable to controls; on the other hand, if only patients who have failed a full course of conservative therapy and who have persistent pain months down the road are treated, 60% to 70% good-excellent results might be very attractive. The current literature cannot specifically support the use of epidural steroids in acute disk herniations, because most patients get better regardless of treatment, and most studies have not adequately separated these patients to allow subgroup analysis.

Comparing results between different regimens is really not possible from the available literature. Groups studied are rarely homogenous, and are usually so poorly described that it is not possible to tell whether or not one patient population is comparable to another. Six factors persist: (1) *Symptom complex*. Patients included may have back pain, leg pain, or both, and most studies did not thoroughly describe the symptoms being treated. Worse, some authors seem to use the terms "back pain" and "sciatica" interchangeably; (2) *Duration*. Many studies contain a broad mix of patients, roughly described as acute, subacute, or chronic. Acute patients tend to be those with sciatica, while chronic patients tend to have back pain, sciatica, and all the problems associated with long-standing low back pain; (3) *Prior treatment*. Many studies include previously operated patients in their treatment groups, but again, these patients and their symptoms are poorly described; (4) *Assessment*. No consistent method of assessing patient improvement has been employed. Many studies rely on the patient or the physician's subjective impression of pain relief. Others have used gross measures such as return to work or sciatic stretch. Significant discrepancies have been seen in studies comparing different outcome measures, and consequently, clinical trials using different outcome measures may reach different conclusions.[83] Few studies have employed any comprehensive measures of outcome; (5) *Follow-up*. Final assessment of patients has been carried out at anywhere from 3 months to 2 years after treatment; (6) *Controls*. Only two studies have compared the results of epidural steroid injections for sciatica to untreated controls, and these have come to opposite conclusions.

The key to determining if steroids are effective in patients with intractable sciatica is to establish well-controlled, randomized, prospective studies.

References

1. Lindblom K, Rexed B: Spinal nerve injury in dorso-lateral protrusions of lumbar disks. *J Neurosurg* 1948;5:413–432.
2. McRae DL: Asymptomatic intervertebral disc protrusions. *Acta Radiol* 1956;46:9–27.
3. Hitselberger WE, Witten RM: Abnormal myelograms in asymptomatic patients. *J Neurosurg* 1968;28:204–206.
4. Boden SD, Davis DO, Dina TS, et al: Abnormal magnetic-resonance scans of the lumbar spine in asymptomatic subjects: A prospective investigation. *J Bone Joint Surg* 1990;72A:403–408.
5. Hakelius A: Prognosis in sciatica: A clinical follow-up of surgical and non-surgical treatment. *Acta Orthop Scand* 1970;129(suppl):1–76.
6. Howe JF, Loeser JD, Calvin WH: Mechanosensitivity of dorsal root ganglia and chronically injured axons: A physiological basis for the radicular pain of nerve root compression. *Pain* 1977;3:25–41.
7. Howe JF: A neurophysiological basis for the radicular pain of nerve root compression, in Bonica JJ, Liebeskind JC, Albe-Fessard DG, et al (eds): *Advances in Pain Research and Therapy*. New York, NY, Raven Press, 1979, vol 3, pp 647–657.
8. Murphy RW: Nerve roots and spinal nerves in degenerative disk disease. *Clin Orthop* 1977;129:46–60.
9. Viner N: Intractable sciatica: The sacral epidural injections. An effective method of giving relief. *Can Med Assoc J* 1925;15:630–634.
10. Evans W: Intrasacral epidural injection in the treatment of sciatica. *Lancet* 1930;2:1225–1229.
11. Liévre JA, Bloch-Michel H, Attali P: L'injection transsacree: Etude clinique et radiologique. *Bull Soc Med Paris* 1957;73:1110–1118.
12. Brown JH: Pressure caudal anesthesia and back manipulation: Conservative method for treatment of sciatica. *Northwest Med* 1960;59:905–909.

13. Goebert HW Jr, Jallo SJ, Gardner WJ, et al: Sciatica: Treatment with epidural injections of procaine and hydrocortisone. *Cleve Clin Quart* 1960;27:191–197.
14. Heyse-Moore GH: A rational approach to the use of epidural medication in the treatment of sciatic pain. *Acta Orthop Scand* 1978;49:366–370.
15. Nelson DA, Vates TS Jr, Thomas RB Jr: Complications from intrathecal steroid therapy in patients with multiple sclerosis. *Acta Neurol Scand* 1973;49:176–188.
16. Roberts M, Sheppard GL, McCormick RC: Tuberculous meningitis after intrathecally administered methylprednisolone acetate. *JAMA* 1967;200:894–896.
17. Shealy CN: Dangers of spinal injections without proper diagnosis. *JAMA* 1966;197:1104–1106.
18. Lindahl O, Rexed B: Histologic changes in spinal nerve roots of operated cases of sciatica. *Acta Orthop Scand* 1951;20:215–225.
19. Berg A: Clinical and myelographic studies of conservatively treated cases of lumbar intervertebral disk protrusion. *Acta Chir Scand* 1952;104:124–129.
20. Green LN: Dexamethasone in the management of symptoms due to herniated lumbar disc. *J Neurol Neurosurg Psychiatry* 1975;38:1211–1217.
21. Marshall LL, Trethewie ER: Chemical irritation of nerve-root in disc prolapse. *Lancet* 1973;2:320.
22. Saal JS, Sibley R, Dobrow R, et al: Cellular response to lumbar disc herniation: An immunohistologic study. *Orthop Trans* 1991;15:316.
23. Di Rosa M, Calignano A, Carnuccio R, et al: Multiple control of inflammation by glucocorticoids. *Agents Action* 1986;17:284–289.
24. Parente L, Flower RJ: Hydrocortisone and "macrocortin" inhibit the zymosan-induced release of lyso-PAF from rat peritoneal leucocytes. *Life Sci* 1985;36:1225–1231.
25. Beutler B, Cerami A: Cachectin: More than a tumor necrosis factor. *N Engl J Med* 1987;316:379–385.
26. Dayer JM, Beutler B, Cerami A: Cachectin/tumor necrosis factor stimulates collagenase and prostaglandin E2 production by human synovial cells and dermal fibroblasts. *J Exp Med* 1985;162:2163–2168.
27. Dinarello CA, Cannon JG, Wolff SM, et al: Tumor necrosis factor (cachectin) is an endogenous pyrogen and induces production of interleukin-1. *J Exp Med* 1985;163:1433–1450.
28. Dinarello CA, Mier JW: Lymphokines. *N Engl J Med* 1987;317:940–945.
29. Cronstein BN, Kimmel SC, Levin RI, et al: A mechanism for the antiinflammatory effects of corticosteroids: The glucocorticoid receptor regulates leukocyte adhesion to endothelial cells and expression of endothelial-leukocyte adhesion molecule-1 and intercellular adhesion molecule-1. *Proc Natl Acad Sci USA* 1992;89:9991–9995.
30. Varani J, Ginsburg I, Schuger L, et al: Endothelial cell killing by neutrophils: Synergistic interaction of oxygen products and proteases. *Am J Pathol* 1989;135:435–438.
31. Ito R: The treatment of low back pain and sciatica with epidural corticosteroids injection and its pathophysiological basis. *Nippon Seikeigeka Gakkai Zasshi* 1971;45:769–777.
32. Holter W, Goldman CK, Casabo L, et al: Expression of functional IL-2 receptors by lipopolysaccharide and interferon-gamma stimulated human monocytes. *J Immunol* 1987;138:2917–2922.
33. Spriggs MK, Lioubin PJ, Slack J, et al: Induction of an interleukin-1 receptor (IL-1R) on monocytic cells: Evidence that the receptor is not encoded by a T cell-type IL-1R mRNA. *J Biol Chem* 1990;265:22499–22505.
34. Rappolee DA, Werb Z: Secretory products of phagocytes. *Curr Opin Immunol* 1988;1:47–55.
35. Ghezzi P, Sipe JD: Dexamethasone modulation of LPS, IL-1, and TNF stimulated serum amyloid A synthesis in mice. *Lymphokine Res* 1988;7:157–166.
36. Pruzanski W, Vadas P: Phospholipase A2, a mediator between proximal and distal effectors of inflammation. *Immunol Today* 1991;12:143–146.

37. Pruzanski W, Vadas P: Secretory synovial fluid phospholipase A2 and its role in the pathogenesis of inflammation in arthritis. *J Rheumatol* 1988;15:1601–1603.

38. Vadas P, Pruzanski W, Kim J, et al: The proinflammatory effect of intra-articular injection of soluble human and venom phospholipase A2. *Am J Pathol* 1989;134:807–811.

39. Franson RC, Saal JS, Saal JA: Human disc phospholipase A2 is inflammatory. *Spine* 1992;17(suppl 6):S129–S132.

40. Saal JS, Franson RC, Dobrow R, et al: High levels of inflammatory phospholipase A2 activity in lumbar disc herniations. *Spine* 1990;15:674–678.

41. Bogduk N: The innervation of the lumbar spine. *Spine* 1983;8:286–293.

42. Konttinen YT, Gronblad M, Antti-Poika I, et al: Neuroimmunohistochemical analysis of peridiscal nociceptive neural elements. *Spine* 1990;15:383–386.

43. Weinstein J, Claverie W, Gibson S: The pain of discography. *Spine* 1988;13:1344–1348.

44. Yoshizawa H, O'Brien JP, Smith WT, et al: The neuropathology of intervertebral discs removed for low-back pain. *J Pathol* 1980;132:95–104.

45. Ashton IK, Roberts S, Jaffray DC, et al: Neuropeptides in the human intervertebral disc. *J Orthop Res* 1994;12:186–192.

46. Coppes MH, Marani E, Thomeer, RT, et al: Letter: Innervation of annulus fibrosis in low back pain. *Lancet* 1990;336:189–190.

47. Hohmann EL, Levine L, Tashjian AH Jr: Vasoactive intestinal peptide stimulates bone resorption via a cyclic adenosine 3',5'-monophosphate-dependent mechanism. *Endocrinology* 1983;112:1233–1239.

48. Zaidi M, Fuller K, Bevis PJ, et al: Calcitonin gene-related peptide inhibits osteoclastic bone resorption: A comparative study. *Calcif Tissue Int* 1987;40:149–154.

49. Kimball ES, Fisher MC: Potentiation of IL-1-induced BALB/3T3 fibroblast proliferation by neuropeptides. *J Immunol* 1988;141:4203–4208.

50. Benzon HT: Epidural steroid injections for low back pain and lumbosacral radiculopathy. *Pain* 1986;24:277–295.

51. Swerdlow M, Sayle-Creer WS: A study of extradural medication in the relief of the lumbosciatic syndrome. *Anaesthesia* 1970;25:341–345.

52. Bush K, Cowan N, Katz DE, et al: The natural history of sciatica associated with disc pathology: A prospective study with clinical and independent radiologic follow-up. *Spine* 1992;17:1205–1212.

53. Dilke TF, Burry HC, Grahame R: Extradural corticosteroid injection in management of lumbar nerve root compression. *Br Med J* 1973;2:635–637.

54. Snoek W, Weber H, Jorgensen B: Double blind evaluation of extradural methylprednisolone for herniated lumbar discs. *Acta Orthop Scand* 1977;48:635–641.

55. Beliveau P: A comparison between epidural anaesthesia with and without corticosteroid in the treatment of sciatica. *Rheumatol Phys Med* 1971;11:40–43.

56. Breivik H, Hesla PE, Molnar I, et al: Treatment of chronic low back pain and sciatica: Comparison of caudal epidural injections of bupivacaine and methylprednisolone with bupivacaine followed by saline, in Bonica JJ, Albe-Fessard DG, Fink BR, et al (eds): *Advances in Pain Research and Therapy*. New York, NY, Raven Press, vol 1, 1976, pp 927–932.

57. Yates DW: A comparison of the types of epidural injections commonly used in the treatment of low back pain and sciatica. *Rheumatol Rehabil* 1978;17:181–186.

58. Ridley MG, Kingsley GH, Gibson T, et al: Outpatient lumbar epidural corticosteroid injection in the management of sciatica. *Br J Rheumatol* 1988;27:295–299.

59. Cuckler JM, Bernini PA, Wiesel SW, et al: The use of epidural steroids in the treatment of lumbar radicular pain: A prospective, randomized, double-blind study. *J Bone Joint Surg* 1985;67A:63–66.

60. Klenerman L, Greenwood R, Davenport HT, et al: Lumbar epidural injections in the treatment of sciatica. *Br J Rheumatol* 1984;23:35–38.

61. Bush K, Hillier S: A controlled study of caudal epidural injections of triamcinolone plus procaine for the management of intractable sciatica. *Spine* 1991;16:572–575.
62. Green PW, Burke AJ, Weiss CA, et al: The role of epidural cortisone injection in the treatment of diskogenic low back pain. *Clin Orthop* 1980;153:121–125.
63. Harley C: Extradural corticosteroid infiltration: A follow-up study of 50 cases. *Ann Phys Med* 1967;9:22–28.
64. Kelman H: Epidural injection therapy for sciatic pain. *Am J Surg* 1944;64:183–190.
65. Kim SI, Sadove MS: Caudal-epidural corticosteroids in post-laminectomy syndrome: Treatment for low-back pain. *Compr Ther* 1975;1:57–60.
66. Warr AC, Wilkinson JA, Burn JM, et al: Chronic lumbosciatic syndrome treated by epidural injection and manipulation. *Practitioner* 1972;209:53–59.
67. Power RA, Taylor GJ, Fyfe IS: Lumbar epidural injection of steroid in acute prolapsed intervertebral discs: A prospective study. *Spine* 1992;17:453–455.
68. Andersen KH, Mosdal C: Epidural application of corticosteroids in low-back pain and sciatica. *Acta Neurochir* 1987;87:52–53.
69. Berman AT, Garbarino JL Jr, Fisher SM, et al: The effects of epidural injection of local anesthetics and corticosteroids on patients with lumbosciatic pain. *Clin Orthop* 1984;188:144–151.
70. Hopwood MB, Abram SE: Factors associated with failure of lumbar epidural steroids. *Reg Anesth* 1993;18:238–243.
71. Ferrante FM, Wilson SP, Iacobo C, et al: Clinical classification as a predictor of therapeutic outcome after cervical epidural steroid injection. *Spine* 1993;18:730–736.
72. Jamison RN, VadeBoncouer T, Ferrante FM: Low back pain patients unresponsive to an epidural steroid injection: Identifying predictive factors. *Clin J Pain* 1991;7:311–317.
73. Renfrew DL, Moore TE, Kathol MH, et al: Correct placement of epidural steroid injections: Fluoroscopic guidance and contrast administration. *Am J Neuroradiol* 1991;12:1003–1007.
74. Gordon J: Caudal extradural injection for the treatment of low back pain. *Anaesthesia* 1980;35:515–516.
75. White AH: Injection techniques for the diagnosis and treatment of low back pain. *Orthop Clin North Am* 1983;14:553–567.
76. Brown FW: Management of discogenic pain using epidural and intrathecal steroids. *Clin Orthop* 1977;129:72–78.
77. Winnie AP, Hartman JT, Meyers HL, et al: Pain clinic II: Intradural and extradural corticosteroids for sciatica. *Anesth Analg* 1972;51:990–1003.
78. Davidson JT, Robin GC: Epidural injections in the lumbosciatic syndrome. *Br J Anaesth* 1961;33:595–598.
79. Carabaza A, Cabre F, Garcia AM, et al: Inhibition of phospholipase A2 purified from human herniated disc. *Biochem Pharmacol* 1993;45:783–786.
80. Marshall LA, Bauer J, Sung ML, et al: Evaluation of antirheumatic drugs for their effect in vitro on purified human synovial fluid phospholipase A2. *J Rheumatol* 1991;18:59–65.
81. Johnson A, Ryan MD, Roche J: Depo-Medrol and myelographic arachnoiditis. *Med J Aust* 1991;155:18–20.
82. Nelson DA: Intraspinal therapy using methylprednisolone acetate: Twenty-three years of clinical controversy. *Spine* 1993;18:278–286.
83. Bowman SJ, Wedderburn L, Whaley A, et al: Outcome assessment after epidural corticosteroid injection for low back pain and sciatica. *Spine* 1993;18:1345–1350.

111

Chapter 8
Surgical Outcomes For Herniated Lumbar Disk

Edward N. Hanley, Jr, MD

Introduction

The symptoms of sciatica resulting from nerve root compression caused by aberrations of a lumbar intervertebral disk have been clearly described. In 1911, Goldthwait[1] noted the occurrence of back pain in association with posterior disk displacement. In 1934, Mixter and Barr[2] confirmed the relationship between sciatic pain and lumbar disk herniation, leading to the development of modern surgical treatment for this condition. In recent years, the outcome of such intervention has been viewed objectively, and factors that influence success or failure have been determined. In addition, more information on the accurate diagnosis of conditions affecting the lumbar spine and more insight into their natural history have been obtained.

Although they are frequently analyzed and discussed together, the "problems" of low back pain and sciatica are vastly different. The magnitude of low back pain in terms of incidence and prevalence, diagnostic and treatment perplexity, impairment and disability, and cost to society is much greater than that of the reasonably well-defined entity of sciatica resulting from a ruptured intervertebral disk.

Kirkaldy-Willis and associates[3] have described the natural aging process of the intervertebral disk from nuclear dehydration through a series of inevitable changes. These "degenerative" changes may be accentuated in predisposed individuals or occur in a much lesser extent in others. With progressive degeneration, herniation of disk material causing nerve root compression may occur, generally between the ages of 30 and 50 years. If this compression is severe and persistent enough to cause pain, the patient may be forced to seek medical attention.

The lifetime prevalence of a herniated disk appears to be in the vicinity of 2%, a small fraction of that of low back pain.[4] It is difficult to determine total costs related to the treatment of herniated disks, but it is reasonable to assume that at least some of the cost is attributed to low back pain conditions, particularly for individuals in whom surgery has failed.

The natural history of sciatica indicates spontaneous improvement. Hakelius'[5] study of patients with sciatica treated with a corset and rest showed that 38% improved in 1 month, 52% by 2 months, and 73% by 3 months. In studying the lifetime prevalence of the disease and those patients with sciatica who have persistent radiculopathy (10% to 25%), it would seem that less than 0.5% of the population should consider surgical treatment. However, the lifetime prevalence for spine surgery in the United States appears to be 3% to 4% with wide regional variation,[4,6,7] whereas it is only 1% in Sweden[8] and Denmark.[4,9] Excision of a lumbar disk is the third most frequently performed orthopaedic surgical procedure, exceeded only by surgical fracture treatment and arthroscopy.[10]

Nonsurgical Treatment

The Quebec Task Force on Spinal Disorders studied the available literature on low back conditions and evaluated 11 diagnostic areas and 13 treatment categories for low back pain and lumbar disk disease.[11] Analysis of treatment methods was reviewed relative to scientific validity. Through 1985, only 50 articles meeting the criteria for well-controlled prospective randomized studies were found.[12,13] In this analysis, only brief bed rest and back school information programs were effective, while nonsteroidal anti-inflammatory medication was implicated as effective by nonrandomized control studies.[11] Saal and Saal,[14] in a nonrandomized retrospective study, have recently reported that more than 90% of patients with disk extrusions and radiculopathy had a successful outcome when treated nonsurgically. It appears that clinical improvements may correlate with disk fragment resorption as demonstrated by magnetic resonance imaging (MRI).[15] In this study, however, both computed tomography (CT) and MRI scans were performed, making valid conclusions difficult.

Although a vast array of nonsurgical treatments exist (braces, heat, ice, biofeedback, traction, manipulation, massage, steroids, acupuncture, psychologic support, etc), there remains no true scientifically valid evidence that such methods improve on the natural history of herniated lumbar disks. These findings are reiterated by the recently published Agency for Health Care Policy and Research Guidelines on Acute Low Back Pain in Adults.[15] The fact that such treatment methods have not been validated as improving on the natural history of the problem does not necessarily mean that they are not helpful nor does it implicate them as being harmful.

Selecting Patients for Surgical Treatment

Long-term studies comparing surgical and nonsurgical treatment for radiculopathy show no statistically significant difference in outcome. Weber[16] found no difference between the two treatment groups at 4-year follow-up. Results after 1 year were better in the surgery group, but this difference diminished with time. Hakelius[5] had similar initial results, but by 6 months there was no discernible difference. In his study, the group treated nonsurgically had more back pain at 7 years. Weber,[16] however, found no clinical difference with reference to low back pain at 10-year follow-up. Thus, the only real benefit from surgery for most patients is quicker relief from sciatic pain. It is, therefore, the clinician's task to select for surgery those patients in whom nonsurgical measures are likely to fail and who can be reasonably expected to have symptomatic relief and a return to relatively normal function after a procedure.

Five clinical criteria have been used to select surgical candidates:[17] (1) impairment of bowel or bladder function; (2) gross motor weakness; (3) evidence of increasing impairment of root conduction; (4) severe sciatic pain persisting or increasing despite a course of bed rest; and (5) recurrent episodes of sciatic pain. Most of these indications would be considered relative by most surgeons.

The only emergent indication for surgery would appear to be cauda equina syndrome related to massive disk herniation.[18] Likewise, patients believed to have a progressive neurologic deficit have usually been treated with early surgery.

Thus, the usual indication for surgery is pain, and the decision to perform surgery is influenced by the patient's desires and needs and the opinion of the evaluating physician/surgeon. If surgery is proposed and carried out, it must be justified by having a reasonably high rate of success, limited risk and complications, and a manageable monetary cost to the patient and society.

McCulloch and associates[19] have described the criteria for the diagnosis of sciatica resulting from a herniated disk and have stated that "before intervening surgically for the acute radicular syndrome resulting from a lumbar disk herniation, it is essential to have an accurate clinical diagnosis of the cause of sciatica, an anatomic level of the lesion, and support for both clinical impressions by clinical investigations. If there is not a perfect union of the patient's clinical presentation, the anatomic level, and the structural lesion as demonstrated on myelography, CT scanning, or MRI, then the potential for a poor result increases dramatically."[19] Their contraindications for surgery include the following: the wrong patient selected (psychologic or compensation problems), the incorrect diagnosis, the incorrect level for surgery, a painless herniated disk, and technical issues.[19]

Prolonged symptoms, abnormal illness behavior, a compensable work situation, cigarette smoking, and age older than 40 years may contribute to a negative surgical outcome and should also be taken into consideration, particularly if more than one of these factors is present.[20-22]

Helpful information concerning poor patient selection and its influence on outcome is presented by Fager and Freidberg.[23] In their study of 105 patients in whom disk surgery had been unsuccessful, they found that 68% of the patients had not had appropriate indications for surgery initially; surgical criteria had not been met or no disk herniation was present preoperatively.

Ruggieri and associates,[24] in their review of 872 patients who underwent surgery, found that a major cause of surgical failure was the performance of such a procedure on patients with a bulging disk. They viewed this diagnosis as "a euphemism to conceal an error in diagnosis."[24]

Results of Surgical Treatment

Although in appropriately selected patients disk excision for sciatic symptoms is often successful, this is not always the case. Approximately 60% of patients will have complete relief of their symptoms.[19,25,26] Of the remaining 40%, roughly 15% will have persistent, disabling symptoms leading to further evaluation, treatment, and possibly surgery. Thus, under the best of situations, 15% of patients undergoing this procedure will fall into the category of "failed back" patients.[4,27]

In the United States, approximately 200,000 surgical procedures involving lumbar disk excision are performed each year.[10,27] If a minimum of 15% of these procedures fail to improve the patients' symptoms or, in fact, make them worse, it is reasonable to assume that at least 30,000 people per year enter the failure group in this manner.

Probably the leading cause for failure of surgical disk excision is the preoperative presence of a major low back pain component. With highly selected patients with severe sciatic symptoms and no major back pain component, over 90% can expect relief of lower extremity pain when the procedure is properly performed.[24,27-29] When leg and back pain are present before surgery, however, sciatica relief approximates 80%, but low back pain relief is only in the 50% range.[30-35]

Although the main reasons for entry into the failure group occur in the selection process, even appropriately selected patients can experience problems. Armstrong[36] listed 12 causes of failure of disk excision, most related to cognitive and technical aspects of the surgery. Greenwood and associates[37] analyzed 67 patients in whom lumbar disk procedures had failed, "requiring" a second procedure. Reasons for failure included a new site of herniation in 16 patients, recurrent disk herniation at the same area in 17, root scarring in 24, missed herniations in four, migrated free fragments of disk in five, and postoperative diskitis in one. Failures of reoperation were predominant in those patients with epidural fibrosis.

A similar study by Macnab[17] in 1971 revealed anatomic factors leading to failure of a first procedure, including unrecognized pedicular kinking, underlying spinal stenosis, and unrecognized lateral disk herniation. Scar tissue was responsible for failure of the procedure in six of the 68 patients studied, and, as in the study of Greenwood and associates,[37] repeat surgery was of limited benefit.

In the 32% of patients in Fager and Freidberg's[23] surgical failure series who were deemed to have been appropriately selected, failures were attributed to retained disk fragments, underlying stenosis, scar tissue formation and, most notably, surgery performed at the wrong level.

Ruggieri and associates[24] showed that 17% of their patients treated with surgery had unsatisfactory outcomes primarily related to patient selection errors (bulging disks and multiple level surgery), low back pain, and scar formation.

Thus, it would appear that one of the major reasons for failure of lumbar disk surgery is the inability to select patients who meet surgical criteria and can be expected to improve when the procedure is properly performed. Additionally, there are a number of cognitive and technical aspects of the surgical procedure that, when not met, may lead to failure and worsening of the condition.

Less Invasive Disk Procedures

Although chymopapain chemonucleolysis remains relatively popular in Europe and other parts of the world, its use as a "noninvasive" tool for the treatment of lumbar disk herniation diminished dramatically in North America in the mid-1980s after a series of adverse events and serious complications.[38] These occurrences, along with technologic advances related to arthroscopic surgery and a persistent desire to avoid the problems of open disk excision surgery, led to the development of other percutaneous techniques for the treatment of this disease. These newer procedures include automated percutaneous suction diskectomy,[39-43] percutaneous laser disk decompression,[42,44-46] and percutaneous "arthroscopic" disk excision.[47,48] Although initial reports by the developers or early proponents of these procedures showed results close to those of open diskectomy or open microdiskectomy, more current experiences by others indicate much lower success rates. Possible reasons for these poorer outcomes include difficulties in patient selection (degenerated but not herniated disks, noncontained disk herniation); the fallacies of indirect decompressions (removal or ablation of disk material remote from the site of herniation), and technical problems related to the equipment or the surgeon (problems entering L5-S1, skill necessary for arthroscopic disk excision). A summary of the principles and evolution of each of these techniques follows.

Percutaneous Suction Diskectomy

The automated percutaneous lumbar diskectomy (APLD) technique developed by Onik and associates[40] uses an aspiration-type probe and rotary cutting device to remove material from the central portion of the disk, theoretically permitting a "contained" disk herniation to collapse, thus relieving pressure on the affected nerve root. Although excellent results have been reported,[41] more recent scientifically designed studies show fewer successes[28] when randomized patients were treated by either chymopapain (61% success), APLD (44% success),[42] or microdiskectomy (80% success) versus APLD (27% success).[49] Moreover, patients in whom APLD failed and who underwent subsequent open surgery did not do as well as those primarily treated by open disk excision.[49] Imaging studies performed after percutaneous diskectomy show little if any change in the size or configuration of the disk herniation and no correlations with clinical outcome.[50]

Percutaneous Laser Diskectomy

Percutaneous laser diskectomy uses ablative laser energy delivered through an optical fiber to the interior of the disk space. The concept of removal of disk material is similar to that of percutaneous suction diskectomy, albeit by vaporization and not mechanically. The volume of disk material removal depends on the wavelength of laser energy and the amount of energy used.[51] A variety of laser types can be used (CO_2, Ho:YAG, Nd:YAG, argon). Two (potassium titanyl phosphate and Ho:YAG) have been approved by the U.S. Food and Drug Administration for lumbar disk applications. Imaging of the disk interior through the endoscope as well as deflection of the laser beam and flexible diskoscopy to gain access to peripheral areas of the disk are possible.[51]

Initial clinical experience with laser disk ablation/decompression as reported by Choy and associates[44] yields good results. As with APLD, however, as more reports emerge, the enthusiasm for this technique, at least at this time, has diminished somewhat. Mathews and associates,[45] early advocates of this technique, recently reported 2-year follow-up of patients treated with a KTP/532 wavelength laser for contained herniated disks, contained herniated disks with degenerative changes, and multilevel degenerated/herniated disks. Although the 3-month success rate was 81%, at 2 years it was only 55%, and 35% underwent reoperation. In a recent retrospective report by Ohnmeiss and associates,[46] of

162 patients from three centers who underwent laser disk decompression, only 35 were found to meet appropriate selection criteria. Of these 35, 69% had a successful outcome. Of those patients who did not meet selection criteria, only 29% had successful results.

Percutaneous Arthroscopic Diskectomy

The percutaneous technique that has generated the most interest in the last 10 years is based on arthroscopic technology.[47,48] Using multiple "ports" and maneuverable instruments, access to the outer areas of the disk and even to extruded disk material within the spinal canal is at least theoretically possible. Kambin and Schaffer[48] have shown that with this technique the spinal nerve root and offending disk material can be visualized directly, assisting in the removal of free fragments of extruded disk material. They report an 87% success rate with the procedure. Whether or not the nuances of this procedure are transferable remains to be seen.

Surgical Failures

What happens when initial surgical treatment for herniated disks is unsuccessful? It would appear that if patients continue to meet the criteria necessary for successful results from initial surgery, then a reasonable outcome from a second procedure may be expected when a frank disk herniation is found and the surgery is properly performed.[27,37,52-54] If repeat surgery involves surgical fusion, treatment of infection, or other pathologic conditions, success rates are not nearly as high.[51]

If the variable of a "compensable work" situation is present in a case of failed initial surgery, the prognosis is poor.[22,27] In Waddell's[22] group of 103 patients, the success rate of a second operation was 50%, with an additional 20% of patients considering themselves in worse condition than before surgery. With a third procedure, the success rate was 30%, and 25% considered themselves worse. After four operations, a 20% success rate was achieved, with 45% of these patients considering themselves worse. Sixty-five percent of this group who were tested psychologically showed evidence of anxiety, depression, hypochondriasis, and conversion reactions, all factors that correlate with a poor surgical outcome. Only 23% of the women and 40% of the men who underwent a second surgical procedure returned to work.

La Rocca[28] has succinctly summarized the factors leading to the occurrence and management of failed lumbar disk surgery. Failure of the initial procedure is almost always related to inappropriate patient selection or treatment, or a technical error at surgery. Factors positively influencing repeat surgery include recurrent surgery after a long asymptomatic interval, a new herniation at a new location, and a separate identifiable and correctable pathologic condition. Negative factors include chronic radiculopathy, a failed previous surgical fusion, and negative psychosocial characteristics. The number of surgical successes clearly diminishes proportional to the number of procedures performed.

The Role of Spinal Fusion in Herniated Disks

The once controversial issue of whether or not to perform a spinal arthrodesis with primary disk excision for radicular symptoms appears to be settled.[26,55-60] Results of multiple studies indicate successful relief of radicular pain in most cases when surgical indications are appropriate. This is true whether a standard laminotomy or microsurgical approach is used. As noted previously, however, certain patients will later experience recurrent radicular lower extremity pain with or without concomitant low back pain and may be candidates for further interventional treatment.[53,61,62]

The correct approach to use for patients with recurrent disk herniation depends on the characteristics of the complaints, the physical findings, the results of imaging studies, and the period of time elapsed and the pain-free interval, if any, since the primary procedure. Those patients with minor lower extremity and/or low back pain that is bothersome but not incapacitating are best managed by accepted nonsurgical measures. For individuals with persistent and severe dermatomal-sclerotomal radicular pain, further evaluation, and possibly more aggressive intervention, may be indicated. The two broad categories into which such patients can be divided are those with radiculopathy only and those with a combination of radiculopathy and low back pain. Those patients with radiculopathy only are best managed by repeat surgical intervention with disk excision alone, with the exception of patients with symptoms related to epidural scar formation, who should be managed nonsurgically.

The treatment of patients with recurrent radiculopathy and low back pain presents more of a challenge. Here the major debate is whether or not back pain symptoms are related to mechanical insufficiency of the disk or to definable instability. Plain radiographs and lateral flexion-extension views may reveal instability caused by degenerative change or iatrogenic spinal destabilization from facet removal, pars interarticularis excision, or fracture. MRI may reveal disk degeneration/dehydration, but this method is believed to be insufficient to assess diskogenic pain from insufficiency. Provocative diskography, although controversial, may be useful in such circumstances.[19]

Although numerous criteria have been proposed for instability or hypermobility, most are either vague or incomprehensible. Probably the most reasonable objective measure of hypermobility is greater than 4 mm of translation and/or more than $10°$ of angular change on lateral motion radiographs.[20]

If no gross hypermobility pattern is present, repeat surgery with disk excision and posterolateral fusion is appropriate, although it has been suggested that the addition of instrumentation or combined anterior disk excision and fusion may be indicated for these situations. Surgery of this magnitude is rarely necessary. The expected outcome in more than 75% of cases should be relief of radicular pain and mild residual low back pain. If the level of recurrence demonstrates frank translational or angular instability, then supplementary fixation-instrumentation may help hold the spine in a stable anatomic position while fusion consolidation occurs. Although not objectively proven in clinical series, the rate of arthrodesis consolidation may be slightly improved with such techniques.[63]

Summary

Lumbar disk herniation resulting in nerve root compression and radicular pain in the lower extremity is a distinctly different entity from idiopathic or diskogenic low back pain. It affects a small percentage of individuals but results in pain and neurologic dysfunction. The pain component, in appropriately selected individuals, has been shown to be often improved by surgery, but this outcome must be weighed against the patient's symptoms and the natural history of the disease process. Failures of surgery are usually the result of inappropriate patient selection, unrelated behavioral characteristics of the patients, or technically related complications.

Fusion is not recommended for individuals undergoing primary disk excision. For patients with recurrent disk herniation with back pain and radicular symptoms, arthrodesis may be appropriate. Instrumentation is indicated only for objectively documented translational or angular instability. For individuals with low back pain occurring after diskectomy, fusion is not generally recommended. A possible exception is patients with stable psychometrics who have exhausted prolonged nonsurgical treatment and exhibit correlative morphologic abnormalities and concordant pain provocation by diskography. If such intervention is contemplated, this procedure should be approached with caution and realistic expectations by both the patient and the surgeon.

Current gaps in knowledge about the surgical treatment of lumbar disk herniation include: (1) scientific refinements in the selection process for candidates for the procedure; (2) indications for and more objective results of less invasive treatment methods for the condition; and (3) more validated information as to the indications and results of fusion procedures for failures after primary disk excision.

References

1. Goldthwait JE: The lumbo-sacral articulation: An explanation of many cases of "lumbago," "sciatica," and "paraplegia". *Bost Med Surg J* 1911;164:365–372.
2. Mixter WJ, Barr JS: Rupture of the intervertebral disc with involvement of the spinal canal. *N Engl J Med* 1934;211:210–215.
3. Kirkaldy-Willis WH, Wedge JH, Yong-Hing K, et al: Pathology and pathogenesis of lumbar spondylosis and stenosis. *Spine* 1978;3:319–328.
4. Frymoyer JW: Epidemiology: Magnitude of the problem, in Weinstein JN, Weisel SW (eds): *The Lumbar Spine*. Philadelphia, PA, WB Saunders, 1990, pp 32–38.
5. Hakelius A: Prognosis in sciatica: A clinical follow-up of surgical and non-surgical treatment. *Acta Orthop Scand* 1970;129(suppl):1–76.
6. Nagi SZ, Riley LE, Newby LG: A social epidemiology of back pain in a general population. *J Chron Dis* 1973;26:769–779.
7. Kolata G: Regional incongruity found in medical costs. *New York Times*, 30 January 1996, p B9.
8. Andersson GBJ, Pope MH, Frymoyer JW: Epidemiology, in Pope MH, Frymoyer JW, Andersson GBJ (eds): *Occupational Low Back Pain*. New York, NY, Praeger, 1984, pp 101–114.
9. Biering-Sorensen F: Low back trouble in a general population of 30-,40-,50-, 60-year-old men and women: Study design, representativeness and basic results. *Dan Med Bull* 1982;29:289–299.
10. Rutkow IM: Orthopaedic operations in the United States, 1979 through 1983. *J Bone Joint Surg* 1986;68A:716–719.

11. Quebec Task Force on Spinal Disorders: Scientific approach to the assessment and management of activity-related spinal disorders: A monograph for clinicians. Report of the Quebec Task Force on Spinal Disorders. *Spine*, 1987;12(suppl 7):S1–S59.

12. Morris RW: A statistical study of papers in the Journal of Bone and Joint Surgery [Br], 1984. *J Bone Joint Surg* 1988;70B:242–246.

13. Rudicel S, Esdaile J: The randomized clinical trial in orthopaedics: Obligation or option? *J Bone Joint Surg* 1985;67A:1284–1293.

14. Saal JA, Saal JS: Nonoperative treatment of herniated lumbar intervertebral disc with radiculopathy: An outcome study. *Spine* 1989;14:431–437.

15. Bigos SJ, Bowyer O, Braen G, et al: *Acute Low Back Problems in Adults.* Clinical Practice Guideline No 14. AHCPR Publication No 95-0642, Rockville, MD, US Department of Health and Human Services, 1994.

16. Weber H: Lumbar disc herniation: A controlled, prospective study with ten years of observation. *Spine* 1983;8:131–140.

17. Macnab I: Negative disc exploration: An analysis of the causes of nerve-root involvement in sixty-eight patients. *J Bone Joint Surg* 1971;53A:891–903.

18. Kostuik JP, Harrington I, Alexander D, et al: Cauda equina syndrome and lumbar disc herniation. *J Bone Joint Surg* 1986;68A:386–391.

19. McCulloch JA, Inoue S, Moriya H, et al: Clinical entities: Surgical indications and techniques, in Weinstein JN, Wiesel SW (eds): *The Lumbar Spine.* Philadelphia, PA, WB Saunders, 1990, pp 393–421.

20. Hanley EN Jr, Phillips ED, Kostuik JP: Who should be fused?, in Frymoyer JW, Ducker TB, Hadler NM, et al (eds): *The Adult Spine: Principles and Practice.* New York, NY, Raven Press, 1991, vol 2, pp 1893–1917.

21. Spurling RG, Grantham EG: The end results of surgery for ruptured lumbar intervertebral discs: A follow-up study of 327 cases. *J Neurosurg* 1949;6:57–64.

22. Waddell G: Epidemiology: A new clinical model for the treatment of low back pain, in Weinstein JN, Weisel SW (eds): *The Lumbar Spine.* Philadelphia, PA, WB Saunders, 1990, pp 38–56.

23. Fager CA, Freidberg SR: Analysis of failures and poor results of lumbar spine surgery. *Spine* 1980;5:87–94.

24. Ruggieri F, Specchia L, Sabalat S, et al: Lumbar disc herniation: Diagnosis, surgical treatment, recurrence. A review of 872 operated cases. *Ital J Orthop Traumatol* 1988;14:15–22.

25. Hanley EN Jr, Shapiro DE: The development of low-back pain after excision of a lumbar disc. *J Bone Joint Surg* 1989;71A:719–721.

26. Spangfort EV: The lumbar disc herniation: A computer-aided analysis of 2,504 operations. *Acta Orthop Scand* 1972;142(suppl):1–95.

27. La Rocca H: Failed lumbar surgery: Principles of management, in Weinstein JN, Wiesel SW (eds): *The Lumbar Spine.* Philadelphia, PA, WB Saunders, 1990, pp 872–881.

28. Finneson BE, Cooper VR: A lumbar disc surgery predictive score card: A retrospective evaluation. *Spine* 1979;4:141–144.

29. Hirsch C, Nachemson A: The reliability of lumbar disk surgery. *Clin Orthop* 1963;29:189–195.

30. Wood EG III, Hanley EN Jr: Lumbar disc herniation and open limited discectomy: Indications, techniques, and results. *Operative Tech Orthop* 1991;1:23–28.

31. Falconer MA, McGeorge M, Begg AC: Surgery of lumbar intervertebral disk protrusion: Study of principles and results based upon 100 consecutive cases submitted to operation. *Br J Surg* 1948;35:225–249.

32. Jackson RK: The long-term effects of wide laminectomy for lumbar disc excision: A review of 130 patients. *J Bone Joint Surg* 1971;53B:609–616.

33. O'Connell JEA: Protrusions of the lumbar intervertebral discs: A clinical review based on five hundred cases treated by excision of the protrusion. *J Bone Joint Surg* 1951;33B:8–30.

34. Saal JA, Saal JS, Herzog RJ: The natural history of lumbar intervertebral disc extrusions treated nonoperatively. *Spine* 1990;15:683–686.

121

35. Spengler DM, Freeman CW: Patient selection for lumbar discectomy: An objective approach. *Spine* 1979;4:129–134.

36. Armstrong JR: The causes of unsatisfactory results from the operative treatment of lumbar disc lesions. *J Bone Joint Surg* 1951;33B:31–35.

37. Greenwood J Jr, McGuire TH, Kimbell F: A study of the causes of failure in the herniated intervertebral disc operation: An analysis of sixty-seven reoperated cases. *J Neurosurg* 1952;9:15–20.

38. Nordby EJ, Wright PH, Schofield SR: Safety of chemonucleolysis: Adverse effects reported in the United States, 1982-1991. *Clin Orthop* 1993;293:122–134.

39. Donaldson WF III, Star MJ, Thorne RP: Surgical treatment for the far lateral herniated lumbar disc. *Spine* 1993;18:1263–1267.

40. Onik G, Helms CA, Ginsburg L, et al: Percutaneous lumbar diskectomy using a new aspiration probe. *Am J Neuroradiol* 1985;6:290–293.

41. Onik G, Mooney V, Maroon JC, et al: Automated percutaneous discectomy: A prospective multi-institutional study. *Neurosurgery* 1990;26:228–233.

42. Revel M, Payan C, Vallee C, et al: Automated percutaneous lumbar discectomy versus chemonucleolysis in the treatment of sciatica: A randomized multicenter trial. *Spine* 1993;18:1–7.

43. Kahanovitz N, Viola K, Goldstein T, et al: A multicenter analysis of percutaneous discectomy. *Spine* 1990;15:713–715.

44. Choy DS, Ascher PW, Ranu HS, et al: Percutaneous laser disc decompression: A new therapeutic modality. *Spine* 1992;17:949–956.

45. Mathews HH, Kyles MK, Fiore SM, et al: Laser disc decompression with KTP 532 wavelength: A two-year follow-up. Proceedings of the American Academy of Orthopaedic Surgeons 61st Annual Meeting, New Orleans, LA. Rosemont, IL, American Academy of Orthopaedic Surgeons, 1994, p 199.

46. Ohnmeiss DD, Hochschuler SH, Guyer RD, et al: Laser disc decompression: The importance of proper patient selection. Proceedings of the North American Spine Society 8th Annual Meeting, San Diego, California. Rosemont, IL, North American Spine Society, 1993, p 160.

47. Kambin P, Gellman H: Percutaneous lateral discectomy of the lumbar spine: A preliminary report. *Clin Orthop* 1983;174:127–132.

48. Kambin P, Schaffer JL: Percutaneous lumbar discectomy: Review of 100 patients and current practice. *Clin Orthop* 1989;238:24–34.

49. Findlay G, Chatterjee S, Foy P: A randomised controlled trial comparing automated percutaneous lumbar discectomy and lumbar microdiscectomy. *Orthop Trans* 1995;19:60–61.

50. Deutsch AL, Delamarter RB, Goldstein TB, et al: Percutaneous lumbar discectomy: Pre- and post-magnetic resonance imaging. Proceedings of the American Academy of Orthopaedic Surgeons 58th Annual Meeting, Anaheim, CA. Park Ridge, IL, American Academy of Orthopaedic Surgeons, 1991, p 59.

51. Sherk HH, Black JD, Prodoehl JA, et al: Laser diskectomy. *Orthopedics* 1993;16:573–576.

52. Barr JS, Riseborough EJ, Freeman PA: Abstract: Failed surgery for low-back and sciatic pain. *J Bone Joint Surg* 1963;45A:1553.

53. Cauchoix J, Ficat C, Girard B: Repeat surgery after disc excision. *Spine* 1978;3:256–259.

54. Kelley JH, Voris DC, Svien HJ, et al: Multiple operations for protruded lumbar intervertebral disk. *Proc Staff Meet Mayo Clin* 1954;29:546–550.

55. Adkins EWO: Lumbo-sacral arthrodesis after laminectomy. *J Bone Joint Surg* 1955;37B:208–223.

56. Frymoyer JW, Matteri RE, Hanley EN, et al: Failed lumbar disc surgery requiring second operation: A long-term follow-up study. *Spine* 1978;3:7–11.

57. Frymoyer JW, Hanley E, Howe J, et al: Disc excision and spine fusion in the management of lumbar disc disease: A minimum ten-year follow-up. *Spine* 1978;3:1–6.

58. Hoover NW: Indications for fusion at time of removal of intervertebral disc. *J Bone Joint Surg* 1968;50A:189–193.

59. Nachlas IW: End-result study of the treatment of herniated nucleus pulposus by excision with fusion and without fusion. *J Bone Joint Surg* 1952;34A:981–988.
60. Turner JA, Ersek M, Herron L, et al: Patient outcomes after lumbar spinal fusions. *JAMA* 1992;268:907–911.
61. de Quervain F, Hoessly H: Operative immobilization of the spine. *Surg Gynecol Obstet* 1917;24:428–436.
62. Edwards CC, Curcin A: Spondyloptosis: Definition and long-term results of reduction and fusion. Proceedings of the North American Spine Society 9th Annual Meeting, Minneapolis, MN. Rosemont, IL, North American Spine Society, 1994, pp 58–59.
63. Zdeblick TA: A prospective, randomized study of lumbar fusion: Preliminary results. *Spine* 1993;18:983–991.

Chapter 9

Cost of Low Back Problems: An Economic Analysis

Douglas A. Conrad, PhD
John P. Holland, MD, MPH
Jilan Liu, MD, MHA
Richard A. Deyo, MD, MPH

Introduction

This chapter discusses the application of economic methodology to estimate treatment costs for persons with low back pain (LBP). The context for this analysis is Clinical Practice Guideline 14: Acute Low Back Problems in Adults[1] from the Agency for Health Care Policy and Research (AHCPR). The general purpose of this guideline and those being developed by the AHCPR for other clinical conditions is to improve the efficiency and effectiveness of management of common health problems by presenting systematic, structured, and evidence-based clinical approaches.

This study addresses the expected cost of health services for persons with acute LBP if a sample strategy for following the AHCPR low back guideline were interpreted and implemented in the manner we describe. Because the guideline has not yet been widely implemented in actual medical practices, the analysis relies on projected ''what if'' scenarios. The analysis also considered what benchmarks might be used in comparing the health services cost of implementing the guideline in a particular way versus standard medical practice.

The low back guideline was not developed for the specific purpose of lowering health care costs, but for maximizing treatment effectiveness. Furthermore, any indirect cost savings and health benefits (or, for that matter, cost increases or health losses) outside the episode of care covered by the guideline could be even more important in evaluating the guideline's impact. These longer term and more indirect consequences are beyond the scope of this analysis, and should be the subject of careful study in their own right.

Previous studies have established the societal impact of LBP. It is the second leading reason for ambulatory care in the United States, and direct medical costs are estimated at over $20 billion per year.[2] Moreover, it is difficult to determine etiology and identify the best strategies for alleviating symptoms. By offering a logically ordered, flexible, and evidence-based approach to the diagnosis and treatment of LBP, the guideline offers the possibility of increased clinical efficiency in diagnosis and treatment.

We sought to determine whether direct health care cost savings might be realized by following a sample strategy based on the AHCPR guidelines. This sample strategy is one of many approaches that might be adopted by clinicians who seek to interpret and implement the low back guideline. We defined a "base case" scenario for this sample strategy, and then tested the sensitivity of estimated costs to changes in our assumptions.

Method

This analysis concentrated on health care payments for persons seeking initial outpatient treatment of acute LBP. Provider reimbursements were the proxy used to estimate health care "costs." Payments for services reflect both the transaction prices and the volume of services delivered to persons with acute LBP.

While one would like to know the opportunity cost of the resources used to diagnose and treat acute LBP (the value of the opportunities that could have been realized if those resources had been employed in their next best alternative use), payments to providers at least capture the visible, "real world" dollars exchanged in the care of this health problem. In the absence of an omniscient observer to calculate opportunity costs or a perfectly competitive, frictionless health services market (in which case payments would equal opportunity costs), health services payments are a useful rough approximation of the actual societal costs of delivering services to persons with acute LBP.[3]

The cost "benchmark" used here for identifying effects attributable to implementation of the guideline is total payments for health services observed under current medical practice. The time period (1988-1989) for calculating payments was chosen to be earlier than the initiation of the guideline panel to preclude "contamination" of prevailing practice patterns by the guideline recommendations, but was sufficiently recent to minimize the technologic changes in diagnosing and treating LBP that might affect the comparison of the guideline to prevailing practice.

Sources of Data

The primary source of data for this study was the Market Scan administrative claims database maintained by MEDSTAT Systems, Inc, in Ann Arbor, Michigan. This database included all the health services claims experience for MEDSTAT clients, who are large employer groups representing 5.3 million insured individuals (employees and their dependents) in 45 major metropolitan areas. Insured persons' workers' compensation claims are not included in this database. Thus, the observations used to estimate costs under standard medical practice are drawn from the non-workers' compensation health insurance claims experience of a working-age population presenting initially for outpatient care of LBP.

The guideline is "costed out" using the average paid amounts per unit of service of a given type (eg, initial office visit, electromyography without computed tomography [CT]) actually recorded on the MEDSTAT database for persons treated for LBP in 1988-1989. The use of payments, rather than billed charges, is meant to capture the actual transaction prices, as opposed to "list prices" (which are paid by only a minority of self-paying patients and a small fraction of commercial insurers) (Table 1).

Table 1 Unit price of various clinical procedures, based on 1988-1989 reimbursements (MEDSTAT data)

Procedure	Unit Price ($)
Initial office visit	86
Follow-up office visit	40
Psychiatric consultation	220
Plain radiograph	54
MRI	834
CT, lumbar spine	273
Bone scan	346
Surgery*	10,112
Urinalysis	10
Complete blood count	16
Erythrocyte sedimentation rate	11
Electromyogram	153
Spinal manipulation (per visit)	58
Physical therapy (per visit)	60

*Weighted average price of all types of lumbar spine surgery (laminectomy, diskectomy, and fusion)

The example strategy for implementing the guideline does not outline the anticipated effect of following its recommendations on the future course of individuals' low back problems. Also, there is no "natural experiment" to simulate the cost savings expected from following the guideline beyond the first 3 months of recommended care. Thus, we refrained from speculating about the "ultimate" cost savings from following the sample strategy of implementing the guideline, and instead present direct estimates of differences in 3-month cost of the example strategy versus "standard" medical practice.

Prices derived from the 1988-89 MEDSTAT database were used for estimating the cost of both the "guideline practice" and "standard medical practice." Thus, any cost differences between the simulated guideline strategy and "standard medical practice" will be the result of the clinical decisions embodied in the simulated strategy versus actual practice as reflected in the MEDSTAT data. The validity of the cost comparison, therefore, depends on the reasonableness of the assumptions used to implement the sample strategy, which represents just one example of how the guideline might be used by practicing physicians.

While an unbiased comparison of the direct costs of health services under prevailing medical practice and a "reasonable" sample strategy for treating LBP according to the guideline have been attempted, there are a number of significant limitations on these estimates. First, the MEDSTAT data do not include workers' compensation cases, and thus a very important segment of the working age population with severe LBP has been omitted from the "benchmark" costs. If the implementation of guideline-based practice were likely to generate relatively greater health care cost savings for the subpopulation with occupational or industrial injuries, the estimates presented here would tend to understate the expected savings.

127

Second, the MEDSTAT data only list one diagnosis per outpatient service record (not necessarily the principal diagnosis, in the case of multiple diagnoses on the original insurance claim), and inpatient service records only list two diagnoses (and without explicitly identifying the principal discharge diagnosis). Thus, it is quite possible that some health services related to LBP will be omitted from the service counts and payments calculated in this analysis.

Third, because the MEDSTAT data are drawn from a time period 5 years prior to development of the guideline for low back problems, it is possible that the costs of following today's prevailing practice relative to guideline-based practice will be overstated in this comparison if the treatment of LBP has already moved in the direction indicated by the guideline during the past 5 years. This upward bias in any estimated health care cost savings associated with the guideline is more likely to the extent that practice patterns have evolved toward the guideline-based strategy.

Fourth, there is a potential bias that is in contrast to the health care cost comparison. Only MEDSTAT inpatient and outpatient service records with a low back-related diagnosis are included in the calculation of ''benchmark costs.'' Thus, any outpatient or inpatient treatment for low back and other health problems for which a diagnosis was not recorded will be missing from the MEDSTAT benchmark costs. This would tend to understate potential health care cost savings from implementing the guideline according to the sample strategy.

This analysis drew exclusively from the 55,083 persons identified on the database, using ICD diagnosis codes and CPT-4 procedure codes, who received their initial, or index, health service for a low back-related diagnosis as an outpatient in 1988, and who had no health services utilization (inpatient or outpatient) with a diagnosis related to the low back in the prior year (1987). A claims history for each person was constructed for 1 year (365 days) from the ''index service,'' or date of the initial outpatient service record associated with the low back in 1988. This allowed us to follow a given individual's health care experience for time intervals of 0 to 3 months, 3 to 6 months, and 6 to 12 months (post-index visit). By choosing individuals without low back-related claims in 1987 and whose initial back-related care was as an outpatient, we intended to identify an ''inception cohort'' (at the point of first entering the medical care system for primary care of a low back episode). Because the example guideline strategy explicitly traced only the clinical decisions for the first 3 months of diagnosis and treatment, this costing focused on the first 3 months post-index visit in its comparisons.

In addition to the MEDSTAT administrative claims data, we used existing literature in developing epidemiologic assumptions about the prevalence of particular ''red flag'' findings (principally for cancer or infection, fracture, or cauda equina syndrome (CES) or rapidly progressing neurologic deficit) and the probabilities of particular treatment choices under various contingencies facing patients and providers under the guideline. The assumptions underlying the differential cost estimates presented for the base case are presented next, along with further details and sources for the probability values used in the costing model.

General Assumptions of the Cost Model

The assumptions used in developing this economic cost model for the AHCPR Low Back Guidelines[1] are taken from several sources. When possible, the assumptions are derived from research-based evidence in the scientific literature, from three types of studies: (1) descriptive epidemiology studies (especially those done in primary care settings); (2) controlled studies evaluating effectiveness of specific medical history questions, physical examination findings, and diagnostic tests in assessing patients with acute low back problems; and (3) randomized controlled trials on the effectiveness of specific treatments.

The collective clinical judgment of three physicians (one orthopaedic surgeon, one general internist, and one occupational medicine physician) was also used to assess the reasonableness of assumptions derived from the literature. When appropriate, literature-based estimates were revised, and when no evidence was found in the literature, values for variables in the model were determined.

In some cases the clinicians suggested that ranges of values were more appropriate than a single number for a variable (for example, the percentage of all patients with LBP who are older than 50 years will vary depending on the clinical setting). When ranges of variables were suggested, sensitivity analyses were done with the model using both the highest and lowest values in the range. If the sensitivity analysis showed little difference in the overall cost result, the midpoint of the range was used for the model; otherwise a "best guess" value within the range was chosen.

This cost model has been developed for an adult outpatient primary care office practice because this was considered to be the most common clinical setting for users of the guideline, and because many of the studies used as a basis for the cost model were done in such settings.

Some variables in the cost model might vary greatly from those seen in other clinical settings. Specifically, the proportions of all patients presenting with acute LBP who are older than 50 years or who have a history of significant trauma will vary greatly depending on the clinical setting (family practice clinic, nursing home, student health center, worksite clinic, or emergency room). However, if desired, the cost model could be adjusted for these other clinical settings by substituting different values for these variables.

Assumptions About Initial Assessment Methods

Based on the guideline, the initial step in assessing adults with acute LBP is to search for certain key medical history and physical examination findings, or "red flags," that suggest serious spinal pathology (ie, spinal fracture, infection, tumor, or CES).

These guideline recommendations are based on a study by Deyo and Diehl[4] that evaluated the effectiveness of using certain red flags to detect serious spinal pathology in 1,975 adults with acute LBP. The percentage of persons with acute LBP who had specific red flag findings at initial assessment was obtained. The percentage is used in this model as reasonable estimate of the proportion of patients presenting with red flags for fracture, cancer, or infection.

According to the Deyo and Diehl study,[4] red flag findings in persons with acute LBP indicated that further diagnostic evaluation was needed to rule out spinal fracture, infection, or tumor. However, after further laboratory and radiographic work-up, only a small fraction of those with red flag findings on initial evaluation actually had serious spinal pathology. In addition, spinal fracture, infection, or tumor were less likely to be the cause of symptoms in persons with acute LBP who had no red flags. Based on this observation, it was suggested that in the absence of red flags, no diagnostic evaluation beyond the initial history and physical examination was needed during the first month of care for adults with acute LBP.

Red Flags for Spinal Fracture

Significant trauma as a red flag for spinal fracture was found in 9% of patients studied.[5] Other studies have shown similar findings. A 1-year survey of all adults in a Danish town found that 12% of men and 6% of women who had LBP during the year reported a blow, bump, or fall preceding its onset.[6] A survey of 7,219 persons in Finland found 15% of those with LBP reported a history of traumatic back injury (ie, sudden pain from a blow, distention, or exceptional or accidental force).[7]

The percentages of patients with acute LBP who had a history of significant trauma are likely to vary between studies because: (1) definitions of what constitutes significant trauma vary; (2) the determination of traumatic injury is somewhat subjective and often depends on the patient's description of the event; and (3) different clinical settings encounter different rates of traumatic injury.

Taking all of this into account, for the cost model we assumed 10% of the original group would have red flags for spinal fracture, and spinal radiographs would be obtained. Of these patients, 10% (1% of the original group) will actually have a spinal fracture found on radiograph.[3]

A history of corticosteroid use (found in 1% of the total group) was a red flag for both spinal fracture and infection. However, to avoid double counting, in the cost model, steroid use is considered a red flag for spinal infection only.

Red Flags for Spinal Cancer or Infection

In the study by Deyo and Diehl,[5] red flags for spinal cancer or infection were analyzed together because many of them were similar, and because spinal cancer is much more common than spinal infection. Of those with acute LBP, 43% had red flags for cancer or infection. The most common red flag (29%) was patient age older than 50 years (indicator for spinal fracture, tumor, and infection). Many had more than one red flag. Deyo and Diehl decided that individuals with a prior history of cancer (2% of the total group) should undergo further diagnostic evaluation. Analysis of erythrocyte sedimentation rate (ESR) was performed in the other 41% of the total group with red flags for spinal tumor or infection.

All of those who were ultimately diagnosed with spinal cancer or infection had either a prior history of cancer, an ESR greater than 20 mm/hr, or more than one red flag. Therefore, Deyo and Diehl[5] recommended that all persons meeting these criteria (which represented 22% of the total group in their study) should undergo radiographic evaluation of the spine to look for serious spinal pathology. In this group of patients, 3% had spinal tumors (0.66% of the total group) and no spinal infections were seen.

Another study[8] concluded that spinal infection (osteomyelitis) is very uncommon and is probably present in less than 1 in 1,000 patients with acute LBP.

In estimating the percentage of persons with red flags for cancer or infection and their clinical outcomes, the cost model uses the same percentages and clinical decision logic as the study by Deyo and Diehl.[4]

Red Flags for Cauda Equina Syndrome

Cauda equina syndrome is a rare condition characterized by severe bilateral sciatica, rapidly progressive motor weakness in the legs, and bowel or bladder dysfunction. It usually involves compression of multiple lumbosacral nerve roots (the cauda equina) in the spinal canal, caused by a large central intervertebral disk herniation, tumor, or other space-occupying lesion. Cauda equina syndrome is a surgical emergency, and early detection is very important.

Estimates of the frequency of CES used in this model are derived from Spangfort,[9] who reviewed a case series of 2,500 consecutive operations for herniated lumbar disks in adults, and found CES in 1.2%. He also combined the results of 31 other published case series of herniated disk operations and found CES in 2.4%.

Frymoyer and associates[10] found that of all men in a family practice who reported ever having LBP, 3.4% had undergone low back surgery. Deyo and Diehl[4] have estimated that about 1% to 4% of those seeking medical attention for acute LBP will go on to have herniated disk surgery. Using these figures, we estimated CES would be found in 1 to 10 out of every 10,000 adults seeking medical attention for acute LBP.

No studies were found that directly evaluated the effectiveness of the red flag findings for CES in actually detecting CES in acute LBP patients. However, the literature consistently cites these findings as effective for detecting CES, and the absence of these findings as evidence that CES is not present. We agree with this logic, and also assume that about 10 patients will have red flags for CES (which would dictate immediate evaluation by a back surgeon) for every one patient who ultimately is found to have CES.

Therefore, for the cost model, we assume that red flags for CES will be seen in 1 in 1,000 (0.1%) of acute LBP patients, and CES will actually be found in 1 in 10,000 (0.01%) of all adults with acute LBP.

Ruling Out Nonspinal Conditions as the Cause of Symptoms

After evaluating possible red flags that may suggest underlying systemic diseases, the guideline asks clinicians to evaluate the patient for clinical evidence of nonspinal pathology as a cause of the patient's acute LBP. This would include referred pain from renal disease, as well as other abdominal and pelvic pathology.

No studies were found that provided appropriate estimates of the frequency of such nonspinal pathology relative to the frequency of acute LBP. Therefore, for the cost model, we estimated 1% of patients presenting with acute LBP would have nonspinal pathology, which would be diagnosed at the time of the initial evaluation. This 1% would be dropped from the guideline algorithms.

131

Summary of Initial Assessment

Therefore, in the cost model, after screening the original group for red flags for serious spinal pathology and evidence of nonspinal pathology, we assume the following will occur: of the original group, 10% will have red flags for spinal fracture, and spinal radiographs will be obtained from all of these patients. Of this group, 10% (1% of the total group) will have fractures and will be dropped from the treatment algorithm. The other 9% of the total group will return to the treatment algorithm.

Of the original group, 43% will have red flags for cancer or infection. All patients in this group will undergo an analysis of ESR. Indications for a spinal imaging test will then be a prior history of cancer (here 2% of the original group), an ESR greater than 20 mm/hr, or more than one red flag finding. We assume 20% of the original group will have such indications for an imaging test. We assume a lumbar radiograph will be obtained from all of these patients. An MRI scan (5% of total group) or bone scan (5% of total group) will be obtained from those patients with suspicious radiographs or with strong suspicion for these conditions despite normal radiographs. After this testing is completed, it is assumed that 1% of the total group will be found to have tumor or infection and will be dropped from the algorithm.

It is assumed that 0.1% of the group will have red flags for CES. All of these patients will have a surgical consultation, including an imaging test (MRI or CT scan). One out of 10 of those evaluated will be found to have CES (0.01% of the total group) and will be dropped from the algorithm. The other 0.09% will continue in the algorithm.

It is assumed that 1% of the total group will have evidence of nonspinal pathology as the cause of their low back symptoms, and this group will be dropped from the algorithm. This assessment is based on clinical examination findings alone; further diagnostic testing to evaluate any nonspinal conditions is beyond the scope of the guideline and the cost model.

In summary, a total of 4% of the original group will be dropped from the guideline algorithm after initial evaluation for red flags (including follow-up laboratory and imaging studies). Another 1% of the original group will be dropped because of evidence of nonspinal pathology as the cause of acute LBP. The remaining 95% of the original group will then proceed to Algorithm 2, on initial treatment methods.

Assumptions About Initial Treatment Methods

There were few studies found that provided useful data on what initial treatment methods are likely to be used by patients with acute LBP. In one study by Deyo and Diehl,[4] however, nonsteroidal anti-inflammatory drugs (NSAIDs) or muscle relaxants were administered to 44% of patients with acute LBP.

Based on the guideline, all patients would receive some education about LBP during their initial office visit, including recommendations about appropriate limitation of activities aimed at minimizing back irritation but avoiding debilitation from inactivity. We assumed 80% of the group would desire help with comfort; of this group we assumed 100% would be given medications, while 25% would try manipulation.

For those receiving medication, we assumed all would receive a 4-week course of NSAIDs, which we estimated would cost $50.00 per patient. We recognized that the actual choices of medication, duration of treatment, and cost will vary significantly between individuals, but this seemed a reasonable average for the cost model. In a similar manner, for those choosing manipulation for pain relief, we assumed four office visits would be made during the initial month of care. Again, this seemed to be a reasonable average although individual experience might be different. We also assumed an average of two follow-up office visits (at the ends of week 2 and week 4) during this first month of care.

In addition, according to the guideline, all patients would be advised to start a program of back conditioning exercises during the first month. We assumed many individuals would want to do this on their own, but in other cases patients or clinicians might prefer a supervised exercise program. Therefore, we assumed that 25% of patients would have four physical therapy visits during the first month of care for instruction and supervision in therapeutic exercises aimed at improving aerobic fitness and specific conditioning of the back muscles. These visits would not include charges for the use of physical therapy modalities or traction, which were not recommended by the guideline.

Proportion of Patients Not Improved at 1 Month

At the end of the first month of care, the guideline suggests the majority of patients with acute LBP will have improved significantly while a smaller group will continue to have symptoms that have not improved. There are various estimates in the literature of what proportion of patients with acute LBP will improve after 1 month of care. In a study of family practice patients with acute LBP, Dixon[11] found 50% of patients were improved at 1 week and 90% were improved at 1 month. In a study of men seen for acute LBP in an occupational medicine clinic over a 6-month period, Goertz[12] found that 1 month after the initial visit 90% of patients were performing at regular capacity, another 8% were on light duty, and only 2% were off work because of LBP. In a study of men with acute LBP in a family practice clinic, Lanier and Stockton[13] found 64% had a good outcome 6 weeks after their initial visit, and 91% had a good outcome at 12-week follow-up.

Other studies show that patients with acute LBP who have sciatica have slower rates of improvement than patients with no radicular symptoms. In a study of patients with acute LBP by Andersson and associates,[14] 10 days after the initial visit complete resolution of symptoms was reported by 60% of those who presented with LBP but no radicular symptoms, compared to 9% of those who had LBP with radiation.

In Chavannes and associates'[15] study of patients of general practitioners in the Netherlands who had acute LBP, after 1 month of care 24% of patients had not improved (including 18% of those who initially had LBP alone and 35% of those who initially had sciatica). However, because there were initially more patients with LBP alone, the group in whom LBP had not improved at 1 month was made up of 46% who initially had LBP alone and 54% who initially had sciatica.

Proportion of Patients Presenting With Sciatica

The percentage of patients who have not improved at 1 month will vary to some degree with the proportion of patients who have sciatica. This is another variable of the cost model that could be represented by a range of values. Various estimates of the frequency of sciatica in groups of patients with acute LBP are as follows.

Andersson and associates[14] found that in evaluating all employed persons in Sweden who had a work absence because of LBP, 16.5% reportedly had sciatica. In Chavannes and associates'[15] study of patients of general practitioners in the Netherlands who had acute LBP, on the initial visit 62% had low back pain, while 38% had sciatica. In a study of all adults in a walk-in clinic with uncomplicated LBP, 40% presented with sciatica.[4] In a population survey, Deyo and Tsui-Wu[16] found that of all persons who reported having had an episode of LBP lasting more than 2 weeks, 12% reported symptoms of sciatica.

In a study of all men seen with acute LBP in an occupational medicine clinic over a 6-month period, 31% had pain below the knee.[12] In a population survey of adult men in Denmark, of those who reported an episode of LBP during a 1-year period of the study, 44% reported pain radiating into the legs.[17] In a population study in Finland, of those adults reporting LBP at the time of the survey, 30% of men and 23% of women had sciatica.[18] In a study of all adult males with acute LBP seen in a family practice clinic over a 1-year period, 27% had radiation of pain into the legs.[13]

Summary of Assumptions About the First Month of Treatment

Taking all of this information into account, we made the following assumptions for the cost model. For those patients who entered Algorithm 2 and received 1 month of initial treatment (ie, 95% of the original group), we assume 90% (or 86% of the original group) will have improved significantly at the end of the first month of care.

For those patients who are improved at 1 month, no further diagnostic evaluation will be needed, although a portion of this group might require additional office visits for continued comfort measures. For the cost model, we assume half of the group that had improved (43% of the original group) will require no further medical care, while the other half (43%) will need an average of 2 additional weeks of medication (at a $25 cost per patient) and will have two more follow-up office visits, but no further visits for manipulation or therapeutic exercise.

The 10% whose condition has not improved after 1 month of care will include a proportionally larger number of those who initially had sciatica. Here the proportions found by Chavannes and associates[15] at 1 month are used in the cost model. Therefore, it is assumed that 10% of those who start Algorithm 2 (9.5% of the original group) will have further diagnostic evaluation as described in Algorithm 3, and of those who have this further evaluation, 46% will have initially presented with nonradicular LBP while 54% will have initially had sciatica.

Assumptions About Further Diagnosis and Treatment, For Those Not Improved at 1 Month

The remainder of the cost model, which corresponds to Algorithms 3 through 5 of the guideline, deals with special diagnostic studies and further treatment methods (both surgical and nonsurgical) for patients who have not improved after 1 month of initial treatment. No studies were found in the scientific literature that provided appropriate estimates for the assumptions used in the remainder of the economic model. This is partly because many of the assumptions in Algorithms 3 through 5 involve clinical judgment about what course of action is appropriate, so descriptive epidemiologic data are not useful. In other cases, data that provided answers to the very specific questions posed by the guideline algorithms (eg, the percentage of those with sciatica not improved after 1 month who have clear evidence of radiculopathy on physical examination) were not found. Therefore, all assumptions used in the remainder of the cost model (Algorithms 3 through 5) are based on our clinical judgment.

Results

We developed a spreadsheet model to estimate the costs of following the guideline. The "base case" probabilities of various clinical findings or events were derived from the epidemiologic and health services research literature where possible, and otherwise were educated guesses.

The base case estimates from the spreadsheet model suggested that the average total payments for health services in the first 3 months after index visit, following the guideline's recommendations, would be $381 per person. The average total payments actually observed from the MEDSTAT file were $612 (Table 2). Thus, under the "base case" parameter values, this comparison suggests that implementation of the guideline using our example would produce direct health care cost savings over the first 3 months of approximately 38% relative to the costs of prevailing medical practice for the diagnosis and treatment of low back problems.

Sensitivity Analysis

Several analyses were performed to test the sensitivity of the 3-month cost projections to changes in probabilities from the "base case" assumptions. Table 3 summarizes the results of the sensitivity analyses, which suggest that the following decisions or probabilities have the strongest influence on cost differences: (1) whether an MRI study is performed on patients with suspicion of cancer or infection after laboratory tests and bone scan; (2) the percentage of persons limited by back problems for more than 4 continuous weeks and experiencing neurologic symptoms in their lower limbs; and (3) the proportion of persons with sciatica persisting after 4 weeks who choose surgery to speed symptom relief. The dollar figures presented in Table 3 represent projected *average* cost for the entire cohort of patients, based on alternative assumptions regarding the values of specific cost model parameters.

The 3-month cost projection is not very sensitive to the following decisions and probabilities: (1) the proportion of patients with "red flag" clinical findings for spinal fracture, cancer or infection; (2) the laboratory test (complete

Table 2 Frequency of various clinical procedures for 55,083 LBP patients (expanded version)*

Procedure	Implied by Sample Strategy (an Interpretation of the Low Back Problems Guideline)	MEDSTAT Database
Initial office visit	55,083	55,083
Follow-up office visit	23,925	23,679
Psychiatric consultation	394	0
Plain radiograph	6,843	19,162
MRI	2,222	801
CT scan	1,121	2,275
Bone scan	1,155	249
Surgery	662	1,525
Urinalysis	1,636	1,627
Complete blood count	1,636	420
Erythrocyte sedimentation rate	24,703	339
Electromyogram	1,874	1,193
Spinal manipulation	12,825	15,337
Exercise therapy (using CPT codes as proxies for exercise and conditioning regimens to improve activity tolerance)	15,672	301

* The actual payments observed in the first 3 months of care for low back problems in the MEDSTAT data for the cohort of 55,083 patients were $571 per person. We have added $51 to that amount to reflect the payments for initial office visits involving low back problems but not coded in MEDSTAT with a diagnosis related to low back problems. The MEDSTAT claims for this cohort of 55,083 actually showed only 12,703 initial office visits with a low back-related diagnosis. We reason that, in fact there were an additional 42,380 (55,083-12,703) initial office visits involving low back problems for that cohort by definition; but since MEDSTAT outpatient service records only list a single diagnosis for each service record, our observed count of initial office visits for low back problems would miss all cases for which low back problems were not listed as the first diagnosis on the service record for the visit. It seems more appropriate to add the payments that would have been incurred for those 42,380 visits to the benchmark cost estimate from MEDSTAT. The $51/person = [42,380 additional initial visits per person × $66/initial visit]/55,083 persons

blood count and urinalysis) frequency for patients with "red flag" clinical findings for cancer or infection; (3) the proportion of patients who require help with comfort options during the initial month of care; (4) the number of follow-up visits (one versus two) during the initial month of care for those not recovering from low back problems after the first visit; and (5) the proportion of patients with symptoms persisting beyond 1 month who undergo a bone scan for suspected cancer or infection.

The comparison of the frequency of procedures and services between the sample strategy and the MEDSTAT "standard medical practice" as shown in Table 2 suggests that our interpretation of the guideline would reduce the use of plain radiographs, surgery, and spinal manipulation. At the same time, the assumptions of the sample strategy are associated with increased use of the eryth-

Table 3 Sensitivity analyses

Cost Model Parameter	Projected Average Cost ($) of 3-Month Treatment*
Important cost drivers:	
Of patients with suspicion of cancer or infection after laboratory tests and bone scan, the percentage who undergo MRI:	
5 (base case scenario)	381
17.5 (alternative scenario 1)	423
27.5 (alternative scenario 2)	457
Of patients limited by either low back or back-related leg symptoms for more than 4 continuous weeks, the percentage who experience neurologic symptoms in their lower limbs:	
54 (base case scenario)	381
34 (alternative scenario 1)	326
74 (alternative scenario 2)	436
Of patients with significant sciatica persisting after 4 weeks, the percentage who consider and receive surgery to speed recovery:	
30 (base case scenario)	381
10 (alternative scenario 1)	301
50 (alternative scenario 2)	464
Negligible cost "drivers":	
Patients (%) initially presenting with "red flag" clinical findings for cancer or infection:	
40 (base case scenario)	381
30 (alternative scenario 1)	375
50 (alternative scenario 2)	387
Patients (%) with "red flag" clinical findings for cancer or infection who receive complete blood count and urinalysis in initial testing:	
5 (base case scenario)	381
25 (alternative scenario 1)	383
50 (alternative scenario 2)	385
Patients (%) with "red flag" clinical findings who require help with comfort options during initial month of low back care:	
80 (base case scenario)	381
60 (alternative scenario 1)	360
100 (alternative scenario 2)	402
Number of follow-up visits during initial month of care for those not recovering after first visit:	
1 (base case scenario)	381
2 (alternative scenario)	388
Patients (%) who receive bone scan as part of evaluation for suspected cancer or infection because of persistent symptoms:	
2 (base case scenario)	381
0 (alternative scenario 1)	381
10 (alternative scenario 2)	383

*These dollar figures are the average cost of 3-month treatment for the entire cohort of patients, given the stated percentages presented as alternative assumptions in the cost model parameter column rocyte sedimentation rate and electromyograms for diagnostic testing and a higher frequency of exercise and conditioning regimens to improve activity tolerance.

On the other hand, use of the guideline-based strategy would result in greater use of MRI and bone scanning. This results from two factors: (1) a relatively high assumed frequency of imaging studies, in general, built into the strategy; and (2) the increased adoption of MRI and bone scan studies (partly in substitution for CT), given the current state-of-the-art for the evaluation and management of low back problems. This also drives the lower frequency of CT scans in the sample strategy compared to prevailing 1988-1989 medical practice.

Discussion

Our "base case" comparison between guideline-recommended practice and actual practice suggests substantial direct health care cost savings during the initial 3-month period of diagnosis and treatment. The existence of probable savings does not seem sensitive to variation in the values of certain key variables in the cost model (at least within the range considered in this study). However, in any such "hypothetical simulation," there is the possibility that important effects on other variables that might occur in actual practice may have been missed.

There are substantial early costs of guideline-based practice (eg, repeat visits to the physician and more imaging studies for certain subsets of persons experiencing LBP), and it may take more than 3 months to realize the cost and health benefits of the practice patterns encouraged by the guideline. These benefits might take the form of faster initial return to work, increased productivity in work for pay and household chores, and the avoidance of future hospitalization, rehospitalization, or surgery for LBP. None of these potential cost reductions would appear in the 3-month differential cost estimates presented here. Thus, the estimates of this study may understate the long run cost savings from implementing the guideline.

On the other hand, the guideline leaves considerable discretion in implementation. While the authors have attempted to isolate the key clinical variables that might be affected by the guideline, it is possible that patient-specific factors and other contingencies in actual practice could lead to higher costs than those estimated in our sample strategy. Only by conducting a controlled trial (preferably randomized) in actual practice can short- or long-term cost savings and health benefits from guideline-based practice for low back problems be determined.

Acknowledgments

The authors would like to acknowledge the excellent assistance of Dr. Stanley Bigos in developing the ideas and methods for this chapter, William Kreuter for his skillful programming support, and Sandra Coke and Merrily Diop for their high-quality word processing efforts.

References

1. Bigos SJ, Bower R, Braen G, et al: Acute low back problems in adults, in *Clinical Practice Guideline 14.* Rockville, MD, US Department of Health and Human Services, AHCPR Publication No. 95-0642, 1994, pp 137–141.
2. Frymoyer JW, Cats-Baril WL: An overview of the incidences and costs of low back pain. *Orthop Clin North Am* 1991;22:263–271.
3. Lave JR, Pashos CL, Anderson GF, et al: Costing medical care: Using Medicare administrative data. *Med Care* 1994;32(suppl 7):JS77–JS89.
4. Deyo RA, Diehl AK: Psychosocial predictors of disability in patients with low back pain. *J Rheumatol* 1988;15:1557–1564.
5. Deyo RA, Diehl AK: Cancer as a cause of back pain: Frequency, clinical presentation, and diagnostic strategies. *J Gen Intern Med* 1988;3:230–238.
6. Biering-Sorensen F: A prospective study of low back pain in a general population: I. Occurrence, recurrence and aetiology. *Scand J Rehabil Med* 1983;15:71–79.
7. Heliovaara M, Makela M, Knekt P, et al: Determinants of sciatica and low-back pain. *Spine* 1991;16:608–614.
8. Deyo RA, McNiesh LM, Cone RO III: Observer variability in the interpretation of lumbar spine radiographs. *Arthritis Rheum* 1985;28:1066–1070.
9. Spangfort EV: The lumbar disc herniation: A computer-aided analysis of 2,504 operations. *Acta Orthop Scand* 1972;142(suppl):1–95.
10. Frymoyer JW, Pope MH, Clements JH, et al: Risk factors in low-back pain: An epidemiological survey. *J Bone Joint Surg* 1983;65A:213–218.
11. Dixon A St. J: Progress and problems in back pain research. *Rheumatol Rehabil* 1973;12:165–175.
12. Goertz MN: Prognostic indicators for acute low-back pain. *Spine* 1990;15:1307–1310.
13. Lanier DC, Stockton P: Clinical predictors of outcome of acute episodes of low back pain. *J Fam Pract* 1988;27:483–489.
14. Andersson GB, Svensson HO, Oden A: The intensity of work recovery in low back pain. *Spine* 1983;8:880–884.
15. Chavannes AW, Gubbels J, Post D, et al: Acute low back pain: Patients' perceptions of pain four weeks after initial diagnosis and treatment in general practice. *J R Coll Gen Pract* 1986;36:271–273.
16. Deyo RA, Tsui-Wu YJ: Descriptive epidemiology of low back pain and its related medical costs in the United States. *Spine* 1987;12:264–268.
17. Gyntelberg F: One year incidence of low back pain among male residents of Copenhagen aged 40-59. *Dan Med Bull* 1974;21:30–36.
18. Heliovaara M, Sievers K, Impivaara O, et al: Descriptive epidemiology and public health aspects of low back pain. *Ann Med* 1989;21:327–333.

Chapter 10

Minimally Invasive Arthroscopic Treatment of Painful Disorders of the Lumbar Spine: Arthroscopic Lumbar Disk Surgery

Parviz Kambin, MD

An arthroscopic posterolateral or paramedial approach to the lumbar spine represents an alternative method for diagnosis and treatment of a variety of painful conditions involving the spinal column. Although this approach is used most often for extraction of herniated lumbar disk fragments, with the advent of improved instrumentation it can also be used for arthroscopic lumbar interbody fusion,[1,2] decompression of lateral recess stenosis, and the diagnosis and treatment of disk space infections. An anterior transperitoneal or retroperitoneal approach to L5-S1 intervertebral disks[3] and a transthoracic approach[4] for the treatment of disk herniations, tumor resections, and drainage of abscesses are rapidly being incorporated into the field of minimally invasive arthroscopic and endoscopic surgery.

Since the introduction of the posterolateral approach to the lumbar spine for nuclear decompression,[5-7] there has been remarkable progress in recognition of the arthroscopic appearance of normal and pathologic structures of the lumbar spine, and in arthroscopic surgical approaches and treatment of spinal disorders.

Anatomic and Pathologic Considerations

The common concern about inflicting injury to the neural structures during the introduction of instruments and resection of nuclear tissue via a posterolateral approach is well founded.[8,9] Knowledge of the anatomy, arthroscopic appearance of the neural structures, and radiographic landmarks of the annulotomy site is essential for safe use of the posterolateral approach to the lumbar spine.

As soon as the exiting nerve root departs from the spinal foramen, it descends distally, anteriorly, and laterally. Its position is then safely anterior to the transverse process of the lower lumbar segments. The anterolateral descent of the spinal nerve creates a triangular working zone[10-13] large enough to accommodate the inserted instruments. This triangular working zone is bordered by the spinal nerve anteriorly, the proximal plate of the lower vertebra inferiorly, the proximal articular process of the lower lumbar segment posteriorly, and the dura and traversing nerve root medially. Great care should be exercised to place the instruments between the sacrospinalis, quadratus lumborum, and psoas major muscles. A far lateral approach increases the chance of passing through the perineum and entering the abdominal cavity. Arteries and veins are located anteriorly and are not usually in the path of the inserted instruments; however, deep penetration of the instruments or periannular slippage of the cannula could cause vascular injury. The design of commonly used instruments permits only 2 cm penetration into the intervertebral disk, thus providing an added margin of safety.

Branches of lumbar veins that lie on the surface of the annular fibers occasionally are injured during annular fenestration with circular cutting instruments. Periannular hemostasis may be performed with the aid of a working channel scope and a radiofrequency coagulator.

Age-related anatomic and pathologic changes in the intervertebral disk have been well described.[14-16] Nuclear degeneration usually is preceded by the development of both circumferential and vertical fissures in the anulus. Subsequently, vascular tissue grows through the vertebral end plate, and fluid loss and collagenation occur in the nucleus pulposus. With further progression of the degenerative process and the influence of external forces, annular tears become more evident, thereby allowing migration of a collagenized nuclear fragment to the periphery of the intervertebral disk. Loss of integrity of the intervertebral disk usually is followed by gradual diminution in its height that commonly is visualized in radiographic studies of the lumbar spine. Narrowing of the disk space contributes to further protrusion and bulging of the disk. Expulsion of a nuclear fragment under the posterior longitudinal ligament causes the classic imaging appearance of disk herniation with a sharply localized extradural defect.[17] Nuclear fragments sequestered inside the disk have been identified in intradiskal arthroscopic examinations.[18] It may be postulated that the periodic peripheral migration of these fragments may be responsible for exacerbations and subsequent remissions of sciatic pain in a clinical setting.

In the early stages of degeneration, the nucleus has a whitish "cotton ball" appearance on arthroscopic examination. Herniated disk fragments are usually rubbery and firm collagenized tissue. Extraction of these fragments by intradiskal access requires articulating instrumentation and excellent arthroscopic visualization.

The annulotomy site within the triangular working zone usually is covered with loosely woven adipose tissue. Fibrous bands on the annular surface may be visualized under arthroscopic magnification and illumination following removal of this fatty tissue. The exiting root also is invariably surrounded by vascular fatty tissue. Routine intraoperative exposure and inspection of the nerve is not advisable. The arthroscope may be passed under the pars interarticularis for inspection and visualization of the dura and the traversing nerve root. When intradiskal access to the spinal canal is being attempted, the thick fibers of the posterior longitudinal ligament may be visualized behind the boundary of the anulus adjacent to the ventral dura.

Are All Arthroscopic Diskectomies the Same?

In 1963, Smith and associates[19] proposed an indirect decompression of the lumbar intervertebral disk by chemonucleolysis. It was postulated that spontaneous reduction of posterior and posterolateral herniated fragments may follow nuclear debulking, thus resulting in decompression of the nerve root. Despite the fact that chemonucleolysis is still being used for the treatment of herniated lumbar disks, controversy concerning the efficacy and safety of this procedure has never ceased. Multiple prospective, randomized, double-blind studies by well-intended investigators have produced inconclusive opposing views. It appears that the lack of uniform understanding of the term ''herniated disk'' by various practitioners led to selection of two groups of patients whose clinical symptoms and imaging studies differed and ultimately resulted in contradictory results.

Schwetschenau and associates[20] and Martins and associates[21] found no appreciable difference between outcomes of patients treated with placebo and chymopapain. In a prospective, randomized, double-blind study of 104 patients, Brown and Daroff[22] obtained the same result. However, they concluded that the study had limitations as a result of early code-breaking and recommended further study of a larger group of patients.

In contrast, Javid and associates[23] followed 53 patients treated with placebo and 55 patients treated with chymopapain for a 6-month period and concluded that chymopapain was more effective than placebo for patients with herniated lumbar disks. Seven institutions participated in this study. One center in this group reported no difference in the outcome of patients treated with chymopapain and those treated with normal saline, whereas another institution reported a better outcome in the placebo group than in drug-injected patients. From the results of a double-blind study conducted at the Royal Adelaide Hospital, Adelaide, Australia, Fraser[24] also concluded that results in chymopapain-injected patients were superior to those in the placebo group. Thirty patients in each group were injected, and the results were determined by questionnaires completed by the patients 2 years after treatment.

Various procedures for mechanical decompression of the nucleus were developed in the early and mid 1970s.[5,6] The cause of mechanical nuclear resection for treatment of herniated lumbar disks was further advanced by introduction of a mechanical suction device in 1985.[25] Satisfactory outcomes varying from 50% to 75% following chemonucleolysis, automated mechanical nucleotomy, and laser nuclear ablation have been reported by various investigators (P Kambin, MD, interdepartmental communication, 1973).[26-29]

However, many investigators' experiences with mechanical nuclear debulking and laser nuclear ablation have been disappointing.[30-32] The limited flexibility of the plastic, disposable scopes that have been used with mechanical nucleotomy devices or laser light does not permit access to posterior and posterolateral herniations. In addition, intradiskal orientation and identification of herniated fragments with the latter instruments are difficult. A minimally invasive, percutaneous diskectomy technique should not be accepted as an alternative treatment for disk herniations unless it can be used to retrieve the herniated fragments similarly to what is accomplished following an open laminotomy.

The concept of intradiskal retrieval of herniated disk fragments through a posterolateral approach was formulated in 1979[5,7] by adapting the posterolateral approach to vertebral bodies used for bone biopsy.[33,34] However, a major modification, both in approach and instrumentation, was made following a series of anatomic studies. The outer diameter (OD) of the cannula was enlarged to 6.9 mm to accommodate the insertion of upbiting and larger tipped forceps. In contrast to biopsy techniques in which the instruments were inserted 6 cm from the midline,[34] a more lateral placement of the skin entry point to the lateral boundary of the paraspinal muscles (10 to 11 cm from the midline) was advocated.[35,36] This placement permitted further medialization of the annulotomy site at the midpedicular region, thus facilitating posterior positioning of the instruments in the intervertebral disk and providing closer access to the posterolateral and midline herniated fragments.

To accommodate the biportal approach for interbody arthrodesis and diskectomy that was introduced in later years, the patient was placed in a prone position. A high negative pressure was used to dislodge the semi-attached collagenized disk fragments. However, with the advent of arthroscopic visualization by a biportal approach, less use has been found for this technique.

In order to make certain that the instruments are posteriorly positioned in the intervertebral disk, the tip of the needle is localized on the surface of the anulus at the onset of the procedure.[5,12,13,35,36] Following a series of cadaver studies, the triangular working zone was identified, and its radiographic landmarks were described.[10,12,37]

In the ensuing years, safe intradiskal use of articulating instruments adjacent to neural structures required arthroscopic visualization of the inserted instruments (Fig. 1) through use of a biportal approach (Fig. 2). This arthroscopic intradiskal visualization required adequate inflow and outflow of saline solution through the surgical field that could not be obtained with a uniportal approach. The knowledge of arthroscopic anatomy of periannular structures, foramina, and

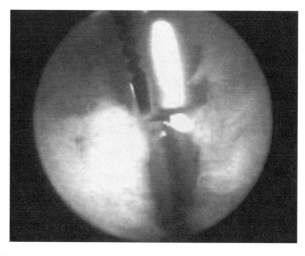

Fig. 1 *Intradiskal arthroscopic view of an articulating instrument that is being used to access the floor of the spinal canal.*

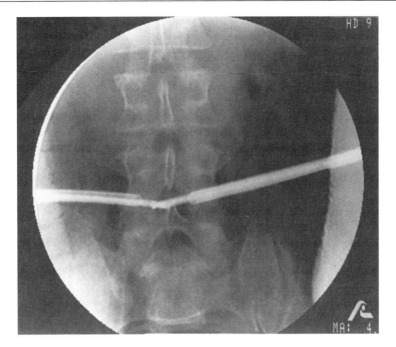

Fig. 2 *Intraoperative anteroposterior fluoroscopy demonstrates bilateral biportal access to L4-L5 intervertebral disk. The deflecting forceps is introduced from one portal and the 70° arthroscope from the opposite side for the removal of a central herniation under arthroscopic control.*

content of the spinal canal became necessary for safe performance of arthroscopic spine surgery.[12,37,38]

In contrast to other nuclear debulking procedures, arthroscopic disk surgery through a 6.4-mm OD cannula represents a percutaneous procedure that simulates open laminotomy techniques in its ability to harvest the offending compressive herniated fragments from the spinal canal (Fig. 3).

Instruments

A variety of instruments (Fig. 4) is available and is currently being used for minimally invasive intradiskal and extra-annular surgery of the lumbar spine through a posterolateral approach.

Needles

An 18-gauge needle or a 0.045-inch Kirschner wire is usually used for fluoroscopic localization of the annulotomy site. Following the proper positioning of the tip of the needle in the triangular working zone, the stylus of the needle may be replaced by a 7-inch long 22-gauge needle for dual needle technique diskography if deemed necessary.

145

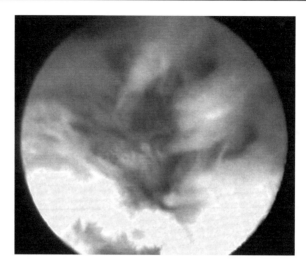

Fig. 3 *Arthroscopic appearance of the ventral dura following removal of a herniated fragment through an intradiskal approach.*

Cannulated Obturator

The cannulated obturators have a blunt end that passes through the muscle fibers when inserted. In my hands, a small-caliber obturator with 4.9-mm OD has proven to be safe for both posterolateral intradiskal and extra-annular spine surgery. The larger obturator with an OD of 9.9 mm is used for arthroscopic facet fusion or arthroscopic access to the pedicles for the insertion of pedicular bolts. The obturators are cannulated to permit precise insertion of the instruments over the previously positioned guide wire into the triangular working zone. An auxiliary obturator may be used with the aid of an obturator jig to develop a broader access to the intervertebral disk in preparation for insertion of an oval cannula.

Access Cannula

I currently use three different access cannulas for minimally invasive spinal surgery. The universal access cannula has an internal diameter (ID) of 5 mm and an OD of 6.4 mm. This cannula accommodates various instruments that are used for arthroscopic retrieval of herniated fragments via intradiskal or extra-annular access. Two sizes of oval cannulas are usually used. The smaller cannula has an ID of 5 × 8 mm, and the larger cannula has an ID of 5 x 10 mm. The oval cannula with the larger diameter is usually used for arthroscopic interbody fusion, whereas the one with the smaller diameter is used for arthroscopic disk extraction or, at times, interbody arthrodesis.

Manual Instruments

Different types of forceps are used for manual extraction of herniated fragments. The straight forceps is used for intradiskal surgery and is capable of retrieving nuclear tissue that is in the path of the inserted cannula. An upbiting

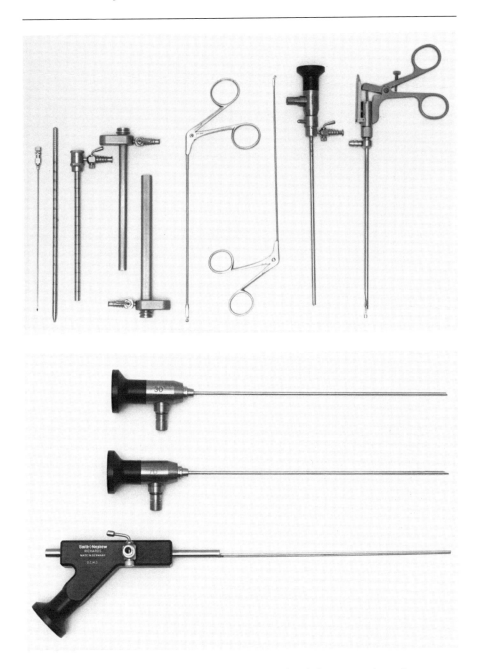

Fig. 4   *Top, From left to right, 18-gauge needle, cannulated obturator, universal access cannula and suction irrigation valve, 5 × 8 mm oval cannula, 5 × 10 mm oval cannula, straight punch forceps, upbiting forceps, 0° arthroscope, and deflecting suction forceps. **Bottom**, 30° arthroscope, 70° arthroscope, and working channel scope.*

forceps allows the surgeon to reach a few millimeters beyond the boundary of the cannula. A flexible tip forceps is used in conjunction with a deflecting tube and allows approximately 45° dorsal angulation of the tip of the inserted forceps. A deflecting suction forceps provides up to 120° dorsal angulation of the tip of the forceps and should be used for intradiskal access to the spinal canal with a biportal arthroscopic approach.

Straight and Curved Power-Driven Instruments (Trimmer Blades)

These instruments are used for nucleotomy and facilitate creation of a cavity behind the inner fibers of the posterior anulus in preparation for extraction of the herniated fragments.

Arthroscopes

Two kinds of arthroscopes usually are used for arthroscopic spinal surgery. Rigid arthroscopes have been used for years to illuminate and magnify internal structures of the joints. These arthroscopes have been modified and elongated for minimally invasive spinal surgery. At the present time, rigid glass arthroscopes provide higher resolution and clearer imaging than disposable plastic arthroscopes. Although the flexibility of the disposable plastic arthroscopes appears to be desirable for intradiskal maneuvering, their limited flexibility and large arc of deflection precludes their use for access to posterior and posterolateral disk herniations.

Working Channel Scope

The working channel scope permits simultaneous visualization of normal and pathologic tissue and, at times, extraction of the offending herniated fragments. This 0° arthroscope permits inspection of the entire annular surface at one glance. To make certain that neither the exiting root, the traversing root (Fig. 5), nor the dural sac are in the path of the inserted cannula, adipose tissue on the surface of the anulus may have to be removed with a forceps for inspection of the annular surface. An extraforaminal, a foraminal, and occasionally an intracanalicular herniation may be extracted with the aid of a working channel scope. Additionally, the working channel scope may be used to develop communication with the opposite portal when a bilateral biportal approach is being used. At times, the forceps and the arthroscope of the working channel scope may be passed under the pars interarticularis to observe and to perform intracanalicular surgery. However, because the working channel scope is a straight instrument, it is of limited use for intradiskal removal of nonmigrated sequestered disk or midline posterior herniations.

An 8-mm oval cannula may be used effectively as a working channel scope for simultaneous visualization and tissue extraction via an ipsilateral approach. The 5- × 8-mm oval cannula accommodates a 0° or 30° arthroscope and a forceps. An oval cannula may be positioned in the foramen to provide either subligamentous intradiskal access to the herniation site or extra-annular access to the spinal canal for visualization of the traversing nerve root, for fenestration of the anulus lateral to the traversing root, and for intradiskal subligamentous evacuation of herniated fragments.

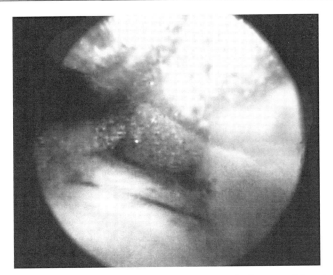

Fig. 5 *Arthroscopic visualization of the spinal canal. On the bottom of the photo, the traversing nerve root is being viewed with the aid of a 30° arthroscope that is passed under the pars interarticularis. The dural sac is covered by epidural adipose tissue and is observed at the top of the photo.*

Management of Pain Associated With Herniated Lumbar Disks

Patient selection for arthroscopic disk surgery is similar to that described in the literature for open laminotomy. Failure to respond to well-planned, nonsurgical management; having greater sciatic pain than back pain; presenting with a positive tension sign and neurologic deficit; and correlative dermatomal distribution of pain and imaging studies are prerequisites for consideration of arthroscopic microdiskectomy. Both contained and uncontained lumbar disk herniations are retrievable by an arthroscopic approach. However, a migrated sequestered fragment cannot be removed by currently available arthroscopic techniques.

Extraforaminal, foraminal, and intracanalicular paramedial herniations may be extracted through a single cannula inserted dorsolaterally from the symptomatic side. Large intracanalicular central herniations, particularly a subligamentous or nonmigrated sequestered herniation, will require a dual approach. At this time, patients with lateral recess stenosis associated with severe facet arthropathy and narrowing of the intervertebral disk are not treatable using arthroscopic techniques.

The removal of a large central or sequestered fragment from the L5-S1 intervertebral disk through a posterolateral approach may be difficult in an individual with a high iliac crest. Retrieval of this type of herniation requires the establishment of two portals on the right and left sides. The iliac crest in this group of patients interferes with adequate intradiskal triangulation between the inserted arthroscope and the instruments. However, arthroscopes may be used via a translaminar approach[39] for localization and extraction of an intracanalicular herniation in the latter group of patients. The 30° or 70° rigid scopes pro-

149

vide an added advantage over the commonly used microscopes for intracanalicular surgery by allowing the inspection of those structures that are proximal or distal to the laminotomy site. Individuals who are involved in medicolegal disputes and those with psychosocial disorders are not good candidates for minimally invasive arthroscopic disk extraction. Patients with long-standing histories of pain and use of controlled analgesics may not respond to arthroscopically assisted disk surgery.

Arthroscopic microdiskectomy is a skill-oriented procedure associated with a learning curve. It should be performed by either an orthopaedic or neurologic surgeon, who is trained and capable of performing open spine procedures. This surgical procedure may be time consuming and should be performed in a surgical suite under a strict sterile environment. The retrieval of a herniated fragment through a posterolateral approach may be accomplished either through an intradiskal or periannular approach.[12,17]

Patients who are selected for minimally invasive arthroscopic spinal surgery should have at least plain anteroposterior (AP) and lateral radiograms of the lumbar spine, including the pelvis. These studies not only help to determine the accessibility of the index level to the posterolateral approach, but also help to rule out the presence of other bony pathologic conditions. Attention should be paid to the height of the intervertebral disk as it is visualized in the lateral radiogram. It may not be possible to insert an access cannula into a severely collapsed, degenerated intervertebral disk. The height of the iliac crest may pose difficulties in accessing the L5-S1 intervertebral disk. When there is a steep angle between the ilium and the proximal plate of the sacrum,[37] it may not be possible to establish bilateral biportal access and triangulate inside the intervertebral disk. When there is a question with regard to instability of the lumbar motion segment, a plain radiographic examination of the lumbar spine should be obtained in flexion and extension.

A preoperative magnetic resonance imaging (MRI) study provides a broad view of the anatomic structures of the lumbar and lower thoracic spine, the status of hydration of the intervertebral disks, and the presence or absence of disk herniation. Preoperative computed tomography (CT) scanning is also useful in demonstrating the presence of calcification in the anulus and posterior longitudinal ligament, facet arthropathy, and marginal osteophytosis. In the institution where I work, my coworkers and I reserve the use of myelography and post-myelogram CTs for patients with severe obesity, claustrophobia, deformities, and those with multiply operated spines.

Preoperatively, the surgeon should determine whether the herniated fragments are retrievable through a single portal or if a biportal or translaminar access is needed. The biportal approach requires longer surgical time and may require the use of a general anesthetic. Prophylactic antibiotics are used for diskectomy and fusion patients. All patients received 1 g of cefazolin sodium intravenously before surgery. This is followed by three additional doses over the next 24 hours. If a patient is allergic to penicillin or cefazolin sodium, vancomycin is used.

Outcome Studies

The outcome of arthroscopic microdiskectomy by a posterolateral approach has been the subject of many publications.[5,12,35,36,40-42] In a recent prospective controlled study,[43] 175 consecutive patients underwent arthroscopic posterolateral disk decompression and fragmentectomy. A biportal approach to the index level was used for retrieval of a large central or sequestered herniated fragment in 59 patients in this group. The length of postoperative follow-up varied from 24 to 78 months. Information was gathered from pre- and postoperative questionnaires that included an analog pain scale and the examining physician's evaluation forms. Of these patients, 88% had overall satisfactory outcomes, a result compatible with those obtained from laminotomy and diskectomy. Past[44] attempts to conclude a double-blind, prospective study on the development of degenerative spondylosis of the lumbar spine after partial diskectomy have not been successful. Although direct arthroscopic visualization and extraction of the herniated fragments may reduce the necessity for such a study, the authors'[36] postoperative imaging studies of the index level have been providing excellent objective evidence of change in the external geometry of the anulus at the herniation site following arthroscopic microdiskectomy. In contrast to open laminotomy, the absence of postoperative bleeding and hematoma formation, particularly in a contained disk herniation, contributes to clear CT delineation of the herniation site in immediate postoperative CT studies.

No neurovascular complications have been encountered in this group of patients.[43] However, four individuals developed postoperative causalgic-type of pain in their involved extremity. This pain responded to the use of anti-inflammatory medication. Postoperative use of Hemovac tubes has eliminated the latter complication.

Discussion

It is not my intention to suggest that arthroscopic disk fragmentectomy represents a better or technologically more advanced modality for the treatment of herniated lumbar disks than the conventional laminotomy procedure, but to introduce an alternative, less invasive way to access and retrieve herniated disk material. Whether a patient should undergo conventional laminotomy and diskectomy or arthroscopic decompression depends largely on the physician's and patient's choice combined with the surgeon's familiarity and skill in performing either surgical procedure.

A distinction must be made between mechanical nucleotomy techniques, laser nuclear ablation, chemonucleolysis, and arthroscopic disk surgery through a uniportal or biportal approach. The latter makes it possible to visualize and remove the offending herniated fragments under arthroscopic magnification and illumination. Although a valid explanation for relief of sciatic pain following extraction of compressive elements has been provided,[45] the mechanism by which nuclear debulking provides relief is not well understood.

The cannulization of the paraspinal muscles via a posterolateral approach minimizes the development of postoperative scar formation and denervation of paraspinal muscles that may lead to chronic fatigue and postoperative pain. The avoidance of entry into the spinal canal and of intraoperative retraction and manipulation of the nerve roots and the protection of the epidural venous system reduces the development of postoperative intraneural and perineural fibrosis.[46-48] The late development of degenerative spondylitis and instability appears to be less common following arthroscopic microdiskectomy at the L4-L5 level than after open laminotomy.[44] When deemed necessary, an arthroscopic translaminar approach may be used for the removal of herniated disk fragments. The spectrum of application of minimally invasive spinal surgical procedures is being broadened by further research and feasibility studies. New, challenging tasks of the future are use of the arthroscope for visual diagnosis of various spinal disorders, therapeutic delivery of inflammatory agent inhibitors, and even intradiskal repair and tissue restoration.

Finally, minimally invasive arthroscopic spine surgery is a skill-oriented procedure and should not be attempted without proper training and exposure to the surgical techniques. In a properly selected patient population, a satisfactory outcome compatible with that in open procedures should be realized.

References

1. Kambin P: Arthroscopic lumbar interbody fusion, in White AH, Schofferman JA (eds): *Spine Care.* St. Louis, MO, Mosby-Year Book, 1995, vol 2, pp 1055–1066.
2. Kambin P: Posterolateral percutaneous lumbar interbody fusion, in Kambin P (ed): *Arthroscopic Microdiscectomy: Minimal Intervention in Spinal Surgery.* Baltimore, MD, Urban & Schwarzenberg, 1991, pp 117–121.
3. Obenchain TG: Laparoscopic lumbar discectomy: Case report. *J Laparoendosc Surg* 1991;1:145–149.
4. Regan JJ, Mack MJ, Picetti GD III: A technical report on video-assisted thoracoscopy in thoracic spinal surgery: Preliminary description. *Spine* 1995;20:831–837.
5. Kambin P, Gellman H: Percutaneous lateral discectomy of the lumbar spine: A preliminary report. *Clin Orthop* 1983;174:127–132.
6. Hijikata S: Percutaneous nucleotomy: A new concept and 12 years' experience. *Clin Orthop* 1989;238:9–23.
7. Kambin P: History of disc surgery, in Kambin P (ed): *Arthroscopic Microdiscectomy: Minimal Intervention in Spinal Surgery.* Baltimore, MD, Urban & Schwarzenberg, 1991, pp 3–8.
8. Onik G, Maroon JC, Jackson R: Cauda equina syndrome secondary to an improperly placed nucleotome probe. *Neurosurgery* 1992;30:412–415.
9. Epstein NE: Surgically confirmed cauda equina and nerve root injury following percutaneous discectomy at an outside institution: A case report. *J Spinal Disord* 1990;3:380–383.
10. Kambin P: Percutaneous lumbar discectomy: Current practice. *Surg Rounds Orthop* 1988;2:31–35.
11. Kambin P: Arthroscopic microdiscectomy laser nucleolysis. *Philadelphia Med* 1991;87:548–549.
12. Kambin P: Arthroscopic microdiscectomy. *Arthroscopy* 1992;8:287–295.
13. Schaffer JL, Kambin P: Percutaneous posterolateral lumbar discectomy and decompression with a 6.9-millimeter cannula: Analysis of operative failures and complications. *J Bone Joint Surg* 1991;73A:822–831.
14. Kirkaldy-Willis WH, Wedge JH, Yong-Hing K, et al: Pathology and pathogenesis of lumbar spondylosis and stenosis. *Spine* 1978;3:319–328.
15. Kambin P, Nixon JE, Chait A, et al: Annular protrusion: Pathophysiology and roentgenographic appearance. *Spine* 1988;13:671–675.

16. Crock HV: Internal disc disruption: A challenge to disc prolapse fifty years on. *Spine* 1986;11:650–653.

17. Kambin P: Arthroscopic microdiscectomy: Lumbar and thoracic, in White AH, Schofferman JA (eds): *Spine Care*. St. Louis, MO, Mosby-Year Book, 1995, pp 1002–1016.

18. Kambin P: The role of minimally invasive spinal surgery in spinal disorders, in Stauffer R, Kostuik JP (eds): *Advances in Operative Orthopaedics*. St. Louis, MO, Mosby-Year Book, 1995, vol 3, pp 147–171.

19. Smith L, Garvin PJ, Gesler RM, et al: Enzyme dissolution of the nucleus pulposus. *Nature* 1963;198:1311–1312.

20. Schwetschenau PR, Ramirez A, Johnston J, et al: Double-blind evaluation of intradiscal chymopapain for herniated lumbar discs: Early results. *J Neurosurg* 1976;45:622–627.

21. Martins AN, Ramirez A, Johnston J, et al: Double-blind evaluation of chemonucleolysis for herniated lumbar discs: Late results. *J Neurosurg* 1978;49:816–827.

22. Brown MD, Daroff RB: The double blind study comparing Discase to placebo: An editorial comment. *Spine* 1977;2:233–236.

23. Javid MJ, Nordby EJ, Ford LT, et al: Safety and efficacy of chymopapain (Chymodiactin) in herniated nucleus pulposus with sciatica: Results of a randomized, double-blind study. *JAMA* 1983;249:2489–2494.

24. Fraser RD: Chymopapain for the treatment of intervertebral disc herniation: The final report of a double-blind study. *Spine* 1984;9:815–818.

25. Onik G, Helms CA, Ginsburg L, et al: Percutaneous lumbar diskectomy using a new aspiration probe. *Am J Roentgenol* 1985;144:1137–1140.

26. Maroon JC, Onik G, Sternau L: Percutaneous automated discectomy: A new approach to lumbar surgery. *Clin Orthop* 1989;238:64–70.

27. Davis GW, Onik G: Clinical experience with automated percutaneous lumbar discectomy. *Clin Orthop* 1989;238:98–103.

28. Suguro T, Oegema TR Jr, Bradford DS: The effects of chymopapain on prolapsed human intervertebral disc: A clinical and correlative histochemical study. *Clin Orthop* 1986;213:223–231.

29. Choy DS, Case RB, Fielding W, et al: Letter: Percutaneous laser nucleolysis of lumbar disks. *N Engl J Med* 1987;317:771–772.

30. Kambin P: Arthroscopic microdiscectomy: Laser nuclear ablation, in Sherk HH (ed): *Laser Discectomy*. Philadelphia, PA, Hanley & Belfus, 1993, pp 95–101.

31. Kahanovitz N, Viola K, Goldstein T, et al: A multicenter analysis of percutaneous discectomy. *Spine* 1990;15:713–715.

32. Revel M, Payan C, Vallee C, et al: Automated percutaneous lumbar discectomy versus chemonucleolysis in the treatment of sciatica: A randomized multicenter trial. *Spine* 1993;18:1–7.

33. Craig FS: Vertebral-body biopsy. *J Bone Joint Surg* 1956;38A:93–102.

34. Ottolenghi CE: Diagnosis of orthopaedic lesions by aspiration biopsy: Results of 1,061 punctures. *J Bone Joint Surg* 1955;37A:443–464.

35. Kambin P, Sampson S: Posterolateral percutaneous suction-excision of herniated lumbar intervertebral discs: Report of interim results. *Clin Orthop* 1986;207:37–43.

36. Kambin P, Schaffer JL: Percutaneous lumbar discectomy: Review of 100 patients and current practice. *Clin Orthop* 1989;238:24–34.

37. Kambin P: Posterolateral percutaneous lumbar discectomy and decompression: Arthroscopic microdiscectomy, in Kambin P (ed): *Arthroscopic Microdiscectomy: Minimal Intervention in Spinal Surgery*. Baltimore, MD, Urban & Schwarzenberg, 1991, pp 67–100.

38. Kambin P: Arthroscopic microdiskectomy. *Semin Orthop* 1991;6:97–108.

39. Kambin P: Arthroscopic techniques for spinal surgery, in McGinty JB, Caspari RB, Jackson RW, et al (eds): *Operative Arthroscopy,* ed 2. Philadelphia, PA, Lippincott-Raven, 1996, pp 1215–1225.

40. Kambin P: Arthroscopic microdiscectomy of the lumbar spine. *Clin Sports Med* 1993;12:143–150.

153

41. Kambin P, Brager MD: Percutaneous posterolateral discectomy: Anatomy and mechanism. *Clin Orthop* 1987;223:145–154.
42. Peterson RH: Posterolateral microdiskectomy in a general orthopaedic practice. *Semin Orthop* 1991;6:117
43. Kambin P, Schaffer JL, Zhou L: Incidence of complications and failures following percutaneous posterolateral arthroscopic disc surgery. *Orthop Trans* 1995;19:404–405.
44. Kambin P, Cohen LF, Brooks M, et al: Development of degenerative spondylosis of the lumbar spine after partial discectomy: Comparison of laminotomy, discectomy, and posterolateral discectomy. *Spine* 1995;20:599–607.
45. Smyth MJ, Wright V: Sciatica and the intervertebral disc: An experimental study. *J Bone Joint Surg* 1958;40A:1401–1418.
46. Parke WW: The significance of venous return impairment in ischemic radiculopathy and myelopathy. *Orthop Clin North Am* 1991;22:213–221.
47. Olmarker K, Rydevik B, Holm S: Edema formation in spinal nerve roots induced by experimental, graded compression: An experimental study on the pig cauda equina with special reference to differences in effects between rapid and slow onset of compression. *Spine* 1989;14:569–573.
48. Hoyland JA, Freemont AJ, Jayson MI: Intervertebral foramen venous obstruction: A cause of periradicular fibrosis? *Spine* 1989;14:558–568.

Directions for Future Research

Study the natural history of disk abnormalities seen on advanced imaging studies.

Imaging studies have shown that disk abnormalities (bulges, annular tears, herniations, dehydration, degeneration) are common in asymptomatic persons. However, it is less clear whether these abnormalities predict the likelihood of future disk herniations, sciatica, or back pain. Even among symptomatic persons, the prognostic significance of these abnormalities is unclear. That is, do these lesions portend worse outcomes or response to therapy? Thus, longitudinal studies are needed to identify persons with and without specific anatomic lesions (by imaging tests such as magnetic resonance imaging (MRI)), and follow them at intervals for development or resolution of anatomic lesions and/or symptoms. Furthermore, such studies could help characterize the symptom complexes (if any) associated with specific anatomic lesions. Knowledge of this natural history could influence the design of preventive strategies, treatments, and the timing of interventions.

Determine the factors that lead to the recurrence of acute herniated nucleus pulposus.

Low back pain and sciatica in subjects with herniated nucleus pulposus (HNP) have a higher recurrence rate than that of unaffected patients. Information gathered from studies of patients after their initial acute episode has resolved would help explain the risk factors for recurrence and provide the basis for preventive approaches.

Specific hypotheses should be developed on factors (for example, patient variables, clinical and diagnostic findings, treatments used) that may predispose a patient to a subsequent acute HNP event. The previous episode should have been resolved for a defined period of time. A 3- to 5-year follow-up with periodic patient evaluations should yield important information.

Conduct randomized, controlled trials to investigate the efficacy of nonsurgical therapy in patients with herniated nucleus pulposus.

Although HNP may result in acute, disabling pain in many patients, its natural history is generally one of spontaneous improvement over time for the majority of patients. A variety of nonsurgical treatments are currently widely prescribed to reduce pain and allow return to function without surgery. Exercise programs, bracing, bed rest, oral medications, and epidural steriod therapy are among treatments currently used. The efficacy, cost-effectiveness, and long-term benefit of these and other treatments have not been determined in well-controlled, randomized, prospective trials. The studies should have clearly defined inclusion and exclusion criteria. The studies must be placebo-controlled to account for the 70% good to excellent results expected with natural history. Cotreatments must be standardized, and follow-up should be at least 1 year to account for deteriorating results (or recurrences) in various treatment groups. Outcomes measures must be clearly defined. Cost comparisons should be made relative to the control groups. Outcomes measures must be clearly defined. Cost comparisons should be made relative to the control groups, and to historical surgical groups as well.

Identify prognostic factors in patients with herniated nucleus pulposus and/or sciatica.

HNP with sciatica is a condition that usually resolves over time. It is unclear what factors (occupational, genetic, socioeconomic, etc) lead to delayed recovery and/or no recovery without surgical intervention. Further, surgical procedures are not always successful, and outcome studies would help better define programs.

The "natural" history of HNP and/or sciatica is not clearly defined; there are no direct obstacles to performing such a study, and the epidemiologic methodology exists. Return to function should be determined at several levels. Previous outcome studies for nonspecific low back pain have included separate patient groups, including those with sciatica, which would be helpful in designing future studies.

Study the accuracy, reproducibility, and validity of parameters used in the diagnosis of herniated disks, including history, physical examination, imaging studies, and electrodiagnostics.

Tests used to confirm the diagnosis of disk herniations have not been well characterized because of the lack of a widely accepted, practical gold standard and anatomic evidence of disk herniations in the absence of clinical symptoms. Careful analysis of the sensitivity, specificity, and predictive value of different diagnostic tests used in patients with disk herniations will result in more appropriate test selection and usage. Studies of reproducibility are needed for most tests currently in use.

Study the reasons for the large variation in surgical treatment that exists between and within countries.

Large variations in surgical rates exist locally, regionally, and across countries. Although the appropriate surgical rates are unknown, the reasons why these differences exist must be determined. Cultural, economic, and educational reasons have been suggested. Differences in treatment expectations, socioeconomic systems, reimbursement, surgical training and philosophy, and pain acceptance are certainly possible reasons that need to be defined and studied using scientific methods.

Determine the optimal timing for diagnostic imaging and therapeutic interventions in patients with lumbar radiculopathy.

Wide variability in timing of imaging and treatment for radiculopathy is observed among different geographic regions and different types of providers. There are few data regarding the optimal timing of diagnostic and therapeutic interventions with regard to impact on clinical outcome and health care costs.

A prospective study should be performed to compare patients with lumbar radiculopathy randomized to receive early imaging (for example, MRI within 2 weeks of symptom onset) or late imaging (MRI only as a preoperative study for patients about to undergo surgery; that is, patients refractory to nonsurgical management). A second group of studies should be designed to determine the optimal timing for various nonsurgical and surgical interventions. Special effort should be made to measure influences of timing on clinical outcome, use of services (referrals, additional tests, treatments), and costs. Costs should include both direct medical costs and the indirect costs of work absenteeism and wage compensation.

Develop randomized, controlled trials of surgical intervention techniques.

Herniated lumbar intervertebral disks are commonly treated with surgery. Despite success rates of approximately 90% with open disk excision, several "less invasive" treatment interventions have been recently introduced. The precise success rates with these techniques are difficult to determine because of variations in indications for surgery, efficacy of technique developers and proponents, differences in timing and technical expertise, nonstandardization of outcome measures, and variable expectations from patients and providers. Additionally, a true measure of the cost of such treatments and the period of functional disability after these treatments are unknown.

Areas that should be studied include comparison of the "new" arthroscopic techniques and percutaneous procedures to standardized limited open diskectomy and microdiskectomy. Additionally, the results of disk excision alone in the treatment of symptomatic recurrent disk herniation should be compared to those of disk excision with fusion.

Prospective, randomized, controlled studies with standardized entry, treatment, and outcome measures are the best way to obtain this information. A by-product of this research would be to identify anatomic or pathologic factors in lumbar disk tissues that influence disk herniation. Many advances in diagnosis and treatment have been based on observations made at autopsy and/or at examination of surgical specimens. Analysis of interventional disk tissue may give insight into pathologic change in the disk, collagen and monopolysaccharide formation and structure, and cellular viability and activity. Cellular response to pharmacologic agents, growth factors, and physical/mechanical parameters may assist in understanding the disease process and lead to its prevention and treatment.

Identify risk factors for disk degeneration and herniation and the approximate magnitude of their effects.

Before prevention approaches can be considered, an understanding of the etiology and risk factors for disk degeneration and herniation is necessary. The value of epidemiologic studies of "symptomatic disk herniation" (and other back-related conditions) has been limited by problems with measurement of both risk factors and outcomes, definition of cases, and failure to adequately control confounding factors. These methodologic issues must be addressed to improve the quality of epidemiologic studies.

One area of particular interest concerns genetic influences. Studies based on familial aggregation suggest that genetic influences may determine disk degeneration and herniation to a substantial degree. Additional investigations are

157

needed, however, to differentiate the effects of genetic influences from those of shared environments, to estimate the general magnitude of these effects, and to investigate possible gene-environment interactions.

The effects of other suspected risk factors, such as specific physical loading conditions and whole-body vibration are also of interest, but improved measurement methods are needed.

Section Two

Basic and Applied Science Issues of Lumbar Radiculopathy

Section Editor:
Björn L. Rydevik, MD, PhD

Raymond W. Colburn, BS
Joyce A. DeLeo, PhD
Marshall Devor, PhD
Kenneth A. Follett, MD, PhD
Gerald F. Gebhart, PhD
Vijay K. Goel, PhD
Hiroshi Hashizume, MD
Mamoru Kawakami, MD, PhD
Shigeru Kobayashi, MD, PhD

Tomofumi Morita, MD, PhD
Robert R. Myers, PhD
Sadaaki Nakai, MD, PhD
Kjell Olmarker, MD, PhD
Naoyuki Shizu, MD
Tetsuya Tamaki, MD, PhD
James N. Weinstein, DO, MS
Hidezo Yoshizawa, MD, PhD

Overview

Peripheral Mechanisms

The initial precipitating event for a herniated nucleus pulposus (HNP) is a change in the internal pressure that results in altered disk kinematics with a concomitant change in internal distribution of mechanical stresses. This change leads to altered fluid flow in the disk, which in turn results in an increase in the physiologic disk bulge. If severe enough, the increase may result in circumferential or radial tears, which lead to changes in the end plate and extrusion of the anulus, followed by extrusion of the nucleus pulposus. The material extruded from the disk includes cells from the anulus and nucleus pulposus as well as from the end plate.

Mechanical Effects of Herniated Nucleus Pulposus on Nerve Roots

Acute compression of a normal nerve or nerve root does not cause more than a brief painful response. The size of the disk herniation does not determine the severity of the pain. Compression of the dura may cause reduced blood flow to the nerve root, but there are insufficient data to state that mechanical deformation of the dura could cause pain.

Ischemia to the nerve and resulting Schwann cell injury leading to demyelination have not been demonstrated to be associated with behavioral changes associated with neuropathic pain. Prolonged or severe ischemia may result in axonal breakdown with wallerian degeneration, which, in animal models, results in pain behavior. Injury to the nerve results in alterations in both anterograde and retrograde axonal transport, as well as changes in the distribution of membrane sodium channels. Direct mechanical compression may injure the myelin sheaths, leading to segmental demyelination. The effects of mechanical deformation on axonal membranes is less well known. Information from imaging studies indicates that direct compression by HNP on dorsal root ganglion is uncommon. Tension of the nerve root may have mechanical effects on the dorsal root ganglion, but the consequences of such effects are not known.

Biochemical Effects of Herniated Nucleus Pulposus on Nerve Roots

A considerable amount of research has been performed recently regarding the release of various biochemical products associated with disk herniation and their effects on nervous tissue. In particular, HNP is associated with the release of a variety of cytokines as well as an apparent increase in the synthesis of certain cytokines as a result of triggering of nucleus pulposus cells. Some cytokines have a direct effect on the structure of the nerve fibers and stimulate Schwann cells/glial cells as well as the release of certain neuropeptides. Substance P can cause changes in blood flow and microvascular permeability. Immunocompetent cells, such as T cells, have been identified in HNP specimens obtained at surgery.

Spinal Cord Mechanisms

Experimental data on the effect of nucleus pulposus-induced nerve root injury on pain mechanisms in the spinal cord are minimal. However, it may be reasonable to extrapolate current knowledge from studies on peripheral pain from other tissues. Certain inferences may be made from the numerous studies on the effect of peripheral nerve injury on the spinal cord. If sensitization following nerve injury occurs in the nerve root in the same manner as in peripheral nerves, pain responses could result from mechanical, ischemic, or chemical stimulation of the nerve fibers rather than from direct nociceptive stimulation.

Brain Stem and Cortical Mechanisms

No information is available on the effects of HNP on brain or brain stem pain mechanisms, and the general knowledge on such mechanisms is sparse. There seems to be increased function in the thalamus, somatosensory cortex, and cingulate gyrus in response to painful peripheral stimulation. Based on observations regarding the strong association between psychological factors and low back pain, especially chronic low back pain syndromes, central mechanisms have been thought to play a greater role in the perception of spinal pain than in the perception of pain from other tissues.

Chapter 11

The Role of Cytokines in Nociception and Chronic Pain

Joyce A. DeLeo, PhD
Raymond W. Colburn, BS

Introduction

Back pain affects 50% to 80% of the adult population at some point in their lives; the cause is unknown in approximately 85% of the cases. Understanding the pathophysiologic mechanisms responsible for the development of low back and leg pain after lumbar disk herniation and lumbar canal stenosis may provide more effective therapy as well as information about possible prevention of the pain. A wealth of experimental and clinical data have been generated in the study of neuropathic pain following peripheral nerve and root injury. These data may be applied to understanding the mechanisms of chronic pain following the compression of nerve roots or dorsal root ganglia (DRG) that occurs in disk herniation and stenosis.

Very recently, basic scientific research has focused on the role of cytokines in acute nociception and the generation of chronic neurogenic pain. A cytokine can generally be defined as any polypeptide that affects the functions of other cells. They are trophic regulatory proteins that can be broadly classified into four major groups: growth factors, interleukins, interferons, and tumor necrosis factors. This chapter will review the accumulating evidence supporting the role of specific cytokines in the establishment of pain states. General information on representative cytokines from each major group will be provided and then data will be discussed in the context of nociception.

Following this overview, experimental data will be presented on neuroimmune responses resulting from two distinct peripheral nerve injuries that produce neuropathic pain in the rat. Our sciatic cryoneurolysis (SCN) model[1] and the chronic constriction injury (CCI) model[2] are both well-established mononeuropathy models with differential behavioral outcomes. SCN is described as a complete, albeit temporary peripheral nerve lesion that results in a delayed but sustained mechanical allodynia (enhanced sensitivity to a non-noxious stimulus) without evidence of thermal hyperalgesia (increased sensitivity to a noxious stimulus). The CCI model involves a partial, chemically generated nerve lesion that results in an almost immediate, but transient mechanical allodynia and thermal hyperalgesia. Differential neuroimmune reactions in these animal models may provide important insight into the mechanisms that generate and maintain neuropathic pain behaviors after different types of nerve injury. These results might then be extrapolated to the study of mechanisms responsible for idiopathic low back pain.

Overview

Background on Cytokines

Cytokines influence a variety of cellular functions including proliferation, differentiation, gene expression, regulation of numerous components of immune and inflammatory responses, and control of synthesis of matrix proteins that are important to cell growth and tissue repair.[3] The role cytokines play in influencing the nervous system is currently under intense scrutiny. For example, following nerve injury, local release of cytokines directs the process of peripheral nerve degeneration and regeneration.[4] Moreover, cytokines may play a role in the generation of neuropathic pain both in the periphery and in the central nervous system (CNS). Following a peripheral nerve injury, polymorphonuclear leukocytes at the site of injury attract monocytes, which differentiate into macrophages.[5,6] Schwann cells, glial cells of the peripheral nervous system, respond to nerve injury by phagocytizing debris and reforming myelin sheaths around damaged axons. The activated macrophages and Schwann cells secrete cytokines and specific growth factors required for nerve regeneration. Although it is unlikely that macrophages or Schwann cells directly invade the CNS, the cytokines they produce may be transported retrograde via axonal or nonaxonal mechanisms.[7] Cytokines can then accumulate in the DRG, dorsal horn neurons, glia, or perivascular structures where they can have profound effects on neuronal activity.

Factors generated at the site of injury are a necessary component to pain behaviors generated by the nerve injury. This indication is supported by the finding that blocking axonal transport by topical colchicine prevents hyperalgesia in the CCI model of neuropathic pain.[8] In response to nerve injury, such as axotomy, cytokines are also produced within the CNS by activated microglia and astrocytes.[9] Microglia are morphologically, immunophenotypically, and functionally related to cells of the macrophage lineage. They are the first cell types to respond to several types of CNS injury. Microglia release, as well as respond to, several cytokines, including interleukin (IL) -1, IL-6, tumor necrosis factor-alpha (TNF-α), interferon-gamma (IFN-γ), and transforming growth factor-beta (TGF-β). These cytokines are instrumental in astrocytic activation, induction of cell adhesion molecule expression, and recruitment of T cells at the lesion site. In addition to the synthesis of inflammatory mediators, microglia act as cytotoxic effector cells by releasing other harmful substances, such as proteases, reactive oxygen intermediates, and nitric oxide.[10]

It is likely that certain cytokines are involved in synaptic plasticity and hyperexcitability due to their ability to produce long-term potentiation.[11,12] We have hypothesized that an imbalance of such peptides may lead to spinal hypersensitization and abnormal peripheral nerve regeneration, the pathologic correlate to chronic neuropathic pain (Fig. 1). Pharmacologic manipulation to prevent or attenuate this sensitization may involve the peripheral or central administration of specific cytokine antagonists in the event of excess produc-

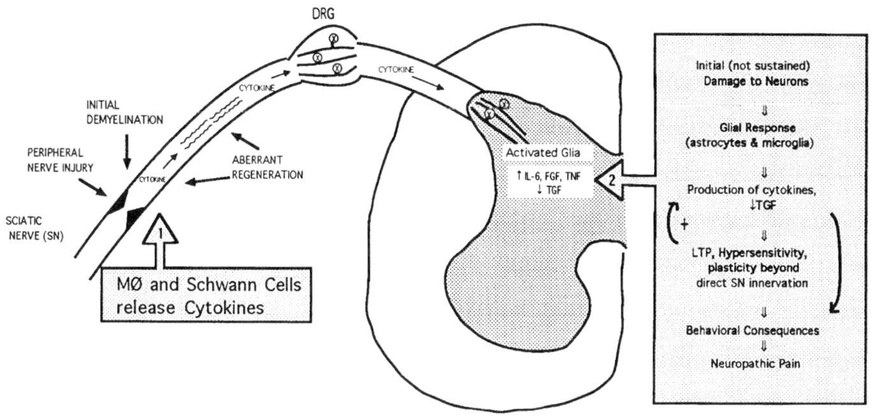

Fig. 1 *Proposed theoretical model of the role of cytokines and neuropathic pain. 1 indicates proposed peripheral mechanism for cytokine and growth factor involvement in neuropathic pain. 2 indicates central glial response as a consequence of dorsal horn neuronal damage following a peripheral nerve injury. MØ = macrophages, DRG = dorsal root ganglion, GF = growth factors, LTP = long-term potentiation, SN = sciatic nerve, IL-6 = interleukin-6, FGF = fibroblast growth factor, TNF = tumor necrosis factor, TGF = transforming growth factor.*

tion or administration of an anticytokine, such as TGF-β or IL-10. This approach has immediate clinical potential because specific cytokines and their neutralizing antibodies have been introduced into clinical trials for the treatment of stroke, Alzheimer's disease, autoimmune diseases, wound healing, and amyotrophic lateral sclerosis.[13-15] Extensive characterization of peripheral and central cytokine profiles is needed following nerve and nerve root injuries in order to focus such therapeutic interventions for the treatment of acute and chronic neurogenic pain.

The following sections will briefly review recent major findings of specific growth factors, interleukins, interferons, and tumor necrosis factors as they relate to the generation of acute and chronic pain. Table 1 summarizes these specific cytokine activities.

Growth Factors

The last 10 years have seen the polypeptide growth factors emerging as a distinct and major subgroup of the cytokines. By definition, growth factors control cell proliferation but they may also regulate many cellular processes, such as differentiation, protein expression, and even cell survival. Most tissues produce and respond to growth factors and the CNS is no exception. A number of different growth factors have been found in the mature and developing CNS, where their occurrence may be due to local synthesis, systemic uptake, or axonal transport from the periphery. This section will review three growth factors: Nerve growth factor (NGF), basic fibroblast growth factor (bFGF) and TGF-β. One of the most important and well-studied of the growth factors is NGF, especially in

Table 1 Summary of cytokines known to play a role in nociception

Family	Members*	Major Finding in Pain Research
Growth factors	NGF	NGF induces hyperalgesia
	bFGF	Increases following peripheral or central injury
	TGF-β	Induced following axotomy, limits glial activation, inhibits proinflammatory cytokines such as IL-6
Interleukins	IL-1	Produces both analgesia and algesia depending on biologic system
	IL-6	Induces pain behaviors, increased in SCN model
	IL-10	Limits cytokine-mediated inflammatory hyperalgesia
Interferons	IFN-γ	Facilitates spinal nociceptor flexor reflex; mechanism may involve nitric oxide
Tumor necrosis factors	TNF-α	TNF-α antagonist eliminates observed hyperalgesia following endotoxin administration

*NGF, nerve growth factor; bFGF, basic fibroblast growth factor; TGF, transforming growth factor; IL, interleukin; IFN, interferon; TNF, tumor necrosis factor; SCN, sciatic cryoneurolysis-neuropathic pain model in the rat

regards to nociception. This growth factor will be discussed in more detail to illustrate receptor and signal transduction mechanisms common to many cytokines.

Nerve Growth Factor NGF is the classic target-derived factor responsible for the survival and maintenance of specific peripheral and central neurons during development and maturation.[16,17] It is known to be active in such processes as inflammatory cell differentiation and axonal phenotype modulation, as well as expression and secretion of neuropeptides, neurotransmitters, ion channel proteins, and other cytokines, both centrally and peripherally. These properties most likely contribute to NGF's newfound identity as a major link between inflammation and hyperalgesia.[18]

The NGF gene family, in addition to NGF, includes brain-derived neurotrophic factor (BDNF) and neurotrophins -3, and -4/5. All are members of a family of neurotrophins that can interact independently with p75 (low affinity neurotrophin receptor) or selectivity with specific members of the *Trk* (tropomyosin receptor kinase) family of receptor tyrosine kinases.[19,20] Binding of neurotrophins to these receptors initiates *Trk* dimerization and autophosphorylation of tyrosine residues, which, in turn, activates cytosolic signaling cascades, retrograde transport of activated factors to the cell body, and regulation of specific gene expression.[21] The role of the p75 neurotrophin receptor is less well understood in that no clear cytosolic or nuclear effector pathway has been delineated, although a sphingomyelin signaling pathway recently has been proposed.[22] The presence of the p75 in conjunction with *TrkA* (specific *Trk* receptor for NGF) is known to modulate *Trk* tyrosine kinase activity, enhance ligand discrimination, and increase the activity for the high affinity NGF site.[23] The highly regulated expression of these two types of receptors (p75 and *Trk*A) in development and in response to injury could provide for marked differential tissue sensitivities to NGF. Recent evidence supports the concept that neurotrophins and their receptors are synthesized within certain neuronal populations and could conceivably exert paracrine or autocrine effects on neuronal survival and excitability.[24]

NGF is produced primarily as a target-derived factor in the periphery and taken up at the terminals of peripheral axonal processes. In this manner, NGF directs sprouting and peripheral innervation in developing sensory and sympathetic neurons.[25] Beyond a critical developmental period, sensory neurons are not dependent on NGF for survival, and NGF is not expressed to a significant extent in adult peripheral nerves. Following nerve injury, there is a massive increase in NGF mRNA in a peripheral nerve just proximal to the lesion, along the distal nerve segment, and in the peripheral target tissue. This rapid increase is followed by a second localized increase (starting at 2 to 3 days) in NGF mRNA that lasts several weeks. The prolonged phase is predominantly due to IL-1 release by macrophages invading the injured nerve. This effect of IL-1 is via both enhanced translation and transcription of NGF that probably occurs in endoneurial fibroblasts or Schwann cells.[26]

Although constitutive levels of NGF are required for axonal maintenance and peripheral innervation adjustments, the effects of a nerve lesion attenuate NGF levels at the DRG and increase NGF in the periphery. Paradoxically, both these situations may ultimately promote pain behaviors. In deafferented spinal nerves, sympathetic postganglionic neurons sprout from perivascular structures to form close associations with medium to large diameter neurons in the DRG.[27] By effectively setting the sensitivity on afferent stimulation, these sympathetic connections provide an anatomic substrate for sympathetically maintained pain.[28] Exogenous NGF delivered to the proximal stump of a transected sciatic nerve ameliorates many of the morphologic, biochemical, and electrophysiologic alterations in the axotomized DRG cell bodies.[29-31]

In the periphery, exaggerated levels of NGF, whether by transgenic overexpression or exogenous application, have been shown to result in thermal and mechanical hyperalgesia.[32,33] Similarly, scenarios that enhance NGF expression, such as partial deafferentation or focal inflammation, are associated with hyperalgesia.[34] Mechanisms of NGF-induced hyperalgesia include: (1) acute sensitization of C fibers to thermal stimuli in the periphery, thereby inducing a rapid hyperalgesia. This sensitization may be due to the degranulation of mast cells, which results in the release of autocoids, such as prostaglandins and bradykinin.[18] In addition, low concentrations of NGF directly prolong action potentials on primary afferent nociceptive neurons.[35] (2) A latent, longer lasting thermal hyperalgesia may be mediated by increased expression of neuropeptides in the DRG, which results in N-methyl-D-aspartate (NMDA)-mediated central sensitization.[18] NGF affects prolonged changes in sensory neuron excitability via tyrosine kinase linked transcription factors and specific gene expression. NGF has been shown to increase the synthesis, axonal transport, and neuronal content in both central and peripheral terminals of the algesic neuropeptides, substance P and calcitonin gene-related peptide,[36,37] as well as to increase Na^+ channel expression.[38] There is also evidence to demonstrate that NGF decreases the inhibitory neurotransmitter gamma-aminobutyric acid (GABA).[39] (3) A mechanical hyperalgesia may be produced by a non-NMDA mediated central sensitization.[33] Unlike other cytokines, eg, IL-1 and IL-6, exogenous NGF administration does not produce allodynic or spontaneous pain behaviors. Therefore, these behaviors must be mediated through other possibly low threshold mechanoreceptor, sympathetic, and/or central mechanisms.

Basic Fibroblast Growth Factor Other growth factors also appear to be involved in the response to nerve injury. The FGF family contains seven different, closely related proteins.[40,41] Two of these, acidic and basic FGF, stimulate mitogenesis and act as neurotrophic factors that promote the survival and regeneration of neurons. bFGF increases after transection of the optic nerve or following CNS injury.[42] We are presently investigating its role in neuropathic pain. Our preliminary data have shown a differential expression of bFGF in our SCN and the CCI models of mononeuropathy.

Transforming Growth Factor-Beta The family of TGF-β comprises five different isoforms (TGF-β1 to -β5). TGF-β1 is found in meninges, choroid plexus, peripheral ganglia, and nerves.[43] Its mRNA is induced following axotomy and may be involved in a negative feedback loop to limit the extent of glial activation.[9] This growth factor inhibits macrophage activation and T cell proliferation to counteract the effects of proinflammatory cytokines, such as IL-6.[15] TGF-β1 also antagonizes nitric oxide production in macrophages.[44] As will be discussed further, nitric oxide has been strongly implicated in the final common pathway of neuropathic pain.[45] Thus, by its anticytokine action, TGF-β1 may prove to be an effective therapy for neuropathic pain.

Interleukins

The interleukins are a family of cytokines, secreted by lymphocytes and mononuclear phagocytes, that mainly induce growth and differentiation. Although there are at least 15 recognized interleukins, this discussion will focus only on IL-1, -6, and -10 due to recent data that support their interaction in pain mechanisms.

IL-1 has multiple roles in inflammation and in the immune response. It has two forms, IL-1α and IL-1β. The latter is the form secreted in plasma and tissue fluids and is the predominant molecule in brain tissue.[12] IL-1β production was enhanced following a crush injury to a peripheral nerve[46] and in the CNS after trauma in microglia and astrocytes.[47] Of particular importance to the role of cytokines in nociception, IL-1β mimics the hyperalgesic action of illness-inducing substances, such as lithium chloride and endotoxin. This hyperalgesia is abolished by the systemic administration of an IL-1 receptor antagonist (IL-1ra).[48,49] Paradoxically, IL-1β also has potent peripheral antinociceptive effects on inflamed but not on noninflamed tissue.[50,51] This action has been explained by the finding that cytokines stimulate the release of endogenous opioid peptides from immune cells.[52] This release subsequently activates opioid receptors on sensory nerves to inhibit nociception. However, IL-1β not only induces the long-term increase of axonally transported opioid receptors, but also enhances the production of substance P, one of the major inflammatory and nociceptive mediators.[53] The final physiologic outcome, ie, analgesia or hyperalgesia, may depend on the exquisite balance and modulation in both the periphery and CNS of these peptides in a given injured state.

IL-6 is synthesized by mononuclear phagocytes, vascular endothelial cells, fibroblasts, and other cells in response to IL-1 and TNF. IL-6 is produced both locally, at the site of peripheral nerve injury, and centrally, in response to nerve damage. In the sciatic nerve, IL-6 production was induced distal to the site of a crush injury, possibly by Schwann cells.[54] Centrally, IL-6 is known to be produced by astrocytes and microglia.[55,56] The presence of IL-6 mRNA is one of the earliest changes observed in the spinal cord following peripheral axotomy.[9] Endogenously produced IL-6 may act as an important early signal for glial activation following nerve injury. This activity may be important because we have observed a delayed, but sustained, astrocytic reaction in the spinal cord in our neuropathic pain animal model. Our laboratory also has immunocytochemical and behavioral data to support a direct involvement of IL-6 in allodynia behavior following a peripheral nerve injury in the rat.

To add to the complexity of cytokine action in biologic systems, certain cytokines inhibit the production of proinflammatory cytokines. IL-10 is one such anticytokine that has been shown to suppress macrophage functions, such as class II expression,[57] cell surface adhesion,[58] and the synthesis of certain cytokines, eg, IL-1β, IL-6, IL-8, and TNF-α.[59-62] In an animal model of mechanical hyperalgesia, the hyperalgesic responses to bradykinin, TNF-α, IL-1β, and IL-6 was inhibited by prior treatment with IL-10.[61] In further studies, this group also demonstrated that IL-10 limited inflammatory hyperalgesia by both inhibition of cytokine production and inhibition of IL-1β-evoked prostaglandin E_2 production.

Interferons

The IFNs are a group of proteins classified as IFN-α, IFN-β, and IFN-γ. Recent attention in the neurosciences has been focused on IFN-γ since the discovery of a distinct neuronal form that is larger than the immune IFN-γ but shares multiple immunologic epitopes.[62] Xu and associates[63] reported that intrathecal IFN-γ facilitated the spinal nociceptive flexor reflex in the rat. It was postulated that IFN-γ released in the CNS following injury may participate in eliciting pain and hyperalgesia. The mechanisms underlying this participation in pain are unknown. However, recent data have demonstrated the coinduction of neuronal IFN-γ and nitric oxide synthase (NOS), the enzyme responsible for the synthesis of nitric oxide in rat motor neurons after axotomy.[64] In addition, Xu and associates[63] have showed that an NOS inhibitor blocked the reflex facilitory effect of IFN-γ, indicating that IFN-γ activated the L-arginine–nitric oxide pathway in the spinal cord. Evidence strongly supports a major role played by the synthesis of nitric oxide in the mediation of prolonged spinal cord excitability. For example, NOS inhibitors have been shown to block the hyperalgesic effect of intrathecal NMDA and behavioral responses in the formalin test.[65]

Tumor Necrosis Factors

The TNFs include TNF-α, also known as cachectin, and TNF-β, also known as lymphotoxin.[66,67] These factors produce a wide variety of similar but not identical biologic effects. One major action of these factors is the ability to kill certain tumor cells from which their names are derived. The TNFs are referred to as "inflammatory cytokines" because they have a role in initiating (along with IL-1) the cascade of other cytokines and factors in the immune response. TNF-α has been implicated in enhancing pain responsivity following administration of illness-inducing substances, such as lithium chloride, lipopolysaccharide (LPS), and endotoxin.[49] When a TNF-α antagonist is administered systemically, the hyperalgesia observed after LPS is completely eliminated, suggesting that TNF, like IL-1, is a critical cytokine for the induction of LPS hyperalgesia.

Summary

This brief review demonstrates the possible role of specific cytokines in nociception and hyperalgesia. The following section will provide data from our laboratory on the peripheral and spinal neuroimmunologic responses following peripheral nerve injury in the rat. The use of experimental neuropathic pain models has provided and will continue to provide invaluable information that may help explain the etiology of clinical back pain. In particular, Kawakami and associates[68,69] have developed an animal model of lumbar radiculopathy. They suggest that the development of lumbar radiculopathy may be due to a local chemical contribution from injured tissue. Clinical studies support this suggestion that a chemical inflammatory reaction within or around nerve roots may be necessary to produce symptoms of radiculopathy.[70-72] We have obtained data to support this suggestion by demonstrating a robust peripheral and spinal immune reaction in a mononeuropathy model in the rat as described below.

Cytokine Implications Using Sciatic Cryoneurolysis as a Model for Neuropathic Pain

We have developed a reliable and reproducible rat mononeuropathy model, SCN, in which a focal peripheral nerve lesion is produced by exposure and freezing of the sciatic nerve (Fig. 2).[1,73] SCN results in abnormal behaviors, such as sustained mechanical allodynia, that mimic human neuropathic pain conditions. Because of predictable resultant behaviors and neurochemical outcomes, this model is useful for the study of peripheral and spinal mechanisms that may be responsible for neuropathic pain.[74-81] Results from peripheral nerve pathology, central glial changes, and the immunocytochemical localization of specific cytokines following SCN strongly supports the involvement of cytokines in the development and maintenance of neuropathic pain. Observations such as these might be extrapolated to help understand the painful sequelae due to lumbar disk herniation and canal stenosis in humans. In addition, we will present behavioral data demonstrating that when IL-6 was administered intrathecally in normal rats, its action mimicked neuropathic pain behaviors.

SCN Peripheral Nerve Pathology

We have characterized the temporal pathologic changes in the sciatic nerve after SCN as compared with those in a sham-control group (nerves exposed but not frozen).[78] Results from these studies, performed in collaboration with Robert Myers, PhD, implicate a potential neuroimmune mechanism in the development of neuropathic pain behaviors following nerve injury. Briefly, the histologic methods used were as follows: semi-thin transverse tissue

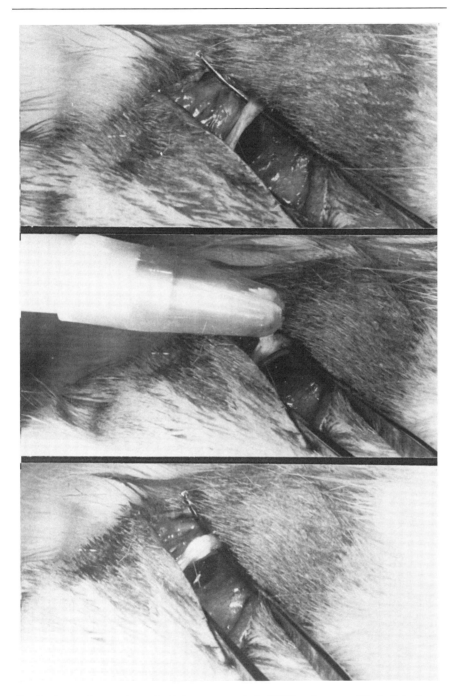

Fig. 2 *Surgical procedure of sciatic cryoneurolysis (SCN) using a modified clinical cryoprobe.* **Top,** *Dissection of the common sciatic nerve proximal to its primary trifurcation. Instruments and surgical approaches are standardized to minimize nerve trauma.* **Center,** *Cryoprobe placement on the sciatic nerve using a freeze-thaw-freeze cycle.* **Bottom,** *transient iceball formation immediately following the freeze. (Reproduced with permission from DeLeo JA, Coombs DW, Willenbring S, et al: Characterization of a neuropathic pain model: Sciatic cryoneuro.* Pain *1994;56:9–16.)*

sections, proximal, distal, and at the lesion site, were prepared and used for the determination of axon diameters by the use of computer-assisted measurements. Grid morphometry was used to categorize endoneurial structures into one of the following: normal myelinated axon, abnormal axon (degenerating or demyelinating), blood vessel, edema (no detectable structure), unmyelinated axonal sprout, or phagocytic cells. This latter category included leukocytes (inferred macrophages), fibroblasts, and Schwann cells.

Major findings consisted of both axonal fiber changes and a significant presence of phagocytic cells. The axonal changes were consistent with expected wallerian degeneration (Fig. 3). Abnormal axons peaked in number at 3 days following SCN and persisted through day 35. By 35 days, axonal morphometry was still abnormal, reflected by an elevation in smaller (2 to 4 mm) diameter axons and a decrease in larger diameter (4 to 6 and 6 to 8 mm) axons. Macrophages and Schwann cell nuclei made up 50% of the fascicular area at 7 and 14 days after SCN, with a second plateau (35%) at 21 and 28 days (Figs. 3 and 4). Autotomy behavior strongly correlated with the presence of phagocytic cells and was inversely correlated with the presence of edema. Mechanical allodynia typically develops in the SCN model between 21 and 28 days. These data suggest that products of macrophages, fibroblasts, and Schwann cells, ie, cytokines, may contribute to abnormal behaviors in this neuropathic pain model.

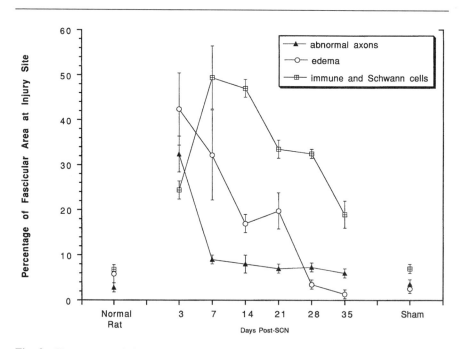

Fig. 3   *Time course of changes in axon diameter following sciatic cryoneurolysis at lesion site and selected grid morphometry data.*

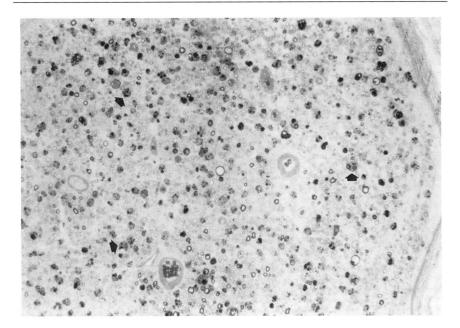

Fig. 4 *Photomicrograph of transverse section of rat sciatic nerve 14 days after sciatic cryoneurolysis. High numbers of phagocytic cells including macrophages are evident at this time (see arrows). Original magnification 100×.*

Central Spinal Changes Following SCN

We have used neuronal and glial staining methods to determine spinal pathologic changes following SCN. Specifically, Nissl staining (1% Cresyl violet) was used to determine viable neuronal cell bodies in lumbar spinal cord after the SCN peripheral nerve lesion. One day after SCN, there were significantly fewer cells in the ipsilateral dorsal horn compared to the contralateral dorsal horn (n = 10 rats, $p < 0.0001$). Nissl staining was not quantitatively different between dorsal horns of the spinal cord in sham-operated animals. Interestingly, these Nissl changes were maximal within 24 hours following SCN and did not increase further over time. This fact possibly reflects an initial, unsustained afferent degeneration.

Glial fibrillary acidic protein (GFAP) immunoreactivity was also used as an astrocytic marker for spinal insult following a peripheral nerve injury.[82-84] Immunoreactive GFAP significantly increased on the ipsilateral side in L2 through L4 segments in SCN rats as compared to the contralateral side (n = 10 rats, $p < 0.05$). As seen in Figure 5, the peak difference between the number of immunoreactive cells in the ipsilateral compared to the contralateral dorsal horn occurred at 14 days. At 42 days, ipsilateral GFAP was further increased. These time periods reflect the two main behavioral windows seen after SCN: autotomy peaks between 11 and 14 days, and by 42 days most animals display significant mechanical allodynia. A slight, nonsignificant decrease in GFAP was observed at 21 days. This is of interest because autotomy has diminished by this time and allodynia is not yet evident.

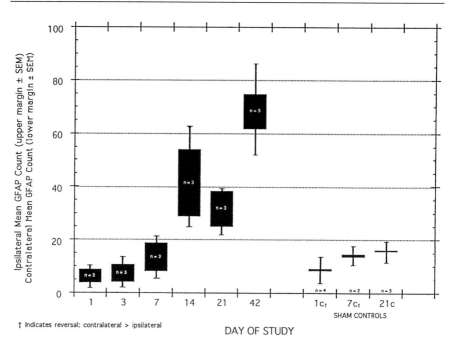

Fig. 5   *Graph depicting the number of glial fibrillary acidic protein (GFAP) immunoreactive cells in the dorsal horn of the spinal lumbar segment L3 at various times following sciatic cryoneurolysis or sham surgery. The upper margin of each bar represents ipsilateral GFAP cell averages (± SEM) and the lower margin of each bar represents contralateral GFAP cell averages (± SEM) for that same group of animals. The height of each bar represents the difference between the ipsilateral and contralateral averages.*

The surprising latent GFAP increase at 42 days was not correlated with neuronal Nissl loss in the spinal cord. This result was unexpected because in other CNS injury models, neuronal damage is also associated with increases in GFAP. Our findings suggest that the glial response is due to mechanisms other than neuronal damage, such as peripherally transported cytokines or spinal cytokine production. New studies have demonstrated that most, if not all, glial cells in vitro and in vivo express both voltage-dependent Na^+ and Ca^{++} channels and ligand gated channels, such as glutamate and GABA-gated ion channels.[85] These findings suggest that glial cells may be more involved in CNS function than has been previously thought. They may not act only as supportive cells for neurons but may actually sense and respond to a large array of neuronal signals.

It has been shown that the inhibition of glial metabolism by fluorocitrate resulted in a marked attenuation of hyperalgesia produced by an intraplantar chemical irritant, zymosan.[86] Murphy and associates[87] have demonstrated the presence of an astrocyte-derived vasorelaxing factor with properties similar to nitric oxide. It has been established that nitric oxide plays a significant role in the mechanisms responsible for hyperalgesia following nerve injury.[45] Glial cells may participate in long-term potentiation by synthesizing and releasing cytokines and arachidonic acid. Both interleukins and arachidonic acid have been demonstrated to induce a long-term, activity-dependent enhancement of synaptic transmission in the hippocampus.[12,88] Because glial cells exhibit a high degree of plasticity in response to neuronal signals, long-term changes in glial cell membrane properties may mediate chronic changes in synaptic function.

Cytokine Immunohistochemical Changes Following SCN

In an initial study, the SCN lesion was examined at 3, 7, 14, 21, 35, 42, and 120 days to correlate potential spinal changes in cytokines with behaviors suggestive of neuropathic pain. These results were compared with results in normal, unoperated control rats. Immunohistochemistry was performed using an avidin-biotin complex (ABC) elite kit (Vector Laboratories, Burlingame, CA) on free-floating sections. A polyclonal antibody to IL-6 (working dilution 1:1000) was purchased from Genzyme, Cambridge, MA, and an antibody to bFGF (working dilution 1:5000) was supplied by Dr. Andrew Baird. Negative controls were done in each run in which the primary antibody was omitted. (For detailed immunohistochemical methodology see Wagner and associates.[76]) As previously described, computer-assisted image analysis was used to quantify immunohistochemical changes.[73,76] The density of IL-6 staining in the medial and lateral substantia gelatinosa was quantified by measuring transmitted light levels in a fixed area sample. Three sections from each rat (n = 3/time period) were sampled, and the mean of each group was determined. A lower number represents decreased transmission of light, which translates into enhanced density of staining.

Interleukin-6 Spinal IL-6 immunoreactivity was minimal in the normal, control rats. Conversely, immunoreactive IL-6 increased incrementally in the medial and lateral substantia gelatinosa and motor neurons up to 35 days after SCN, the time point when allodynia is most pronounced (Fig. 6). In rats in which allodynia had subsided (120 days after SCN), IL-6 expression was markedly reduced. As shown in Figure 7, cytoplasmic staining was observed in what appeared to be both glia and neurons. Further studies are currently underway to determine the exact cell type by double labeling methods. As shown in Table 2, the quantitative data verify the descriptive observations of increased IL-6 immunoreactivity over time following SCN. There was a significant increase of IL-6 staining in the ipsilateral, dorsal horns of the spinal cord in rats as early as 3 days after SCN as compared to normal, control rats. The contralateral dorsal horn also demonstrated a significant increase by 14 days after SCN as compared with the control group.

Basic Fibroblast Growth Factor In normal, unoperated rats minimal immunoreactive bFGF was seen in the dorsal horn and motoneurons. At 3 days post-SCN, intense bFGF immunoreactivity was present in the ipsilateral ventral horn, specific to motoneurons (Fig. 8). There was also evidence of white matter glial staining and increased dorsal horn staining at this time. At 7 and 14 days post-SCN there was increased contralateral dorsal horn staining. By 42 days post-SCN, bFGF immunoreactivity was more variable between animals, with staining observed in ipsilateral and contralateral dorsal horns and ventral horn motoneurons.

These immunohistochemical results demonstrate that two distinct cytokines, IL-6 and bFGF, are both increased in the spinal segments innervated by the injured sciatic nerve. The dorsal horn localization and the time course of expres-

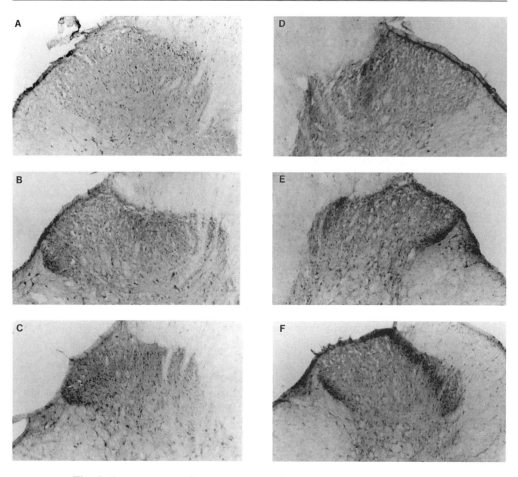

Fig. 6 *Representative photomicrographs of ipsilateral dorsal horn interleukin-6 immunore-activity in normal rats (**A**) and at 3 (**B**), 7 (**C**), 14 (**D**) , 21 (**E**), and 35 (**F**) days after sciatic cryoneurolysis. Original magnification 40×.*

sion imply that these polypeptides may play a role either in the development or maintenance of neuropathic pain behaviors. The cellular sources of these two cytokines in this scenario have not yet been defined. Results from these experiments may differentiate peripheral and central mechanisms in the generation of acute and chronic pain states.

Cytokine Immunohistochemical Changes Following Chronic Constriction Injury

With the collaborative efforts of Dr. Gerald Gebhart, immunohistochemistry was performed on spinal cords from rats following CCI. Analysis of the differential spinal expression of specific cytokines in the distinct SCN and CCI mononeuropathy models provides information on both the type of nerve lesion and the subsequent behavioral modality observed. Further, the chemical toxicity of chromic gut (as opposed to silk suture) is required for the robust devel-

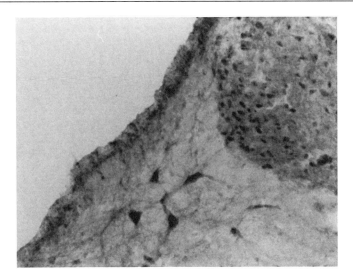

Fig. 7 *Interleukin-6 staining in white matter 3 days after sciatic cryoneurolysis. Original magnification 100×.*

Table 2 Computer analysis of spinal operated and unoperated dorsal horn interleukin-6 immunoreactivity over time following SCN[*]

Group (N=3 per time)	Unoperated Dorsal Horn[‡]	Operated, Ipsilateral Dorsal Horn§
Normal	105.39 ± 1.17	105.78 ± 0.11
3 days after SCN	103.50 ± 1.25	98.50 ± 1.42[¶]
7 days after SCN	104.67 ± 0.79	98.83 ± 1.17[¶]
14 days after SCN	100.06 ± 0.47[¶]	96.56 ± 1.00[¶]
21 days after SCN	97.16 ± 2.62[¶]	94.83 ± 2.75[¶]
35 days after SCN	88.72 ± 1.65**	83.22 ± 1.02**

[*]A lower number represents decreased transmission of light, which translates into enhanced density of staining
[‡] $p < 0.001$ using analysis of variance (F=17.84, 17 df) for analysis of means on unoperated dorsal horn by group
§ $p < 0.001$ using analysis of variance (F=25.33, 17 df) for analysis of means on unoperated dorsal horn by group
[¶] $p < 0.05$ using linear regression with normal group as reference category
** $p < 0.001$ using linear regression with normal group as reference category

opment of abnormal behaviors observed following CCI.[89] This implicates a chemical inflammatory response that may involve the production of cytokines. IL-6 and bFGF immunohistochemistry was performed by the methods described above in lumbar spinal cords from hyperalgesic rats euthanized on day 6 following CCI surgery.

Interleukin-6 The localization and density of IL-6 immunoreactivity in lumbar segments following CCI was very similar to IL-6 staining in SCN rat spi-

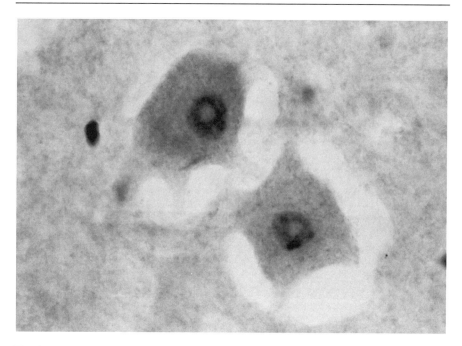

Fig. 8   *Representative photomicrograph of basic fibroblast growth factor immunoreactivity in motoneurons 3 days after sciatic cryoneurolysis. Original magnification 400×.*

nal cord (Fig. 9). A robust increase was noted in the ipsilateral dorsal horn as compared with minimal staining in normal rats. There was also evidence of dense motoneuron IL-6 staining in both ventral horns.

Basic Fibroblast Growth Factor In contrast to bFGF increases in the SCN model, there appeared to be no obvious staining differences in lumbar spinal cord following CCI as compared with normal rats. The staining density and location was similar to that in the control group.

Interpretation of these immunohistochemical data raise interesting questions. Using two different animal models of neuropathic pain provides the capability to dissect mechanisms pertaining to the type of nerve lesion and the expression of differential behaviors. Is the bFGF increase observed in SCN related to regenerative changes[90] following a complete nerve lesion and not related to painful behavioral sequelae? Is it possible to discover a unifying cascade of events in the establishment of chronic neurogenic pain or are distinct peripheral and spinal changes unique to specific nerve lesions? For these questions to be answered, further research needs to be performed using different animal models of neuropathy with further in-depth studies of neuroimmune actions.

Intrathecal Delivery of IL-6 in Normal and SCN Rats

Following the immunohistochemical results with IL-6, we wanted to determine whether intrathecally administered IL-6 would mimic neuropathic pain behaviors in normal, untreated rats (n = 6). Recombinant human IL-6 (R & D Sys-

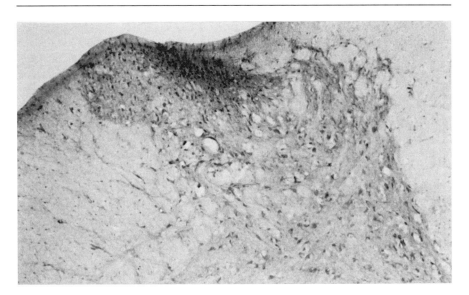

Fig. 9 *Representative photomicrograph of ipsilateral dorsal horn interleukin-6 immunoreactivity 6 days after chronic constriction injury nerve lesion. Original magnification 40×.*

tems, Minneapolis, MN) at a dose of 100 ng in a total volume of 10 μl followed by a 10 μl saline flush was administered via previously implanted intrathecal catheters.[91] Individual rats were placed under inverted mice cages that were on a raised wire mesh for a 1-hour observation period.

Within 10 minutes following administration, significant touch-evoked allodynia (TEA) was observed, which was more accentuated in the hind quarters. TEA was associated with vocalization and guarding of hind quarters. Visceral writhing was occasionally observed. Heightened exploratory activity was intermixed with posturing and crouching. Rats would always right themselves when prompted, indicating no gross motor effects. In an additional study, rats with previous SCN nerve lesions were administered IL-6 intrathecally at the same dose as above. The behavior in SCN rats was similar to that in normal rats administered IL-6; however, TEA was much more focused to hind paws with increased chewing and guarding. The previously SCN-injured hind paw was lifted and clenched with obvious avoidance of any contact with the mesh floor. These rats displayed increased grooming directed at the scrotum and face.

The immunohistochemical data provide evidence that IL-6 is altered in the spinal cord following a peripheral nerve lesion that reliably results in neuropathic behaviors. The finding that immunoreactive IL-6 was only substantially increased in allodynic versus nonallodynic rats following SCN lends further support to the concept that cytokines may indeed be involved in chronic pain processes. Finally, the behavioral data described above provide direct evidence that spinally administered IL-6 is capable of mimicking and even potentiating pain behaviors that are observed following peripheral nerve injury.

Conclusion

This review has highlighted only a fraction of the available data on the interactions of cytokines in the nervous system. Cytokines and their mechanisms of action in the peripheral and central nervous systems are only beginning to be understood. It is surprising that although these peptides have been implicated in a wide variety of disease states, their role in normal physiology is largely undefined. Numerous recent findings have implicated a very complex view of cytokine involvement in the CNS. There exists an apparent redundancy of cytokine action, as well as evidence that cytokines exert opposing actions depending on their concentration, site, and duration of action and the presence of other cytokines, hormones, neurotransmitters, and so forth in the microenvironment. Cytokines have several, distinct actions on the nervous system: as communicators to the brain following systemic injury, infection, and inflammation; as modulators of responses to peripheral nerve injury; as neuromodulators (maybe even neurotransmitters) in the CNS response to disease and injury; and as substances that mediate or mitigate neurodegeneration and repair of the brain and spinal cord.[92]

The understanding of the potential role of cytokines in chronic neurogenic pain is only in its infancy. The pace of this research has accelerated in the recent past, and it may possibly afford a clearer picture in the next few years. Although there has been an increase in studies addressing the role of cytokines in nociception, information about biologic activity, eg, the pharmacokinetics and pharmacodynamics of cytokines, are lacking. For example, IL-1β inhibits long-term potentiation at lower concentrations, and actually causes the release of nitric oxide and arachidonic acid at higher concentrations, enhancing long-term potentiation.[11,93] Before extensive cytokine agonism or antagonism dose-response studies are initiated to attenuate experimental neuropathic behaviors, data are needed to determine cytokine responses in nerve injury. In addition, the behavioral effects of specific cytokines administered via different routes in normal animals at relevant biologic doses should be known.

In idiopathic low back pain, abnormal spinal mechanics may directly lead to structural and biochemical changes. These changes, either directly or indirectly, may sensitize nociceptors, leading to a painful state. This sensitization may be due to inflammatory mediators, direct chemical irritation, and/or neuroimmunologic factors. The functional spinal unit includes nerve roots, the dorsal root ganglion, and peripheral nerves. It is easily conceivable that an imbalance of cytokines at any or all of these sites would potentiate painful sequelae following injury to the intervertebral disk. In addition, immunologic factors may be present or possibly even produced in the nucleus pulposus. The presence of abundant macrophages, IL-1β-expressing cells, bFGF, and TGF-βs have been demonstrated in disk herniation tissue.[94] Thus, it is plausible that cytokines may initiate or propagate hypersensitivity in chronically irritated nerves following lumbar disk herniation and lumbar canal stenosis. A better understanding of cytokine processes in the development and maintenance of acute and chronic pain, as well as the advent of superior methodology in the detection and manipulation of cytokines may eventually lead to the discovery of novel, nonopioid therapeutic potential for both the prevention and treatment of refractory pain syndromes.

Acknowledgments

The authors would like to graciously thank Mark E. Splaine, MD, for statistical consultation and editorial assistance; Rochelle Wagner, PhD, Robert Myers, PhD, and Gerald Gebhart, PhD, for their scientific contributions reviewed in this chapter; Dr. Andrew Baird for the generous contribution of bFGF antibody; and Bonnie Twitchell, Michelle Nichols, Amit Malhotra, and Cara Cargill for their technical and secretarial support.

References

1. DeLeo JA, Coombs DW, Willenbring S, et al: Characterization of a neuropathic pain model: Sciatic cryoneurolysis in the rat. *Pain* 1994;56:9–16.
2. Bennett GJ, Xie YK: A peripheral mononeuropathy in rat that produces disorders of pain sensation like those seen in man. *Pain* 1988;33:87–107.
3. Logan A: CNS growth factors. *Br J Hosp Med* 1990;43:428–437.
4. Zelena J (ed): *Nerves and Mechanoreceptors: The Role of Innervation in the Development and Maintenance of Mammalian Mechanoreceptor.* London, England, Chapman & Hall, 1994.
5. Olsson Y, Sjostrand J: Origin of macrophages in Wallerian degeneration of peripheral nerves demonstrated autoradiographically. *Exp Neurol* 1969;23:102–112.
6. Bruck W, Bruck Y, Maruschak B, et al: Mechanisms of macrophage recruitment in Wallerian degeneration. *Acta Neuropathol* 1995;89:363–367.
7. Streit WJ: Microglial-neuronal interactions. *J Chem Neuroanat* 1993;6:261–266.
8. Yaksh, TL, Yamamoto T, Myers RR: Pharmacology of nerve compression-evoked hyperesthesia, in Willis WD Jr (ed): *Hyperalgesia and Allodynia.* New York, NY, Raven Press, 1992, pp 245–258.
9. Kiefer R, Lindholm D, Kreutzberg GW: Interleukin-6 and transforming growth factor-beta 1 mRNAs are induced in rat facial nucleus following motoneuron axotomy. *Eur J Neurosci* 1993;5:775–781.
10. Gehrmann J, Matsumoto Y, Kreutzberg GW: Microglia: Intrinsic immuneffector cell of the brain. *Brain Res Brain Res Rev* 1995;20:269–287.
11. Patterson PH, Nawa H: Neuronal differentiation factors/cytokines and synaptic plasticity. *Cell* 1993;72(suppl):123–137.
12. Rothwell NJ: Functions and mechanisms of interleukin-1 in the brain. *Trends Pharmacol Sci* 1991;12:430–436.
13. Cotman CW, Gomez-Pinilla F. Basic fibroblast growth factor in the mature brain and its possible role in Alzheimer's disease. *Ann N Y Acad Sci* 1991;638:221–231.
14. Mazue G, Bertolero F, Jacob C, et al: Preclinical and clinical studies with recombinant human basic fibroblast growth factor. *Ann N Y Acad Sci* 1991;638:329–340.
15. Roberts AB, Sporn MB: Physiological actions and clinical applications of transforming growth factor-beta (TGF-beta). *Growth Factors* 1993;8:1–9.
16. Levi-Montalcini R, Hamburger V: Selective growth stimulating effects of mouse sarcoma on the sensory and sympathetic nervous system of the chick embryo. *J Exp Zool* 1951;116:321–361.
17. Thoenen H, Barde YA: Physiology of nerve growth factor. *Physiol Rev* 1980;60:1284–1335.
18. Lewin GR, Ritter AM, Mendell LM: Nerve growth factor-induced hyperalgesia in the neonatal and adult rat. *J Neurosci* 1993;13:2136–2148.
19. McMahon SB, Armanini MP, Ling LH, et al: Expression and co-expression of Trk receptors in subpopulations of adult primary sensory neurons projecting to identified peripheral targets. *Neuron* 1994;12:1161–1171.
20. Verge VM, Merlio JP, Grondin J, et al: Colocalization of NGF binding sites, trk mRNA, and low-affinity NGF receptor mRNA in primary sensory neurons: Responses to injury and infusion of NGF. *J Neurosci* 1992;12:4011–4022.
21. Curtis R, Adryan KM, Stark JL, et al: Differential role of the low affinity neurotrophin receptor (p75) in retrograde axonal transport of the neurotrophins. *Neuron* 1995;14:1201–1211.

22. Dobrowsky RT, Werner MH, Castellino AM, et al: Activation of the sphingomyelin cycle through the low-affinity neurotrophin receptor. *Science* 1994;265:1596–1599.

23. Chao MV, Hempstead BL: p75 and Trk: A two-receptor system. *Trends Neurosci* 1995;18:321–326.

24. Acheson A, Conover JC, Fandl JP, et al: A BDNF autocrine loop in adult sensory neurons prevents cell death. *Nature* 1995;374:450–453.

25. Rich KM, Yip HK, Osborne PA, et al: Role of nerve growth factor in the adult dorsal root ganglia neuron and its response to injury. *J Comp Neurol* 1984;230:110–118.

26. Heumann R, Lindholm D, Bandtlow C, et al: Differential regulation of mRNA encoding nerve growth factor and its receptor in rat sciatic nerve during development, degeneration, and regeneration: Role of macrophages. *Proc Natl Acad Sci USA* 1987;84:8735–8739.

27. McLachlan EM, Janig W, Devor M, et al: Peripheral nerve injury triggers noradrenergic sprouting within dorsal root ganglia. *Nature* 1993;363:543–546.

28. Devor M, Janig W, Michaelis M: Modulation of activity in dorsal root ganglion neurons by sympathetic activation in nerve-injured rats. *J Neurophysiol* 1994;71:38–47.

29. Fitzgerald M, Wall PD, Goedert M, et al: Nerve growth factor counteracts the neurophysiological and neurochemical effects of chronic sciatic nerve section. *Brain Res* 1985;332:131–141.

30. Otto D, Unsicker K, Grothe C: Pharmacological effects of nerve growth factor and fibroblast growth factor applied to the transectioned sciatic nerve on neuron death in adult rat dorsal root ganglia. *Neurosci Lett* 1987;83:156–160.

31. Kinnman E, Levine JD: Sensory and sympathetic contributions of nerve injury-induced sensory abnormalities in the rat. *Neuroscience* 1995;64:751–767.

32. Davis BM, Lewin GR, Mendell LM, et al: Altered expression of nerve growth factor in the skin of transgenic mice leads to changes in response to mechanical stimuli. *Neuroscience* 1993;56:789–792.

33. Lewin GR, Rueff A, Mendell LM: Peripheral and central mechanisms of NGF-induced hyperalgesia. *Eur J Neurosci* 1994;6:1903–1912.

34. Woolf CJ, Safieh-Garabedian B, Ma QP, et al: Nerve growth factor contributes to the generation of inflammatory sensory hypersensitivity. *Neuroscience* 1994;62:327–331.

35. Shen KF, Crain SM: Nerve growth factor rapidly prolongs the action potential of mature sensory ganglion neurons in culture, and this effect requires activation of Gs-coupled excitatory kappa-opioid receptors on these cells. *J Neurosci* 1994;14:5570–5579.

36. Toledo-Aral JJ, Brehm P, Halegoua S, et al: A single pulse of nerve growth factor triggers long-term neuronal excitability through sodium channel gene induction. *Neuron* 1995;14:607–611.

37. Fanger GR, Jones JR, Maue RA: Differential regulation of neuronal sodium channel expression by endogenous and exogenous tyrosine kinase receptors expressed in rat pheochromocytoma cells. *J Neurosci* 1995;15:202–213.

38. Devor M, Govrin-Lippmann R, Angelides K: Na+ channel immunolocalization in peripheral mammalian axons and changes following nerve injury and neuroma formation. *J Neurosci* 1993;13:1976–1992.

39. Bevan S, Winter J: Nerve growth factor (NGF) differentially regulates the chemosensitivity of adult rat cultured sensory neurons. *J Neurosci* 1995;15:4918–4926.

40. Baird A, Klagsbrun M (eds): The fibroblast growth factor family. *Ann NY Acad Sci* 1991;638.

41. Logan A, Frautschy SA, Baird A: Basic fibroblast growth factor and central nervous system injury. *Ann N Y Acad Sci* 1991;638:474–476.

42. Eckenstein FP, Shipley GD, Nishi R: Acidic and basic fibroblast growth factors in the nervous system: Distribution and differential alteration of levels after injury of central versus peripheral nerve. *J Neurosci* 1991;11:412–419.

43. Unsicker K, Flanders KC, Cissel DS, et al: Transforming growth factor beta isoforms in the adult rat central and peripheral nervous system. *Neuroscience* 1991;44:613–625.
44. Ding A, Nathan CF, Graycar J, et al: Macrophage deactivating factor and transforming growth factors-beta 1, -beta 2 and -beta 3 inhibit induction of macrophage nitrogen oxide synthesis by IFN-gamma. *J Immunol* 1990;145:940–944.
45. Meller ST, Gebhart GF: Nitric oxide (NO) and nociceptive processing in the spinal cord. *Pain* 1993;52:127–136.
46. Rotshenker S, Aamar S, Barak V: Interleukin-1 activity in lesioned peripheral nerve. *J Neuroimmunol* 1992;39:75–80.
47. Yan HQ, Banos MA, Herregodts P, et al: Expression of interleukin (IL)-1 beta, IL-6 and their respective receptors in the normal rat brain and after injury. *Eur J Immunol* 1992;22:2963–2971.
48. Maier SF, Wiertelak EP, Martin D, et al: Interleukin-1 mediates the behavioral hyperalgesia produced by lithium chloride and endotoxin. *Brain Res* 1993;623:321–324.
49. Watkins LR, Wiertelak EP, Goehler LE, et al: Characterization of cytokine-induced hyperalgesia. *Brain Res* 1994;654:15–26.
50. Schafer M, Carter L, Stein C: Interleukin-1 beta and corticotropin-releasing factor inhibit pain by releasing opioids from immune cells in inflamed tissue. *Proc Natl Acad Sci USA* 1994;91:4219–4223.
51. Czlonkowski A, Stein C, Herz A: Peripheral mechanisms of opioid antinociception in inflammation: Involvement of cytokines. *Eur J Pharmacol* 1993;242:229–235.
52. Stein C: The control of pain in peripheral tissue by opioids. *N Engl J Med* 1995;332:1685–1690.
53. Jeanjean AP, Moussaoui SM, Maloteaux JM, et al: Interleukin-1 beta induces long-term increase of axonally transported opiate receptors and substance P. *Neuroscience* 1995;68:151–157.
54. Bolin LM, Verity AN, Silver JE, et al: Interleukin-6 production by Schwann cells and induction in sciatic nerve injury. *J Neurochem* 1995;64:850–858.
55. Frei K, Malipiero UV, Leist TP, et al: On the cellular source and function of interleukin-6 produced in the central nervous system in viral diseases. *Eur J Immunol* 1989;19:689–694.
56. Le JM, Vilcek J: Interleukin-6: A multifunctional cytokine regulating immune reactions and the acute phase protein response. *Lab Invest* 1989;61:588–602.
57. de Waal Malefyt R, Haanen J, Spits H, et al: Interleukin-10 (IL-10) and viral IL-10 strongly reduce antigen-specific human T cell proliferation by diminishing the antigen-presenting capacity of monocytes via downregulation of class II major histocompatibility complex expression. *J Exp Med* 1991;174:915–924.
58. Fiorentino DF, Zlotnik A, Mosmann TR, et al: IL-10 inhibits cytokine production by activated macrophages. *J Immunol* 1991;147:3815–3822.
59. Bogdan C, Vodovotz Y, Nathan C: Macrophage deactivation by interleukin-10. *J Exp Med* 1991;174:1549–1555.
60. Oswald IP, Wynn TA, Sher A, et al: Interleukin-10 inhibits macrophage microbicidal activity by blocking the endogenous production of tumor necrosis factor alpha required as a costimulatory factor for interferon gamma-induced activation. *Proc Natl Acad Sci USA* 1992;89:8676–8680.
61. Poole S, Cunha FQ, Selkirk S, et al: Cytokine-mediated inflammatory hyperalgesia limited by interleukin-10. *Br J Pharmacol* 1995;115:684–688.
62. Olsson T, Kelic S, Edlund C, et al: Neuronal interferon-gamma immunoreactive molecule: Bioactivities and purification. *Eur J Immunol* 1994;24:308–314.
63. Xu XJ, Hao JX, Olsson T, et al: Intrathecal interferon-gamma facilitates the spinal nociceptive flexor reflex in the rat. *Neurosci Lett* 1994;182:263–266.
64. Kristensson K, Aldskogius M, Peng ZC, et al: Co-induction of neuronal interferon -gamma and nitric oxide synthase in rat motor neurons after axotomy: A role in nerve repair or death? *J Neurocytol* 1994;23:453–459.

183

65. Malmberg AB, Yaksh TL: Spinal nitric oxide synthesis inhibition blocks NMDA-induced thermal hyperalgesia and produces antinociception in the formalin test in rats. *Pain* 1993;54:291–300.

66. Carswell EA, Old LJ, Kassel RL, et al: An endotoxin-induced serum factor that causes necrosis of tumors. *Proc Natl Acad Sci USA* 1975;72:3666–3670.

67. Beutler B, Greenwald D, Hulmes JD, et al: Identity of tumour necrosis factor and the macrophage-secreted factor cachectin. *Nature* 1985;316:552–554.

68. Kawakami M, Weinstein JN, Spratt KF, et al: Experimental lumbar radiculopathy: Immunohistochemical and quantitative demonstrations of pain induced by lumbar nerve root irritation of the rat. *Spine* 1994;19:1780–1794.

69. Kawakami M, Weinstein JN, Chatani K, et al: Experimental lumbar radiculopathy: Behavioral and histologic changes in a model of radicular pain after spinal nerve root irritation with chromic gut ligatures in the rat. *Spine* 1994;19:1795–1802.

70. Greenbarg PE, Brown MD, Pallares VS, et al: Epidural anesthesia for lumbar spine surgery. *J Spinal Disord* 1988;1:139–143.

71. Kuslich SD, Ulstrom CL, Michael CJ: The tissue origin of low back pain and sciatica: A report of pain response to tissue stimulation during operations on the lumbar spine using local anesthesia. *Orthop Clin North Am* 1991;22:181–187.

72. Marshall LL, Trethewie ER, Curtain CC: Chemical radiculitis: A clinical, physiological and immunological study. *Clin Orthop* 1977;129:61–67.

73. DeLeo JA, Coombs DW: Autotomy and decreased spinal substance P following peripheral cryogenic nerve lesion. *Cryobiology* 1991;28:460–466.

74. Fromm C, DeLeo JA, Coombs DW, et al: The ganglioside GM1 decreases autotomy but not substance P depletion in a peripheral mononeuropathy rat model. *Anesth Analg* 1993;77:501–506.

75. Serpell MG, DeLeo JA, Coombs DW, et al: Intrathecal catheterization alone reduces autotomy after sciatic cryoneurolysis in the rat. *Life Sci* 1993;53:1887–1892.

76. Wagner R, DeLeo JA, Coombs DW, et al: Spinal dynorphin immunoreactivity increases bilaterally in a neuropathic pain model. *Brain Res* 1993;629:323–326.

77. Wagner R, DeLeo JA, Coombs DW, et al: Gender differences in autotomy following sciatic cryoneurolysis in the rat. *Physiol Behav* 1995;58:37–41.

78. Wagner R, DeLeo JA, Heckman HM, et al: Peripheral nerve pathology following sciatic cryoneurolysis: Relationship to neuropathic behaviors in the rate. *Exp Neurol* 1995;133:256–264.

79. Willenbring S, DeLeo JA, Coombs DW: Differential behavioral outcomes in the sciatic cryoneurolysis model of neuropathic pain in rats. *Pain* 1994;58:135–140.

80. Willenbring S, Beauprie IG, DeLeo JA: Sciatic cryoneurolysis in rats: A model of sympathetically independent pain: Part 1. Effects of sympathectomy. *Anesth Analg* 1995;81:544–548.

81. Willenbring S, DeLeo JA, Coombs DW. Sciatic cryoneurolysis in rats: A model of sympathetically independent pain: Part 2. Adrenergic pharmacology. *Anesth Analg* 1995;81:549–554.

82. Tetzlaff W, Graeber MB, Bisby MA, et al: Increased glial fibrillary acidic protein synthesis in astrocytes during retrograde reaction of the rat facial nucleus. *Glia* 1988;1:90–95.

83. Garrison CJ, Dougherty PM, Kajander KC, et al: Staining of glial fibrillary acidic protein (GFAP) in lumbar spinal cord increases following a sciatic nerve constriction injury. *Brain Res* 1991;565:1–7.

84. Hajos F, Csillik B, Knyihar-Csillik E: Alterations in glial fibrillary acidic protein immunoreactivity in the upper dorsal horn of the rat spinal cord in the course of transganglionic degenerative atrophy and regenerative proliferation. *Neurosci Lett* 1990;117:8–13.

85. Barres BA: New roles for glia. *J Neurosci* 1991;11:3685–3694.

86. Meller ST, Dykstra C, Grzybycki D, et al: The possible role of glia in nociceptive processing and hyperalgesia in the spinal cord of the rat. *Neuropharmacology* 1994;33:1471–1478.

87. Murphy S, Minor RL Jr, Welk G, et al: Evidence for an astrocyte-derived vasorelaxing factor with properties similar to nitric oxide. *J Neurochem* 1990;55:349–351.
88. Williams JH, Errington ML, Lynch MA, et al: Arachidonic acid induces a long-term activity-dependent enhancement of synaptic transmission in the hippocampus. *Nature* 1989;341:739–742.
89. Maves TJ, Pechman PS, Gebhart GF, et al: Possible chemical contribution from chromic gut sutures produces disorders of pain sensation like those seen in man. *Pain* 1993;54:57–69.
90. Sugimoto T, Bennett GJ, Kajander KC: Transsynaptic degeneration in the superficial dorsal horn after sciatic nerve injury: Effects of a chronic constriction injury, transection, and strychnine. *Pain* 1990;42:205–213.
91. Yaksh TL, Rudy TA: Chronic catheterization of the spinal subarachnoid space. *Physiol Behav* 1976;17:1031–1036.
92. Hopkins SJ, Rothwell NJ: Cytokines and the nervous system I: Expression and recognition. *Trends Neurosci* 1995;18:83–88.
93. Rothwell NJ, Relton JK: Involvement of cytokines in acute neurodegeneration in the CNS. *Neurosci Biobehav Rev* 1993;17:217–227.
94. Gronblad M, Virri J, Tolonen J, et al: A controlled immunohistochemical study of inflammatory cells in disc herniation tissue. *Spine* 1994;19:2744–2751.

Chapter 12

Pain Arising From the Nerve Root and the Dorsal Root Ganglion

Marshall Devor, PhD

Introduction

Joints, bone, ligaments, and muscles cannot, by themselves, give rise to pain. Only nerve tissue can do so. To understand low back pain, it is necessary to focus on those processes associated with low back pain that cause the relevant *neurons* to fire. The relevant neurons are those central nervous system (CNS) cells whose pattern of activity defines pain sensation in a conscious brain. Because there is no way at present to delimit this central cell assembly, this chapter will focus on the peripheral afferent neurons that drive it.

The primary afferent neurons responsible for low back pain would classically be defined as those A delta (Aδ) and C nociceptors that innervate low back tissues. Limiting one's purview to nociceptors, however, is no longer tenable. There is now excellent evidence, based on studies of both acute laboratory-induced pain and chronic neuropathic pain, in animals and in man, that impulses in low threshold A beta (Aβ) afferents can provoke a sensation of pain. Such Aβ touch-evoked pain occurs when the spinal cord is in a hyperexcitable state called "central sensitization." Central sensitization in the spinal cord can be triggered by relatively modest noxious input, such as simple pain-provoking stimuli, inflammation, or frank tissue injury, and it persists for as long as that input continues. Therefore, in any condition in which nociceptive afferents are activated, including low back pain, central sensitization is likely to play a role.

I will begin this chapter by noting the sources of primary afferent activity most likely to be responsible for low back pain. Then, I will discuss pathophysiologic processes that cause axons of the nerve roots and neurons of the dorsal root ganglion (DRG) to come onto this list. Finally, I will provide a brief summary of the evidence for Aβ-evoked pain, and of the presumed mechanism of central sensitization. This last section is for the benefit of readers who are not yet familiar with the concept of central sensitization and its likely importance for low back pain.

Sources of Primary Afferent Activity Responsible for Low Back Pain

Transduction of sensory signals (force, temperature, irritant chemicals) normally occurs at the sensory terminal of the primary afferent neuron. The cell membrane in this distal few tens of micrometers of the axon's length is specialized for this purpose.[1,2] In the remainder of the axon, that is, the remaining 99.9% of its length, electrical properties are inappropriate for the generation of repetitive firing in response to natural (slowly depolarizing) stimuli. This fact is easily demonstrated by simply pressing over the course of your own median nerve. Pressure is felt at the location where you press because the skin there is invested with sensory endings. Median nerve axons, however, are not activated. If they were, a sensation would be felt in the median distribution of the hand.

It is important to stress that the afferent axon end itself is the sensory transducer element. There are no definite examples of nonneural transduction cells driving afferents as do hair cells in the auditory and vestibular systems (the Merkel cell remains the one potential exception). It is true that the sensory axon end may be wrapped by nonneural cells to form a specialized apparatus, such as the pacinian corpuscle, but the axon end itself remains the transducer. Whenever sensory impulses arise at locations other than the normal sensory axon ending, they arise ectopically. Ectopic discharge can be evoked by firmly tapping on a nerve as it runs over a bony promontory. It also arises as a result of nerve injury.

Because of these basic considerations, peripheral sources of neural discharge in low back pain can be divided into two main categories: afferent transducer endings and ectopic sources. Impulse activity in nociceptive Aδ and C afferents can be expected to evoke back pain whether it arises normally in the sensory ending or ectopically. Likewise, nociceptive impulses can trigger and maintain central sensitization whether they arise normally or ectopically. Finally, in the presence of central sensitization, impulses in Aβ touch afferents can evoke pain whether they arise normally or ectopically.[3] The potential sources of afferent activity in low back pain are summarized in Outline 1.

An analysis of low back pain must consider all six of these potential sources (actually, eight because the last source listed in Outline 1 includes three distinct origins of Aβ ectopia). Knowledge of which of these sources is active in any given case of low back pain is usually lacking. The stress that most authors, including those in the present volume, place on sensitized nociceptor endings (the second source listed) is not necessarily justified.

Outline 1 Potential sources of afferent activity in low back pain

Afferent sensory endings innervating low back tissues
  Sensory endings of normal Aδ and C nociceptors
  Sensory endings of nociceptors sensitized by inflammation
  Sensory endings of normal low threshold Aβ afferents in the presence of
    central sensitization
Ectopic firing (ectopia) in injured afferents
  Ectopia originating in injured nociceptor axons in the spinal nerve or root
  Ectopia originating in nociceptor neuron somata in the DRG
  Ectopia originating in injured low threshold Aβ afferents (nerve, root or
    DRG) in the presence of central sensitization

Normal Sensory Endings and Sensitized Nociceptors

Sensory Receptor Endings

The detailed mechanism of normal sensory reception is still poorly understood, mostly because of the objective difficulty of studying the very fine axonal endings involved. The same is true of mechanisms of peripheral sensitization.[4] These subjects are dealt with elsewhere in this volume (see chapters 11, 17, and 35). I will restrict this section to a few issues that form essential background for the later discussion of ectopic impulse sources. Sensory reception in afferent endings involves two distinct processes: signal transduction and stimulus encoding (Fig. 1).

Signal Transduction Stimuli generate a transmembrane current and, hence, the sensory generator potential. For mechanical stimuli, the generator current is due to ion flow through ''stretch activated'' (SA) or ''mechanosensitive'' (MS) channels. These channels are unique transmembrane proteins that are found in virtually all cells including prokaryotes, but are enriched in mechanoreceptive afferents.[5] Na^+ is the major inward current carrier. MS channels rather than voltage-sensitive Na^+ channels are involved, however, so the generator current is not tetrodotoxin (TTX)-sensitive.[1] It is not known whether the distinction between mechanonociceptors and low threshold mechanoreceptors lies in the gating properties of MS channels, their density, or posttransduction encoding.

The mechanism of thermal transduction (warm and cold) is not yet known, but it probably involves either transmembrane proteins or intracellular effector molecules with a high temperature coefficient (Q_{10}).

Chemoreception (in polymodal C fibers) is presumed to be based on specific receptor-effector molecules analogous to neurotransmitter and olfactory receptor molecules. There are probably many types. A few are exteroceptors of pH and certain plant and animal toxins (for example, vanilloid receptors for capsaicin, the hot in hot peppers). Evolutionarily, the mucous membranes of the oral cavity are the probable biologic target tissue, but afferents serving skin and deep tissues are also responsive. Most chemoreceptive C afferents are interoceptors designed to detect the array of intrinsic mediators of inflammation.

Stimulus Encoding The transduction process yields a decremental generator potential, the effect of which is limited to the distal few hundred micrometers of the axon end. For sensation to occur, the generator potential must be ''encoded'' into a spike train. This occurs in a nearby patch of membrane, the encoder, that is presumably rich in voltage-sensitive Na^+ channels and functions like the axon hillock-initial segment zone of CNS projection neurons (Fig.1, *top left*). In contrast to transduction, the encoding process is TTX-sensitive.

Encoding is a nonlinear process (Fig.1, *top right*). There is always a threshold value below which no spikes are generated (single spike threshold). Many afferent types also have a second, higher, ''threshold for repetitive firing.''[6,7] The value of the threshold for repetitive firing could, in principle, determine whether an afferent responds as a nociceptor or as a low-threshold mechanoreceptor, independent of the generator potential. Correspondingly, a shift in the repetitive firing threshold toward lower stimulus values would sensitize the ending, much like an increase in generator potential (Fig. 1, *bottom*). This appears to be what happens in the case of nerve injury.

189

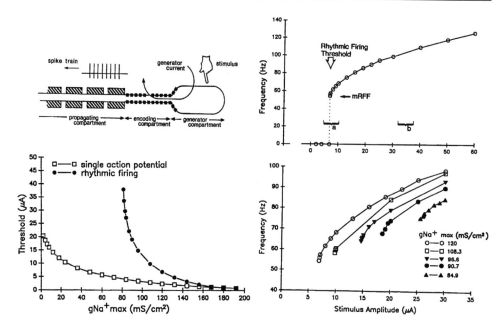

Fig. 1 *Principles of rhythmic electrogenesis in sensory endings.* **Top left,** *Representation of the generator, encoding, and propagating compartments of the axon end, intact or chronically severed.* **Top right** *and* **bottom,** *Computer simulation of repetitive firing in response to a prolonged depolarizing generator current, based on the Hodgkin-Huxley equations for the squid giant axon.* **Top right,** *Frequency-current (f-I) relationship (encoding function). At threshold, firing rate increases stepwise from zero to the fiber's minimum rhythmic firing frequency (mRFF). Note that a small change in stimulus strength around threshold (region (a)) has a much larger effect on firing frequency than the same change in region (b). (Reproduced with permission from Matzner O, Devor M: Na^+ conductance and the threshold for repetitive neuronal firing. Brain Res 1992;597:92–98.)* **Bottom right,** *A family of f-I curves using gradually increasing Na^+ channel density (gNa^+_{max}). As Na^+ channels are added, repetitive firing threshold decreases, as does the mRFF.* **Bottom left,** *The change in rhythmic firing threshold, and the threshold for evoking a single spike, as a function of Na^+ channel density. Note that with the parameters adopted,[7] repetitive firing cannot be elicited below about 80 ms/cm^2 no matter how strong the stimulus. (Reproduced with permission from Devor M, Lomazov P, Matzner O: Na^+ channel accumulation in injured axons as a substrate for neuropathic pain, in Boivie J, Hansson P, Lindblom U (eds): Touch, Temperature and Pain in Health and Disease: Mechanisms and Assessments. Seattle, WA, IASP Press, 1994, pp 207–230.)*

Peripheral Sensitization by Inflammatory Mediators

Inflammation increases the sensitivity of nociceptive endings in peripheral tissues by means of a complex soup of mediator molecules (see chapters 11, 17, and 35).[4] Some act directly on afferent endings, while others evoke the release of direct-acting mediators. Inflammatory mediators activate nociceptor endings and, in addition, make them prone to activation by weak touch stimuli. This action yields ongoing pain (stinging, burning) and abnormal sensitivity on movement. These two effects may be independent. Some mediators, for example, do not induce ongoing pain, but do sensitize. As many as one third of nociceptors cannot normally be activated by even strong noxious stimuli. These "silent" nociceptors are engaged only in the presence of inflammation.[8]

Despite the dearth of direct evidence, it is widely assumed that the main action of inflammatory mediators is to depolarize the membrane of nociceptor endings, bringing them closer to threshold.[4,8] Another possibility, rarely mentioned, is that they lower the repetitive firing threshold itself, ie, shift the encoding function to the left (Fig. 1, *top right* and *bottom*).[9]

Peripheral sensitization of C-nociceptors in inflamed tissue contributes to pain in two ways: (1) The ongoing and movement-evoked nociceptive barrage it occasions yields pain directly, and (2) this barrage triggers central sensitization. As a result, normal Aβ afferent endings might contribute to low back pain even though they themselves are only minimally affected by inflammatory mediators.

Ectopic Firing in Injured Afferents

Many of the chapters in this volume document the fact that herniation of the nucleus pulposus, or other forms of spinal injury, can apply compression and traction forces to the spinal nerve, the DRG, and the dorsal roots (DRs) of the spine. As already noted, forces of this sort do not trigger impulses in normal axons (nerve or DR) although they may activate DRG cells. Therefore, compression or traction in and of itself is probably not an important source of low back pain. However, if compression and traction forces are applied over hours and days, the basic electric properties of axons gradually change. The midnerve part of the axon develops the ability to generate impulses on weak mechanical, thermal, and chemical stimulation. That is, the nerve injury site becomes a locus of ectopic impulse generation.

Conversion of Axons to Sources of Ectopic Firing: The Severed Axon

The relatively blunt forces of intervertebral disk herniation do not sever spinal nerves completely leaving a nerve end neuroma. However, compression and traction forces, when applied for hours or days, cause many axons to be, in effect, severed as a result of slow pathophysiologic processes, such as necrosis and phagocytosis. In a rat model of painful nerve entrapment, for example, the sciatic nerve is loosely constricted. Depending on the duration of entrapment, within a few days most or all A fibers, and also many C fibers, begin undergoing anterograde (wallerian) degeneration,[10-14] which is a result of their having been severed at the injury site.

When an axon is severed, its end rapidly seals off and forms a terminal swelling or endbulb. It may also die retrogradely for up to a few millimeters. The myelin sheath near the cut end is invariably disrupted, as is myelin in many of the variable number of axons that are not severed.[15,16] In neonates, most axotomized DRG cells die, but in adults the majority survive. Within 24 hours, fine processes (axonal sprouts), emerge from the retracted endbulb. Under optimal conditions, when injury has occurred peripheral to the DRG, these regenerating sprouts may elongate and eventually reach their peripheral target, restoring sensory function.[10,15] When forward growth is blocked, however, terminal endbulbs and aborted sprouts persist.[16]

Thus, depending on the location, duration, and magnitude of the compressive and/or traction forces involved, disk herniation might leave a variable mix of intact through-conducting axons, axons with local demyelination, regenerating axons, and trapped sprouts and endbulbs. This bruised stretch of spinal nerve or root is a ''neuroma-in-continuity.'' Sprouts that do begin to regenerate may subsequently get caught up distal to the injury site, forming disseminated microneuromas scattered along the nerve trunk, its tributary branches, the spinal cord entry zone, and peripheral target tissue. Nerve injury also triggers the collateral sprouting of nearby intact afferents.[17]

Axonal endbulbs and sprouts that form in association with nerve and root entrapment may become a source of hyperexcitability and ectopic firing (Fig. 2, *right*). The abnormal firing involves Aδ and C afferents as well as Aβ afferents.[18-23] Ectopic hyperexcitability means both spontaneous firing and abnormal sensitivity to a range of physical, chemical, and metabolic challenges. For example, by exploring the surface of the nerve injury site with fine probes, it is usually possible to demonstrate localized ''hotspots'' of mechanosensitivity (Fig. 3).

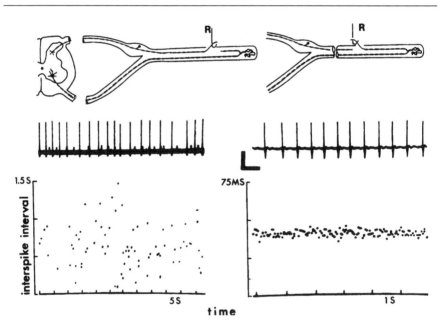

Fig. 2   *Spontaneous ectopic discharge is generated in chronically injured sensory neurons.[23] Alternative sources are the DRG (**left**) and the nerve injury site (**right**). The dot displays below the sample spike trains illustrate two of the most common firing patterns: slow irregular (**left**, the most common pattern in DRGs and neuroma C fibers), and rapid rhythmic, with highly regular intervals between consecutive impulses (**right**, the most common pattern in neuroma A fibers). (Reproduced with permission from Devor M: The pathophysiology of damaged peripheral nerve, in Wall PD, Melzack R, Bonica JJ (eds): Textbook of Pain, ed 3. Edinburgh, Scotland, Churchill Livingstone, 1994, pp 79–100.)*

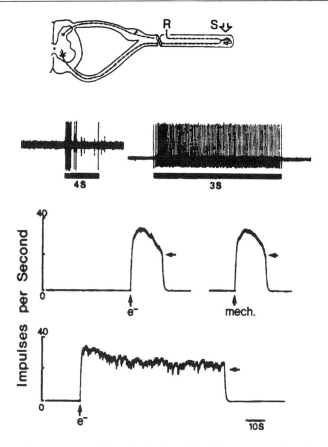

Fig. 3 *Abnormal mechanosensitivity of injured peripheral nerve axons.* **Top,** *Recordings were made from sensory axons (R) in chronically injured rat sciatic nerve.*[23] **Center,** *Many fibers responded to sustained displacement at the injury site (S) with a rapidly (left) or slowly adapting (right) impulse discharge.* **Bottom,** *Some fibers responded with a prolonged discharge burst that long outlasted the momentary stimulus applied, e⁻= electrical, and mech. = mechanical. (Reproduced with permission from Devor M: The pathophysiology of damaged peripheral nerve, in Wall PD, Melzack R (eds):* Textbook of Pain, *ed 3. Edinburgh, Scotland, Churchill Livingstone, 1994, pp 79–100.)*

The functional consequences of axotomy due to compression and traction depend on where along the axon the injury occurred. If the injury occurred in the DR, between the DRG and the spinal cord (for example, in many disk herniations and in spinal stenosis), the axon segment between the injury site and the spinal cord is disconnected from the cell soma and, therefore, degenerates. This may yield true deafferentation effects. However, any ectopic firing that may develop in the surviving parts of the sensory neuron has no direct access to the sensorium. On the other hand, if the injury occurred within or distal to the DRG, the proximal axon stump remains in continuity with the DRG and the CNS, and whatever ectopic firing occurs there can enter the spinal cord with obvious consequences for sensation.

Conversion of Axons to Sources of Ectopic Firing: Demyelination

Axons that have been demyelinated locally, but are otherwise in continuity, may also become hyperexcitable. As with severed axons, this hyperexcitability is reflected in spontaneous impulse discharge and mechanosensitivity.[24-27] Disk herniation and spinal stenosis can cause extensive demyelination in spinal roots and, hence, functionally significant demyelination-related ectopia. It is not known whether ectopic firing develops in unmyelinated (C) axons that remain in continuity through zones of compression in which A fibers suffer demyelination. Even if it does not, ectopia in Aβ axons can be painful in the presence of central sensitization.

Spontaneous Ectopic Discharge

Different sensory receptor types contribute unequally to the overall ectopic barrage.[28-30] In rats, at least, A fibers are most active in the first few weeks following injury, during which time as many as 25% of the afferents fire spontaneously. Later, ectopia in C fibers predominates.[23] Early signs of emerging ectopic mechanosensitivity are present within 4 hours of injury, although spontaneous firing becomes prominent only after 2 to 3 days.[20,23,29,31] There are some indications that deep (muscle and joint) afferents may be more prone to generating ectopia than cutaneous afferents.[30]

Most spontaneously active neuroma A-afferents (about 90% in rats) discharge rhythmically, with highly regular intervals between adjacent impulses within a train (Fig. 2, *right*). This is the firing pattern expected of intrinsic electrogenesis at a single active pacemaker site, "autorhythmicity."[7] Interspike interval for individual fibers usually falls within the range of 65 to 35 ms, which translates to an instantaneous discharge rate in the range of 15 to 30 Hz.[20,23] Such rates represent a substantial sensory stimulus in normal nerve. In just over a third of autorhythmic fibers, the discharge is interrupted by silent pauses, resulting in a burst-like on-off pattern. The remaining A fibers have a slow irregular firing pattern (0.1 to 10 Hz). Curiously, nearly all spontaneously active C fibers, in rat neuromas at least, fire slowly and irregularly. This implies an interesting and perhaps exploitable difference in the mechanism of electrogenesis in A versus C fibers.

Mechano-, Thermo-, and Chemosensitivity

Ectopic hyperexcitability is also reflected in abnormal sensitivity to a broad range of presumably depolarizing stimuli. For example, as already noted, many spontaneously active fibers, and previously silent ones as well, are excited by mechanical probing. The evoked discharge is usually limited to the time of stimulation.[23] Sometimes, however, discharge continues for an extended period of time after the end of the stimulus (mechanical afterdischarge; Fig. 3, *bottom*).

In man, mechanosensitivity is reflected in the Tinel sign and in "trigger points" at sites of neuroma-in-continuity. Locations in which nerves run adjacent to tendon and bone (carpal tunnel, spinal and cranial foramina) or those in which small branches cross over tough fascial planes are prone to developing consistently located mechanosensitive tender spots (as in fibromyalgia). Afferents running in the dorsal rami and serving paraspinal tissues appear to be particularly at risk. Acquired damage of dorsal ramus axons in tissue retraction during laminectomy may be an important reason for recurrent pain following low back surgery.

A practical example of the role of ectopia in the realm of back pain was given recently by Kuslich and associates.[32] They performed lumbar spine decompression operations for spinal stenosis and disk herniation using progressive local anesthesia. Briefly, each subsequent tissue layer was infiltrated, permitting mechanical, thermal, and electrical stimulation of the underlying tissue in which the innervation remained at least partially functional. Noxious stimulation of most tissues, including ligaments, bone, facet synovium and cartilage, muscle, epidural fat, and vasculature, sometimes produced sharp, localized pain, but rarely if ever the dull ache of low back pain (lumbago) and never shooting pain in the leg (sciatica). In contrast, in most patients, stimulation of the anulus fibrosus, and occasionally the adjacent posterior longitudinal ligament, produced low back pain similar in quality to the pain that brought the patient to surgery. Likewise, the application of local anesthetic obliterated the pain. Pain referral was topographic. The central anulus and posterior longitudinal ligament produced pain in the central back. Stimulation to the right or left of center produced pain on the corresponding side. Initiation of pain in the buttock required simultaneous manipulation of the nerve root and the outer anulus fibrosus. Pressure on intact nerves was always painless. However, the authors were consistently able to reproduce the patients' sciatica by stimulating a traumatized region of nerve root or its DRG, or by applying traction to the dural sleeve that would be transmitted to these tissues. The sciatic pain so evoked was consistently eliminated by local anesthetic block in the area of nerve injury.

The clear and consistent relation between sciatic reference and stimulation of the nerve root and DRG suggests that in the case of the anulus fibrosus, too, it might not only be local nerve endings in the anulus that caused the pain referral, but also transmission of a stretch stimulus to small bundles of traumatized dorsal ramus tributaries that innervate the corresponding low back tissue and buttock.

Using microneurographic recording in awake humans, Nystrom and Hagbarth[33] documented ongoing discharge in the peroneal nerve in a lower extremity amputee. The patient had ongoing phantom foot pain that was augmented by percussion of the neuroma. The same percussion elicited an intense burst of spike activity, mostly in slow-conducting axons. This burst was eliminated, along with the evoked pain, by local anesthetic block of the neuroma. Most of the ongoing discharge persisted, indicating that it arose upstream, perhaps in the DRG, and reached the recording electrode by propagating antidromically. In a related study, dysesthesias referred to the foot were triggered by straight-leg lifting (Lasègue's sign) in a patient with radicular pain related to surgery for disk herniation. This maneuver evoked ectopic bursts in the sural nerve, the intensity of which waxed and waned in close correlation with the abnormal sensation.[34] Once again, nerve blocks suggested that the ectopic source was in the injured root or DRG. Corresponding data were obtained in patients with positive sensory signs associated with nerve entrapment and multiple sclerosis.

In addition to physical stimuli, metabolic and chemical factors that influence membrane potential can excite ectopic discharge. Examples include ischemia, changes in blood gases and ion concentrations, pharmacologic blockade of K^+

conductances, inflammatory mediators, catecholamines, peptides, and various other endogenous neuroactive substances.[23] For example, nerve fibers damaged as a result of disk herniation are likely to come into contact with inflammatory mediators, both at the injury site and during regeneration into injured and inflamed tissue of the lower spine. These substances (for example, histamine and prostaglandins) are known to selectively excite injured C fibers.[35,36] The injection of excitatory substances into an ectopic focus in experimental animals augments firing and evokes pain, whereas the injection of membrane stabilizing drugs (for example, lidocaine) suppresses them.[23] Some of these observations have recently been verified in humans. Specifically, Chabal and associates[37,38] showed that the injection of K[+] channel blockers and of adrenoreceptor agonists into nerve end neuromas produces severe acute pain that can be relieved by subsequent infiltration of local anesthetics.

Ectopic Electrogenesis in Dorsal Root Ganglia

The development of ectopic firing capability in injured axons reflects a pathophysiologic change in membrane electrical properties. In contrast, some sensory cell somata in DRGs and cranial nerve ganglia are intrinsically rhythmogenic in the intact organism. For example, in intact animals some DRG cells fire repetitively on direct depolarization and are sensitive to mechanical probing and to various chemical mediators.[39-41] Mechanosensitivity, at least, is normally latent because DRGs are protected within a solid bony cavity. However, DRG mechanosensitivity probably is an important substrate for the immediate, acute pain of disk herniation and other injuries that apply traction or compressive forces directly to ganglia. A small percentage of DRG neurons fire spontaneously (Fig. 2, *left*). The magnitude of DRG discharge is significantly augmented by chronic nerve injury, including nerve transection and nerve constriction.[19,39-42] The nerve injury site and the DRG appear to be near-equal partners in the generation of ectopia.

Sympathetic-Sensory Coupling

A particularly significant source of enhanced neuropathic ectopia is sympathetic efferent activity. In experimentally injured afferent A and C fibers, repetitive discharge is often evoked or enhanced by systemic or close arterial injection of adrenaline or noradrenaline and by electrical stimulation of postganglionic sympathetic efferents (Fig. 4). The use of receptor-selective pharmacologic agents has revealed that these responses are mediated primarily by α_2-adrenoreceptors.[18,23,43-45] Sympathetic-sensory coupling also develops in the DRG following nerve injury.[46] This functional coupling is accompanied by sprouting of postganglionic efferent axons within the DRG.[47] The effect of sympathetic activity is not due to vasoconstrictor-induced cooling or ischemia; rather, it most likely reflects a direct action of α-agonists on adrenoreceptive endbulbs, sprouts, and/or DRG somata.[23,46]

Little work has been done to date on the possible involvement of sympathetic enhanced ectopic discharge in low back pain. However, there is good evidence that afferent excitation by sympathetics plays a major role in certain other chronic pain states, such as reflex sympathetic dystrophy.[23,43] In these, systemically injected phentolamine, an α-adrenoreceptor antagonist, has proved to be a useful diagnostic test for the sympathetic dependence of the pain.[48,49]

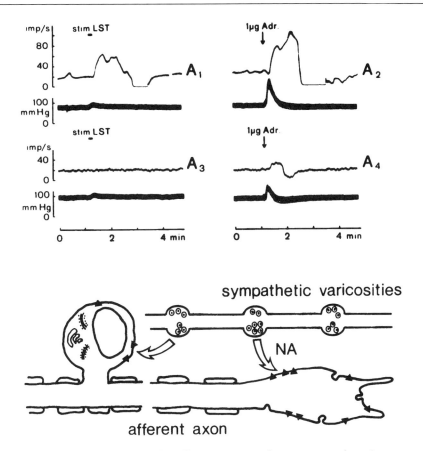

Fig. 4 *Sympathetic-sensory coupling.* **Top,** *Excitation of a spontaneously active neuroma afferent following stimulation of sympathetic efferent fibers in the lumbar sympathetic trunk (LST, A1), and following systemic injection of adrenaline (A2). Both responses are attenuated by the α-adrenoreceptor antagonist phentolamine (10 µg iv, A3 and A4). Simultaneous arterial pressure records are also shown. (Reproduced with permission from Devor M, Janig W: Activation of myelinated afferents ending in a neuroma by stimulation of the sypathetic supply in the rat.* Neurosci Lett *1981;24:43–47.)* **Bottom,** *A model of the underlying mechanism: noradrenaline (NA) released from nearby sympathetic efferent fibers binds to α-adrenoreceptors (filled triangles) on the injured afferent, evoking depolarization and ectopic firing.*

Cross-Excitation at Sites of Ectopic Electrogenesis

In healthy nerves, individual afferents constitute independent sensory conduction channels. In the event of injury, crosstalk of various sorts may emerge. The best known example, although not necessarily the most important from a functional point of view, is ephaptic crosstalk.[23,50,51] Both severed axons and adjacent demyelinated ones may become coupled ephaptically. In each case, ephaptic crosstalk is thought to result from close apposition between adjacent axons in the absence of the normal glial insulation.[51,52] Because coupled fibers are frequently of different types, this is a mechanism whereby nociceptors might be activated by low-threshold afferents or even efferents.

The signature of ephaptic crosstalk is high safety-factor, bidirectional coupling in which a single impulse in an active fiber evokes a single impulse in its neighbor. Lisney and Devor[53] discovered a completely different form of cross-excitation called crossed afterdischarge. Here, single impulses have no effect, but repetitive activity excites passive neighbors to repetitive autonomous firing. In contrast to ephaptic crosstalk, crossed afterdischarge develops soon after nerve injury, depends less on close axonal apposition, occurs also in the DRG, and comes to involve a much larger proportion of afferents.[23,53]

The process of crossed afterdischarge at nerve injury sites and DRGs raises the possibility of a striking functional consequence. Triggered by an afferent volley resulting from a sudden movement, excitatory coupling could enter a positive feedback mode. The initial volley would cross-excite close neighbors, and these would cross-excite more distant neighbors, and so forth, setting off a chain reaction. Such an excitatory explosion that involved the entire nerve or DRG might be felt as a paroxysmal shock-like pain.[54]

What Causes the Development of Ectopic Hyperexcitability in Injured Axons and Axotomized DRG Cells?

The development of ectopia in the hours and days following axotomy and demyelination is thought to be due to remodeling of the axon membrane's local electrical properties.[9,23] The principal underlying mechanism appears to be the accumulation of excess voltage-sensitive Na^+ channels in terminal swellings (neuroma endbulbs) and sprouts in the region of injury and in patches of demyelination (Fig. 5). Na^+ channels, like other membrane-bound proteins, are synthesized in the cell soma in the DRG, transported down the axon by antero-

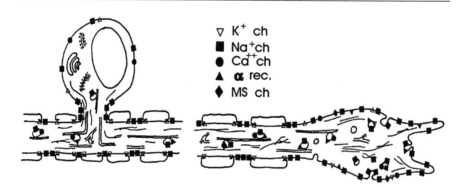

∇ K^+ ch
■ Na^+ch
● Cd^{++}ch
▲ α rec.
◆ MS ch

Fig. 5 *Working hypothesis of the mechanism of hyperexcitability of injured axons. Various ion channels and receptors, notably Na^+ channels, are transported anterogradely along the axon and incorporated in excess into the axon membrane near the injury site. K^+ch = potassium channels; Na^+ ch = sodium channels; Ca^{++} ch = calcium channels; αrec. = α-adrenoreceptors; MS ch = mechanosensitive channels. (Adapted with permission from Devor M: The pathophysiology of damaged peripheral nerve, in Wall PD, Melzack R (eds): Textbook of Pain, ed 3. Edinburgh, Scotland, Churchill Livingstone, 1994, pp 79–100.)*

grade axoplasmic flow, and incorporated into the axolemma by exocytotic vesicle fusion. At midnerve sites in intact axons, Na^+ channel density is too low to support electrogenesis. Nerve injury-induced channel accumulation apparently results from elimination of the factors that normally exclude Na^+ channels from the midnerve axolemma (particularly myelin) and from the damming up of channels originally destined for downstream targets.[9,23] Axonal injury also appears to trigger the upregulation of channel synthesis in the cell soma in the DRG and to induce the expression of previously silent Na^+ channel types.[55,56] Nerve injury sites are rich in nerve growth factor (NGF) released by local non-neural cells.[57] In vitro, exposure to NGF has been shown to trigger upregulation of Na^+ channel synthesis in neurons.[58,59]

Numeric simulation indicates that both increased Na^+ conductance (Fig.1, *bottom*) and decreased K^+ conductance[9] shift the threshold for repetitive firing in the direction of hyperexcitability. As expected, K^+ channel blockers excite already established ectopic sources and evoke pain.[23,37] Elimination of K^+ channels, however, cannot be a primary cause of ectopia because the application of K^+ channel blockers to acutely cut axons, even in the presence of enhanced Na^+ conductance, is insufficient to elicit firing.[60] On the other hand, the reduction in K^+ channel-related afterhyperpolarization in the cell soma may play a primary role in ectopia originating in axotomized DRG neurons.

The accumulation of excess Na^+ channels at neuroma endbulbs and patches of demyelination confers on these sites the characteristics of a sensory encoder. Still, to generate ectopic discharge, there must be an adequate generator current. This current appears to be provided by passive membrane leak or by transducer receptors and channels as in normal sensory endings (for example, MS channels). Like Na^+ channels, these other receptors and channels are synthesized in the DRG neuron and transported distally. Thus, they too may accumulate at sites of axotomy and demyelination. The presence of abnormal types or concentrations of receptors and channels is indicated by the fact that ectopic firing sites respond in a specific manner to mechanical displacement (Fig. 3), temperature changes, and relevant chemical mediators, including inflammatory mediators and adrenergic agonists.[23] Indeed, there is evidence that individual axons recapitulate the specific sensitivities and adaptation characteristics that they expressed at their normal transducer ending before axotomy.[28,29]

Ectopic electrogenesis originating at nerve injury sites and the DRG is suppressed by Na^+ channel blockers (membrane stabilizers) at concentrations far lower than those required to block nerve conduction.[61] This observation has prompted the increased clinical use of systemically and regionally administered membrane stabilizers (for example, systemic lidocaine, carbamazepine, mexiletine, and others) in the management of subacute and chronic pain.[62,63] Analgesic effectiveness has been demonstrated in a considerable range of conditions, including diabetic neuropathy, postherpetic neuralgia, cranial nerve neuralgias, multiple sclerosis, adiposis dolorosa, burn pain, rheumatoid arthritis, postsurgical pain, some cancer pains, thalamic pain, anesthesia dolorosa, and arachnoiditis. Membrane stabilizing drugs applied systemically or regionally might prove to be efficacious in the treatment of disk pain as well, especially in forms associated with ectopic hyperexcitability.

Central Sensitization

Ectopic firing may develop in both low threshold Aβ afferents and in Aδ and C nociceptors. When only Aβ fibers are active the result is nonpainful paresthesias.[64] However, as with inflammatory pain, ectopic firing in nociceptors contributes to pain in two ways. First, it evokes pain directly. Second, it evokes central sensitization, thereby initiating tenderness in tissues with residual Aβ innervation and augmenting spontaneous and movement-evoked pain from ectopically active Aβ and nociceptive afferents. All of these sources probably contribute to low back pain. What is the evidence for central sensitization?

Central Sensitization and Secondary Hyperalgesia

The reality of central sensitization is best illustrated by the example of localized inflammation of the skin, but the same process also is very likely to occur in deep tissues of the lumbar spine. Following localized skin trauma, tenderness (mechanical allodynia) spreads for a considerable distance from the area of trauma, including into areas where there is no detectable inflammation. Tenderness at a distance from the area of trauma is secondary hyperalgesia. An important historic debate centered on whether secondary hyperalgesia is due to nociceptors sensitized by diffusion of algogenic substances or by axon reflex activity, or whether it is due to altered processing of impulses entering the CNS along normal low threshold Aβ touch afferents.[65,66]

Evidence tilting the scale toward the latter hypothesis has been obtained only recently. There are four main lines of evidence.[67-71] First, on use of cuff and anesthetic procedures that block A and C fibers (relatively) selectively, secondary hyperalgesia fades with block of A-fiber conduction, and returns only when A-fiber conduction is restored. Second, the stimulus to response latency of touch-evoked pain corresponds to conduction at A-fiber velocity. Third, intraneural and transcutaneous electrical stimulation of Aβ axons, which bypasses their sensory ending, elicits pain in the zone of secondary hyperalgesia (and also in the zone of primary hyperalgesia) but not in intact skin. Finally, recording experiments have failed to yield evidence of nociceptor sensitization away from the area of obvious inflammation. The same types of evidence indicate that in many cases of neuropathy, allodynic pain is evoked by activity in Aβ afferents.[68,71,72] The central sensitization responsible for Aβ-evoked pain appears to be triggered by C-fiber input generated, alternatively, by noxious stimulation of intact skin (or deep tissue), stimulation of sensitized C nociceptors in inflamed tissue, or ectopic firing of C afferents at the site of nerve injury and associated DRGs.

Central Sensitization and Neuropathic Pain

The dual role of nociceptor ectopia in the generation of chronic pain is best illustrated in conditions in which a well-localized ectopic focus can be specifically identified. Sheen and Chung,[73] for example, severed the spinal nerve of DRGs L5 and L6 in rats, creating a focus of ectopic discharge in the L5 and L6 neuromas and DRGs. This lesion is akin to what might occur with disk herniation. The result was behavioral signs of ongoing pain, presumably due directly to the ectopia, and allodynia in the hindlimb skin served by the L4 root, presumably due to central sensitization (Fig. 6). Eliminating the ectopia by secondarily cutting the L5 and L6 dorsal roots eliminated the ongoing discomfort

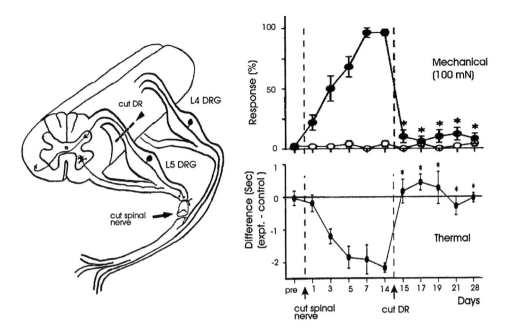

Fig. 6 *Evidence that ectopia originating at sites of nerve injury and associated dorsal root ganglia (DRGs) contributes to cutaneous hypersensitivity.[73] Graphs on the right plot withdrawal responses of rats to mechanical probing and to radiant heat projected onto the plantar surface of the foot.* **Upper graph,** *Percentage of trials on which there was a withdrawal response; open circles-intact side, filled circles-operated side.* **Lower graph,** *Response latency calculated as operated side minus control side. Negative values reflect excess sensitivity on the operated side. (See text for explanation.)*

and also normalized sensation in the L4 territory. Gracely and associates[72] demonstrated similar events in humans. One of their neuropathic pain patients, for example, had a focally painful scar near the knee and allodynia extending up the thigh and down the calf. Local anesthetic block of the scar eliminated the scar pain and also the extended allodynia for the duration of the block. In the lumbar spine, ectopic and inflammatory sources of noxious input probably often set up central sensitization. Subsequently, sensory input evoked by gentle movement, activating only Aβ afferents, would contribute to low back pain.

Neural Mechanism of Central Sensitization

Central sensitization, as manifest behaviorally and psychophysically, has its counterpart in spinal cord electrophysiology. Within a few minutes of delivering a brief (seconds) noxious conditioning stimulus to afferent C fibers in acute experiments in rats and in monkeys, a transient hyperexcitability state develops in postsynaptic neurons in the dorsal horn representation of the corresponding body part. The indicators of emerging hyperexcitability are windup (stimulus-to-stimulus increase in response magnitude) on repetitive C-fiber stimulation, expansion of cutaneous receptive fields, and the acquisition by nociceptive-selective neurons of wide dynamic range (WDR) properties.[74,75] In each case

Aβ afferents come to drive postsynaptic neurons that they were previously in-effective at driving. The exaggerated postsynaptic responses persist for tens of minutes and up to more than an hour in the case of conditioning on a muscle nerve. Correspondingly, awake animals show the expected behavioral hyper-sensitivity.[71,73]

The mechanism thought to account for central sensitization is illustrated in Figure 7. Briefly, spinal terminals of Aβ touch afferents normally activate WDR neurons by releasing glutamate. This drives the neurons modestly, via non-N-methyl-D-aspartate (NMDA) glutamate receptors. NMDA glutamate receptors, present postsynaptically, are blocked at normal membrane potentials by Mg^{2+} ions. C nociceptors release glutamate and peptide neurotransmitters, notably sub-stance P (SP). Adequately intense C input produces prolonged (tens of seconds) SP-evoked depolarization, which displaces the Mg^{2+} block, enabling the NMDA receptors and rendering them responsive to Aβ touch afferents. Because the Aβ

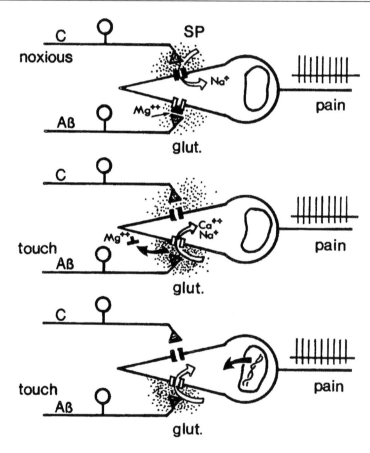

Fig. 7 *Schematic diagram of the proposed neural mechanism of central sensitization. (See text for explanation.) The idea (**bottom**) that Ca^{++} entry through NMDA receptors may al-ter gene expression in a way that makes central sensitization permanent and independent of ongoing nociceptor drive remains speculative.*

fibers now act via NMDA as well as non-NMDA receptors, they drive WDR neurons more effectively than before, and hence elicit allodynia. The persistence of sensitization beyond the duration of the SP-evoked depolarization is thought to be due to Ca^{2+} entry through the NMDA receptor channels. This activates a Ca^{2+}-dependent protein kinase and phosphorylates ion channels, sustaining the sensitized state.[75]

The Time-Constant (Persistence) of Central Sensitization

Central sensitization can apparently be sustained indefinitely if the noxious conditioning input is maintained, such as in chronic inflammatory diseases or sustained ectopic firing in neuropathy. However, when the sustaining noxious input is eliminated, for example, by cooling or use of local anesthetics, Aβ pain disappears rapidly, usually within minutes.[68,72] For this reason, the primary noxious focus is said to both trigger and maintain central sensitization. It is possible that amplification due to central sensitization might be prevented using pharmacologic antagonists to NMDA-receptors. Several trials of this approach are currently in progress. Another strategy being tested in an attempt to lessen postoperative pain is preemptive analgesia.[76] The idea here is to prevent the central sensitizing effects of noxious input during surgery by supplementing general anesthetics with regional block or opiates.

Beyond the nociceptor-initiated central sensitization phenomenon just discussed, injury to peripheral nerves triggers a spectrum of long-term CNS changes.[77] In principle, any of these could form the basis for a persistent type of central sensitization.

Summary and Perspective

To understand low back pain, it is essential to focus on those processes that induce abnormal firing in the primary afferent neurons that innervate low back tissue. Herniation of the nucleus pulposus, spinal stenosis, vertebral trauma, and other forms of spinal injury and disease apply compression and traction forces to the spinal nerve, the DRG, and the DRs of the spine. Blunt forces of this sort are incapable of triggering impulses in normal axons in nerves or DRs, although they may activate some DRG cells. Thus, acute nerve/root compression or traction per se is probably not a direct cause of low back pain. DRG compression may be. However, the continuous or repeated application of compression and traction forces over hours and days brings about a gradual neuropathic change in the affected axons including demyelination and frank axotomy. These changes are responsible for the emergence of spontaneous ectopic firing and hypersensitivity to weak mechanical stimulation, such as is generated in the lower back during movement. Ectopic hyperexcitability is also reflected in the abnormal sensitivity of afferents to a broad range of other presumably depolarizing stimuli that potentially are present at or near the site of injury. These include ischemia and hypoxia, chemical mediators of inflammation, and sympathetic efferent activity. Injured afferent axons and axotomized sensory cell bodies within the DRG are also subject to various forms of neuron-to-neuron cross-excitation. All of these factors contribute to the ectopic impulse barrage arising from the nerve roots and the DRG. Both low threshold Aβ afferents and Aδ and C nociceptors are involved.

It is no longer tenable to presume that if pain is felt, it must be a direct reflection of activity in Aδ or C nociceptive afferents. In the presence of central sensitization, impulses in Aβ touch afferents may also give rise to pain. Central sensitization can be triggered by C nociceptor input. Therefore, whenever nociceptor activity is present, Aβ touch fibers as well as Aδ and C nociceptors are likely to contribute to pain. For example, when spinal trauma triggers inflammation in tissues of the lower back, Aδ and C nociceptors may become sensitized (peripheral sensitization), giving rise to a painful afferent barrage. In addition, however, this input may trigger central sensitization with the result that normal and ectopic low threshold Aβ input generated at rest and by movement augments the pain. By the same token, ectopic firing in nociceptors contributes to pain in two ways. It evokes pain directly, and it evokes central sensitization, thereby initiating tenderness in paraspinal tissues with residual normal Aβ innervation and augmenting spontaneous and movement-evoked pain from ectopically active Aβ and nociceptive afferents. The emerging understanding of the neural mechanisms of ectopic hyperexcitability in injured afferent neurons and the knowledge that normal and ectopic Aβ touch input, as well as Aδ and C-nociceptor input, contribute to subacute and chronic pathophysiologic pain states, suggests previously unanticipated possibilities for clinical pain control. These include the systemic and regional use of membrane stabilizers, including the development of ones with greater selectivity for nociceptors; targeting of DRG ectopia; more circumspect surgery; block of sympathetic-sensory coupling; use of NMDA receptor antagonists; and preemptive maneuvers.

Acknowledgments

The author's work on this subject is supported primarily by the US-Israel Binational Science Foundation (BSF), the German-Israel Foundation for Research and Development (GIF), the Israel Science Foundation, the Israel Ministry of Science and Arts, and the Hebrew University Center for Research on Pain.

References

1. Loewenstein WR: Mechano-electric transduction in the Pacinian corpuscle: Initiation of sensory impulses in mechanoreceptors, in Autrum H (ed): *Handbook of Sensory Physiology.* Berlin, Germany, Springer-Verlag, 1971, vol 1, pp 267–290.
2. Hille B (ed): *Ionic Channels of Excitable Membranes*, ed 2. Sunderland, MA, Sinauer Associates, 1992.
3. Devor M, Basbaum AI, Bennett GJ, et al: Mechanisms of neuropathic pain following peripheral injury, in Basbaum AI, Besson JMR (eds): *Towards a New Pharmacotherapy of Pain.* Chichester, England, John Wiley & Sons, 1991, pp 417–440.
4. Levine J, Taiwo Y: Inflammatory pain, in Wall PD, Melzack R, Bonica JJ (eds): *Textbook of Pain*, ed 3. Edinburgh, Scotland, Churchill Livingstone, 1994, pp 45–56.
5. Sachs F: Biophysics of mechanoreception. *Mem Biochem* 1986;6:173–195.
6. Jack JJB, Noble D, Tsien RW (eds): *Electric Current Flow in Excitable Cells.* Oxford, England, Clarendon Press, 1983.
7. Matzner O, Devor M: Na⁺ conductance and the threshold for repetitive neuronal firing. *Brain Res* 1992;597:92–98.

8. Schmidt RF, Schaible H-G, Meslinger K, et al: Silent and active nociceptors: Structure, functions, and clinical implications, in Gebhart GF, Hammond DL, Jensen TS (eds): *Progress in Pain Research and Management.* Seattle, WA, IASP Press, 1994, vol 2, pp 213–250.

9. Devor M, Lomazov P, Matzner O: Na$^+$ channel accumulation in injured axons as a substrate for neuropathic pain, in Boivie J, Hansson P, Lindblom U (eds): *Touch, Temperature and Pain in Health and Disease: Mechanisms and Assessments.* Seattle, WA, IASP Press, 1994, pp 207–230.

10. Guilbaud G, Gautron M, Jazat F, et al: Time course of degeneration and regeneration of myelinated nerve fibres following chronic loose ligatures of the rat sciatic nerve: Can nerve lesions be linked to the abnormal pain-related behaviours? *Pain* 1993;53:147–158.

11. Basbaum AI, Gautron M, Jazat F, et al: The spectrum of fiber loss in a model of neuropathic pain in the rat: An electron microscopic study. *Pain* 1991;47:359–367.

12. Nuytten D, Kupers R, Lammens M, et al: Further evidence for myelinated as well as unmyelinated fibre damage in a rat model of neuropathic pain. *Exp Brain Res* 1992;91:73–78.

13. Nitz AJ, Matulionis DH: Ultrastructural changes in rat peripheral nerve following pneumatic tourniquet compression. *J Neurosurg* 1982;57:660–666.

14. Mosconi T, Kruger L: Fixed-diameter polyethylene cuffs applied to the rat sciatic nerve induce a painful neuropathy: Ultrastructural morphometric analysis of axonal alterations. *Pain* 1996;64:37–57.

15. Fawcett JW, Keynes RJ: Peripheral nerve regeneration. *Annu Rev Neurosci* 1990;13:43–60.

16. Fried K, Govrin-Lippmann R, Rosenthal F, et al: Ultrastructure of afferent axon endings in a neuroma. *J Neurocytol* 1991;20:682–701.

17. Devor M, Schonfeld D, Seltzer Z, et al: Two modes of cutaneous reinnervation following peripheral nerve injury. *J Comp Neurol* 1979;185:211–220

18. Wall PD, Gutnick M: Ongoing activity in peripheral nerves: The physiology and pharmacology of impulses originating from a neuroma. *Exp Neurol* 1974;43:580–593.

19. Kirk EJ: Impulses in dorsal spinal nerve rootlets in cats and rabbits arising from dorsal root ganglia isolated from the periphery. *J Comp Neurol* 1974;155:165–176.

20. Papir-Kricheli D, Devor M: Abnormal impulse discharge in primary afferent axons injured in the peripheral versus the central nervous system. *Somatosens Motor Res* 1988;6:63–77.

21. Habler H-J, Janig W, Koltzenburg M: Activation of unmyelinated afferents in chronically lesioned nerves by adrenaline and excitation of sympathetic efferents in the cat. *Neurosci Lett* 1987;82:35–40.

22. Xie Y-K, Xiao W-H: Electrophysiological evidence for hyperalgesia in the peripheral neuropathy. *Sci China B* 1990;33:663–672.

23. Devor M: The pathophysiology of damaged peripheral nerve, in Wall PD, Melzack R, Bonica JJ (eds): *Textbook of Pain,* ed 3. Edinburgh, Scotland, Churchill Livingstone, 1994, pp 79–100.

24. Calvin WH, Devor M, Howe JF: Can neuralgias arise from minor demyelination? Spontaneous firing, mechanosensitivity and after-discharge from conducting axons. *Exp Neurol* 1982;75:755–763.

25. Rasminsky M: Hyperexcitability of pathologically myelinated axons and positive symptoms in multiple sclerosis, in Waxman SG, Ritchie JM (eds): *Demyelinating Diseases: Basic and Clinical Electrophysiology.* New York, NY, Raven Press, 1981, pp 289–297.

26. Smith KJ, McDonald WI: Spontaneous and mechanically evoked activity due to central demyelinating lesion. *Nature* 1980;286:154–155.

27. Burchiel KJ: Ectopic impulse generation in focally demyelinated trigeminal nerve. *Exp Neurol* 1980;69:423–429.

28. Devor M, Keller CH, Ellisman MH: Spontaneous discharge of afferents in a neuroma reflects original receptor tuning. *Brain Res* 1990;517:245–250.

205

29. Koschorke GM, Meyer RA, Tillman DB, et al: Ectopic excitability of injured nerves in monkey: Entrained responses to vibratory stimuli. *J Neurophysiol* 1991;65:693–701.

30. Johnson RD, Munson JB: Regenerating sprouts of axotomized cat muscle afferents express characteristic firing patterns to mechanical stimulation. *J Neurophysiol* 1991;66:2155–2158.

31. Michaelis M, Blenk K-H, Janig W, Vogel C: Development of spontaneous activity and mechanosensitivity in axotomized afferent nerve fibers during the first hours after nerve transection in rats. *J Neurophysiol* 1995;74:1020–1027.

32. Kuslich SD, Ulstrom CL, Michael CJ: The tissue origin of low back pain and sciatica: A report of pain response to tissue stimulation during operations on the lumbar spine using local anesthesia. *Orthop Clin North Am* 1991;22:181–187.

33. Nystrom B, Hagbarth KE: Microelectrode recordings from transected nerves in amputees with phantom limb pain. *Neurosci Lett* 1981;27:211–216.

34. Nordin M, Nystrom B, Wallin U, et al: Ectopic sensory discharges and paresthesiae in patients with disorders of peripheral nerves, dorsal roots and dorsal columns. *Pain* 1984;20:231–245.

35. Welk E, Leah JD, Zimmermann M: Characteristics of A- and C-fibers ending in a sensory nerve neuroma in the rat. *J Neurophysiol* 1990;63:759–766.

36. Devor M, White DM, Goetzl EJ, et al: Eicosanoids, but not tachykinins, excite C-fiber endings in rat sciatic nerve-end neuromas. *Neuroreport* 1992;3:21–24.

37. Chabal C, Jacobson L, Russell LC, et al: Pain responses to perineuromal injection of normal saline, gallamine, and lidocaine in humans. *Pain* 1989;36:321–325.

38. Chabal C, Jacobson L, Russell LC, et al: Pain responses to perineuromal injection of normal saline, epinephrine, and lidocaine in humans. *Pain* 1992;49:9–12.

39. Howe JF, Loeser JD, Calvin WH: Mechanosensitivity of dorsal root ganglia and chronically injured axons: A physiological basis for the radicular pain of nerve root compression. *Pain* 1977;3:25–41.

40. Wall PD, Devor M: Sensory afferent impulses originate from dorsal root ganglia as well as from the periphery in normal and nerve-injured rats. *Pain* 1983;17:321–339.

41. Burchiel KJ: Spontaneous impulse generation in normal and denervated dorsal root ganglia: Sensitivity to alpha-adrenergic stimulation and hypoxia. *Exp Neurol* 1984;85:257–272.

42. Kajander KC, Wakisaka S, Bennett GJ: Spontaneous discharge originates in the dorsal root ganglion at the onset of a painful peripheral neuropathy in the rat. *Neurosci Lett* 1992;138:225–228.

43. Janig W, Koltzenburg M: What is the interaction between the sympathetic terminal and the primary afferent fiber? in Basbaum AI, Besson J-MR (eds): *Towards a New Pharmacotherapy of Pain.* Chichester, England, John Wiley & Sons, 1991, pp 331–352.

44. Devor M, Janig W: Activation of myelinated afferents ending in a neuroma by stimulation of the sympathetic supply in the rat. *Neurosci Lett* 1981;24:43–47.

45. Chen Y, Michaelis M, Janig W, et al: Adrenoreceptor subtype mediating sympathetic-sensory coupling in injured sensory neurons. *J Neurophysiol*, in press.

46. Devor M, Janig W, Michaelis M: Modulation of activity in dorsal root ganglion neurons by sympathetic activation in nerve-injured rats. *J Neurophysiol* 1994;71:38–47.

47. McLachlan EM, Janig W, Devor M, et al: Peripheral nerve injury triggers noradrenergic sprouting within dorsal root ganglia. *Nature* 1993;363:543–546.

48. Arner S: Intravenous phentolamine test: Diagnostic and prognostic use in reflex sympathetic dystrophy. *Pain* 1991;46:17–22.

49. Raja SN, Treede R-D, Davis KD, et al: Systemic alpha-adrenergic blockade with phentolamine: A diagnostic test for sympathetically maintained pain. *Anesthesiology* 1991;74:691–698.

50. Seltzer Z, Devor M: Ephaptic transmission in chronically damaged peripheral nerves. *Neurology* 1979;29:1061–1064.

51. Rasminsky M: Ephaptic transmission between single nerve fibres in the spinal nerve roots of dystrophic mice. *J Physiol* 1980;305:151–169.

52. Fried K, Govrin-Lippmann R, Devor M: Close apposition among neighbouring axonal endings in a neuroma. *J Neurocytol* 1993;22:663–681.
53. Lisney SJ, Devor M: Afterdischarge and interactions among fibers in damaged peripheral nerve in the rat. *Brain Res* 1987;415:122–136.
54. Rappaport ZH, Devor M: Trigeminal neuralgia: The role of self-sustaining discharge in the trigeminal ganglion. *Pain* 1994;56:127–138.
55. Waxman SG, Kocsis JD, Black JA: Type III sodium channel mRNA is expressed in embryonic but not adult spinal sensory neurons, and is reexpressed following axotomy. *J Neurophysiol* 1994;72:466–470.
56. Rizzo MA, Kocsis JD, Waxman SG: Selective loss of slow and enhancement of fast Na+ currents in cutaneous afferent DRG neurons following axotomy. *Neurobiology of Disease,* in press.
57. Heumann R, Lindholm D, Bandtlow C, et al: Differential regulation of mRNA encoding nerve growth factor and its receptor in rat sciatic nerve during development, degeneration, and regeneration: Role of macrophages. *Proc Natl Acad Sci USA* 1987;84:8735–8739.
58. Zur KB, Oh Y, Waxman SG, et al: Differential up-regulation of sodium channel α- and μ1-subunit mRNAs in cultured embryonic DRG neurons following exposure to NGF. *Brain Res Mol Brain Res* 1995;30:97–105.
59. Toledo-Aral JJ, Brehm P, Halegoua S, et al: A single pulse of nerve growth factor triggers long-term neuronal excitability through sodium channel gene induction. *Neuron* 1995;14:607–611.
60. Matzner O, Devor M: Hyperexcitability at sites of nerve injury depends on voltage-sensitive Na+ channels. *J Neurophysiol* 1994;72:349–359.
61. Devor M, Wall PD, Catalan N: Systemic lidocaine silences ectopic neuroma and DRG discharge without blocking nerve conduction. *Pain* 1992;48:261–268.
62. Glazer S, Portenoy RK: Systemic local anesthetics in pain control. *J Pain Symptom Manage* 1991;6:30–39.
63. Tanelian DL, Victory RA: Sodium channel-blocking agents: Their use in neuropathic pain conditions. *Pain Forum* 1995;4:75–80.
64. Ochoa JL, Torebjork HE: Paraesthesiae from ectopic impulse generation in human sensory nerves. *Brain* 1980;103:835–853.
65. Lewis T: *Pain.* New York, NY, MacMillan, 1942.
66. Hardy JD, Wolf HG, Goodell H: *Pain Sensations and Reactions.* Baltimore, MD, Williams & Wilkins, 1952.
67. Meyer RA, Campbell JN, Raja SN: Peripheral neural mechanisms of nociception, in Wall PD, Melzack R, Bonica JJ (eds): *Textbook of Pain,* ed 3. Edinburgh, Scotland, Churchill Livingstone, 1994, pp 13–44.
68. Koltzenburg M, Torebjork HE, Wahren LK: Nociceptor modulated central sensitization causes mechanical hyperalgesia in acute chemogenic and chronic neuropathic pain. *Brain* 1994;117:579–591.
69. Torebjork HE, Lundberg LE, LaMotte RH: Central changes in processing of mechanoreceptive input in capsaicin-induced secondary hyperalgesia in humans. *J Physiol* 1992;448:765–780.
70. LaMotte RH, Shain CN, Simone DA, et al: Neurogenic hyperalgesia: Psychophysical studies of underlying mechanisms. *J Neurophysiol* 1991;66:190–211.
71. Coderre TJ, Katz J, Vaccarino AL, et al: Contribution of central neuroplasticity to pathological pain: Review of clinical and experimental evidence. *Pain* 1993;52:259–285.
72. Gracely RH, Lynch SA, Bennett GJ: Painful neuropathy: Altered central processing maintained dynamically by peripheral input. *Pain* 1992;51:175–194.
73. Sheen K, Chung JM: Signs of neuropathic pain depend on signals from injured nerve fibers in a rat model. *Brain Res* 1993;610:62–68.
74. Cook AJ, Woolf CJ, Wall PD, et al: Dynamic receptive field plasticity in rat spinal cord dorsal horn following C-primary afferent input. *Nature* 1987;325:151–153.

75. Woolf CJ: Excitability changes in central neurons following peripheral damage: Role of central sensitization in the pathogenesis of pain, in Willis WD Jr (ed): *Hyperalgesia and Allodynia*. New York, NY, Raven Press, 1992, pp 221–243.
76. Woolf CJ, Chong M-S: Preemptive analgesia: Treating postoperative pain by preventing the establishment of central sensitization. *Anesth Analg* 1993;77:362–379.
77. Devor M: Central changes mediating neuropathic pain, in Dubner R, Gebhart GF, Bond MR (eds): *Pain Research and Clinical Management*. Amsterdam, The Netherlands, Elsevier, 1988, vol 3, pp 114–128.

Chapter 13

The Difference in Nociceptive Potential of the Nucleus Pulposus and the Anulus Fibrosus

Mamoru Kawakami, MD, PhD
James N. Weinstein, DO, MS
Tetsuya Tamaki, MD, PhD
Hiroshi Hashizume, MD

Introduction

The underlying mechanisms for pain secondary to a lumbar disk herniation associated with low back and radicular symptoms remain an enigmatic clinical problem. It remains clear that mechanical compression alone generally is not the sole cause of radicular pain and dysfunction.[1,2] Recently, a reliable animal model for experimental radiculopathy in rats has been created.[3] In this model, rats treated with chromic gut ligatures, and not rats in which the nerves were mechanically compressed with a hemoclip or those treated with silk ligatures, showed a time-dependent, reversible thermal hyperalgesia.[3] This work suggests that the mechanisms underlying thermal hyperalgesia in this model of lumbar radiculopathy probably are not due to a mechanical compression or deformity of the nerve roots, but are due to a local chemical contribution.[4]

There are few reports on the pathomechanisms of radiculopathy due to lumbar disk herniation. Nerve root irritation produced by the effect of proteoglycans released from a disk,[5] an autoimmune reaction from exposure to disk tissues,[6-8] and/or an increased concentration of lactic acid and a lower pH around the nerve roots[9] have been suggested as stimuli associated with the clinical signs of radiculopathy. In addition, production of phospholipase A_2 (PLA_2),[10] infiltration of immune response cells,[11] cytokines such as interleukin (IL),[12,13] and generation of nitric oxide (NO)[12] in lumbar herniated disk materials have been reported.

The purpose of this chapter is to review whether intervertebral disk materials have nociceptive potential, whether there is a difference in nociceptive potential of the nucleus pulposus and the anulus fibrosus (AF), and if nociceptive chemicals are produced within the disk materials and correlate with the pain-related behaviors. We hope that this chapter will further elucidate the pathomechanisms of radicular pain caused by lumbar disk herniation.

Nociceptive Potentials of the Intervertebral Disk Materials

There have been few evaluations of lumbar radiculopathy in animal models. Olmarker and associates[8] have reported that in a porcine model, the application of nucleus pulposus (NP) to the epidural space caused a delay in nerve conduction velocity of nerve roots without mechanical compression of the dural sac. This report indicates that it is possible for nucleus pulposus itself to produce nerve root damage. However, both the NP and the AF are involved in surgically resected herniated disk materials in humans, and it is unknown if isolated intervertebral disk materials, such as NP and AF, produce radicular pain. In an experimental rat model, application of intervertebral disk materials on the lumbar epidural space was evaluated for pain-related behaviors, that is, hyperalgesia.[14,15] In this model, application of NP alone (NP group) produced evidence of a mechanical hyperalgesia at 1 and 2 weeks postoperatively (PO), and rats in this group returned to normal thresholds by 4 weeks PO. Conversely, there was evidence of a mechanical hypoalgesia at 1 week PO in the animals subjected to application of NP and AF (NP+AF group). The hypoalgesia resolved by 2 weeks PO without evidence of hyperalgesia. However, rats in the NP+AF group showed evidence of hypersensitivity to thermal nociceptive stimulation at 1 and 2 weeks PO. The magnitude of the thermal hyperalgesia was maximal at 2 weeks PO. The hyperalgesia resolved 4 weeks after surgery. Rats in the NP group did not show evidence of thermal hyperalgesia or hypoalgesia. In all rats in which adipose tissue (control) was allografted on the lumbar epidural space, there was no evidence of hyperalgesia or hypoalgesia to either mechanical or thermal stimuli.

In models of painful peripheral neuropathies, mechanical and/or thermal hyperalgesia have been reported following loose ligation of the sciatic nerve[16] and it has been suggested that this hyperalgesia is one of a number of pain-related behaviors seen in the rats. We also observed evidence of similar pain-related behaviors, which indicate that these allograft materials of the NP and AF may produce radicular pain. It was identified that the NP and AF produce different nociceptive potentials to the nerve root (Table 1).

Table 1 Relationships among pain-related behavior and histologic findings

Allograft Material*	Sensitivity to Stimuli		Histology†		
	Mechanical	Thermal	IL-1α	PLA$_2$	NO
Fat	normal	normal	+	−	±
NP	hyper	normal	+	+	±
NP+AF	hypo	hyper	+	+	+

*NP = nucleus pulposus; AF = anulus fibrosus
†IL-1α = interleukin-1alpha; PLA$_2$ = phospholipase A$_2$; NO = nitric oxide; − = negative; ± = slightly positive; + = positive

Mechanisms of the Different Nociceptive Potentials of the Intervertebral Disk

In recent pharmacologic studies, investigators have evaluated mechanisms associated with hyperalgesia in other models and found that hyperalgesia is produced and/or mediated by chemicals such as NO, PLA_2, protein kinase C, and soluble guanylate cyclase.[17,18] In the experimental models in which intervertebral disk materials and adipose tissues were allografted onto the lumbar epidural space, IL-1, PLA_2, and NO have been observed in and around the applied intervertebral disk material and adipose tissue with use of immunohistochemistry[14] and in situ hybridization techniques.[15] IL-1α, PLA_2, and nitric oxide synthase (NOS) were not detected in normal intervertebral disk or adipose tissue.

IL-1α immunoreactivity was detected in the fat, NP, and NP+AF groups. IL-1 has been shown to enhance prostaglandin E_2 production in rheumatoid synovial cells.[19,20] It is thought that prostaglandin E_2 depolarizes primary afferent neurons and produces pain.[21] In this experimental model, rats with allografted fat did not show any evidence of hyperalgesia, although IL-1α immunoreactivity was observed in the applied fat tissue. This suggests that although IL-1α immunoreactivity was observed in the other experimental groups, cytokines such as IL-1α do not play a role in the pathomechanism of hyperalgesia related to radicular pain.

The potential role for other mediators that have been reported to be associated with hyperalgesia, PLA_2, and NO, have also been explored.[18] The reported significant increase in PLA_2 content in herniated disk materials provides biochemical evidence of inflammation at the site of lumbar disk herniations.[10] Consistent with this, in the experimental model described above, we did not find PLA_2 immunoreactivity in normal NP and AF, but did clearly observe increases in PLA_2 immunoreactivity in applied NP and AF tissue at 1 and 2 weeks PO. Results of recent pharmacologic studies have suggested that PLA_2 mediates mechanical hyperalgesia but not thermal hyperalgesia.[18] Ozaktay and associates[22] showed that PLA_2 injected into the facet joint caused acute changes in nerve discharge in the rabbit. Collectively, these data suggest that mechanical hyperalgesia observed in the rat with NP applied into the epidural space may be directly related to an increase in PLA_2 immunoreactivity.

There is increasing interest in the role of NO as a novel intra- and intercellular messenger. Recently, Meller and associates[17] reported that NO mediates the thermal hyperalgesia produced in the rat by loose ligation of the sciatic nerve with chromic gut sutures. Therefore, the possible role of NO in the hyperalgesia produced by tissue allografts has been examined. In the NP+AF group, NO was detected in some disk-surrounding cells at 1 and 2 weeks PO. Notwithstanding that various cells (macrophage, endothelium, etc) produce NO, allografted NP and AF demonstrated an associated thermal hyperalgesia, but not a mechanical hyperalgesia. Therefore, thermal hyperalgesia produced by the intervertebral disk may be related to NO production. Kang and associates[12] reported that herniated lumbar intervertebral disk specimens in culture were able to produce NO. Therefore, it is thought that NO may also be involved in radicular pain found in the lumbar disk herniation patients.

PLA_2 immunoreactivity was also observed in the applied AF and NP. However, rats in the NP+AF group did not show evidence of mechanical hyperal-

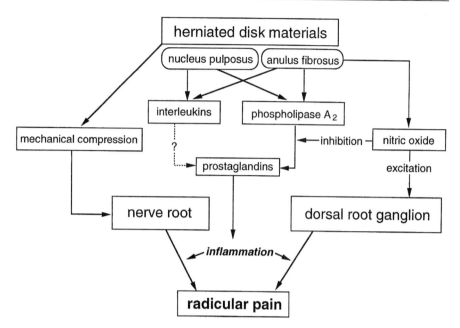

Fig. 1   *Possible mechanisms of radicular pain secondary to lumbar herniated disk.*

gesia. Zhuo and associates[23] demonstrated that intrathecal administration of the cholinergic muscarinic receptor antagonist atropine produced a dose-dependent decrease in the mechanical threshold for tail withdrawal, which was reversed rapidly by subsequent intrathecal administration of the NO precursor, L-arginine. The production of endogenous NO is required for tonic inhibition of spinal nociceptive mechanical transmission. NO production around the AF may inhibit the mechanical hyperalgesia produced by PLA_2 in the NP and AF of the applied intervertebral disks.

Although an immune response to a foreign body and the presence of cytokines (IL-1α) do not appear to be involved in the pathomechanism of diskogenic radicular pain, production of PLA_2 and NO may play an important role in the pathomechanisms of radicular pain in lumbar disk herniation (Fig. 1).

Conclusion

The NP and AF produce different forms of hyperalgesia (mechanical versus thermal) with different and distinct histologic changes. It is possible that radicular pain of a lumbar disk herniation results from chemicals, such as PLA_2 and NO.

References

1. Boden SD, Davis DO, Dina TS, et al: Abnormal magnetic-resonance scans of the lumbar spine in asymptomatic subjects: A prospective investigation. *J Bone Joint Surg* 1990;72A:403–408.

2. Boumphrey FR, Bell GR, Modic M, et al: Computed tomography scanning after chymopapain injection for herniated nucleus pulposus: A prospective study. *Clin Orthop* 1987;219:120–123.
3. Kawakami M, Weinstein JN, Spratt KF, et al: Experimental lumbar radiculopathy: Immunohistochemical and quantitative demonstrations of pain induced by lumbar nerve root irritation of the rat. *Spine* 1994;19:1780–1794.
4. Kawakami M, Weinstein JN, Chatani K, et al: Experimental lumbar radiculopathy: Behavioral and histologic changes in a model of radicular pain after spinal nerve root irritation with chromic gut ligatures in the rat. *Spine* 1994;19:1795–1802.
5. MacNab I: The mechanisms of spondylotic pain, in Hirsch C, Zotterman Y (eds): *Cervical Pain*. Oxford, England, Pergamon Press, 1972, pp 88–95.
6. Bobechko WP, Hirsch C: Auto-immune response to nucleus pulposus in the rabbit. *J Bone Joint Surg* 1965;47B:574–580.
7. Gertzbein SD, Tile M, Gross A, et al: Autoimmunity in degenerative disc disease of the lumbar spine. *Orthop Clin North Am* 1975;6:67–73.
8. Olmarker K, Rydevik B, Nordborg C: Autologous nucleus pulposus induces neurophysiologic and histologic changes in porcine cauda equina nerve roots. *Spine* 1993;18:1425–1432.
9. Nachemson A: Intradiscal measurements of pH in patients with lumbar rhizopathies. *Acta Orthop Scand* 1969;40:23–42.
10. Saal JS, Franson RC, Dobrow R, et al: High levels of inflammatory phospholipase A_2 activity in lumbar disc herniations. *Spine* 1990;15:674–678.
11. Nohara Y, Tohmura T: Fate of epidurally sequestrated disk: An immuno-histological study of herniated nucleus pulposus of the lumbar spine. *Orthop Trans* 1994;18:836–837.
12. Kang JD, Georgescu HI, McIntyre L, et al: Herniated lumbar intervertebral discs make neutral metalloproteases, nitric oxide, and interleukin-6. *Orthop Trans* 1995;19:53.
13. Yamagishi M, Nemoto O, Kikuchi T, et al: Ruptured human disc tissues produce metalloproteinase and interleukin-1. *Trans Orthop Res Soc* 1992;17:190.
14. Kawakami M, Tamaki T, Weinstein JN, et al: Disc materials produce pain-related behavior in the rat: The role of pH, immune response and chemicals. *Trans Orthop Res Soc* 1995;20:666.
15. Kawakami M, Tamaki T, Weinstein JN, et al: Pathomechanism of pain-related behavior produced by allografts of intervertebral disc in the rat. *Spine*, in press.
16. Bennett GJ, Xie YK: A peripheral mononeuropathy in rat that produces disorders of pain sensation like those seen in man. *Pain* 1988;33:87–107.
17. Meller ST, Pechman PS, Gebhart GF, et al: Letter: Nitric oxide mediates the thermal hyperalgesia produced in a model of neuropathic pain in the rat. *Neuroscience* 1992;50:7–10.
18. Meller ST: Thermal and mechanical hyperplasia: A distinct role for different excitatory amino acid receptors and signal transduction pathways? *J APS* 1994;3:214–231.
19. Dayer JM, Zavadil-Grob C, Ucla C, et al: Induction of human interleukin 1 mRNA measured by collagenase- and prostaglandin E2-stimulating activity in rheumatoid synovial cells. *Eur J Immunol* 1984;14:898–901.
20. Mizel SB, Dayer JM, Krane SM, et al: Stimulation of rheumatoid synovial cell collagenase and prostaglandin production by partially purified lymphocyte-activating factor (interleukin 1). *Proc Natl Acad Sci USA* 1981;78:2474–2477.
21. Yanagisawa M, Otsuka M, Garcia-Arraras JE: E-type prostaglandins depolarize primary afferent neurons of the neonatal rat. *Neurosci Lett* 1986;68:351–355.
22. Ozaktay AC, Kallakuri S, Li QH, et al: Electrophysiological changes induced by phospholipase A_2 in rabbit lumbar facet joint and adjacent tissues. *Trans Orthop Res Soc* 1995;20:112.
23. Zhuo M, Meller ST, Gebhart GF: Endogenous nitric oxide is required for tonic cholinergic inhibition of spinal mechanical transmission. *Pain* 1993;54:71–78.

Chapter 14

Mechanical and Biochemical Injury of Spinal Nerve Roots: An Experimental Perspective

Kjell Olmarker, MD, PhD

Although injuries of the lumbosacral spinal nerve roots in the spinal canal have been recognized for over six decades as the primary cause of the symptoms of sciatica, the basic pathophysiologic mechanisms are still poorly understood.[1] However, interest in this topic has increased over the last decade, perhaps as a result of the powerlessness faced by the medical profession in treatment of this common and societally costly condition. Recent research has thus been aimed at defining basic pathophysiologic events involved in the nerve root injury at the cellular or subcellular level in order to design better and more specific treatment modalities. In this chapter, I will review the current knowledge about these mechanisms and propose some hypotheses about the pathophysiology of the symptoms of sciatica.

Symptomatology of Sciatica

The symptoms of sciatica may be divided into two main categories, pain and nerve dysfunction. Sciatic pain typically is radiating pain, the distribution of which usually may be referred to a specific nerve root and which commonly extends to the calf or foot. If the pain is sharp and clearly linked to a specific nerve root, it may be called "radicular pain" but if it is more dull and does not relate to a certain nerve root, it may instead be called "referred pain."[2] If the sciatic pain is the result of excessive axonal traffic in the roots and spinal cord, then nerve dysfunction is the result of a reduction in the axonal traffic. Dysfunction may be present in both motor and sensory nerves. Although pain and nerve dysfunction are assumed to be opposites, they usually coincide, which indicates the pathophysiology is very complex. However, it is necessary to consider pain and dysfunction separately because they may result from different pathophysiologic events.

Pathophysiologic Mechanisms

Two specific pathophysiologic mechanisms—mechanical deformation of the nerve roots and biologic or biochemical activity of the disk tissue with effects on the roots—may be separated at the tissue level. The mechanical deformation theory, the oldest concept of nerve root injury induced by herniated disk tissue, can be traced to some clinical observations made at the turn of the century regarding injuries in the lumbosacral junction with subsequent leg pain.[1,3-5] However, the theory that biologic activity of the disk tissue can injure the nerve roots was confirmed experimentally in 1993.[6] These two mechanisms will be discussed separately.

Mechanical Effects

Enclosed by the vertebral bones, the spinal nerve roots are relatively well protected from external trauma (Fig. 1). However, because they do not have the

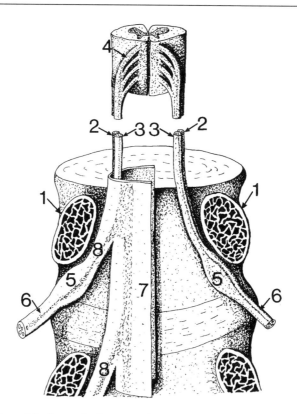

Fig. 1 *Drawing of the intraspinal course of a human lumbar spinal nerve root segment. The vertebral arches have been removed by cutting the pedicles (1), and the opened spinal canal can be viewed from behind. The ventral (2) and dorsal (3) nerve roots leave the spinal cord as small rootlets (4) that caudally converge into a common nerve root trunk. Just prior to leaving the spinal canal, there is a swelling of the dorsal nerve root called the dorsal root ganglion (5). Caudal to the dorsal root ganglion, the ventral and the dorsal nerve roots mix and form the spinal nerve (6). The spinal dura encloses the nerve roots both as a central cylindrical sac (7) and as separate extensions called root sleeves (8). (Reproduced with permission from Olmarker K:* Spinal Nerve Root Compression. *Gothenburg, Sweden, Gothenburg University, 1990. Thesis.)*

same amounts and organization of protective connective tissue sheaths as do the peripheral nerves, the spinal nerve roots may be particularly sensitive to mechanical deformation resulting from intraspinal disorders, such as disk herniations/protrusions, spinal stenosis, degenerative disorders, and tumors.[7,8] There has been moderate interest in the study of nerve root compression in experimental models. Gelfan and Tarlov,[9] in 1956, and Sharpless,[10] in 1975, performed some initial experiments on the effects of compression on nerve impulse conduction. Although the compression devices used were not calibrated, the results of both experiments indicated that nerve roots were more susceptible to compression than peripheral nerves.[9,10] During recent years, however, interest in nerve root pathophysiology has increased considerably.

Experimental Nerve Root Compression   Olmarker and associates[11,12] presented a model that, for the first time, allowed for experimental, graded compression of cauda equina nerve roots in pigs at known pressure levels. In this model, the cauda equina was compressed by an inflatable, translucent balloon fixed to the spine (Fig. 2). This model made it possible to study the flow in the intrinsic nerve root blood vessels at various pressure levels.[13] The experiment was designed so that the pressure in the compression balloon was increased by 5 mm Hg every 20 seconds. The blood flow and vessel diameters of the intrinsic vessels could simultaneously be observed through the balloon, using a vital microscope. The average occlusion pressure for the arterioles was found to be slightly below and directly related to the systolic blood pressure. The blood flow

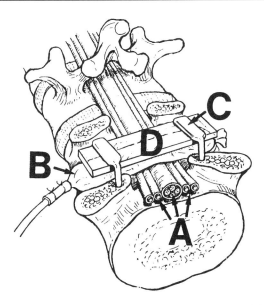

Fig. 2 *Schematic drawing of experimental nerve root compression model. The cauda equina (A) is compressed by an inflatable balloon (B) that is fixed to the spine by two L-shaped pins (C) and a Plexiglas plate (D). (Reproduced with permission from Olmarker K, Holm S, Rosenqvist A-L, et al: Experimental nerve root compression: A model of acute, graded compression of the porcine cauda equina and an analysis of neural and vascular anatomy. Spine 1991;16:61–69.)*

in the capillary networks was intimately dependent on the blood flow of the adjacent venules. This corroborates the assumption, which has been suggested as one mechanism in the carpal tunnel syndrome, that venular stasis may induce capillary stasis and thus changes in the microcirculation of the nerve tissue.[14] There were large variations in the mean occlusion pressures for the venules; however, a pressure of 5 to 10 mm Hg was found to be sufficient for inducing venular occlusion. It is not unreasonable to assume that the capillary blood flow also will be affected as a result of retrograde stasis.

The effects of gradual decompression, after initial acute compression maintained for a short while, were studied using the same experimental setup.[15] The average pressure for starting the blood flow was slightly lower for arterioles, capillaries, and venules. However, with this protocol, the blood flow was not fully restored until the compression was lowered from 5 mm Hg to 0 mm Hg. This observation supports the previous impression that there is vascular impairment even at low pressure levels.

Compression-induced impairment of the microcirculation may, thus, be one mechanism for nerve root dysfunction because it affects the nutrition of the nerve root. However, the nerve roots also are nourished by diffusion of nutrients from the cerebrospinal fluid (CSF).[16] To assess compression-induced effects on nerve root nutrition, an experiment was designed in which systemically injected ^{3}H-labeled methylglucose could be transported to the nerve tissue in the compressed segment via both blood vessels and CSF diffusion.[17] The results showed that no compensatory mechanism from CSF diffusion could be expected at the low pressure levels. In fact, 10 mm Hg compression was sufficient to induce a 20% to 30% reduction in the transport of methylglucose to the nerve roots, as compared to control.

Compression also may induce an increase in the vascular permeability, leading to intraneural edema.[18] Such edema may increase the endoneurial fluid pressure, which, in turn, may impair the endoneurial capillary blood flow and, thus, jeopardize the nutrition of the nerve roots.[19-22] Because the edema usually persists for some time after removal of a compressive agent, it may negatively affect the nerve root for a longer period than the compression itself. The presence of intraneural edema also is related to subsequent intraneural fibrosis,[23] and it thus may contribute to the slow recovery seen in some patients with nerve compression disorders. To determine if intraneural edema in nerve roots also results from compression, the distribution of Evans-blue labeled albumin in the nerve tissue was analyzed after compression at various pressures and at various durations.[24] The study showed that edema occurred even at low pressure levels. The predominant location was at the edges of the compression zone.

Nerve root function has been studied using direct electrical stimulation and recordings either on the nerve itself or in the corresponding muscular segments.[25-28] During a 2-hour compression period, a critical level for inducing a reduction in mean arterial pressure seems to be between 50 and 75 mm Hg. Higher pressures (100 to 200 mm Hg) may induce a total conduction block with varying degrees of recovery after compression release. To study the effects of compression on sensory nerve fibers, the electrodes in the sacrum were used to record a compound nerve action potential after stimulating the sensory nerves in the tail (distal to the compression zone). The results showed that the sensory fibers are slightly more susceptible to compression than the motor fibers.[27,28] Also, the nerve roots are more susceptible to compression injury if the blood pressure is lowered pharmacologically.[26] These data substantiate the importance of the blood supply for maintaining the functional properties of the nerve roots.

Onset Rate of Compression   The onset rate, ie, the time from initiation of compression to full compression, may vary clinically from fractions of seconds in traumatic conditions to months or years in degenerative processes. There even may be a wide variation among the clinically rapid onset rates. The model described above (Fig. 2) allowed variation in the onset rate of compression. Two onset rates have been investigated. In one, the pressure was preset and compression started by flipping the switch of the compressed-air system used to inflate the balloon; in the other, the compression pressure level was slowly increased over 20 seconds. The first onset rate was measured to be 0.05 to 0.1 seconds, a rapid compression onset.

The rapid onset rate was found to have more pronounced effects than the slow onset rate on edema formation,[24] methylglucose transport,[17] and impulse propagation.[25] Methylglucose levels within the compression zone are more pronounced after rapid onset than after slow onset to corresponding pressure levels. There was also a striking difference in the segments outside the compression zones. In the slow onset series, the levels approached baseline values closer to the compression zone than in the rapid onset series. This difference may indicate the presence of a more pronounced edge-zone edema in the rapid onset series, with a subsequent reduction in nutrient transport in the nerve tissue adjacent to the compression zone.

For rapid onset compression, which would be more closely related to spine trauma or disk herniation than to spinal stenosis, a pressure of 600 mm Hg maintained for only 1 second is sufficient to induce a gradual impairment of nerve conduction during the 2 hours studied after the compression was ended.[29] Overall, the mechanisms for the pronounced differences between measured parameters at the different onset rates are not clear; these differences may be a result of differences in the rates of displacement of the compressed nerve tissue toward the uncompressed parts as a result of the viscoelastic properties of the nerve tissue.[8] Such phenomena may lead not only to structural damage to the nerve fibers, but also to structural changes in the blood vessels, with subsequent edema formation. The gradual formation of intraneural edema also may be related closely to the described observations of a gradually increasing difference in nerve conduction impairment between the two onset rates.[24,25]

Multiple Levels of Nerve Root Compression   Patients with double levels of spinal stenosis seem to have more pronounced symptoms than patients with a stenosis only at one level.[30] The model was modified to address this interesting clinical question. Using two balloons at two adjacent disk levels, with a 10-mm uncompressed nerve segment between the balloons, resulted in a much more pronounced impairment of nerve impulse conduction than had been found at corresponding pressure levels.[31] For instance, a pressure of 10 mm Hg in each of two balloons resulted in a 60% reduction of nerve impulse amplitude during 2 hours of compression, whereas there was no reduction with 50 mm Hg in one balloon.

The mechanism for the difference between single and double compression may not be based simply on the fact that the nerve impulses have to pass more than one compression zone at double-level compression. There may also be a mechanism based on the local vascular anatomy of the nerve roots. Although they exist in peripheral nerves, there are no regional nutritive arteries from surrounding structures to the intraneural vascular system in spinal nerve roots.[11,32-35] Therefore, compression at two levels might result in a nutritionally impaired region between the two compression sites, and the segment affected by the compression would be widened from one balloon diameter (10 mm) to two balloon diameters plus the nerve segment between them (30 mm). This hypothesis was partly confirmed in an experiment on continuous analyses of the total blood flow in the uncompressed nerve segment between two compression balloons. There was a 64% reduction in total blood flow when both balloons were inflated to 10 mm Hg.[36] At a pressure close to the systemic blood pressure, there was complete ischemia in the nerve segment. Preliminary data from a study on nutritional transport to the nerve tissue at double compression demonstrated a reduction in transport to the uncompressed nerve segment between the two compression balloons that was similar to the reduction within the two compression sites.[37] These data indicate that nutrition to a nerve root segment located between two compression sites is severely impaired, although the nerve segment itself is uncompressed.

It was also evident that increasing the distance between the compression balloons from one vertebral segment to two segments enhanced the effects on nerve conduction.[31] However, this was not the case in the nutritional transport study. The methylglucose levels in the compression zones and in the uncompressed intermediate segment were similar whether double compression was over one or two vertebral segments.[37] Thus, nutrition to the uncompressed nerve segment between two compression sites is affected almost as much as at the compression sites, regardless of the distance between them, whereas functional impairment may be directly related to the distance between the two compression sites. Impairment of nutrition to the nerve segment between the two compression balloons seems to be more important than the fact that the nerve impulses have to overcome two compression sites in double level compression.

Chronic Experimental Nerve Root Compression This discussion of compression-induced effects on nerve roots has been dealing with acute compression, ie, compression that lasts for some hours with no survival of the animal. To better mimic the clinical situation, compression must be applied over longer periods of time. Many changes in nerve tissue, such as adaptation of axons and vasculature, that probably occur in patients cannot be studied in experimental models using only 1 to 6 hours of compression. Furthermore, onset time may be very slow in clinical syndromes with nerve root compression. For instance, the gradual remodeling of the vertebrae that results in spinal stenosis probably requires an onset time of many years. It is, of course, difficult to mimic such a situation in an experimental model. It also is impossible to control the pressure acting on the nerve roots in chronic models because of the remodeling and adaptation of the nerve tissue to the applied pressure. However, knowing the exact pressures is probably less important in chronic than in acute compression situations. Study of chronic models requires controlled compression with a slow onset time that is easily reproducible. Such models may be well suited for studies of pathophysiologic events and for studies of intervention by surgery or drugs.

Delamarter and associates[38,39] presented a model on the dog cauda equina in which they applied a constricting plastic band that was tightened around the thecal sac to induce a 25%, 50%, or 75% reduction of the cross-sectional area. The band was left in place for various times. Analyses showed both structural and functional changes that were proportional to the degree of constriction.

To induce a slower onset and more controlled compression, Cornefjord and associates (unpublished data, 1995) used a constrictor to compress nerve roots in the pig. The constrictor was initially intended for inducing vascular occlusion in experimental ischemic conditions in dogs. It consists of an outer metal shell that is covered on the inside with a material called ameroid that expands when in contact with fluids. Because of the metal shell, the ameroid expands inward with a maximum of expansion after 2 weeks, resulting in the compression of a nerve root placed in the central opening of the constrictor. Compression of the first sacral nerve root in the pig using a constrictor with a defined original diameter has resulted in axonal injuries and a significant reduction of nerve conduction velocity. An increase in substance P in the nerve root and the dorsal root ganglion has also been found following such compression.[40] Substance P is a neurotransmitter that is related to pain transmission. The study may thus provide experimental evidence that compression of nerve roots produces pain. The constrictor model has also been used to study blood flow changes in the nerve root vasculature.[41] It then was observed that the blood flow not only is reduced just inside the compression zone, but also is significantly reduced in parts of the nerve roots located outside the constrictor.

In clinical nerve root compression, the compression level probably is not stable but varies as the result of changes in posture and movements.[42,43] After evaluating the normal anatomy and the effects of acute compression using compressed air,[44] Konno and associates[45] introduced a model in which the pressure could be changed after a period of initial chronic compression. An inflatable balloon was introduced under the lamina of the seventh lumbar vertebra in the dog evaluated. By slowly (over 1 hour) inflating the balloon with a viscous substance that hardens in the balloon, the cauda equina was compressed at a known initial pressure level. The initial compression was verified by myelography. Because the balloon under the lamina comprised a twin set of balloons, the second balloon could be connected to a compressed-air system and used to further compress the cauda equina.

Mechanical Deformation and Pain Some experimental observations indicate that mechanical deformation per se may induce impulses that might be interpreted by the central nervous system as pain. Howe and associates[46] found that mechanical stimulation of nerve roots or peripheral nerves resulted in nerve impulses of short duration, and that these impulses were prolonged if the nerve tissue had been exposed for mechanical irritation by a chromic gut ligature for 2 to 4 weeks. The same results were obtained recently using rabbit nerve roots in an in vitro system.[47] However, in this setup it was also evident that the dorsal root ganglion (DRG) was more susceptible to mechanical stimulation than the nerve roots. The DRG has drawn special interest in this regard, and increased levels of neurotransmitters related to pain transmission have been found in the DRG in response to full body vibration of rabbits.[48,49] A similar increase has also been seen in the DRG and nerve root after local constriction of the same nerve root.[40]

Biologic/Biochemical Effects

The clinical picture of sciatica with a characteristic distribution of pain and nerve dysfunction, but in the absence of herniated disk material both at radiologic examination and at surgery, has indicated that the mechanical component may not be the only mechanism present. It therefore has been suggested that the disk tissue per se may have some injurious properties of pathophysiologic significance.[7,8] However, it was only recently confirmed in an experimental setup that local, epidural application of autologous nucleus pulposus in the pig, with no mechanical deformation, induces significant changes in both structure and function of the adjacent nerve roots.[6] This finding has opened up a new field of research; the current knowledge is reviewed below.

Biologic Activity of Disk Tissue (Nucleus Pulposus) In a rabbit model, autologous nucleus pulposus obtained from a lumbar disk was placed onto the tibial nerve.[50] No changes in nerve function or structure were observed. However, differences in the microscopic anatomy and vascular permeability of peripheral nerves and nerve roots make the comparison difficult. McCarron and associates[51] applied autologous nucleus pulposus from disks of the dog's tail in the epidural space of the animal. They found an epidural inflammatory reaction that did not occur when a saline control was injected. However, the nerve tissue was not assessed in this study.[51]

Olmarker and associates[6] demonstrated that application of autologous nucleus pulposus on the pig cauda equina may cause both a reduction in nerve conduction velocity and light microscopic structural changes (Fig. 3). However, these axonal changes had a focal distribution, and the quantity of injured axons was too low to be responsible for the significant neurophysiologic dysfunction observed. A follow-up study of areas of the nerve roots that were exposed to nucleus pulposus and appeared to be normal under the light microscope revealed that there were significant injuries of the Schwann cells with vacuolization and disintegration of the Schmidt-Lanterman incisures (Fig. 4).[52] The Schmidt-Lanterman incisures are essential for the normal exchange of ions between the axon and the surrounding tissues; therefore, an injury to this structure would be likely to interfere with the normal impulse conduction properties of the axons. However, the distribution of changes also was too limited to fully explain the neurophysiologic dysfunction observed. The potency of the nucleus pulposus was further emphasized in an experiment using a dog model. In that experiment, incisure of the anulus fibrosus, with minimal leakage of nucleus pulposus, was enough to induce significant changes in structure and function of the adjacent nerve root (S Kayama, S Konno, K Olmarker, unpublished data, 1995).

Data from these initial experiments suggest that nucleus pulposus can injure the nerve roots after local application. However, the mechanisms for the nucleus pulposus-induced nerve root injury currently are not fully understood. Indications in the studies described above that inflammatory reactions were present, at least epidurally, led to initiation of a study in which a potent anti-inflammatory agent, methylprednisolone, was administered intravenously at different times after nucleus pulposus application.[53] The nucleus pulposus-induced reduction in nerve conduction velocity was eliminated if methylprednisolone was administered within 24 hours of application. If methylprednisolone was administered within 48 hours, the effect was not eliminated but was significantly lower than

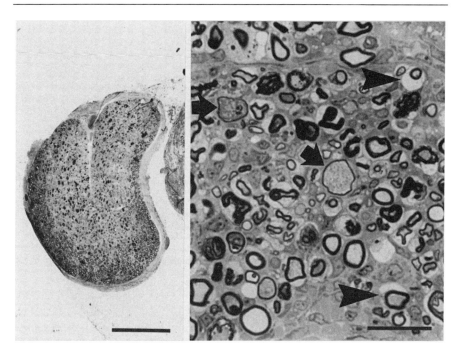

Fig. 3 *Porcine nerve roots that were exposed to autologous nucleus pulposus.* **Left**, *Nerve root with a characteristic central injury. In the periphery the axons look normal but in the center and the top of the nerve root, there are signs of nerve injury. (Richardson, Bar 260 μm).* **Right**, *Axons in a higher magnification, 3 days after epidural exposure to autologous nucleus pulposus. There are axons with increased axonal density (arrows) and axons with swellings of the Schwann cells (arrowheads). (Richardson, Bar 26 μm). (Reproduced with permission from Olmarker K, Rydevik B, Nordborg C: Autologous nucleus pulposus induces neurophysiologic and histologic changes in porcine cauda equina nerve roots.* Spine *1993;18:1425–1432.)*

if no drug was used. This observation indicates that the negative effect does not occur immediately, but will develop during the first 24 hours after application. However, if methylprednisolone is administered within 24 hours, areas in the nerve roots, which have normal impulse conduction properties, have the same amount of light microscopic axonal changes as in the previous study.[6] These data further corroborate the impression that the structural nerve injury inducing nerve dysfunction must be sought at the subcellular level.

Although methylprednisolone affected the pathophysiologic events of the nucleus pulposus-induced nerve root injury, it was not clear if its effects were due to the anti-inflammatory properties of the methylprednisolone or to some other property. To determine whether the presence of autologous nucleus pulposus could initiate a leukotactic response from the surrounding tissues, a study was initiated that assessed the potential inflammagenic properties of the nucleus pulposus.[54] Autologous nucleus pulposus and autologous retroperitoneal fat were placed in separate, small perforated titanium chambers and placed subcutaneously, together with a sham chamber, in the pig. Seven days later, the number

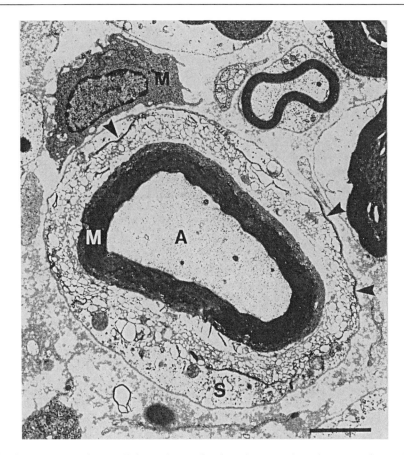

Fig. 4 *An axon in the pig, 7 days after epidural application of autologous nucleus pulposus. There is a prominent vesicular swelling of the Schmidt-Lanterman incisure. Note the mononuclear cell (black M) in close contact with the nerve fiber. Also indicated are a well-preserved and probably uninjured axon (A), myelin sheath (white M), outer Schwann cell cytoplasm (S), and myelin sheath layers outside the Schmidt-Lanterman incisure (arrowheads). (Bar-2.5 μm). (Reproduced with permission from Olmarker K, Rydevik B, Nordborg C: Ultrastructural changes in spinal nerve roots induced by autologous nucleus pulposus. Spine, in press.)*

of leukocytes in each chamber was measured. The same number of leukocytes were found in the fat and the sham chambers. However, the nucleus pulposus-containing chambers had a number of leukocytes that exceeded the others by 250%. Also, when nucleus pulposus was injected in contact with the microvasculature of the hamster cheek pouch, it caused an increase in macromolecular permeability that did not occur if the animals were simultaneously treated with indomethacin (J Blomquist, J Strömberg, P Zachrisson, unpublished data, 1995).[54] In another experiment, autologous nucleus pulposus and muscle in GoreTex tubes were placed subcutaneously in rabbits.[55] After 2 weeks, there was an accumulation of macrophages, T helper cells, and T suppressor cells in the tube with nucleus pulposus; the accumulation persisted the full observation time of 4 weeks. These data support the impression that autologous nucleus pulposus may elicit inflammatory or immunologic reactions when outside the intervertebral disk space.

Two studies were undertaken to assess the possibility that nucleus pulposus can induce pain. In an in vitro experimental setup, Cavanaugh and associates[47] observed that local application of nucleus pulposus onto the DRG in prepared specimens from rabbits produced nerve discharges that sometimes lasted several minutes. The responding units were mainly A delta and A beta fibers. These discharges may be interpreted as pain transmission elicited from stimulation of either the ganglion cells or the capsule of the DRG. Kawakami and associates[56] placed homologous fat tissue, nucleus pulposus, and nucleus pulposus/anulus fibrosus in the spinal canal of rats. The mechanical withdrawal threshold and the thermal withdrawal threshold were evaluated. Nucleus pulposus caused lowered mechanical thresholds and the combination nucleus pulposus/anulus fibrosus increased the mechanical thresholds but lowered the thermal thresholds. These observations indicate that disk material in the spinal canal may be correlated to pain.

Components of the Nucleus Pulposus of the Intervertebral Disks   The nucleus pulposus comprises mainly proteoglycans, collagen, and cells.[57,58] Therefore, the observed effects of local application of nucleus pulposus probably are related to one or more of these components. Glycoproteins have been suggested to have a direct irritating effect on nerve tissue.[59-61] Neither the collagen or cells have been suggested to be of pathophysiologic importance. However, recent studies have shown that the cells of the nucleus pulposus are capable of producing metalloproteases, such as collagenase or gelatinase, as well as interleukin-6 and prostaglandin E_2, and do so spontaneously in culture.[62] Using the pig model described above, Olmarker and associates[63] have assessed the possible role of nucleus pulposus cells in nucleus pulposus-induced nerve injury. In a blinded fashion, autologous nucleus pulposus was subjected to 24 hours of freezing at -20°C, digestion by hyaluronidase, or a heating box at 37°C for 24 hours. The treated nucleus pulposus was reapplied after 24 hours, and analyses were performed 7 days later. There were no changes in nerve conduction velocity after application of nucleus pulposus that had been frozen (and the cells thus killed); whereas, in the other two series, the results were similar to those in the previous study.[6] Therefore, it seems reasonable to believe that the cells have been responsible in some way for inducing the nerve injury and that the structural molecules should be less important. However, which substances are produced by the cells is not yet clear, but the substances may be related to those described by Kang and associates.[62] Immunoglobulin G, hydrogen ions, and phospholipase A_2 have also been suggested and must be considered.[64-67]

Mechanisms and Transport Routes   Three pathologic mechanisms that act below the tissue level seem reasonable: (1) a direct neurotoxic effect on the nerve tissue, (2) a vascular impairment, and (3) inflammatory or immunologic reactions.

It is difficult to relate the observed histologic changes in nerve tissue induced by nucleus pulposus to direct neurotoxicity. Observations have indicated that the changes are focal and mainly found in the center of the nerve roots and that they resemble a mononeuritis simplex, which is induced by nerve infarction caused by embolism of the intraneural vessels.[6,52,68] The work of Jayson and

225

associates,[69] and others,[70-72] which indicates an impairment of the venous outflow from the nerve roots caused by periradicular vascular changes, increases interest in vascular impairment. Even relatively large molecules deposited in the epidural space may be found in the intraneural vessels of the adjacent nerve roots within seconds after application.[73] The relevance of vascular impairment is increased by the possibility that epidurally placed substances can penetrate the relatively impermeable dura, cross over the CSF, and then diffuse through the root sheath and into the axons. Nucleus pulposus seems to have some inflammatory properties.[6,54,55,62] Because many of the inflammatory mediators are involved in vascular and rheologic phenomena, such as coagulation, vascular impairment of the nerve root may be the result of vascular embolism. In fact, it has been observed that the presence of nucleus pulposus may induce thrombus formation in micro vessels.[54] Inflammatory mediators might also exert a direct effect on the myelin sheaths, as indicated by an electron microscopic study of nerve roots exposed to autologous nucleus pulposus in the pig.[52] There were significant injuries of the Schwann cells with vacuolization and disintegration of the Schmidt-Lanterman incisures, which closely resembles the injury pattern of inflammatory nerve disease.[74,75]

It has also been suggested that, because the nucleus pulposus is avascular and thus "hidden" from the systemic circulation, application of the nucleus pulposus could result in an autoimmune reaction directed to antigens present in the nucleus pulposus, and that bioactive substances from this reaction may injure the nerve tissue.[76-83] It also is possible to hypothesize that there could be autoimmune reactions, not only to the disk, but also to nerve tissue components, such as basic myelin protein, that are released as the result of injury. However, at present, no clear data exist as to whether the immunologic mechanisms are a clinical reality.

Symptomatology of Sciatica

Nerve Dysfunction

Based on the data presented above, it seems reasonable to believe that nerve dysfunction may be the result of both mechanical deformation and the presence of nucleus pulposus. Mechanical deformation, ie, compression or tension, may affect normal nerve conduction either directly by mechanical effects, such as separation of the nodes of Ranvier at higher pressures (> 400 mm Hg), or indirectly by vascular impairment, which may occur at much lower pressures.[13,84-88] The mechanisms for the nucleus pulposus-induced nerve dysfunction are not known but may be based on direct neurotoxic effects, vascular impairment, or the action of inflammatory agents.

Pain

Pain obviously is much more difficult to assess in controlled experimental studies. The available literature indicates that pain may be induced by both mechanical and nucleus pulposus-mediated factors. The role of the nucleus pulposus in this context is particularly interesting in view of patients who have obvious symptoms of disk herniation but no visible herniation at radiologic examination or surgery.[89,90] Existing data suggest that communication between the intradiskal space and the epidural space is sufficient for inducing effects on the nerve roots, thereby indicating that annular disruption with a discrete leakage of nucleus pulposus material into the spinal canal, with no visible herniation, could be sufficient enough to induce symptoms. The potential of nucleus pulposus material to induce pain is also indicated in one clinical study, which showed that noncontained herniations (the nucleus pulposus was in contact with the epidural space), were much more painful and had a more pronounced effect on straight leg raising (SLR) than contained herniations.[91]

It can be hypothesized that mechanical or biologic factors may induce pain either by direct stimulation of axons or by neuroischemia. Vascular impairment, with a nutritional deficit of the nerve tissue resulting in ischemia of the nerve, seems a likely pain mechanism, and it could probably be induced by both mechanical and biologic factors.

In studies in which pain was suspected to be caused by direct stimulation of the nerve roots, the nucleus pulposus material was primarily in contact with the surrounding meninges rather than the axons.[47,56,91] Moreover, in a study where locally anesthetized patients re-experienced their sciatic pain after local stimulation of the nerve root, it could be argued that the meninges was the actual tissue being stimulated.[92] The spinal dura mater is known to contain nerve endings, and its stimulation has been suggested as a mechanism for sciatic pain.[93-95] Irritation or stimulation of the dura is an interesting theory that could explain many clinical features of sciatica. If the dura is assumed to be segmentally innervated (Fig. 5) and the sensory nerves travel in a caudal/lateral direction and are connected to the corresponding nerve root by the nerve of Luschka,[96-98] stimulation of the dura at a point where the dorsolateral herniations appear should be recorded by the corresponding nerve root. However, at this location the irritation may spread medially to the contralateral segment, producing bilateral symptoms, or laterally, producing symptoms from the level above. Similarly, a lateral disk herniation could produce symptoms in the lower level (Fig. 5). If the pain of the SLR test is the result of dura irritation due to friction to the herniated mass, the phenomenon of ''crossed SLR'' may be based on simultaneous stimulation of the contralateral dura. Such a ''radiculitis'' or ''local meningitis'' could probably be regarded as similar to peritonitis, in which there usually is a muscle contraction over the affected area. An analogue for this ''local meningitis'' could be the ipsilateral contraction of the spinal muscles, producing the ''sciatic scoliosis'' or lateral bending of the spine at the level of herniation.

It is possible to speculate further that the deep visceral pain presented earlier as referred pain may be related to painful conditions in the nerve, and that the sharp, distinct pain presented as radicular pain may be related to dura irritation. However, the view of spinal pain may change dramatically over the coming years based on new ideas and concepts as well as on the rapidly increasing knowledge of the molecular events active in the pathophysiology of sciatica.

Conclusion

Sciatica is a complex condition in which a number of different pathophysiologic mechanisms are responsible for the symptoms (Fig. 6). Although the pain

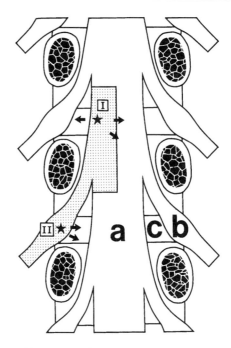

Fig. 5 *Suggested area of innervation by one recurrent sinuvertebral nerve (nerve of Luschka). Disk herniation at location I may be recorded by the same nerve and also by the nearby innervation areas, laterally and contralaterally, as indicated by the arrows. At location II, a lateral herniation of the disk one level below may affect the same nerve root and the root one level below, located medial to this root, as indicated by the arrows.*

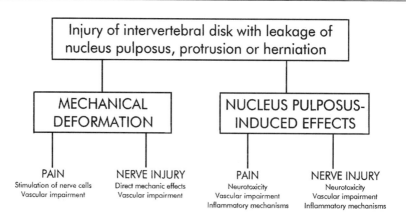

Fig. 6 *The pathophysiologic events in disk herniation. The two mechanisms at the tissue level, mechanical deformation and nucleus pulposus-induced effects, may both induce pain and nerve injury.*

and the nerve dysfunction are different characteristics, they may be based on similar events. It is evident that mechanical deformation of a nerve root is significantly linked to the symptoms of sciatica. In addition, the potency of disk-derived materials has not been fully recognized. In fact, it seems that mere leakage of these substances is sufficient for initiating pathophysiologic events.

References

1. Mixter WJ, Barr JS: Rupture of the intervertebral disc with involvement of the spinal canal. *N Engl J Med* 1934;211:210–215.
2. Olmarker K, Hasue M: Classification and pathophysiology of spinal pain syndromes, in Weinstein JN, Rydevik BL, Sonntag VKH (eds): *Essentials of the Spine*. New York, NY, Raven Press, 1995, pp 11–25.
3. Sachs B, Fraenkel J: Progressive ankylotic rigidity of the spine (spondylose rhizomélique). *J Nerv Ment Dis* 1900;27:1–15.
4. Bailey P, Casamajor L: Osteo-arthritis of the spine as a cause of compression of the spinal cord and its roots, with reports of five cases. *J Nerv Ment Dis* 1911;38:588–609.
5. Goldthwait JE: The lumbo-sacral articulation: An explanation of many cases of "lumbago," "sciatica" and "paraplegia." *Boston Med Surg J* 1911;164:365–372.
6. Olmarker K, Rydevik B, Nordborg C: Autologous nucleus pulposus induces neurophysiologic and histologic changes in porcine cauda equina nerve roots. *Spine* 1993;18:1425–1432.
7. Murphy RW: Nerve roots and spinal nerves in degenerative disk disease. *Clin Orthop* 1977;129:46–60.
8. Rydevik B, Brown MD, Lundborg G: Pathoanatomy and pathophysiology of nerve root compression. *Spine* 1984;9:7–15.
9. Gelfan S, Tarlov IM: Physiology of spinal cord, nerve root and peripheral nerve compression. *Am J Physiol* 1956;185:217–229.
10. Sharpless SK: Susceptibility of spinal nerve roots to compression block: The research status of spinal manipulative therapy, in Goldstein M (ed): *NINCDS Monograph No. 15*. Bethesda, MD, US Department of Health, Education and Welfare, 1975, pp 155–161.
11. Olmarker K: Spinal nerve root compression: Nutrition and function of the porcine cauda equina compressed in vivo. *Acta Orthop Scand* 1991;242(suppl):1–27.
12. Olmarker K, Holm S, Rosenqvist A-L, et al: Experimental nerve root compression: A model of acute, graded compression of the porcine cauda equina and an analysis of neural and vascular anatomy. *Spine* 1991;16:61–69.
13. Olmarker K, Rydevik B, Holm S, et al: Effects of experimental graded compression on blood flow in spinal nerve roots: A vital microscopic study on the porcine cauda equina. *J Orthop Res* 1989;7:817–823.
14. Sunderland S: The nerve lesion in the carpal tunnel syndrome. *J Neurol Neurosurg Psychiatry* 1976;39:615–626.
15. Olmarker K, Holm S, Rydevik B, et al: Restoration of intrinsic blood flow during gradual decompression of the porcine cauda equina: A vital microscopic study. *Neuro-Orthop* 1991;10:83–87.
16. Rydevik B, Holm S, Brown MD, et al: Diffusion from the cerebrospinal fluid as a nutritional pathway for spinal nerve roots. *Acta Physiol Scand* 1990;138:247–248.
17. Olmarker K, Rydevik B, Hansson T, et al: Compression-induced changes of the nutritional supply to the porcine cauda equina. *J Spinal Disord* 1990;3:25–29.
18. Rydevik B, Lundborg G: Permeability of intraneural microvessels and perineurium following acute, graded experimental nerve compression. *Scand J Plast Reconstr Surg* 1977;11:179–187.
19. Low PA, Dyck PJ: Increased endoneurial fluid pressure in experimental lead neuropathy. *Nature* 1977;269:427–428.
20. Lundborg G, Myers R, Powell H: Nerve compression injury and increased endoneurial fluid pressure: A "miniature compartment syndrome." *J Neurol Neurosurg Psychiatry* 1983;46:1119–1124.

229

21. Myers RR, Mizisin AP, Powell HC, et al: Reduced nerve blood flow in hexachlorophene neuropathy: Relationship to elevated endoneurial fluid pressure. *J Neuropathol Exp Neurol* 1982;41:391–439.

22. Myers RR, Powell HC: Galactose neuropathy: Impact of chronic endoneurial edema on nerve blood flow. *Ann Neurol* 1984;16:587–594.

23. Rydevik B, Lundborg G, Nordborg C: Intraneural tissue reactions induced by internal neurolysis: An experimental study on the blood-nerve barrier, connective tissues and nerve fibres of rabbit tibial nerve. *Scand J Plast Reconstr Surg* 1976;10:3–8.

24. Olmarker K, Rydevik B, Holm S: Edema formation in spinal nerve roots induced by experimental, graded compression: An experimental study on the pig cauda equina with special reference to differences in effects between rapid and slow onset of compression. *Spine* 1989;14:569–573.

25. Olmarker K, Holm S, Rydevik B: Importance of compression onset rate for the degree of impairment of impulse propagation in experimental compression injury of the porcine cauda equina. *Spine* 1990;15:416–419.

26. Garfin SR, Cohen MS, Massie JB, et al: Nerve-roots of the cauda equina: The effect of hypotension and acute graded compression on function. *J Bone Joint Surg* 1990;72A:1185–1192.

27. Rydevik BL, Pedowitz RA, Hargens AR, et al: Effects of acute, graded compression on spinal nerve root function and structure: An experimental study of the pig cauda equina. *Spine* 1991;16:487–483.

28. Pedowitz RA, Garfin SR, Massie JB, et al: Effects of magnitude and duration of compression on spinal nerve root conduction. *Spine* 1992;17:194–199.

29. Olmarker K, Lind B, Holm S, et al: Continued compression increases impairment of impulse propagation in experimental compression of the porcine cauda equina. *Neuro-Orthop* 1991;11:75–81.

30. Porter RW, Ward D: Cauda equina dysfunction: The significance of two-level pathology. *Spine* 1992;17:9–15.

31. Olmarker K, Rydevik B: Single- versus double-level nerve root compression: An experimental study on the porcine cauda equina with analyses of nerve impulse conduction properties. *Clin Orthop* 1992;279:35–39.

32. Lundborg G: Structure and function of the intraneural microvessels as related to trauma, edema formation, and nerve function. *J Bone Joint Surg* 1975;57A:938–948.

33. Parke WW, Gammell K, Rothman RH: Arterial vascularization of the cauda equina. *J Bone Joint Surg* 1981;63A:53–62.

34. Parke WW, Watanabe R: The intrinsic vasculature of the lumbosacral spinal nerve roots. *Spine* 1985;10:508–515.

35. Petterson CÅ, Olsson Y: Blood supply of spinal nerve roots: An experimental study in the rat. *Acta Neuropathol* 1989;78:455–461.

36. Takahashi K, Olmarker K, Holm S, et al: Double-level cauda equina compression: An experimental study with continuous monitoring of intraneural blood flow in the porcine cauda equina. *J Orthop Res* 1993;11:104–109.

37. Cornefjord M, Takahashi K, Matsui H, et al: Impairment of nutritional transport at double level cauda equina compression: An experimental study. *Neuro-Orthop* 1992;13:107–112.

38. Delamarter RB, Bohlman HH, Dodge LD, et al: Experimental lumbar spinal stenosis: Analysis of the cortical evoked potentials, microvasculature and histopathology. *J Bone Joint Surg* 1990;72A:110–120.

39. Delamarter RB, Sherman JE, Carr JB: Cauda equina syndrome: Neurologic recovery following immediate, early, or late decompression. *Spine* 1991;16:1022–1029.

40. Cornefjord M, Olmarker K, Farley DB, et al: Neuropeptide changes in compressed spinal nerve roots. *Spine* 1995;20:670–673.

41. Sato K, Olmarker K, Cornefjord M, et al: Effects of chronic nerve root compression on intra radicular blood flow: An experimental study in pigs. *Neuro-Orthop* 1994;16:1–7.

42. Takahashi K, Miyazaki T, Takino T, et al: Epidural pressure measurements: Relationship between epidural pressure and posture in patients with lumbar spinal stenosis. *Spine* 1995;20:650–653.
43. Konno S, Olmarker K, Byröd G, et al: Intermittent cauda equina compression: An experimental study of the porcine cauda equina with analyses of nerve impulse conduction properties. *Spine* 1995;20:1223–1226.
44. Sato K, Konno S, Yabuki S, et al: A model for acute, chronic, and delayed graded compression of the dog cauda equina: Neurophysiologic and histologic changes induced by acute, graded compression. *Spine* 1995;20:2386–2391.
45. Konno S, Yabuki S, Sato K, et al: A model for acute, chronic, and delayed graded compression of the dog cauda equina: Presentation of the gross, microscopic, and vascular anatomy of the dog cauda equina and accuracy in pressure transmission of the compression model. *Spine* 1995;20:2758–2764.
46. Howe JF, Loeser JD, Calvin WH: Mechanosensitivity of dorsal root ganglia and chronically injured axons: A physiological basis for the radicular pain of nerve root compression. *Pain* 1977;3:25–41.
47. Cavanaugh JM, Özaktay AC, Vaidyanathan S: Mechano- and chemosensitivity of lumbar dorsal roots and dorsal root ganglia: An in vitro study. *Trans Orthop Res Soc* 1994;19:109.
48. Weinstein J: Mechanisms of spinal pain: The dorsal root ganglion and its role as a mediator of low-back pain. *Spine* 1986;11:999–1001.
49. Weinstein J, Pope M, Schmidt R, et al: Effects of low frequency vibration on the dorsal root ganglion. *Neuro-Orthop* 1987;4:24–30.
50. Rydevik B, Brown MD, Ehira T, et al: Abstract: Effects of graded compression and nucleus pulposus on nerve tissue: An experimental study in rabbits. *Acta Orthop Scand* 1983;54:670–671.
51. McCarron RF, Wimpee MW, Hudkins PG, et al: The inflammatory effect of nucleus pulposus: A possible element in the pathogenesis of low-back pain. *Spine* 1987;12:760–764.
52. Olmarker K, Rydevik B, Nordborg C: Ultrastructural changes in spinal nerve roots induced by autologous nucleus pulposus. *Spine* 1996;21:411–414.
53. Olmarker K, Byröd G, Cornefjord M, et al: Effects of methylprednisolone on nucleus pulposus-induced nerve root injury. *Spine* 1994;19:1803–1808.
54. Olmarker K, Blomquist J, Strömberg J, et al: Inflammatogenic properties of nucleus pulposus. *Spine* 1995;20:665–669.
55. Takino T, Takahashi K, Miyazaki T, et al: Immunoreactivity of nucleus pulposus. Transactions of the International Society for the Study of the Lumbar Spine, Helsinki, Finland, 1995, p 107.
56. Kawakami M, Weinstein JN, Hashizume H, et al: Pathomechanisms of pain-related behaviour produced by intervertebral disc in the rat. Transactions of the International Society for the Study of the Lumbar Spine, Helsinki, Finland, 1995, p 53.
57. Eyre D, Benya P, Buckwalter J, et al: The intervertebral disk: Basic science perspectives, in Frymoyer JW, Gordon SL (eds): *New Perspectives on Low Back Pain*. Park Ridge, IL, American Academy of Orthopaedic Surgeons, 1989, pp 147–207.
58. Bayliss MT, Johnstone B: Biochemistry of the intervertebral disc, in Jayson MIV (ed): *The Lumbar Spine and Back Pain*. Edinburgh, Scotland, Churchill Livingstone, 1992, pp 111–131.
59. Naylor A: The biochemical changes in the human intervertebral disc in degeneration and nuclear prolapse. *Orthop Clin North Am* 1971;2:343–358.
60. Marshall LL, Trethewie ER: Chemical irritation of nerve-root in disc prolapse. *Lancet* 1973;2:320.
61. Marshall LL, Trethewie ER, Curtain CC: Chemical radiculitis: A clinical, physiological and immunological study. *Clin Orthop* 1977;129:61–67.
62. Kang JD, Georgescu HI, Larkin L, et al: Herniated lumbar and cervical intervertebral discs spontaneously produce matrix metalloproteinases, nitric oxide, interleukin-6, and prostaglandin E2. *Trans Orthop Res Soc* 1995;20:350.

231

63. Olmarker K, Yabuki S, Nordborg C, et al: The effects of normal, frozen and hyaluronidase digested nucleus pulposus on nerve root function. *Spine*, in press.

64. Diamant B, Karlsson J, Nachemson A: Correlation between lactate levels and pH in discs of patients with lumbar rhizopathies. *Experientia* 1968;24:1195–1196.

65. Nachemson A: Intradiscal measurements of pH in patients with lumbar rhizopathies. *Acta Orthop Scand* 1969;40:23–42.

66. Pennington JB, McCarron RF, Laros GS: Identification of IgG in the canine intervertebral disc. *Spine* 1988;13:909–912.

67. Saal JS, Franson RC, Dobrow R, et al: High levels of inflammatory phospholipase A2 activity in lumbar disc herniations. *Spine* 1990;15:674–678.

68. Dyck PJ, Karnes J, Lais A, et al: Pathologic alterations of the peripheral nervous system of humans, in Dyck PJ, Thomas PK, Lambert EH, et al (eds): *Peripheral Neuropathy*, ed 2. Philadelphia, PA, WB Saunders, 1984, vol 1, pp 760–780.

69. Jayson MI, Keegan A, Million R, et al: A fibrinolytic defect in chronic back pain syndromes. *Lancet* 1984;2:1186–1187.

70. Klimiuk PS, Pountain GD, Keegan AL, et al: Serial measurements of fibrinolytic activity in acute low back pain and sciatica. *Spine* 1987;12:925–928.

71. Hoyland JA, Freemont AJ, Jayson MI: Intervertebral foramen venous obstruction: A cause of periradicular fibrosis? *Spine* 1989;14:558–568.

72. Cooper RG, Freemont AJ, Hoyland JA, et al: Herniated intervertebral disc-associated periradicular fibrosis and vascular abnormalities occur without inflammatory cell infiltration. *Spine* 1995;20:591–598.

73. Byröd G, Olmarker K, Konno S, et al: A rapid transport route between the epidural space and the intraneural capillaries of the nerve roots. *Spine* 1995;20:138–143.

74. Dalcanto M, Wisniewski HM, Johnson AB, et al: Vesicular disruption of myelin in autoimmune demyelination. *J Neurol Sci* 1975;24:313–319.

75. Hahn AF, Gilbert JJ, Feasby TE: Passive transfer of demyelination by experimental allergic neuritis serum. *Acta Neuropathol* 1980;49:169–176.

76. Naylor A: The biophysical and biochemical aspects of intervertebral disc herniation and degeneration. *Ann R Coll Surg Engl* 1962;31:91–114.

77. Bobechko WP, Hirsch C: Auto-immune response to nucleus pulposus in the rabbit. *J Bone Joint Surg* 1965;47B:574–580.

78. LaRocca H: New horizons in research on disc disease. *Orthop Clin North Am* 1971;2:521–531.

79. Naylor A, Happey F, Turner RL, et al: Enzymic and immunological activity in the intervertebral disk. *Orthop Clin North Am* 1975;6:51–58.

80. Gertzbein SD, Tile M, Gross A, et al: Autoimmunity in degenerative disc disease of the lumbar spine. *Orthop Clin North Am* 1975;6:67–73.

81. Bisla RS, Marchisello PJ, Lockshin MD, et al: Auto-immunological basis of disk degeneration. *Clin Orthop* 1976;121:205–211.

82. Gertzbein SD: Degenerative disk disease of the lumbar spine: Immunological implications. *Clin Orthop* 1977;129:68–71.

83. Gertzbein SD, Tait JH, Devlin SR: The stimulation of lymphocytes by nucleus pulposus in patients with degenerative disk disease of the lumbar spine. *Clin Orthop* 1977;123:149–154.

84. Bentley FH, Schlapp W: The effects of pressure on conduction in peripheral nerve. *J Nerv Ment Dis* 1943;38:588–609.

85. Fowler TJ, Danta G, Gilliatt RW: Recovery of nerve conduction after a pneumatic tourniquet: Observations on the hind-limb of the baboon. *J Neurol Neurosurg Psychiatry* 1972;35:638–647.

86. Ochoa J, Fowler TJ, Gilliatt RW: Anatomical changes in peripheral nerves compressed by a pneumatic tourniquet. *J Anat* 1972;113:433–455.

87. Rydevik B, Lundborg G, Bagge U: Effects of graded compression on intraneural blood flow: An in vivo study on rabbit tibial nerve. *J Hand Surg* 1981;6A:3–12.

88. Rydevik B, Nordborg C: Changes in nerve function and nerve fibre structure induced by acute, graded compression. *J Neurol Neurosurg Psychiatry* 1980;43:1070–1082.

89. Macnab I: Negative disc exploration: An analysis of the causes of nerve-root involvement in sixty-eight patients. *J Bone Joint Surg* 1971;53A:891–903.
90. Crock HV: Observations on the management of failed spinal operations. *J Bone Joint Surg* 1976;58B:193–199.
91. Jönsson B: *Lumbar Nerve Root Compression Syndromes. Symptoms, Signs and Surgical Results.* Lund, Sweden, University of Lund, 1995. Thesis.
92. Kuslich SD, Ulstrom CL, Michael CJ: The tissue origin of low back pain and sciatica: A report of pain response to tissue stimulation during operations on the lumbar spine using local anesthesia. *Orthop Clin North Am* 1991;22:181–187.
93. El-Mahdi MA, Abdel Latif FY, Janko M: The spinal nerve root "innervation" and a new concept of the clinicopathological interrelations in back pain and sciatica. *Neurochirurgie* 1981;24:137–141.
94. Olmarker K, Rydevik B: Pathophysiology of sciatica. *Orthop Clin North Am* 1991;22:223–234.
95. Rydevik B, Olmarker K: Pathophysiology of the nerve roots in the lumbar spine, in Holtzman RNN, McCormick P, Farcy J-PC (eds): *Contemporary Perspectives in Neurosurgery: Spinal Instability.* New York, NY, Springer-Verlag, 1993, pp 55–61.
96. Rudinger N (ed): *Die Gelenknerven des menschlichen Körpers.* Erlangen, Germany, Ferdinand Enke, 1857.
97. Edgar MA, Nundy S: Innervation of the spinal dura mater. *J Neurol Neurosurg Psychiatry* 1966;29:530–534.
98. Kaplan EB: Recurrent meningeal branch of the spinal nerves. *Bull Hosp Joint Dis* 1947;8:108–109.

Chapter 15

Intraradicular Edema Formation as a Basic Factor in Lumbar Radiculopathy

Hidezo Yoshizawa, MD, PhD
Sadaaki Nakai, MD, PhD
Shigeru Kobayashi, MD, PhD
Tomofumi Morita, MD, PhD
Naoyuki Shizu, MD

Introduction

Mixter and Barr[1] were the first to describe prolapse of the intervertebral disk as a causative agent in the production of low back and leg pain. It now is commonly acknowledged that derangements of the intervertebral disk lead to many cases of low back pain and sciatica. However, acute compression of a normal nerve root does not always cause pain; instead, it can cause numbness, paresthesia, and motor weakness. Compressed nerve roots can exist without causing any pain. These facts suggest that some secondary changes in and around the nerve root may be a critical factor in radicular pain.

Nerve Root Enhancement With Gd-DTPA

In recent years, gadolinium diethylenetriaminepentaacetic acid (Gd-DTPA)-enhanced magnetic resonance imaging (MRI) has been of great value in delineating intraradicular edema resulting from increased permeability of blood capillaries in which the blood–nerve barrier is broken down by compression.[2-9] MR images enhanced 42 nerve roots in 37 patients with disk herniation who underwent microsurgery and were followed up in our clinic for more than 1 year. Most of the patients came to our clinic within a month after the start of radicular symptoms. However, it is difficult to know when the herniated disk began to compress the nerve root. All the cases became symptom-free within a few weeks after surgery.

The condition of the affected nerve root at surgery was classified as follows: type 1, only mechanical deformation of the nerve root; type 2, inflammatory changes in the nerve root, such as redness, swelling, and slight adhesion to the surrounding tissue; and type 3, atrophy and heavy adhesion of the nerve root (Fig. 1). Among the 42 affected nerve roots, 22 (52.4%) were type 1, 15 (35.7%) were type 2, and five (11.9%) were type 3.

Before surgery and 3, 6, and 12 months after surgery, 5-mm thick T1- and T2-weighted spin-echo images were obtained in the sagittal and axial planes,

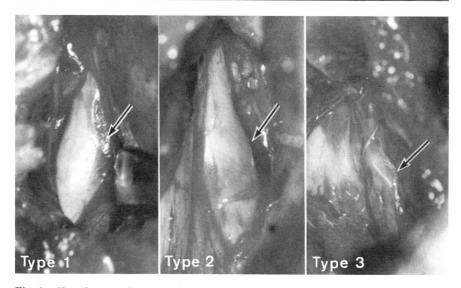

Fig. 1 *Classification of surgical findings around the affected nerve root. Type 1, mechanical deformation only; type 2, inflammatory changes in the nerve root; and type 3, atrophy and heavy adhesion of the nerve root.*

Gd-DTPA (0.2 mmol/kg) was administered, and T1-weighted images were obtained in the same plane (Fig. 2). All type 2 and 3 nerve roots were enhanced by Gd-DTPA before surgery, whereas 14 type 1 nerve roots (63.6%) were not enhanced. The enhancement rate of types 1, 2, and 3 nerve roots were 27.3%, 66.7%, and 100%, respectively, 3 months after surgery and 13.6%, 33.3%, and

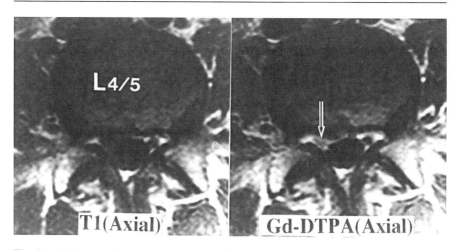

Fig. 2 *Axial magnetic resonance images of type 2 nerve root before surgery. The left L5 root (black arrow) is enhanced with gadolinium diethylenetriaminepentaacetic acid (Gd-DTPA).*

80.0%, respectively, 6 months after surgery (Fig. 3). The pathologic status in nerve roots lasts more than 6 months after removal of mechanical compression to the nerve root. By 12 months after surgery, no nerve roots were enhanced with Gd-DTPA.

Anatomic Structure of the Nerve Root

The nerve root, which is surrounded by cerebrospinal fluid, has a sheath that is composed only of scanty connective tissue. It lacks epineurium and perineurium, which are well developed in the peripheral nerve. In the transition zone near the dorsal root ganglion, between the nerve root and the spinal nerve, the epineurium of the spinal nerve is in direct continuity with the dura mater (dural sleeve).[10] Most of the perineurium of the spinal nerve passes outward between the dura mater and the arachnoid. A few deeper perineurial cell layers continue on to the nerve root to become part of the nerve root sheath.[10-12]

The nerve root sheath is loosely constructed, with generous, often empty intercellular spaces punctuated by intercellular junctions. The only coherent structural barrier between the endoneurium and the subarachnoid space is the basement membrane.[13] This membrane is open near the junction with the spinal cord, forming an open-ended tube.[12] The superficial layer of the arachnoid curves onto the nerve root at the subarachnoid angle,[14] which is the lateralmost extension of the subarachnoid space, and forms the superficial layer of the nerve root sheath. The nerve root sheath is continuous with the pia mater at the junction with the spinal cord. The subarachnoid space appears to communicate with the endoneurial space of the nerve root[14] (Fig. 4).

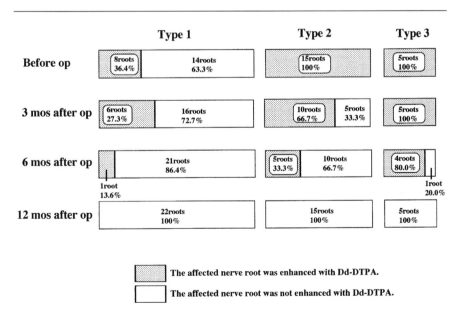

Fig. 3   *Gadolinium diethylenetriaminepentaacetic acid (Gd-DTPA) enhancement rate of the affected nerve root before and after surgery.*

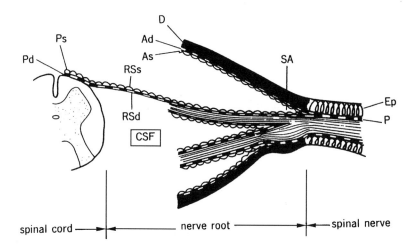

Fig. 4 *Anatomic structure of the nerve root. D, dura mater; As, superficial layer of arachnoid; Ad, deep layer of arachnoid; RSs, superficial layer of nerve root sheath; RSd, deep layer of nerve root sheath; Ps, superficial layer of pia mater; Pd, deep layer of pia mater; Ep, epineurium; P, perineurium; SA, subarachnoid angle; and CSF, cerebrospinal fluid. (Reproduced with permission from Yoshizawa H, Kobayashi S, Nakai S: Structure anatomique et vascularisation des racines L4L5S1, in Gastambide D (ed): Instabilities Vertebrales Lombaires. Paris, France, Expansion Scientifique, 1995, pp 20–34.)*

Normally, the internal milieu of peripheral nerve fascicles is controlled by the combined barrier action of the endoneurial blood vessels[15-20] and the perineurium. In the case of the nerve root, however, the function of the diffusion barrier exists only in the deep layer of the perineurial epithelium of the arachnoid membrane[21-30] and not in the nerve root sheath.

The nerve fibers in spinal nerve roots, as well as peripheral nerves, depend on a continuous supply of oxygen and other nutrients to maintain proper function. In general, the blood supply of nerve roots is less well developed than that of peripheral nerves.[31-33] Rydevik and associates,[18,34] working with isotopes, indicated that the nerve roots seem to derive some of their nutrition not only from the microvascular system inside the nerve root, but also via diffusion from cerebrospinal fluid. My coworkers and I[33,35] also demonstrated partial oxygen pressure of cerebrospinal fluid to be much higher than for the nerve root. Additionally, protein tracers injected into the subarachnoid space permeate into the endoneurial space of the nerve root and drain into the capillary lumen[33] (Fig. 5).

Pulsating cerebrospinal fluid surrounding the nerve root is thus important for normal function of the nerve root, and disturbance of cerebrospinal fluid flow due to mechanical compression may have an adverse effect on the intraradicular circulation.[33-36]

Blood–Nerve Barrier

The structural and physiologic aspects of the permeability of blood capillaries have been studied extensively[37-40] since the development of the electron mi-

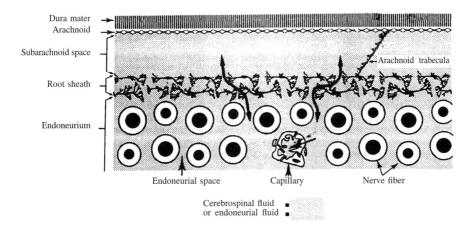

Fig. 5   *The relation between the cerebrospinal fluid and the endoneurial tissue fluid. The cerebrospinal fluid communicates with the endoneurial tissue fluid in the nerve root through the nerve root sheath, which has no diffusion barrier. The endoneurial tissue fluid can be carried into the capillary lumen. (Reproduced with permission from Kobayashi S, Yoshizawa H, Hachiya Y, et al: Vasogenic edema induced by compression injury to the spinal nerve root: Distribution of intravenously injected protein tracers and gadolinium-enhanced magnetic resonance imaging.* Spine *1993;18:1410–1424.)*

croscope. Bennet and associates[37] proposed morphologic classification of capillaries based on (1) the presence or absence of continuous basement membrane, (2) the nature of the endothelial cell, and (3) the presence or absence of a complete investment of pericytes. These structural features of the capillary may be relevant to problems related to the exchange of materials between blood plasma and parenchymal cells.

In general, capillaries are classified into three types: continuous, fenestrated, and discontinuous (Fig. 6). Continuous capillaries are further divided into brain type and muscle type. Brain type capillaries are located mainly in the central and peripheral nervous systems where the blood–brain (nerve) barrier is present. The blood–nerve barrier has analogous functions to the blood–brain barrier, but there is less restraint to the penetration of materials and less selectivity in the blood–nerve barrier than in the blood–brain barrier.[41-43] The blood–nerve barrier consists of tight junctions (zonulae occludentes) between adjacent endothelial cells with a very small number of endothelial vesicles.

The capillaries in the endoneurial space of the nerve root, except in the dorsal root ganglion (DRG), are all continuous type capillaries, as in the case of peripheral nerves.[44,45] There are tight junctions between their endothelial cells, showing the existence of a blood–nerve barrier. Pinocytotic vesicles related to transport of nutrients and waste matter are more abundant in endothelial cells of capillaries in the nerve roots than in those of capillaries in peripheral nerves. Also, the capillaries of nerve roots have a pericyte that is less well developed than that of peripheral nerves. Protein tracers injected into the subarachnoid space pass through the nerve root sheath and enter into the vessels in the endoneurial space. There is no extravasation of the tracers injected intrave-

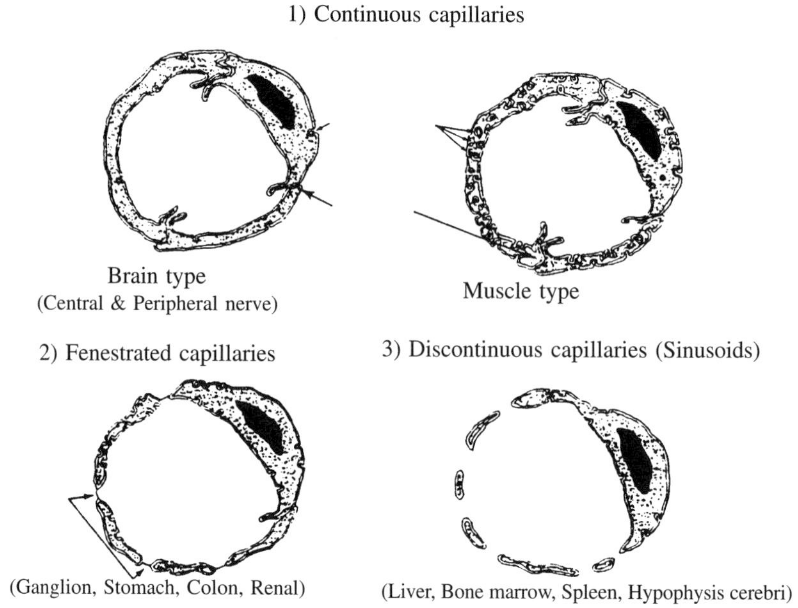

1) Continuous capillaries

Brain type
(Central & Peripheral nerve)

Muscle type

2) Fenestrated capillaries

3) Discontinuous capillaries (Sinusoids)

(Ganglion, Stomach, Colon, Renal)

(Liver, Bone marrow, Spleen, Hypophysis cerebri)

Fig. 6 *Classification of the capillary. (Reproduced with permission from Kobayashi S, Yoshizawa H, Hachiya Y, et al: Vasogenic edema induced by compression injury to the spinal nerve root: Distribution of intravenously injected protein tracers and gadolinium-enhanced magnetic resonance imaging.* Spine *1993;18:1410–1424.)*

nously.[33] Wagner and associates[46] have pointed out that the existence of a blood–brain barrier does not necessarily imply the existence of a brain–blood barrier. These structural features of capillaries in the nerve root indicate that the blood–nerve barrier is not as tight as that of peripheral nerves.

In the DRG there are both continuous and fenestrated capillaries. Endothelial cells of the continuous type capillaries in the DRG are linked with gap junctions (endothelial intercellular clefts, zonulae adherens) between adjacent endothelial cells. The fenestrated capillaries have a fenestration with a diaphragm in an endothelial cell. Data from protein tracer studies[9,47-51] indicate that these fenestrations and gap junctions are the most important routes of the tracer leakage. That is, there is no blood–nerve barrier in the DRG. In the endoneurial space of the DRG, macrophages are often seen both in the perivascular space and between nerve cells and nerve fibers. These macrophages seem to be concerned with important mechanisms for elimination of foreign proteins from the endoneurial space.

Chronic Nerve Root Compression

In 1948 Lindblom and Rexed[52] reported on macroscopic and histologic postmortem examination of intervertebral disk protrusions in 17 cases. They observed that the changes in the nerves caused by the compression consisted of a slight increase in connective tissue elements in the perineurium and of a mixture of degeneration and regeneration of the nerve fibers themselves, which looked like a whorl of small newly formed fibers and bulblike structures, in addition to the purely mechanical deformation. The bulblike structures are formed by proliferated Schwann cells and endoneurial fibroblasts in the degenerating ventral root.

Lindahl and Rexed[53] histologically investigated biopsy specimens from the nerve roots in patients operated on for sciatica. Chronic nerve compression was

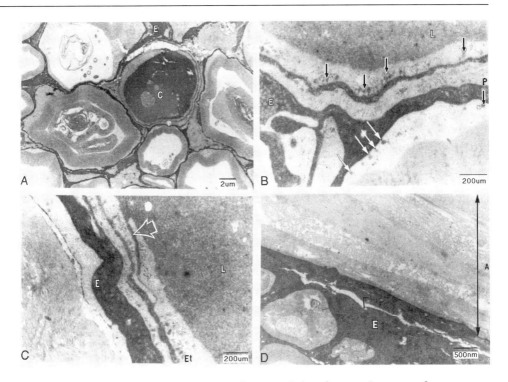

Fig. 7 *Transverse sections of a nerve root seen under transmission electron microscope after intravenous injection of horseradish peroxidase.* **A,** *After 1 month of tubing, the dark reaction products of horseradish peroxidase leak out of capillaries (c) and are present in the endoneurial space (original magnification × 5000).* **B,** *Many pinocytotic vesicles appear to carry the reaction products of horseradish peroxidase away from the capillary lumen (transcellular transport; black arrows). The pinocytotic vesicles in the Schwann cell containing the reaction product are noted (white arrows) (original magnification × 30,000).* **C,** *The tight junction between two endothelial cells is broken down and filled with reaction products of horseradish peroxidase (paracellular transport, open arrow) (original magnification × 30,000).* **D,** *The reaction products of horseradish peroxidase do not get through A, showing that the arachnoid membrane acts as a diffusion barrier (original magnification × 10,000). A, arachnoid membrane; C, capillary; E, endoneurial space; Et, endothelium; L, capillary lumen; P, pericyte. (Reproduced with permission from Yoshizawa H, Kobayashi S, Morita T: Chronic nerve root compression: Pathophysiologic mechanism of nerve root dysfunction. Spine 1995;20:397–407.)*

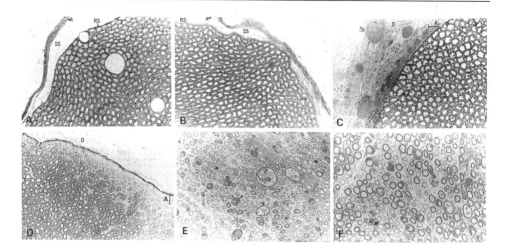

Fig. 8 *Light micrographs of a transverse section of the nerve root wrapped with a Silastic tube (toluidine blue, original magnification × 40). A, The control section. B, After 2 weeks of tubing, the nerve root is essentially normal. C, After 1 month of tubing, the dura mater and arachnoid membrane are thickened. The endoneurium looks normal. D, After 3 months of tubing, a fallout in the large myelinated fiber population at the periphery of the nerve root is noted. E, After 6 months of tubing, fewer fibers are noted and a shift in fiber population to smaller and more thinly myelinated fibers is seen. F, After 12 months of tubing, the myelin sheaths are more regenerated than destroyed. A, arachnoid membrane; D, dura mater; RS, root sheath; and SS, subarachnoid space. (Reproduced with permission from Yoshizawa H, Kobayashi S, Morita T: Chronic nerve root compression: Pathophysiologic mechanism of nerve root dysfunction. Spine 1995;20:397–407.)*

associated with connective tissue changes, initially hyperplasia of the perineurium (dural and arachnoidal sheath) and ultimately endoneurial fibrosis. With these connective tissue changes, there was a decrease in the large myelinated fibers situated in the periphery of the fascicle and, eventually, wallerian degeneration.

We have recently reported on a pathophysiologic mechanism of nerve root dysfunction caused by using an experimental model of chronic compression after application of a siliconized rubber tube to the lumbar nerve root of a dog.[54] The earliest abnormal finding was the thickening of the dural sleeve and arachnoid membrane due to scar formation around the affected nerve root. The capillaries in the scar had leaky tight junctions and large intercellular gaps.[55] However, the histologic and electrophysiologic status of the nerve fibers at this stage were essentially normal. The thickening of the arachnoid membrane corresponded to the breakdown of the blood–nerve barrier function in the endoneurial vessels, electron microscopically indicating that paracellular transport was induced by opening of tight junctions and increased transcellular vesicular transport. Disappearance of the subarachnoid space around the nerve root, breakdown of the blood–nerve barrier in the endoneurial space, and persistence of the diffusion barrier in the perineurial epithelium of the arachnoid membrane may result in edema within the nerve root and increased endoneurial fluid pressure, with subsequent replacement of nerve root tissues by fibrosis.[56] Edema in the nerve root was observed after 1 to 12 months of application of siliconized rubber tubing (Fig. 7). After 3 months of nerve root tubing, definite histologic changes in the nerve fibers were noted, with a decrease in large myelinated fibers and an increase in small, newly formed fibers along the periphery of the fascicle. These changes were similar to those observed in human specimens[52,53] (Fig. 8).

The earliest electrophysiologic abnormality was observed at this stage; it showed a decrease in compound action potential amplitudes corresponding with a decrease in large myelinated fibers. The nerve conduction velocity did not decrease as long as some of the large myelinated fibers remained, but obviously decreased after 12 months of tubing when the large myelinated fibers disappeared completely (Fig. 9).

Conclusion

The clinical and experimental data from our studies indicate that the Gd-DTPA enhancement in and around the compressed nerve root seen in patients with disk herniations reflects intraradicular edema resulting from breakdown of the blood–nerve barrier in the nerve root. Scar formation around the nerve root correlates reasonably well with the surgical and pathologic findings. Mechanical compression blocks cerebrospinal fluid flow around the nerve root, and the diffusion barrier, which is in the perineurial epithelium of the arachnoid membrane, blocks the edema diffusion into the cerebrospinal fluid. Persistence of this chronic condition may lead to subsequent replacement of normal components of the nerve tissues with fibrosis. This change may occur as a basis of radiculopathy, provoking ectopic discharges that create radicular pain.

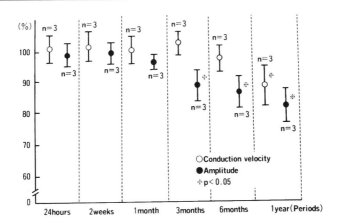

Fig. 9 *Nerve conduction studies. (Reproduced with permission from Yoshizawa H, Kobayashi S, Morita T: Chronic nerve root compression: Pathophysiologic mechanism of nerve root dysfunction.* Spine *1995;20:397–407.)*

References

1. Mixter WJ, Barr JS: Rupture of the intervertebral disk with involvement of the spinal canal. *N Engl J Med* 1934;211:210–215.
2. Brasch RC, Weinmann HJ, Wesbey GE: Contrast-enhanced NMR imaging: Animal studies using gadolinium: DTPA complex. *Am J Roentgenol* 1984;142:625–630.
3. Hueftle MG, Modic MT, Ross JS et al: Lumbar spine: Postoperative MR imaging with Gd-DTPA. *Radiology* 1988;167:817–824.
4. Ross JS, Blaser S, Masaryk TJ, et al: Gd-DTPA-enhancement of posterior epidural scar: An experimental model. *Am J Neuroradiol* 1989;10:1083–1088.
5. Ross JS, Masaryk TJ, Schrader M, et al: MR imaging of the postoperative lumbar spine: Assessment with gadopentetate dimeglumine. *Am J Neuroradiol* 1990;11:771–776.
6. Jinkins JR: MR of enhancing nerve roots in the unoperated lumbosacral spine. *Am J Neuroradiol* 1993;14:193–202.
7. Jinkins JR, Osborn AG, Garrett D Jr, et al: Spinal nerve enhancement with Gd-DTPA: MR correlation with the postoperative lumbosacral spine. *Am J Neuroradiol* 1993;14:383–394.
8. Toyone T, Takahashi K, Kitahara H et al: Visualisation of symptomatic nerve roots: Prospective study of contrast-enhanced MRI in patients with lumbar disk herniation. *J Bone Joint Surg* 1993;75B:529–533.
9. Kobayashi S, Yoshizawa H, Hachiya Y, et al: Vasogenic edema induced by compression injury to the spinal nerve root: Distribution of intravenously injected protein tracers and gadolinium-enhanced magnetic resonance imaging. *Spine* 1993;18:1410–1424.
10. Key A, Retzius G (eds): *Studien in der Anatomie des Nervensystems und des Bindegewebes.* Stockholm, Sweden, Samon & Wallin, 1876.
11. Haller FR, Low FN: The fine structure of the peripheral nerve root sheath in the subarachnoid space in the rat and other laboratory animals. *Am J Anat* 1971;131:1–19.
12. Haller FR, Haller C, Low FN: The fine structure of cellular layers and connective tissue space at spinal nerve root attachments in the rat. *Am J Anat* 1972;133:109–123.
13. McCaabe JS, Low FN: The subarachnoid angle: An area of transition in peripheral nerve. *Anat Rec* 1969;164:15–33.
14. Himango WA, Low FN: The fine structure of a lateral recess of the subarachnoid space in the rat. *Anat Rec* 1971;171:1–19.
15. Pedowitz RA, Rydevik BL, Hargens AR, et al: Neurophysiologic and histologic changes induced by acute, graded compression of the pig cauda equina. *Orthop Trans* 1988;12:626.
16. Putti V: New conceptions in the pathogenesis of sciatic pain. *Lancet* 1927;2:53–60.
17. Rydevik B, Lundborg G: Permeability of intraneural microvessels and perineurium following acute, graded experimental nerve compression. *Scand J Plast Reconstr Surg* 1977;11:179–187.
18. Rydevik B, Holm S, Brown MD, et al: Nutrition of spinal nerve roots: The role of diffusion from the cerebrospinal fluid. *Trans Orthop Res Soc* 1984;9:276.
19. Rydevik B, Brown MD, Lundborg G: Pathoanatomy and pathophysiology of nerve root compression. *Spine* 1984;9:7–15.
20. Sunderland S: The connective tissues of peripheral nerves. *Brain* 1965;88:841–854.
21. Kristensson K, Olsson Y: The perineurium as a diffusion barrier to protein tracers: Differences between mature and immature animals. *Acta Neuropathol* 1971;17:127–138.
22. Lundborg G, Nordborg C, Rydevik B, et al: The effect of ischemia on the permeability of the perineurim to protein tracers in rabbit tibial nerve. *Acta Neurol Scand* 1973;49:287–294.
23. Nabeshima S, Reese TS, Landis DM, et al: Junctions in the meninges and marginal glia. *J Comp Neurol* 1975;164:127–169.
24. Oldfors A, Sourander P: Barriers of peripheral nerve towards exogenous peroxidase in normal and protein deprived rats. *Acta Neuropathol* 1978;43:129–134.

25. Olsson Y, Kristensson K: The perineurium as a diffusion barrier to protein tracers following trauma to nerves. *Acta Neuropathol* 1973;23:105–111.

26. Shanthaveerappa TR, Bourne GH: A perineural epithelium. *J Cell Biol* 1962;14:343–346.

27. Shanthaveerappa TR, Hope J, Bourne GH: Electron microscopic demonstration of the perineural epithelium in rat peripheral nerve. *Acta Anat* 1963;52:193–201.

28. Shanthaveerappa TR, Bourne GH: Perineural epithelium: A new concept of its role in the integrity of the peripheral nervous system. *Science* 1966;154:1464–1467.

29. Sima A, Sourander P: The effect of perinatal undernutrition on perineurial diffusion barrier to exogenous protein: An experimental study on rat sciatic nerve. *Acta Neuropathol* 1973;24:263–272.

30. Soderfeldt B, Olsson Y, Kristensson K: The perineurium as a diffusion barrier to protein tracers in human peripheral nerve. *Acta Neuropathol* 1973;25:120–126.

31. Kobayashi S: Experimental study on the blood flow disturbance in nerve root. *Bull Fujita Gakuen Med Soc* 1990;8:107–142.

32. Parke WW, Gammell K, Rothman RH: Arterial vascularization of the cauda equina. *J Bone Joint Surg* 1981;63A:53–62.

33. Yoshizawa H, Kobayashi S, Hachiya Y: Blood supply of nerve roots and dorsal root ganglia. *Orthop Clin North Am* 1991;22:195–211.

34. Rydevik B, Holm S, Brown MD, et al: Diffusion from the cerebrospinal fluid as a nutritional pathway for spinal nerve roots. *Acta Physiol Scand* 1990;138:247–248.

35. Ukai T: Effect of stagnant cerebrospinal fluid on spinal cord. *Bull Fujita Gakuen Med Soc* 1991;10:155–176.

36. Yoshizawa H, Kobayashi S, Kurose J: Various problems around nerve roots: Nutrition and adhesion of the nerve root. *Spine Spinal Cord* 1990;3:883– 839.

37. Bennett HS, Luft JH, Hampton JC: Morphological classification of vertebrate blood capillaries. *Am J Physiol* 1959;196:381–390.

38. Karnovsky MJ: The ultrastructural basis of capillary permeability studied with peroxidase as a tracer. *J Cell Biol* 1967;35:213–236.

39. Majno G: Ultrastructure of the vascular membrane, in Hamilton WF, Dow P (ed): *Handbook of Physiology: Section 2. Circulation.* Washington, DC, American Physiology Society, 1965, vol 3, pp 2293–2375.

40. Palade GE: Abstract: Fine structure of blood capillaries. *J Appl Phys* 1953;24:1424.

41. Arvidson B: Cellular uptake of exogenous horseradish peroxidase in mouse peripheral nerve. *Acta Neuropathol* 1977;37:35–41.

42. Fukuhara N: Blood-nerve barrier. *Shinkei Kenkyu no Shimpo* 1979;23:152–169.

43. Welch K, Davson H: The permeability of capillaries of the sciatic nerve of the rabbit to several materials. *J Neurosurg* 1972;36:21–26.

44. Kobayashi S, Yoshizawa H, Hachiya Y, et al: Fine structure of lumbosacral spinal nerve root: Transmission electron microscopical study. *Cent Jpn J Orthop Traumatol* 1991;34:463–465.

45. Kobayashi S, Yoshizawa H, Hachiya Y, et al: Pathophysiology of spinal nerve root compression. *Spine Spinal Cord* 1991;4:109–120.

46. Wagner HJ, Pilgrim C, Brandl J: Penetration and removal of horseradish peroxidase injected into the cerebrospinal fluid: Role of cerebral perivascular spaces, endothelium and microglia. *Acta Neuropathol* 1974;27:299–315.

47. Arvidson B: Distribution of intravenously injected protein tracers in peripheral ganglia of adult mice. *Exp Neurol* 1979;63:388–410.

48. Doinikow B: Histologische und histopathologische Untersuchungen am peripheren Nervensystem mittels vitaler Färbung. *Folia Neurobiol* 1913;7:731–749.

49. Jacobs JM, Macfarlane RM, Cavanagh JB: Vascular leakage in the dorsal root ganglia of the rat, studied with horseradish peroxidase. *J Neurol Sci* 1976;29:95–107.

50. Kobayashi S, Yoshizawa H, Hachiya Y, et al: Blood permeability of dorsal root ganglion. *J Japan Med Soc Paraplegia* 1992;5:126–127.

51. Olsson Y: Topographical differences in the vascular permeability of the peripheral nervous system. *Acta Neuropathol* 1968;10:26–33.

245

52. Lindblom K, Rexed B: Spinal nerve injury in dorso-lateral protrusions of lumbar disks. *J Neurosurg* 1948;5:413–432.

53. Lindahl O, Rexed B: Histologic changes in spinal nerve roots of operated cases of sciatica. *Acta Orthop Scand* 1951;20:215–225.

54. Yoshizawa H, Kobayashi S, Morita T: Chronic nerve root compression: Pathophysiologic mechanism of nerve root dysfunction. *Spine* 1995;20:397–407.

55. Ross JS, Delamarter R, Hueftle MG et al: Gadolinium-DTPA-enhanced MR imaging of the postoperative lumbar spine: Time course and mechanism of enhancement. *Am J Neuroradiol* 1989;10:37–46.

56. Lundborg G: Structure and function of the intraneural microvessels as related to trauma, edema formation, and nerve function. *J Bone Joint Surg* 1975;57A:938–948.

Chapter 16

The Neuropathology of Nerve Injury and Pain

Robert R. Myers, PhD

Introduction

The direct relationship between nerve injury and pain seems clear, at least in the acute sense when physical forces disrupt nerve fibers and cause aberrant electrophysiologic activity. But what is known about the pathogenesis of low back pain in the absence of magnetic resonance imaging (MRI) findings? Is low-grade nerve injury painful? What is known about the pathogenesis of chronic neuropathic pain states arising after nerve injury? Is there a relationship between the pathology of the peripheral injury and central changes in sensory systems predisposing to hyperalgesia? What are the roles of ischemic and inflammatory factors in the pathogenesis of pain? Should the traditional belief that the type of nerve fiber injury relates to the behavioral manifestations of pain be expanded to include general roles for toxic, inflammatory, and immunologic variables in the pathogenic mechanisms of low back pain? Answers to these questions are being sought in new studies of experimental neuropathology that combine modern techniques for quantifying the structure of injured nerves with characterizations of tissue immunochemistry and molecular biology. Taken together, data from these studies are beginning to define a new understanding of afferent sensory processing and pain behavior.

Traditionally, investigators have focused on compression and stretch nerve injuries as the major cause of low back pain, but the lack of chronic animal models of the human condition has limited the progress of research. The development of a porcine model of cauda equina compression in 1989[1] represented a major advance in low back pain research by permitting controlled compression of nerve roots during extended periods of electrophysiologic measurements. Use of the model has revealed important changes in neural and vascular anatomy that have been correlated with electrophysiologic dysfunction.[1-4] The advantages of the model include (1) the close anatomic resemblance of the porcine cauda equina to the human lumbosacral cauda equina, (2) the ease of surgical exposure, and (3) the bioengineering sophistication of the nerve compression device that allows for controlled, graded compression of the cauda equina. The acute pathology of this model will be reviewed in this chapter and in the chapter by Dr. Olmarker, who discusses the pathophysiology of nerve root compression versus tension. The primary limitation of the model is that it has been used to date only in acute experiments in anesthetized pigs, a use that restricts the ability of the neuropathologist to explore the temporal links between insult, injury, and pain. Recently developed models of neuropathic pain in the rat,[5,6] however, are not limited in this way and have proven useful in exploring the relationship between chronic compressive nerve injuries and the development and resolution of neuropathic pain syndromes. These rodent models, in combination with the porcine model, allow for an array of complementary research paradigms that have stimulated collaborative multidisciplinary studies of nerve injury.

The purpose of this chapter is to illustrate the neuropathologic changes in experimental nerve injury and to outline the results of recent laboratory investigations of the pathogenesis of neuropathic pain. The intent is to identify pathologic features common to painful focal neuropathies. The review is focused on experimental studies of nerve root injury but includes discussions of major pathogenic mechanisms of peripheral nerve injury that may hold keys to understanding the pathogenesis of low back pain.

Relationship of Nerve Injury to Pain

A historic approach to the study of the relationship between structural changes in human nerve and pain is provided by Dyck and associates,[7] who conducted a large retrospective clinical study at the Mayo Clinic, in which they sought to correlate morphology and pain. They found evidence of a relationship between acute nerve fiber breakdown and the degree and frequency of pain, but no correlation between pain and the ratio of large to small intact myelinated fibers. Although other studies of selected human populations do not always support these findings,[8] there is increasing experimental evidence, discussed below, to confirm that acute injuries involving the integrity of the axon, as opposed to predominantly demyelinating injuries, are key factors in the pathogenesis of neuropathic pain states.[9] Data from quantitative laboratory experiments also support the clinical finding that there is no correlation between pain and the ratio of large to small myelinated fibers surviving the injury, as might be predicted by the gate theory of pain,[10] although the electrophysiologic viability of some unmyelinated fibers[11] seems to be a necessary prerequisite to establishment of chronic neuropathic pain states.[12]

Recently developed animal models, such as the chronic constriction injury (CCI) model of Bennett and Xie,[5] are crucial for exploring the relationship between peripheral nerve injury and the development of chronic pain states because mechanisms producing complex behaviors such as pain cannot be extrapolated from noninvasive studies of humans nor studies of cell culture systems. CCI nerve injury is a well-established experimental model of peripheral neuropathy. Data from studies using this model suggest that the process of peripheral nerve degeneration following injury is responsible for secondary changes in the neuroaxis thought to drive chronic pain behaviors. CCI involves loose constriction of the sciatic nerve, which causes wallerian degeneration of affected fibers but leaves some fibers intact in the endoneurium.[13,14] Rats display abnormal behaviors, such as allodynia (innocuous mechanical stimuli perceived as noxious) and hyperalgesia (an exaggerated response to a noxious stimulus), which are suggestive of human neuropathic pain.[5,15] The chronology of peripheral nerve degeneration is strongly linked with the expression of hy-

peralgesia and allodynia behaviors,[9,13,14] and full regeneration of injury resolves abnormal behavior.[5,6,14] The link between degeneration and pain-like behaviors is further supported by studies of OLA/WLD mice. This mouse strain
demonstrates histologically delayed peripheral nerve degeneration,[16] which has
been correlated to the deferred expression of neuropathic behaviors following
CCI.[17]

Insight into the mechanistic links between nerve fiber degeneration and the
genesis of neuropathic pain has developed from recent studies of neuroimmunologic events: (1) In an important study, Yamamoto and Yaksh[18] applied
colchicine, which inhibited axonal transport but not electrical activity, proximal to CCI nerve injury and prevented the development of hyperalgesia. (2)
A preliminary study[19] further suggested that one such factor may be tumor
necrosis factor-alpha (TNF-α), a macrophage and Schwann cell-derived cytokine. In this study, inhibition of the production of TNF with thalidomide
resulted in attenuated hyperalgesia in CCI rats. (3) Macrophages are essential
to the degeneration of injured neural processes, because recruited macrophages actively invade injured tissue and phagocytose damaged cellular components.[20] Furthermore, peak percentages of these phagocytic cells precede the
development of allodynia in a time frame consistent with retrograde axonal
transport. (4) In a study by Watkins and associates,[21] cytokines produced by
macrophages have been shown to affect the behavior of normal, uninjured rats.
The authors showed that immunologic peptides, such as interleukin-1β, can
mediate thermal hyperalgesia in rats. Watkins and associates[21] propose that
immunologic peptides, which are produced during fever, may account for the
hyperalgesia that frequently is observed during illness. It is well-known that
reactive substances produced during injury and inflammation are nociceptive.
For example, tachykinins produced following injury have been shown experimentally to result in pain-like behavior.[22-24] Therefore, the production of immunologic peptides appears to link peripheral nerve degeneration following
injury to the expression of neuropathic behaviors.

Thus, it is suggested that the pathogenesis of hyperalgesia in neuropathic pain
syndromes depends on wallerian-like degeneration of nerve fibers in an environment of activated macrophages and glial cells, which together affect the integrity and function of sensory axons. This hypothesis provides a pathologic basis to compare the potential for pain syndromes arising from different classes
of nerve injury, including the major etiologies of ischemia, compression, and
toxic insults to the nerve roots. This hypothesis is discussed in more detail at
the end of the chapter, after a review of the vascular anatomy of nerves and the
pathology of compressive, ischemic, and toxic nerve injuries.

Vascular Anatomy of Nerves and Nerve Roots

The vascular anatomy of nerves[25] and nerve roots[26] has been described in
detail (Fig. 1). Each has a dual circulation comprising radicular, extrinsic vessels running longitudinally outside the nerve bundles and an intrinsic plexus of
primarily capillary-sized vessels within the endoneurium. The extrinsic circulation consists of adrenergically innervated arterioles[27,28] and small arteries and
veins. The intrinsic circulation lacks this sympathetic control and effective metabolic control of vascular diameter such that endoneurial blood flow is not ef-

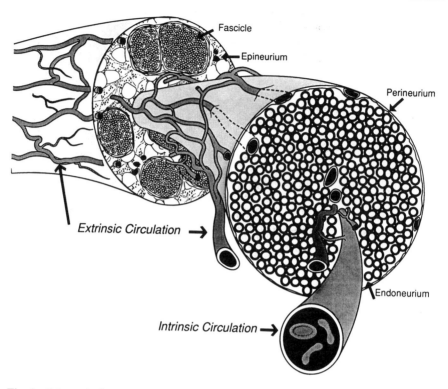

Fig. 1 *Schematic drawing of circulation. Nerve bundles contain a dual circulation consisting of adrenergically innervated extrinsic vessels in the epineurial space and an intrinsic circulation in the endoneurium, which lacks innervation and consists primarily of capillary-sized vessels. Endoneurial blood flow is not autoregulated. These two circulations are connected by anastomic transperineurial vessels that are subject to compression by increased endoneurial fluid pressure. (Reproduced with permission from Myers RR, Heckman HM, Galbraith JA, et al: Subperineurial demyelination associated with reduced nerve blood flow and oxygen tension after epineurial vascular stripping.* Lab Invest *1991;65:41–50.)*

fectively autoregulated. However, because there is anastomotic communication between the extrinsic and intrinsic circulation through transperineurial vessels, epinephrine and other vasoactive drugs coming into contact with extrinsic vessels can reduce endoneurial blood flow.[29]

In peripheral nerves, removal of the extrinsic circulation by stripping away a 2-cm length of the epineurium reduces nerve blood flow by 50% and subperineurial oxygen tension by 38%.[30] Although nerves have a metabolic reserve that allows for periods of reduced blood flow, a 50% reduction in blood flow for extended periods is a critical level associated with injury to nerve fibers. The extrinsic vasculature is less dense in nerve roots than in peripheral nerves (Fig. 2). This difference may exist because the cerebrospinal fluid provides spinal nerve roots with a nutritional pathway,[31] which reduces the importance of the extrinsic circulation in this tissue. Another independent indication that transperineurial permeability may be an important mechanism of nutrition

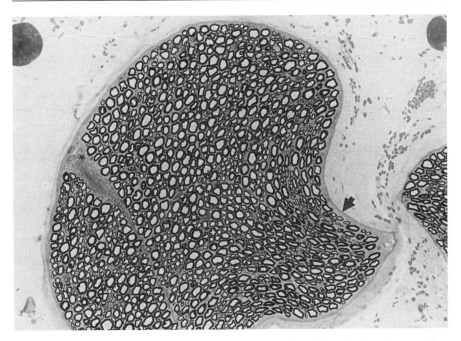

Fig. 2 *Normal pig cauda equina. The extrinsic epineurial circulation is less dense and less closely associated with fascicles in nerve roots than in peripheral nerves. Note the relatively thin perineurial sheath (arrow) that may permit diffusion of materials from cerebrospinal fluid into the endoneurium and densely packed myelinated fibers in the endoneurial space. The collapsed vessel in the endoneurium is an occasional normal finding without pathologic significance.*

and macromolecular transport in nerve roots is the finding that the nerve root sheath is permeable to protein tracers injected into the intrathecal space.[32] In the nerve, the tight junctions between perineurial cells excludes protein transport and represents an important structural component of the blood–nerve barrier. The other component of the blood–nerve barrier is the tight junctions between endothelial cells; both nerve roots and peripheral nerves have tight endothelial junctions that exclude extravasation of macromolecules, but vessels in the dorsal root ganglia (DRG) are leaky to macromolecules. Protein osmolytes regulating endoneurial hydration arise from the focal deficit in the blood–nerve barrier at the level of the DRG.

Ischemic Nerve Root Injury

Ischemic nerve injury is a ubiquitous insult that can produce a wide range of neuropathologic consequences, depending on the magnitude and duration of the ischemic event.[30,33] Ischemic injury to nerves produces predominantly demyelinating injuries, although prolonged ischemia can also interfere with axonal transport mechanisms,[34] causing axonal injury and wallerian-like degeneration of the nerve fiber (Fig. 3). The cause of ischemic nerve root injury is often compression of the extrinsic circulation.

Vascular damage and fibrosis are common within the vertebral canal and intervertebral foramen, and this vascular damage is significantly related to the severity of degenerative disk disease.[35] Disk protrusion may lead to compression of epidural veins with dilation of noncompressed veins. Jayson[35] notes a significant statistical relationship between evidence for venous obstruction, perineural fibrosis, and neural atrophy. Fibrosis may further impede nutrient transfer to endoneurial fibers and predispose to nerve stretch injuries.

In an experimental study by Olmarker and associates[36] on the effects of experimental graded compression on blood flow in the porcine cauda equina, intravital microscopy showed a direct relationship between arterial pressure and the pressures required to stop flow in arterioles. Balloon compression pressures of approximately 50 mm Hg stopped flow in capillaries, whereas pressures of less than 50 mm Hg interrupted flow in venules. Based on comparisons with results of a previous study of peripheral nerves,[37] the authors noted that the pressures required to stop the flow in the venules and capillaries are lower in nerve roots than in peripheral nerves. In another study, Lind and associates[38] showed that hypertension significantly decreased the susceptibility of the spinal nerve roots to compression at and below 100 mm Hg compressive force.

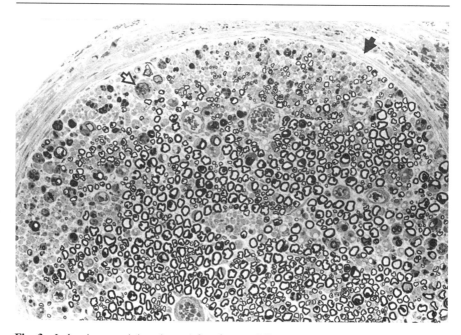

Fig. 3 *Ischemic nerve injury in peripheral nerve following removal of a short segment of extrinsic circulation. Note the perineurium is thicker in this tissue than in nerve roots (arrow), phagocytic cells (open arrow), and demyelinated axon (star).*

Pathology of Nerve Compression and Ischemic Injuries

Nerve compression injuries are associated with several distinct pathologic findings, some of which are thought to be secondary to ischemic injury and activation of fibroblasts and other endoneurial support cells and others to direct mechanical injury. It is not entirely clear which mechanisms are dominant in different forms of compression injury, ie, low-grade chronic compression or large amplitude acute compression. Each can result in neuropathic pain syndromes.

Compression of peripheral nerves can injure the tissue in two ways. Large pressure forces in which there is a sharp gradient between the focal insult and adjacent tissue can cause longitudinal displacement of the compressed tissue that mechanically disrupts its continuity.[39] This problem of tissue stretching has been explored in detail because it is relevant in experimental studies in which fixed-length compression chambers are inflated around nerves.[39] The second way in which compression may cause nerve injury is through ischemia secondary to occlusion of vessels in the extrinsic circulation. This mechanism alone can account for all of the pathologic findings associated with compression neuropathies.[40] Nerve fibers adjacent to the perineurium and in the immediate subperineurial space depend on oxygen from the extrinsic circulation to support metabolic activity, whereas nerve fibers located deeper in the fascicle depend on the circulation provided by the intrinsic vasculature. Reduction of blood flow by physical or functional removal of the extrinsic circulation causes subperineur-

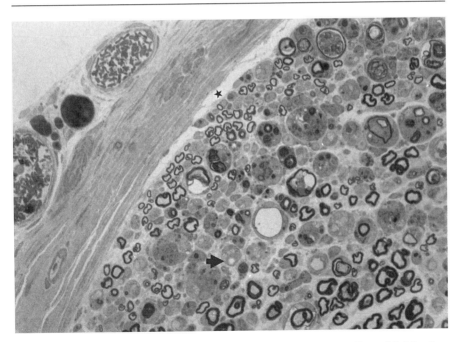

Fig. 4 *Nerve injury caused by circumferential cuff inflated to 30 mm Hg and left in place for 2 hours. Edema, which is especially evident in subperineurial space (star), and demyelination (arrow) dominate the pathology. Hypertrophied Schwann cell cytoplasm and phagocytosis are primary findings in this rat sciatic nerve harvested 7 days after injury.*

ial cellular injury.[30,40] Figure 4 shows significant injury to subperineurial fibers in the rat sciatic nerve following 2 hours of experimental compression at 30 mm Hg. Similar results are seen with epineurial devascularization.[30] Note the sparing of nerve fibers toward the center of the fascicle, which is perfused primarily by the vessels of the intrinsic circulation. Central fascicular fibers are selectively injured by ischemia secondary to microthrombi or other particulate matter, such as experimental microspheres, that occludes the capillaries of the intrinsic circulation.[41]

Demyelination dominates the pathology of these low-grade compressive lesions. It has been shown by electron microscopy (Fig. 5) that the demyelination is associated with Schwann cell necrosis. Thus, the primary mechanism of demyelination in this neuropathy is Schwann cell destruction, with subsequent disintegration of the myelin sheath. This finding may also explain paranodal demyelination, the earliest change in the myelin sheath after Schwann cell injury.[40] The relationship between Schwann cell injury and external compression was first noted by Dyck,[42] who reported that repeated external compression induced Schwann cell proliferation with characteristic "onion bulb" formations of concentric Schwann cell basal lamina.

Compression forces of larger amplitude and/or longer duration may injure the axon. In this instance, the process of wallerian-like degeneration dominates the pathologic findings and is more likely to lead to states of neuropathic pain (Fig. 6).

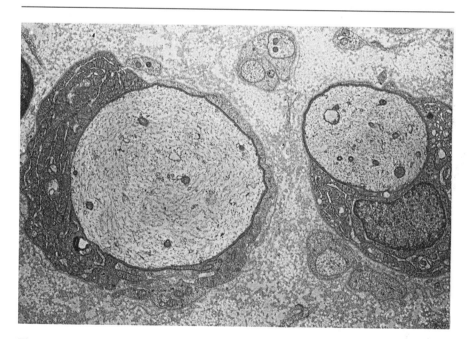

Fig. 5 *Demyelination caused by focal nerve compression at a pressure of 30 mm Hg for 2 hours. Note the normal-appearing axons. Schwann cell necrosis is responsible for loss of myelin. Normal C fibers are encased in Schwann cell cytoplasm at the top center of the electron micrograph.*

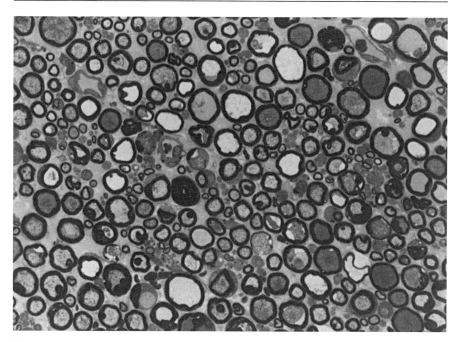

Fig. 6 *Severe axonal injury 24 hours after nerve was compressed at 80 mm Hg for 6 hours. Initial changes appear as dark-staining axoplasm that is retracted from myelin. Wallerian degeneration is the pathologic process that follows and includes further disintegration of the axon, Schwann cells, and myelin sheaths. This process affects the nerve fiber from the site of injury distally to its termination. Axonal regeneration will occur but depends on macrophage phagocytosis of degenerative debris and other factors.*

In a recent study of dog nerve root compression by Yoshizawa and associates[43] in which a Silastic band was placed around an L7 root, there was selective injury to nerve fibers in the periphery of the fascicle. Injury was delayed several months, presumably as inflammation and fibrosis further increased the compressive forces and interfered with the nutritive supply of the nerve fibers subjacent to the Silastic band. Dural fibrosis and arachnoid thickening were early findings. Schwann cell injury, demyelination, and eventually, wallerian degeneration with prominent macrophage activity were observed throughout the fascicles. The preponderance of small myelinated fibers in the subperineurial space at 1 year after placement of the Silastic band is an indication of nerve fiber regeneration following wallerian degeneration. Although behavioral tests of sensory function were not performed, this may prove to be an excellent model of human lumbar spinal stenosis causing pain.[44]

Renaut bodies are often reported to be associated with chronic compression injuries,[43,45] yet their pathogenesis and significance are controversial because they occasionally are seen in normal human nerves. Renaut bodies are whorls of fibroblasts that are filled with loosely textured amorphous and fibrillar material as well as collagen. They always lie in a subperineurial disposition attached to the perineurium. Although they occur with increased frequency in

255

nerves naturally subject to compression, they are also observed in other neuropathies.[46] It is reasonable to assume that they have pathologic significance as reactive fibroblasts. Renaut bodies occupy significant space and may increase endoneurial fluid pressure. Adjacent nerve fibers appear to be normal, however, and Renaut himself thought that the bodies were structures that cushioned the nerve against compression injury. Renaut bodies observed in nerve roots of the normal pig cauda equina (Fig. 7) suggest that this species should be included, along with horses and donkeys, as a species in which Renaut bodies are more prominent than in humans.

Pathology of Toxic Nerve Injury: Phospholipase A$_2$

Neurotoxicology is a broad discipline that relies heavily on neuropathology as a means to identify the mechanisms of nerve injury.[47] Although the nucleus pulposus and several potential chemical and neurotoxic agents liberated from degenerating disks have been proposed to play a role in the pathogenesis of nerve root injury and pain,[48-50] only the effects of nucleus pulposus and phospholipase A$_2$ (PLA$_2$) have been studied histologically.[51] Olmarker and associates[51] have shown that autologous nucleus pulposus applied to porcine cauda equina nerve roots causes nerve injury. Pathologic changes included swelling of the

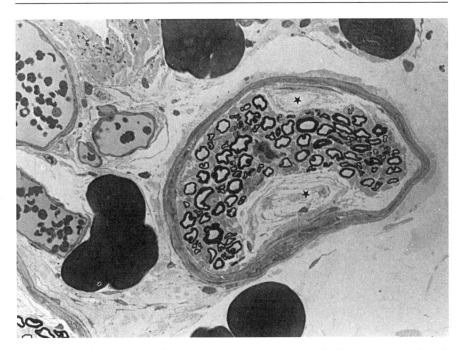

Fig. 7   *Renaut bodies in normal pig cauda equina (star) composed of loosely organized swirls of fibroblasts, collagen, and other material. Nerve fibers are normal. Large dark-staining structures in the epineurium are fat cells. Note the large diameter veins at left and the adjacent nerve root at lower left.*

Schwann cell cytoplasm and axonal vacuolization in association with electro-physiologic deficits.

The key toxic component in degenerating spines may be PLA$_2$, although other irritating substances have been found in disk tissue.[52] In collaboration with Drs. Franson, Saal, Garfin, and Sommer, my coworkers and I have tested the neurotoxic potential of human PLA$_2$ on rat peripheral nerve bundles. Injection of 15 μl of PLA$_2$ into rat sciatic nerve produced primarily demyelination, although axonal injury was also observed (Fig. 8). Twenty-four hours after injection there

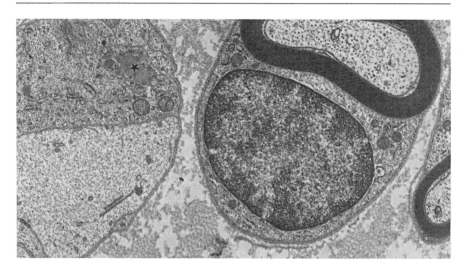

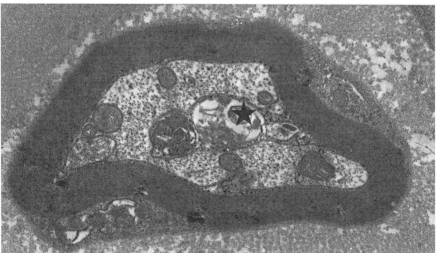

Fig. 8   **Top,** *Electron micrograph showing demyelination caused by phospholipase A$_2$ (PLA$_2$) on the left and a normal axon and Schwann cell on the right. Lipid droplets (star) are seen in the Schwann cell cytoplasm of the demyelinated axon; axoplasm appears normal.* **Bottom,** *Axonal injury caused by PLA$_2$ 24 hours after injection into rat peripheral nerve. Large vesicular inclusion (star). Lipid droplets are seen in other axons. Schwann cell injury is also apparent at the lower left of this electron micrograph.*

were numerous lipid droplets in Schwann cells, macrophages, and in the endothelium of blood vessels in both the epineurium and endoneurium. Lipid droplets are a nonspecific neurotoxic finding associated with myelin degeneration. Vesicular disintegration of the myelin was observed and started at the Schmidt-Lanterman incisures and at the paranodal region. Large filamentous axonal inclusions were also seen but are of unknown significance. Tissue studied 7 days postinjury showed numerous macrophages containing myelin debris and an increase in the number of endoneurial macrophages. This pattern of activated macrophage phagocytic activity is the expected result of the apparent direct, initial PLA_2-induced injury to myelin and may be associated with pain if significant axonal degeneration is present or developing. Early signs of remyelination could be seen at 7 days. Dr. DeLeo presents a more extensive review of the role of PLA_2 in low back pain elsewhere in this book.

Role of Edema in Nerve Injury

Edema is an early pathologic finding in many nerve injuries and is an important component of wallerian degeneration. Edema is a common cause of increases in endoneurial fluid pressure (EFP).[53] Interference with the patency of the blood–nerve barrier can lead to edema, but edema may also be generated by alterations in endoneurial osmotic forces in the presence of an intact blood–nerve barrier.[54] Because the endoneurium lacks lymphatic channels, osmolytes are transported along with endoneurial fluid to the distal terminals of the nerve bundle where the perineurium terminates and endoneurial fluid communicates with systemic interstitial fluid. This transport is driven by a proximodistal gradient in endoneurial fluid pressure.[55]

Edema is initially seen in subperineurial and perivascular spaces in which the endoneurial matrix is less rigid, and it may eventually be manifest diffusely throughout the fascicle separating individual nerve fibers. Mild cases of edema, such as might be caused by mild ischemia or topical application of local anesthetic solutions on nerve, resolve without associated neurologic sequela. Severe edema, however, can interfere with nerve blood flow by compressing transperineurial vessels, and this compression may cause a vicious cycle of inflammation and ischemia.[56]

Compression of the dorsal root ganglion produces an increase in EFP and pain.[57] This "closed compartment syndrome in nerve roots" may be painful because the innervated perineurium is stretched or because of the direct mechanical pressure exerted by EFP on DRG neurons. Vasogenic edema induced by compression injury to spinal nerve roots is reflected as high intensity on gadolinium-enhanced MRI. Yoshizawa and associates[43] conclude from their study of chronic nerve root compression that intraradicular edema caused by alteration of the blood–nerve barrier is the most important factor in the nerve root dysfunction due to chronic compression. The pathologic mechanism of nerve injury is likely ischemia secondary to increased endoneurial fluid pressure.

Role of Inflammation in the Pathogenesis of Neuropathic Pain

As has been discussed, inflammation, as manifested by edema, increased endoneurial fluid pressure, ischemia, nerve injury, immune cell invasion, and macrophage activation, appears to play a critical role in the pathogenesis of neuropathic pain. Extensive use of the Bennett and Xie model[5] of CCI to rat peripheral nerves has aided investigations of these factors. In this model, several chromic gut ligatures are placed loosely around the rat sciatic nerve and left in place during subsequent periods of behavioral testing (Fig. 9). The animals are allodynic, protect the injured limb, and are hyperalgesic to thermal stimuli by the third postoperative day. Allodynia presents early in the course of the neuropathy and is persistent, whereas thermal hyperalgesia peaks during postoperative days 5 to 9 and slowly resolves during the following month.

The CCI technique is sensitive and reproducible within a single laboratory. Variations between laboratories in the extent of the nerve injury and the corresponding behavioral hyperalgesia are most likely related to the tightness of the ligatures and possibly to the ligature material and its preparation. Proper placement of the ligatures corresponds to constriction of the epineurial circulation and an initial reduction in nerve blood flow of 50%.[9] My coworkers and I have used silk and chromic sutures in separate groups of animals and obtained identical behavioral results, suggesting that the ligature material is not the important variable. Sutures that have an added chemotactic inflammatory potential[58] would be expected to potentiate the nerve injury and cause more pain.

The pathology of CCI is striking. Within 7 days, nearly all myelinated nerve fibers are degenerating (Fig. 10, *top*). The process begins with substantial increases in endoneurial edema and ischemic injury causing mixed pathologies of demyelination and axonal degeneration that is best appreciated at the electron mi-

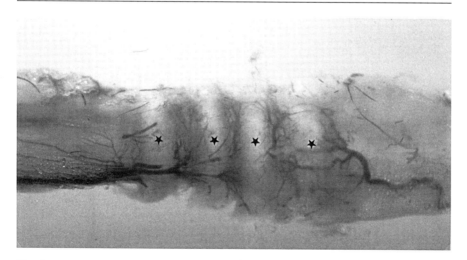

Fig. 9 *Appearance of rat sciatic nerve following removal of four chromic constriction injury ligatures left in place for 7 days. Note the extensive swelling of tissue between ligature sites (stars) and engorging of vessels. This is an important model of an ischemic inflammatory mononeuropathy that is widely used in studies of neuropathic pain.*

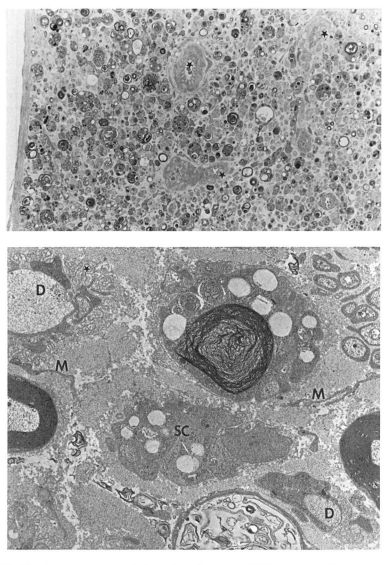

Fig. 10   Top, *Rat sciatic nerve 7 days after placement of CCI ligatures. Perineurium is at left. Note the endothelial hypertrophy and immune cells adherent to the lumen (stars). Essentially all myelinated fibers are degenerating, and there is active phagocytosis of myelin and axonal debris throughout the endoneurium.* **Bottom,** *Electron micrograph of chronic compression injury 7 days after placement of the ligatures. Demyelinated axons (D) are seen in a field with severe Schwann cell injury (SC) and ruffled basal lamina (star), a finding consistent with Schwann cell injury. Schwann cells contain lipid debris. Myelin disintegration is actively proceeding in the large fiber at the top of the micrograph. Note macrophage processes (M) probing the tissue.*

croscopic level (Fig. 10, *bottom*). Axonal injury is associated with invasion of activated hematogeneous macrophages beginning approximately 3 days after placement of the loose ligatures and with wallerian degeneration of the distal nerve fibers. There is immediate activation of endothelial cells with hypertrophy and expression of cytokines such as TNF. Fibroblasts are also activated and are seen in increasing numbers in both perivascular and subperineurial regions. The phagocytic function of macrophages cleans the tissue of debris and prepares it for regeneration. Axonal sprouts are noted distally by 7 days postinjury and regeneration occurs in association with resolution of hyperalgesia. By 23 days postinjury, numerous regenerated fibers are visible by light microscopy as small, thinly myelinated fibers in a field in which there are still observable pathologic changes in endothelial cells and in nerve fibers (Fig. 11).

Using the CCI model and several other nerve injury models, my coworkers and I have concluded that the degree of axonal injury and the subsequent process of wallerian degeneration are the key factors in the pathogenesis of hyperalgesia. We believe that cytokine events associated with activated macrophages and glia participate in the pathogenesis of hyperalgesia following nerve injury by being retrogradely transported to the cell body where they may signal functional changes in afferent processing. Thalidomide-induced inhibition of TNF-α production by macrophages reduces the magnitude and duration of hyperalgesia[19] and it may be this cytokine or a secondary effect of cytokines, such

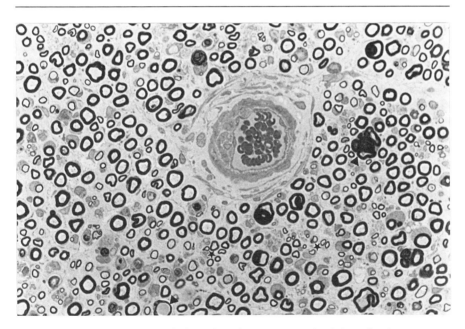

Fig. 11   *Rat peripheral nerve 23 days after chronic constriction injury showing regeneration characterized by small, thinly myelinated nerve fibers (star). Endothelial cells are still abnormal with fibroblasts in the immediate perivascular space. Occasional myelin and axonal abnormalities are also evident (arrowheads).*

as expression of growth factors, that signals neuronal changes leading to hyperalgesia.

A recent therapeutic study that inhibited inflammation (and macrophage production of TNF) with methylprednisolone following nucleus pulposus-induced nerve root injury[59] showed an acute electrophysiologic benefit of the therapy. Continued studies focused on the role of inflammatory factors in the pathogenesis of low back pain may lead to improved understanding and treatment of this debilitating condition.

References

1. Olmarker K, Holm S, Rosenqvist AL, et al: Experimental nerve root compression: A model of acute, graded compression of the porcine cauda equina and an analysis of neural and vascular anatomy. *Spine* 1991;16:61–69.
2. Garfin SR, Cohen MS, Massie JB, et al: Nerve-roots of the cauda equina: The effect of hypotension and acute graded compression on function. *J Bone Joint Surg* 1990;72A:1185–1192.
3. Rydevik BL, Pedowitz RA, Hargens AR, et al: Effects of acute, graded compression on spinal nerve root function and structure: An experimental study of the pig cauda equina. *Spine* 1991;16:487–493.
4. Pedowitz RA, Garfin SR, Massie JB, et al: Effects of magnitude and duration of compression on spinal nerve root conduction. *Spine* 1992;17:194–199.
5. Bennett GJ, Xie YK: A peripheral mononeuropathy in rat that produces disorders of pain sensation like those seen in man. *Pain* 1988;33:87–107.
6. Kim SH, Chung JM: An experimental model for peripheral neuropathy produced by segmental spinal nerve ligation in the rat. *Pain* 1992;50:355–363.
7. Dyck PJ, Lambert EH, O'Brien PC: Pain in peripheral neuropathy related to rate and kind of fiber degeneration. *Neurology* 1976;26:466–471.
8. Llewelyn JG, Gilbey SG, Thomas PK, et al: Sural nerve morphometry in diabetic autonomic and painful sensory neuropathy: A clinicopathological study. *Brain* 1991;114:867–892.
9. Myers RR, Yamamoto TY, Yaksh TL, et al: The role of focal nerve ischemia and Wallerian degeneration in peripheral nerve injury producing hyperesthesia. *Anesthesiology* 1993;78:308–316.
10. Melzack R, Wall PD: Pain mechanisms: A new theory. *Science* 1965;150:971–979.
11. Xie YK, Xiao WH: Electrophysiological evidence for hyperalgesia in the peripheral neuropathy. *Sci China (B)* 1990;33:663–672.
12. Sommer C, Lalonde A, Heckman HM, et al: Quantitative neuropathology of a focal nerve injury causing hyperalgesia. *J Neuropathol Exp Neurol* 1995;54:635–643.
13. Coggeshall RE, Dougherty PM, Pover CM, et al: Is large myelinated fiber loss associated with hyperalgesia in a model of experimental peripheral neuropathy in the rat? *Pain* 1993;52:233–242.
14. Sommer C, Galbraith JA, Heckman HM, et al: Pathology of experimental compression neuropathy producing hyperesthesia. *J Neuropath Exp Neurol* 1993;52:223–233.
15. Attal N, Jazat F, Kayser V, et al: Further evidence for "pain-related" behaviours in a model of unilateral peripheral mononeuropathy. *Pain* 1990;41:235–251.
16. Ludwin SK, Bisby MA: Delayed wallerian degeneration in the central nervous system of Ola mice: An ultrastructural study. *J Neurol Sci* 1992;109:140–147.
17. Myers RR, Sommer C, Powell HC: Abstract: The role of Wallerian degeneration in the pathogenesis of neuropathic pain: Studies with OLA mice. *J Neuropathol Exp Neurol* 1993;52:310.
18. Yamamoto T, Yaksh TL: Effects of colchicine applied to the peripheral nerve on the thermal hyperalgesia evoked with chronic nerve constriction. *Pain* 1993;55:227–233.
19. Sommer C, Myers RR: Thalidomide inhibition of TNF reduces hyperalgesia in neuropathic rats. *Regional Anesthesia* 1994;19(2 suppl):1.

20. Monaco S, Gehrmann J, Raivich G, et al: MHC-positive, ramified macrophages in the normal and injured rat peripheral nervous system. *J Neurocytol* 1992;21:623–634.

21. Watkins LR, Wiertelak EP, Goehler LE, et al: Characterization of cytokine-induced hyperalgesia. *Brain Res* 1994;654:15–26.

22. Ferreira SH: Prostaglandins, aspirin-like drugs and analgesia. *Nature New Biology* 1972;240:200–203.

23. Holzer P: Local effector functions of capsaicin-sensitive sensory nerve endings: Involvement of tachykinins, calcitonin gene-related peptide and other neuropeptides. *Neuroscience* 1988;24:739–768.

24. Nakamura-Craig M, Smith TW: Substance P and peripheral inflammatory hyperalgesia. *Pain* 1989;38:91–98.

25. Bell MA, Weddell AG: A descriptive study of the blood vessels of the sciatic nerve in the rat, man and other mammals. *Brain* 1984;107:871–898.

26. Petterson CA, Olsson Y: Blood supply of spinal nerve roots: An experimental study in the rat. *Acta Neuropathol* 1989;78:455–461.

27. Lundborg G: Ischemic nerve injury: Experimental studies on intraneural microvascular pathophysiology and nerve function in a limb subjected to temporary circulatory arrest. *Scand J Plast Reconstr Surg* 1970;6(suppl):3–113.

28. Hara H, Kobayashi S: Adrenergic innervation of the vasa nervorum in the cranial nerves and spinal roots in the subarachnoid space. *Exp Neurol* 1987;98:673–676.

29. Myers RR, Heckman HM: Effects of local anesthesia on nerve blood flow: Studies using lidocaine with and without epinephrine. *Anesthesiology* 1989;71:757–762.

30. Myers RR, Heckman HM, Galbraith JA, et al: Subperineurial demyelination associated with reduced nerve blood flow and oxygen tension after epineurial vascular stripping. *Lab Invest* 1991;65:41–50.

31. Rydevik B, Holm S, Brown MD, et al: Diffusion from the cerebrospinal fluid as a nutritional pathway for spinal nerve roots. *Acta Physiol Scand* 1990;138:247–248.

32. Kobayashi S, Yoshizawa H, Hachiya Y, et al: Vasogenic edema induced by compression injury to the spinal nerve root: Distribution of intravenously injected protein tracers and gadolinium-enhanced magnetic resonance imaging. *Spine* 1993;18:1410–1424.

33. Nukada H, Powell HC, Myers RR: Spatial distribution of nerve injury after occlusion of individual major vessels in rat sciatic nerves. *J Neuropathol Exp Neurol* 1993;52:452–459.

34. Ochs S, Brimijoin WS: Axonal transport, in Dyck PJ, Thomas, PK, Griffin JW, et al (eds): *Peripheral Neuropathy,* ed 3. Philadelphia, PA, WB Saunders, 1993, vol 1, pp 331–360.

35. Jayson MI: The role of vascular damage and fibrosis in the pathogenesis of nerve root damage. *Clin Orthop* 1992;279:40–48.

36. Olmarker K, Rydevik B, Holm S, et al: Effects of experimental graded compression on blood flow in spinal nerve roots: A vital microscopic study on the porcine cauda equina. *J Orthop Res* 1989;7:817–823.

37. Rydevik B, Lundborg G, Bagge U: Effects of graded compression on intraneural blood flow: An in vivo study on rabbit tibial nerve. *J Hand Surg* 1981;6A:3–12.

38. Lind B, Massie JB, Lincoln T, et al: The effects of induced hypertension and acute graded compression on impulse propagation in the spinal nerve roots of the pig. *Spine* 1993;18:1550–1555.

39. Rydevik B, Lundborg G, Skalak R: Biomechanics of peripheral nerves, in Nordin M, Frankel VH (eds): *Basic Biomechanics of the Musculoskeletal System.* Philadelphia, PA, Lea & Febiger, 1989, pp 75–87.

40. Powell HC, Myers RR: Pathology of experimental nerve compression. *Lab Invest* 1986;55:91–100.

41. Nukada H, Dyck PJ: Microsphere embolization of nerve capillaries and fiber degeneration. *Am J Pathol* 1984;115:275–287.

42. Dyck PJ: Experimental hypertrophic neuropathy: Pathogenesis of onion-bulb formations produced by repeated tourniquet applications. *Arch Neurol* 1969;21:73–95.

263

43. Yoshizawa H, Kobayashi S, Morita T: Chronic nerve root compression: Pathophysiologic mechanism of nerve root dysfunction. *Spine* 1995;20:397–407.
44. Ciricillo SF, Weinstein PR: Lumbar spinal stenosis. *West J Med* 1993;158:171–177.
45. Asbury AK, Johnson PC (eds): *Pathology of Peripheral Nerve.* Philadelphia, PA, WB Saunders, 1978, pp 2–42.
46. Asbury AK: Renaut bodies: A forgotten endoneurial structure. *J Neuropathol Exp Neurol* 1973;32:334–343.
47. Spencer PS, Bischoff MC, Schaumburg HH: Neuropathological methods for the detection of neurotoxic disease, in Spencer PS, Schaumburg HH (eds): *Experimental and Clinical Neurotoxicology.* Baltimore, MD, Williams & Wilkins, 1980, pp 743–757.
48. Pennington JB, McCarron RF, Laros GS: Identification of IgG in the canine intervertebral disk. *Spine* 1988;13:909–912.
49. Saal JS, Franson RC, Dobrow R, et al: High levels of inflammatory phospholipase A2 activity in lumbar disk herniations. *Spine* 1990;15:674–678.
50. Marshall LL, Trethewie ER, Curtain CC: Chemical radiculitis: A clinical, physiological and immunological study. *Clin Orthop* 1977;129:61–67.
51. Olmarker K, Rydevik B, Nordborg C: Autologous nucleus pulposus induces neurophysiologic and histologic changes in porcine cauda equina nerve roots. *Spine* 1993;18:1425–1432.
52. Liu J, Roughley PJ, Mort JS: Identification of human intervertebral disk stromelysin and its involvement in matrix degradation. *J Orthop Res* 1991;9:568–575.
53. Myers RR, Powell HC: Endoneurial fluid pressure in peripheral neuropathies, in Hargens AR (ed): *Tissue Fluid Pressure and Composition.* Baltimore, MD, Williams & Wilkins, 1981, pp 193–207.
54. Mizisin AP, Kalichman MW, Myers RR, et al: Role of the blood-nerve barrier in experimental nerve edema. *Toxicol Pathol* 1990;18:170–185.
55. Myers RR, Rydevik BL, Heckman HM, et al: Proximodistal gradient in endoneurial fluid pressure. *Exp Neurol* 1988;102:368–370.
56. Myers RR, Murakami H, Powell HC: Reduced nerve blood flow in edematous neuropathies: A biomechanical mechanism. *Microvasc Res* 1986;32:145–151.
57. Rydevik BL, Myers RR, Powell HC: Pressure increase in the dorsal root ganglion following mechanical compression: Closed compartment syndrome in nerve roots. *Spine* 1989;14:574–576.
58. Kawakami M, Weinstein JN, Spratt KF, et al: Experimental lumbar radiculopathy: Immunohistochemical and quantitative demonstrations of pain induced by lumbar nerve root irritation of the rat. *Spine* 1994;19:1780–1794.
59. Olmarker K, Byrod G, Cornefjord M, et al: Effects of methylprednisolone on nucleus pulposus-induced nerve root injury. *Spine* 1994;19:1803–1808.

Chapter 17

Associated Neurogenic and Nonneurogenic Pain Mediators That Probably Are Activated and Responsible for Nociceptive Input

Mamoru Kawakami, MD, PhD
James N. Weinstein, DO, MS

Introduction

To treat a patient with low back and/or leg pain, it is very important to understand where the pain comes from. Information about the pain mechanism is needed to clarify the pathomechanism of low back pain and radicular pain secondary to lumbar disorders. The purpose of this chapter is to review the associated neurogenic and nonneurogenic pain mediators that are thought to be activated by and, in part, responsible for nociceptive input.

According to clinical imaging studies[1-3] and an experimental model,[4] mechanical compression is not always the sole cause of radicular pain. Pain originating in the lumbar spine typically arises from mechanical and/or chemical irritation of primary sensory neurons. There are many sensory nerve fibers in the anulus fibrosus, spinal ligament, and facet joint capsule in the lumbar spine,[5-8] and nociceptors are the peripheral terminal endings of the sensory neurons that are selectively responsive to potentially or overtly harmful injuries in the lumbar spine. Lesions, such as a herniated nucleus pulposus, can result in stimulation or irritation of these sensory neurons and be clinically manifested as pain.

Nociceptive afferent neurons are sensitive to a variety of different kinds of noxious stimulus (thermal, mechanical, chemical) and contain and release a wide variety of neuropeptides. Many inflammatory mediators secondary to tissue injury cause excitation or enhance responsiveness of nociceptive afferent terminals, and the neuropeptides released from the terminals accentuate the inflammatory response. Cytokines and growth factors, such as nerve growth factor, may play an important role in the functional changes of nociceptive neurons associated with various chronic pain states.[9] In other types of chronic pain, sympathetic nerve terminals also play an important role. It has been reported that the pain threshold was increased and the number of these sympathetic nerve fibers was reduced by sympathectomy.[10] Thus, sympathetic nerves may be important for generation of low back pain.

Chemical Mediators of Pain

Nonneurogenic Pain Mediators

A variety of endogenous chemicals, which are released from nonneural tissues, have pain-producing capabilities; many agents influence chemical excitation and sensitization of sensory neurons. In this chapter, we will describe the influence of low pH, adenosine triphosphate (ATP), glutamate, bradykinin, 5-hydroxytryptamines (5-HT), histamine, arachidonic acid metabolites, nitric oxide (NO), and cytokines. The pH of the extracellular environment follows pathophysiologic conditions, such as hypoxia/anoxia, as well as inflammation. A low pH evokes prolonged activation of sensory neurons. Membrane depolarization is the most likely basis for the prolonged sensory neuron activation associated with low pH solutions.[11] Although our group[12] could not demonstrate a change in pH of the applied disk materials within the lumbar epidural space, allografted intervertebral disk materials did produce pain-related behavior such as hyperalgesia in the rat. However, a reduction in pH of the lumbar disk may be associated with low back pain or radiculopathy in humans[13] and a change in pH may result in thermal hyperalgesia like that produced by loose ligation of the sciatic nerve with chromic gut sutures.[14] These studies suggest that lowering of pH contributes, in part, to the perception of low back pain in humans and pain-related behavior, such as hyperalgesia, in animal models.

ATP released by tissue damage acts on the surrounding cells, including sensory neurons. ATP receptors are found on inflammatory cells, especially macrophages. Macrophage activation by ATP causes release of various cytokines and prostanoids that can act to sensitize sensory neurons.[9] Glutamate, one of the excitatory amino acids, depolarizes sensory neurons by directly opening ion transport channels.[15] Although local injection of glutamate produces inflammation and hyperalgesia,[16] the physiologic significance has not been established. Bradykinin is an important inflammatory mediator that is known to stimulate nociceptive nerve terminals and cause pain.[17] 5-HT is released from platelets and mast cells during tissue damage and can act in several ways on sensory neurons. Sensitization by 5-HT is known to lower the threshold of primary afferent nociceptors to other noxious stimuli.[18]

Histamine is released from mast cells and acts through sensory neurons to evoke the sensations of itch and pain. In general, it is thought that low concentrations of histamine induce itch, whereas higher concentrations cause pain.[19]

Inflamed tissues contain high concentrations of prostaglandins. A major effect of prostaglandins is to sensitize afferent neurons to noxious chemical agents, to heat, and to mechanical stimulation.[20] The nociceptive fibers in the nerve root may be sensitized by various proinflammatory mediators, in particular various prostanoids (for example, prostaglandins G_2, H_2, I_2, E_2, and thromboxane A_2) produced from the arachidonic acid that is released from cell membrane phospholipids by local phospholipase A_2 (PLA$_2$). Results of recent pharmacologic studies have suggested that PLA$_2$ produces mechanical hyperalgesia but not thermal hyperalgesia.[21] It has been suggested that PLA$_2$ activity may be extremely important in the presence of a clinical radiculopathy associated with a herniated nucleus pulposus.[22] Consistent with this, we did not find PLA$_2$ immunoreactivity in normal nucleus pulposus and anulus fibrosus, but did clearly observe increases 1 and 2 weeks after application of nucleus pulposus and anulus fibrosus tissues on the epidural space.[12] PLA_2 injected into the facet joint causes acute changes in nerve discharge in the rabbit model.[23] Collectively, these studies suggest that mechanical hyperalgesia observed in the rat with nucleus pulposus applied into the epidural space may be directly related to increase in PLA_2 immunoreactivity. It is possible that the intervertebral disk materials sensitize afferent nerve terminals through production of PLA_2. PLA_2 extracted from human lumbar disk has powerful inflammatory activity in vivo.[24] Although prostaglandins rarely activate cutaneous nociceptive afferents directly and do not evoke pain when injected intradermally into human skin, prostaglandin (PGE_1) and prostacyclin (PGI_2) have been shown to increase the activity of nociceptors in rat articular nerve.[9] Therefore, it is possible that prostanoids could contribute directly to the activation of afferent neurons in inflammatory conditions, such as arthritis or a herniated nucleus pulposus.

NO is an unstable molecule considered to be important in intercellular communication in peripheral tissue and in the nervous system,[24] including nociceptive pathways. NO is formed from L-arginine following the activation of nitric oxide synthase (NOS) by calcium and other cofactors.[25] NO then alters cellular processes through the activation of guanylate cyclase and the production of cyclic guanosine 3,5'-monophosphate (cGMP). Dorsal root ganglion (DRG) neurons are able to make NO. An increase in cGMP has been measured in DRG satellite cells following stimulation with an NO donor such as nitroprusside.[26] There is little evidence for direct activation of sensory neurons by NO,[27] but NO indirectly alters their excitability. Paradoxically, a number of NOS inhibitors prevent the peripheral antinociceptive action of acetylcholine and morphine.[28,29]

It has been reported that NO mediates the thermal hyperalgesia produced by loose ligation of the sciatic nerve with chromic gut sutures in the rat.[30] Our group[12] has examined the possible role of NO in the hyperalgesia produced by tissue allografts on the lumbar epidural space in the rat. Using NADPH diaphorase histochemistry and in situ hybridization, we detected NOS in some cells surrounding grafted disk tissue 1 and 2 weeks after application of the nucleus pulposus and anulus fibrosus on the lumbar epidural space. We[12] also found that application of the nucleus pulposus and anulus fibrosus on the lumbar epidural space caused a thermal hyperalgesia, but not a mechanical hyperalgesia in the tail in spite of the fact that various cells produce NO. NO production around the anulus fibrosus may also inhibit the mechanical hyperalgesia produced by PLA_2 in the nucleus pulposus and anulus fibrosus of the intervertebral disks. Therefore, thermal hyperalgesia produced by the intervertebral disk may, in part, be related to NO production. It has been suggested that herniated lumbar intervertebral disk specimens in culture can produce amounts of NO and that NO may also be involved in radicular pain found in lumbar disk herniation patients.[31]

Phagocytic and antigen-producing cells of the immune system are also known to release a variety of cytokines–interleukins (IL), interferons, and tumor necrosis factor (TNF). These molecules are important inflammatory agents and are able to influence the activity of sensory neurons. They probably act by indirect routes that involve products of other cell types.

IL-1β, IL-6, and IL-8 have all been reported to induce hyperalgesia in animals.[32-35] It is thought that IL-1β and IL-6, but not IL-8, evoke the release of prostaglandins from cells, such as mononuclear leukocytes and fibroblasts, and that the prostaglandins in turn act on sensory nerves.[32,34-36] TNF-α also induces hyperalgesia, which can be attenuated by antisera to IL-1, IL-6, and IL-8.[35] IL-1 has been shown to enhance PGE_2 production in rheumatoid synovial cells.[37,38] It is thought that PGE_2 depolarizes primary afferent neurons and produces pain.[39] Cytokines, such as IL, have been detected in lumbar herniated disk materials in humans.[31,40] Our group[12] has demonstrated that rats with allografted fat did not show any evidence of hyperalgesia, although IL-1 immunoreactivity was observed in applied fat tissues.[12] Thus, IL-1 does not appear to play a role in the pathomechanisms of hyperalgesia related to radicular pain. Further studies of the inflammatory reaction in the lumbar spinal lesion, such as herniated nucleus pulposus, are necessary in order to further elucidate the mechanisms of spinal pain.

Neurogenic Pain Mediators

A large number of primary afferent neurons with small and intermediate diameters produce neuropeptides, such as substance P and somatostatin.[41] Vasoactive intestinal peptide (VIP), cholecystokinin, neurotensin, calcitonin gene-related peptide (CGRP), substance P, somatostatin, dynorphin, enkephalin, angiotensin II, bombesin-gastric relating peptide, galanin, and basic fibroblast growth factor (bFGF)[9,42] have been found in anatomic studies of neuropeptides in DRG cells or small sensory neurons. Most immunoreactive substances, such as neuropeptides resembling substance P (approximately 80%), are produced within DRG cell bodies of primary afferent neurons. However, only 20% of these substances are transported along dorsal root afferent fibers to terminals located in lamina I and II in the dorsal part of the dorsal horn, whereas 80% are transported peripherally.[43] Substance P probably acts as a neuromodulator of pain signals at synapses in the region of the substantia gelatinosa where pain perception is first integrated in the spinal cord.[44-46] Somatostatin is released after thermal noxious stimulation and may also play a role in nociceptor transmission and inflammation. VIP increases in the DRG and areas of the dorsal horn of the spinal cord from which other neuropeptides are depleted following peripheral axotomy of the sciatic nerve.[47] It is a neuropeptide that plays a role in reorganization of the nervous system following injury and that has been shown to affect bone mineralization.[48] Peripheral terminals with CGRP-like immunoreactivity are found in tissues in which sensory stimulation is usually painful,[49] suggesting a role for this peptide in nociceptive processing. The functional role of most neuropeptides still remains unclear.

An animal model was used to gain a more basic understanding of the cause (vibration) and effect (back pain) relationship. The localized decrease in substance P and increased VIP seen following frequency vibration are compatible with results following peripheral injury.[50,51] Peptides released from the DRG, when exposed to whole body vibration, may have more than just pain-modulating effects. The degenerative changes manifested by low-frequency vibration may result directly or indirectly from DRG stimulation and the release of these neuropeptides.

In the canine model, diskography has been reported to elevate the DRG concentrations of substance P and VIP, and injection of local anesthesia into the disk has been reported to reduce substance P concentration to a greater degree than it affects VIP.[5] Therefore, pain response during diskography may in part be related to the chemical environment within the intervertebral disk and the sensitized state of its annular nociceptors.

An experimental mechanical stimulation of DRG and nerve roots increased amounts of substance P in DRG cell bodies and in the substantia gelatinosa of the spinal dorsal horn.[52] Thus, substance P may modulate nociception when lumbar nerve roots are stimulated mechanically. In an immunohistochemical study, substance P-containing nerve endings were decreased after chronic and continuous compression of the cauda equina, and somatostatin nerve terminals were reduced and aminergic fibers and serotonin immunoreactivities enhanced after acute and chronic mechanical compression of the cauda equina in the rat.[53] In addition, quantitative analysis revealed that the levels of norepinephrine and serotonin, which are concerned with the descending inhibitory pathways, remained elevated after mechanical compression of the cauda equina.[53] These findings suggest that these neuropeptides and amines have a complicated relationship to pain perception and modulation.

We[4] have demonstrated that loosely tying ligatures of the L4 to L6 spinal nerve roots proximal to the DRGs with chromic gut produced a time-dependent and reversible thermal hyperalgesia.[4] In this experiment, there were also increases in c-*fos* expression in the spinal cord; c-*fos* is one of the proto-oncogenes involved in long-term responses of spinal cord cells to noxious stimuli. In addition, substance P, CGRP, and VIP in the ipsilateral DRGs increased after surgery.[4] The correlation of changes in behavior with changes in c-*fos* expression and neuropeptide content suggests a role for c-*fos*, but not the neuropeptides, in the maintenance of thermal hyperalgesia. Thermal hyperalgesia also occurred in rats with only exposure of the DRG and in rats with loose ligation of the DRG, and was accompanied by an increase in c-*fos* expression and in substance P in the ipsilateral DRG.[54] These experimental models reliably produced a disorder resembling sciatica and should help the understanding of pathomechanisms of radicular pain after irritation of the nerve root and DRG.

The neurogenic and nonneurogenic mediators play a fundamental role in the perception and modulation of pain.[55] The interrelationships between the neurogenic and nonneurogenic mediators in the injury and repair process are important when considering the degenerative spiral of osteoarthritis.[56] Tissue injury activates nerve endings, which send messages and cause release of neurogenic mediators, such as substance P, CGRP, and so forth. These medical mediators act centrally within the spinal cord and peripherally in conjunction with inflammatory cells, such as polymorphonuclear leukocytes and mast cells, to further the inflammatory process (Fig. 1). Thus, the two systems work synergistically in the injury and repair process.

The chemical, inflammatory, and immunologic alterations have been linked directly to proteolytic and collagenolytic enzymes known to cause cartilage matrix degradation and osteoarthritis. In the injury and repair cascade, the matrix cells attempt to increase synthesis by increasing cellular proliferation.[57] The ''degenerative spiral'' hypothesis may help explain the interactions of biomechanics and biochemistry that affect a biologic response. This model is as follows: The release of neuropeptides from the DRG, induced by environmental and structural factors (that is, vibrations), mediates a progressive degeneration of the

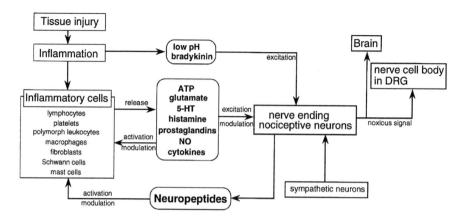

Fig. 1   *Schematic diagram of the interaction between peripheral tissue injury and the central neurogenic components. This scheme demonstrates how neurogenic mediators can affect nonneurogenic (chemical) mediators through the stimulation of inflammatory cells. ATP = adenosine triphosphate, 5-HT = 5-hydroxytryptamine, NO = nitric oxide, DRG = dorsal root ganglion.*

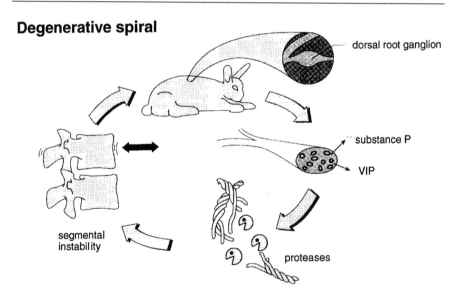

Fig. 2   *The functional spinal unit may undergo degeneration as a result of the interaction of mechanical and chemical stimuli seen in an injured or environmentally stimulated functional spinal unit. VIP = vasoactive intestinal peptide. (Reproduced with permission from Weinstein JN: Anatomy and neurophysiologic mechanism of spinal pain, in Frymoyer JW, Ducker TB, Hadler NM, et al (eds):* The Adult Spine: Principles and Practice. *New York, NY, Raven Press, 1991, vol 1, pp 593–610.)*

functional spinal unit structures by stimulating the synthesis of inflammatory agents (for example, cytokines, PGE_2) and degradative enzymes (for example, proteases, collagenase). As a direct or indirect result of these chemical interactions, secondary changes in mechanical properties occur that then perpetuate this "degenerative or aging spiral" (Fig. 2).[55]

Nonneurogenic and neurogenic pain mediators mutually participate in pathomechanisms of spinal pain through inflammatory reaction secondary to tissue injuries of the spinal unit involving the nerve root and DRG. Chemicals and neurotransmitters play a significant role in pathomechanisms of low back pain and radicular pain. It is very important in the treatment of low back pain and radiculopathy to understand these mechanisms of pain.

References

1. Wiesel SW, Tsourmas N, Feffer HL, et al: A study of computer-assisted tomography: I. The incidence of positive CAT scans in an asymptomatic group of patients. *Spine* 1984;9:549–551.
2. Boumphrey FR, Bell GR, Modic M, et al: Computed tomography scanning after chymopapain injection for herniated nucleus pulposus: A prospective study. *Clin Orthop* 1987;219:120–123.
3. Boden SD, Davis DO, Dina TS, et al: Abnormal magnetic-resonance scans of the lumbar spine in asymptomatic subjects: A prospective investigation. *J Bone Joint Surg* 1990;72A:403–408.
4. Kawakami M, Weinstein JN, Spratt KF, et al: Experimental lumbar radiculopathy: Immunohistochemical and quantitative demonstrations of pain induced by lumbar nerve root irritation of the rat. *Spine* 1994;19:1780–1794.
5. Weinstein J, Claverie W, Gibson S: The pain of discography. *Spine* 1988;13:1344–1348.
6. Coppes MH, Marani E, Thomeer RT, et al: Letter: Innervation of anulus fibrosis in low back pain. *Lancet* 1990;336:189–190.
7. Gronblad M, Weinstein JN, Santavirta S: Immunohistochemical observations on spinal tissue innervation: A review of hypothetical mechanisms of back pain. *Acta Orthop Scand* 1991;62:614–622.
8. Kawakami M, Chatani K, Weinstein JN: Anatomy, biochemistry, and physiology of low-back pain, in White AH, Schofferman JA (eds): *Spine Care: Diagnosis and Treatment.* St. Louis, MO, Mosby-Year Book, 1995, vol 1, pp 84–103.
9. Rang HP, Bevan S, Dray A: Nociceptive peripheral neurons: Cellular properties, in Wall PD, Melzack R, Bonica JJ (eds): *Textbook of Pain*, ed 3. New York, NY, Churchill Livingstone, 1994, pp 57–78.
10. Sekiguchi Y, Konnai Y, Kikuchi S, et al: An anatomical study of neuropeptide immunoreactivities in the lumbar dura matter after sympathectomy. *Trans Orthop Res Soc* 1996;21:162.
11. Steen KH, Reeh PW, Anton F, et al: Protons selectively induce lasting excitation and sensitization to mechanical stimulation of nociceptors in rat skin, in vitro. *J Neurosci* 1992;12:86–95.
12. Kawakami M, Tamaki T, Weinstein JN, et al: Pathomechanism of pain-related behavior produced by allografts of intervertebral disc in the rat. *Spine*, in press.
13. Nachemson A: Intradiscal measurements of pH in patients with lumbar rhizopathies. *Acta Orthop Scand* 1969;40:23–42.
14. Maves TJ, Pechman PS, Gebhart GF, et al: Continuous infusion of acidified saline around the rat sciatic nerve produced thermal hyperalgesia. *Neurosci Lett* 1995;194:45–48.
15. Huettner JE: Glutamate receptor channels in rat DRG neurons: Activation by kainate and quisqualate and blockade of desensitization by Con A. *Neuron* 1990;5:255–266.

16. Follenfant RL, Nakamura-Craig M: Abstract: Glutamate induces hyperalgesia in the rat paw. *Br J Pharmacol* 1992;106(suppl):49P.

17. Manning DC, Raja SN, Meyer RA, et al: Pain and hyperalgesia after intradermal injection of bradykinin in humans. *Clin Pharmacol Ther* 1991;50:721–729.

18. Taiwo YO, Levine JD: Serotonin is a directly-acting hyperalgesic agent in the rat. *Neuroscience* 1992;48:485–490.

19. Simone DA, Alreja M, LaMotte RH: Psychophysical studies of the itch sensation and itchy skin ('alloknesis') produced by intracutaneous injection of histamine. *Somatosens Mot Res* 1991;8:271–279.

20. Birrell GJ, McQueen DS, Iggo A, et al: PGI2-induced activation and sensitization of articular mechanonociceptors. *Neurosci Lett* 1991;124:5–8.

21. Meller ST: Differential mechanisms for thermal and mechanical hyperalgesia. *APS J* 1994;3:215–231.

22. Saal JS, Franson RC, Dobrow R, et al: High levels of inflammatory phospholipase A2 activity in lumbar disc herniations. *Spine* 1990;15:674–678.

23. Ozaktay AC, Kallakuri S, Li QH, et al: Electrophysiological changes induced by phospholipase A2 in rabbit lumbar facet joint and adjacent tissues. *Trans Orthop Res Soc* 1995;20:112.

24. Franson RC, Saal JS, Saal JA: Human disc phospholipase A2 is inflammatory. *Spine* 1992;17(suppl 6):S129–132.

25. Moncada S, Palmer RM, Higgs EA: Nitric oxide: Physiology, pathophysiology, and pharmacology. *Pharmacol Rev* 1991;43:109–142.

26. Morris R, Southam E, Braid DJ, et al: Nitric oxide may act as a messenger between dorsal root ganglion neurones and their satellite cells. *Neurosci Lett* 1992;137:29–32.

27. McGehee DS, Goy MF, Oxford GS: Involvement of the nitric oxide-cyclic GMP pathway in the desensitization of bradykinin responses of cultured rat sensory neurons. *Neuron* 1992;9:315–324.

28. Duarte ID, Lorenzetti BB, Ferreira SH: Peripheral analgesia and activation of the nitric oxide-cyclic GMP pathway. *Eur J Pharmacol* 1990;186:289–293.

29. Ferreira SH, Duarte ID, Lorenzetti BB: The molecular mechanism of action of peripheral morphine analgesia: Stimulation of the cGMP system via nitric oxide release. *Eur J Pharmacol* 1991;201:121–122.

30. Meller ST, Pechman PS, Gebhart GF, et al: Letter: Nitric oxide mediates the thermal hyperalgesia produced in a model of neuropathic pain in the rat. *Neuroscience* 1992;50:7–10.

31. Kang JD, Georgescu HI, McIntyre L, et al: Herniated lumbar intervertebral discs make neutral metalloproteases, nitric oxide, and interleukin-6. *Orthop Trans* 1995;19:53.

32. Ferreira SH, Lorenzetti BB, Bristow AF, et al: Interleukin-1 beta as a potent hyperalgesic agent antagonized by a tripeptide analogue. *Nature* 1988;334:698–700.

33. Follenfant RL, Nakamura-Craig M, Garland LG: Sustained hyperalgesia in rats evoked by 15-hydroperoxyeicosatetraenoic acid is attenuated by the protein kinase inhibitor H-7. *Br J Pharmacol* 1990;99:289P.

34. Cunha FQ, Lorenzetti BB, Poole S, et al: Interleukin-8 as a mediator of sympathetic pain. *Br J Pharmacol* 1991;104:765–767.

35. Cunha FQ, Poole S, Lorenzetti BB, et al: The pivotal role of tumour necrosis factor alpha in the development of inflammatory hyperalgesia. *Br J Pharmacol* 1992;107:660–664.

36. Schweizer A, Feige U, Fontana A, et al: Interleukin-1 enhances pain reflexes: Mediation through increased prostaglandin E2 levels. *Agents Actions* 1988;25:246–251.

37. Dayer JM, Zavadil-Grob C, Ucla C, et al: Induction of human interleukin 1 mRNA measured by collagenase- and prostaglandin E2-stimulating activity in rheumatoid synovial cells. *Eur J Immunol* 1984;14:898–901.

38. Mizel SB, Dayer JM, Krane SM, et al: Stimulation of rheumatoid synovial cell collagenase and prostaglandin production by partially purified lymphocyte-activating factor (interleukin 1). *Proc Natl Acad Sci U S A* 1981;78:2474–2477.

39. Yanagisawa M, Otsuka M, Garcia-Arraras JE: E-type prostaglandins depolarize primary afferent neurons of the neonatal rat. *Neurosci Lett* 1986;68:351–355.
40. Yamagishi M, Nemoto O, Kikuchi T, et al: Ruptured human disc tissues produce metalloproteinase and interleukin-1. *Trans Orthop Res Soc* 1992;17:190.
41. Hokfelt T, Elde R, Johansson O, et al: Immunohistochemical evidence for separate populations of somatostatin-containing and substance P-containing primary afferent neurons in the rat. *Neuroscience* 1976;1:131–136.
42. Salt TE, Hill RG: Neurotransmitter candidates of somatosensory primary afferent fibres. *Neuroscience* 1983;10:1083–1103.
43. Barbut D, Polak JM, Wall PD: Substance P in spinal cord dorsal horn decreases following peripheral nerve injury. *Brain Res* 1981;205:289–298.
44. Marx JL: Brain peptides: Is substance P a transmitter of pain signals? *Science* 1979;205:886–889.
45. Naftchi NE, Abrahams SJ, St. Paul HM, et al: Localization and changes of substance P in spinal cord of paraplegic cats. *Brain Res* 1978;153:507–513.
46. Naftchi NE, Abrahams SJ, St. Paul HM, et al: Substance P and leucine enkephalin changes in spinal cord of paraplegic rats and cats, in Naftchi NE (ed): *Spinal Cord Injury*. Jamaica, NY, Spectrum, 1982, pp 85–101.
47. Shehab SA, Atkinson ME: Vasoactive intestinal polypeptide increases in areas of the dorsal horn of the spinal cord from which other neuropeptides are depleted following peripheral axotomy. *Exp Brain Res* 1986;62:422–430.
48. Hohmann EL, Elde RP, Rysavy JA, et al: Innervation of periosteum and bone by sympathetic vasoactive intestinal peptide-containing nerve fibers. *Science* 1986;232:868–871.
49. Kruger L, Silverman JD, Mantyh PW, et al: Peripheral patterns of calcitonin-gene-related peptide general somatic sensory innervation: Cutaneous and deep terminations. *J Compar Neurol* 1989;280:291–302.
50. Weinstein J: Mechanisms of spinal pain: The dorsal root ganglion and its role as a mediator of low-back pain. *Spine* 1986;11:999–1001.
51. Weinstein J, Pope M, Schmidt R, et al: Effects of low frequency vibration on the dorsal root ganglion. *Neuro-Orthop* 1987;4:24–30.
52. Badalamente MA, Dee R, Ghillani R, et al: Mechanical stimulation of dorsal root ganglia induces increased production of substance P: A mechanism for pain following nerve root compromise? *Spine* 1987;12:552–555.
53. Kawakami M, Tamaki T: Morphologic and quantitative changes in neurotransmitters in the lumbar spinal cord after acute or chronic mechanical compression of the cauda equina. *Spine* 1992;17(suppl 3):S13–S17.
54. Chatani K, Kawakami M, Weinstein JN, et al: Characterization of thermal hyperalgesia, c-fos expression, and alterations in neuropeptides after mechanical irritation of the dorsal root ganglion. *Spine* 1995;20:277–290.
55. Weinstein JN: Anatomy and neurophysiologic mechanisms of spinal pain, in Frymoyer JW, Ducker TB, Hadler NM, et al (eds): *The Adult Spine: Principles and Practice*. New York, NY, Raven Press, 1991, vol 1, pp 593–610.
56. Weinstein JN: The role of neurogenic and non-neurogenic mediators as they relate to pain and the development of osteoarthritis: A clinical review. *Spine* 1992;17(suppl 10):S356–S361.
57. Pedrini-Mille A, Weinstein JN, Found EM, et al: Stimulation of dorsal root ganglia and degradation of rabbit anulus fibrosus. *Spine* 1990;15:1252–1256.

Chapter 18

Experimental Models for Study of the Pathophysiology and Modulation of Effects of Herniated Intervertebral Disk at the Spinal Level

Kenneth A. Follett, MD, PhD
Gerald F. Gebhart, PhD

The applicability of current models and the development of new models for studying the question of whether the pain or sensation caused by herniated intervertebral disk (HIVD) can be perceived (ie, signaled) at the level of the spinal cord are hampered by our lack of understanding of the pathophysiology of the dysfunction associated with intervertebral disk herniation. Few data from studies of humans exist to guide the development of laboratory models and investigations. For example, we do not know conclusively the site of the lesion in symptomatic HIVD in humans (eg, spinal nerve, root, dorsal root ganglion [DRG]), the nature of the insult in humans (eg, compression, ischemia, inflammation), the severity of injury required to elicit symptoms (eg, neurapraxia, axonotmesis), or the physiologic, pharmacologic, or anatomic effects of HIVD in humans at the level of the spinal nerve, root, DRG, or cord. In the absence of human data that address these issues, we cannot know whether our models mimic the effects of HIVD in humans.

Data from human necropsy studies suggest that the neural structures injured most commonly by HIVD are the DRG and proximal spinal nerve.[1,2] Clinically, patients can have similar symptoms and signs regardless of the site of compression (central, posterolateral, or lateral disk herniation injuring root, DRG, or nerve), suggesting that the site of injury may not be a critical factor in determining the response of the nervous system. However, patients with lateral herniation (DRG) reportedly have more acute pain that is resistant, in some cases, to nonsurgical care. In the absence of good data from human studies indicating that the effects of injury to the root, DRG, or spinal nerve differ significantly from one another, models involving experimental manipulation at any of these sites may be equally applicable.

Compression of a neural structure may not be required for HIVD to be symptomatic, and by itself may be insufficient to provoke symptoms. In humans, simple compression (traction) of a normal nerve does not evoke pain or paresthesias; symptoms are produced only by manipulation of nerves that have been subject to prior insult.[3] Acute compressive lesions of peripheral nerves (eg, "Saturday night palsy'') are generally painless.[4] Limb ischemia induced by tourniquet causes paresthesias, and corresponding ectopic activity can be recorded in the nerves supplying the symptomatic dermatomes.[5] Most practitioners have encountered patients with overt radicular signs and symptoms in whom a compressive lesion cannot be identified. Attributing the effects of HIVD to simple mechanical compression and distortion of a root or nerve, or to the resulting disruption of myelin sheaths or axons, may be an overly simplistic view of the pathophysiology of HIVD. Chemical, inflammatory, and/or ischemic mechanisms may account for some of the dysfunction associated with HIVD[6] and should be considered in models of HIVD.

We do not know the magnitude of injury required in humans to provoke a response in the peripheral or central nervous system. Simple neural compression by HIVD may be insufficient, but complete transection is not required to produce symptoms. Necropsy studies in humans indicate that demyelination with partial loss of fibers, proliferation of Schwann cells, and increased endoneurial fibrosis are common findings that accompany compressive lesions of HIVD or spondylosis. The degree of anatomic derangement correlates with the severity of impingement of the neural structure.[1,2] Anatomic data from symptomatic humans are not available, and we lack data from humans indicating whether the electrophysiologic, anatomic, or pharmacologic responses of neurons at the level of the spinal cord are different in axonotmetic (eg, compression) versus neurotmetic lesions. In the absence of such data, we cannot determine whether simple nerve compression models are more applicable than nerve ligation or transection models in studying the effects of HIVD.

Finally, human data concerning the structural and functional responses of nerve and spinal cord to the effects of symptomatic HIVD are virtually nonexistent. Ectopic and antidromically-conducted activity can be recorded in peripheral nerves in humans who have paresthesias in corresponding dermatomes, paresthesias at rest are accompanied by spontaneous neuronal activity, and interventions that increase the paresthesias (eg, straight leg raising, neck flexion to evoke Lhermitte's sign, or eliciting Tinel's sign) increase neuronal discharges.[5,7] Ectopic activity and pain associated with a peripheral nerve neuroma are not abolished by infiltration of the neuroma with local anesthetic.[8] These data suggest that symptoms (paresthesias) of HIVD result from ectopic activity, the source of which may be proximal to the injury site (eg, located proximal on the nerve, within the DRG, or within the spinal cord). Segmental hyperactivity of spinal cord dorsal horn neurons has been demonstrated in a paraplegic patient with chronic deafferentation pain,[9] suggesting a spinal cord source of ectopic impulse generation. These data provide a basis for the development and validation of some models of HIVD, but the paucity of human data concerning physiologic responses to neural injury relevant to HIVD and the lack of human data regarding anatomic and pharmacologic changes in symptomatic HIVD render it difficult to know what changes a model should produce to mimic HIVD in humans.

In summary, the ability to develop models to determine whether the sensory effects of HIVD can be signaled or perceived at the level of the spinal cord is impaired by the lack of understanding of the pathophysiology of HIVD symptoms and a lack of human data on which to base laboratory models. The additional difficulty of validating models of pain has been illustrated by Sweet,[10] who noted that autotomy in an animal (a common measure of ''pain'') is not proof of pain; some patients with congenital analgesia "autotomize," and rhizotomy in humans does not always relieve pain in the deafferentated area. Most likely, no currently available laboratory model mimics precisely the effects of HIVD. The ideal model would permit assessment of the effects of a compressive lesion placed at the level of the nerve root, DRG, and/or spinal nerve, all potential sites of compression by HIVD. It would take into account any chemical and/or inflammatory mediators of the symptoms of HIVD, and it would mimic the pathologic changes seen in symptomatic HIVD. The model would produce quantitatively or qualitatively consistent results on neurophysiologic, anatomic, pharmacologic, or behavioral measures.

Currently available models that can be applied to the study of spinal cord responses to HIVD are based on stimulation or lesioning of neural structures, typically outside the spinal canal, in a fashion that simulates the physiologic or anatomic effects of HIVD. Models are of three general types: (1) acute compression models, (2) neuroma (transection) models, and (3) chronic constriction models. Most of the models relevant to HIVD have been used to study nerve, DRG, or root, rather than spinal cord, but most of them can be applied to studies of anatomic, physiologic, and pharmacologic changes within the spinal cord. None of the existing models is known to mimic the effects of acute or chronic HIVD in humans because of the limitations addressed above.

Compression Models

Most models of nerve compression have been developed to study nerve entrapment syndromes or peripheral neuropathy rather than HIVD. Few studies[4,11] have sought specifically to mimic the effects of HIVD. Effects of acute compression can be studied by simple mechanical manipulation of roots, DRG, or nerves, all potential sites of impingement by HIVD.[4] This approach has been used to demonstrate that dorsal root fibers are relatively resistant to the effects of acute mechanical compression but compression of DRG evokes an intense, slowly adapting discharge. Minor chronic injury to the roots results in spontaneous activity in the roots and renders them abnormally sensitive to mechanical stimulation. These observations correlate with human data suggesting that HIVD may be symptomatic if it compresses the DRG (rather than root or nerve), and whereas acute compression may not have an effect on roots, chronic irritation or injury may result in abnormal activity.[3]

Quantitative data can be obtained using graded mechanical compression models. Granit and associates[11] sought specifically to mimic the effects of HIVD by mechanically compressing sciatic nerve in cats against an ebonite platform. Using this model, they demonstrated that pressure as low as 50 mm Hg causes attenuation of the compound action potential produced by stimulation of the nerve, and abnormal orthodromic and antidromic impulses are generated at the site of compression. An air-driven mechanical compression device has been used to study the effects of graded pressure on peripheral nerve, spinal roots, and spinal cord in dogs, and data demonstrate that roots and spinal cord are more sensitive to the effects of compression than is peripheral nerve, and large fibers are more sensitive than small fibers.[12]

Graded compression of nerves may also be performed using an inflatable cuff. This model has been applied to the sciatic nerve to study the histopathologic effects of mechanical compression and ischemia,[13] which are characterized by endoneurial edema with axonal degeneration, demyelination with Schwann cell necrosis, fibrin deposition, cellular proliferation, inflammation, and hemorrhage. This model also has been used to study the effects of nerve compression at the level of the ganglion.[14] In the rabbit, compression of the vagus nerve at a pressure as low as 30 mm Hg induced changes in the morphology of nodose ganglion cells.[14] This is a clinically relevant pressure because carpal canal pressures in carpal tunnel syndrome have been measured at 30 mm Hg in humans.[15] This model offers the potential to study late responses to acute, transient compression by performing the compression, removing the chamber, and later studying the effects of acute compression on the nerve, DRG, root, or spinal cord. This model may be the most accurate of any available model in simulating the mechanical effects of HIVD, but we do not know what pressure is required to mimic HIVD.

A graded compression model has been developed for studies of roots of the cauda equina.[16] In this model, the cauda equina is exposed via laminectomy, and the roots are compressed between a balloon and a Plexiglass plate. The model has been applied to study the effect of compression on blood flow in the roots and demonstrates histologic effects qualitatively similar to those observed in peripheral nerve, but pressures required to impair blood flow are lower for the cauda equina roots than for peripheral nerve. These data, together with those of Gelfan and Tarlov,[12] indicate that the effects of compression may vary with the site of compression.

Nonquantitative chronic compression has been applied by constricting peripheral nerve with polythene tubing.[17] After 2 to 5 weeks, constriction results in endoneurial edema, possibly from compromise of the vasa nervorum, with histologic changes that are similar to those produced by other chronic constriction models (see below). Conduction velocity is reduced in the nerve, and the general features of the condition are similar to those seen in human nerve entrapment syndromes.

Most of the compression models have been used to study the morphologic effects of nerve compression and typically demonstrate intraneural edema and demyelination, changes that are seen in most other models. Unlike other models of nerve injury, the compression models permit studies of responses to acute and/or transient nerve compression. These models provide the flexibility to study responses in the nerve, root, or spinal cord. A major limitation of these models is that we do not know what force is exerted on a neural structure in cases of symptomatic HIVD. Pressures associated with disk herniation have been calculated in a cadaver model[18] and have been measured in nerve entrapment syndromes,[15] but we do not know whether these data reflect the situation in symptomatic HIVD in humans.

Neuroma (Transection) Models

Neuroma models have been used extensively to study the effects of nerve injury. In 1930, Adrian[19] reported that acute nerve transection produced spontaneous neuronal activity that might be a source of pain following nerve injury. These observations, later refuted,[20] laid the foundation for a laboratory model of nerve injury. Transection may be performed at any level: root, spinal nerve, or peripheral nerve. The effects of lesions vary somewhat according to the site of injury,[21] but it is not known whether a lesion at one site more accurately reflects the effects of HIVD than a lesion elsewhere.

A widely studied model is the neuroma model advanced by Wall and associates:[20,22,23] Sectioning or crushing a nerve produces an immediate high-frequency injury discharge followed by a period of electrical silence, after which ectopic spontaneous activity develops. Ectopic activity, related to alterations in membrane structure and function,[24,25] can originate in the DRG, neuroma, or demyelinated nerve.[26] The abnormal activity becomes detectable about 3 to 5 days after nerve section, peaks in 12 days, and returns to a lower level by 30 days.[27] The development of electrical abnormalities parallels the time course of autotomy behavior observed in the animals,[22,28] with the maximal incidence of autotomy coinciding with the period of maximum barrage of afferent activity from the transected nerve.[29] Ectopic activity is increased by mechanical, chemical, and cold stimulation of the neuroma.[22] Ectopic activity as demonstrated in the neuroma model may account for the positive sensory phenomena (paresthesias) patients report following nerve injury.[26]

The effects of rhizotomy have not been characterized as fully as those of peripheral nerve transection. Rhizotomy results in the development of spontaneous neuronal activity that can be recorded centrally,[21,30-32] but the effects of rhizotomy may differ from those of more peripheral nerve transection. Autotomy is more intense following rhizotomy than after peripheral neurectomy, and the latency of autotomy varies with the location of the lesion along the root or nerve.[21] Autotomy occurs earliest in animals that undergo transection of the nerve just distal to the DRG, compared to rhizotomy or peripheral nerve transection,[21] and the latency to onset of autotomy following rhizotomy is longer than that for peripheral nerve section.[28] Dorsal root fibers degenerate before the onset of autotomy in rhizotomy models, suggesting that peripheral fibers cannot be the source of pain, as they might be in the neuroma models. Rhizotomy appears to result in abnormalities localized within the central nervous system[28] in contrast to more peripheral lesions in which the source of abnormal activity may be either central or peripheral. In particular, abnormal spontaneous activity in the DRG may be a significant contributing factor to pain after peripheral nerve injury.[21]

The effects of rhizotomy are often studied in the lumbar region, but similar responses occur in the trigeminal nerve system and may be easier to study in that location.[32] The trigeminal system offers the advantage that the fibers are almost purely sensory, are in a large bundle, and the target is clearly defined within the brainstem, simplifying studies of the central effects. The applicability of the trigeminal rhizotomy model to studies of the effects of HIVD is not known.

The central and peripheral histologic and physiologic effects of nerve transection have been well characterized, rendering this a useful model for nerve injury. The applicability of transection models to studies of the effects of HIVD is not clear because transection represents a special form of nerve injury. HIVD does not result in physical nerve transection, and we do not know whether axonotmesis and complete transection produce similar effects in humans. Neuroma models may have general applicability in that similar results may be seen in any nerve that has sustained an axonotmetic injury (eg, compression, partial transection, traction), which may produce a neuroma-in-continuity without complete transection of the nerve.[33]

Chronic Constriction Injury Models

Nerve ligation models have been used by numerous investigators to study responses to neural injury.[4,11,17,34,35] In a few instances,[4,11,34] ligation models have been used to extend studies of the effects of compressive lesions on neuronal function. In general, ligation models have been used to study partial nerve injuries that produce neuropathic pain, a condition that may not be modeled adequately by neuroma models.[36]

The most widely studied chronic constriction injury (CCI) model is that of Bennett and Xie.[36] In this model, placement of four 4-0 chromic gut ligatures around the sciatic nerve leads to development of intraneural edema and compression within 24 hours. The intraneural edema has been related to partial occlusion of the nerve's vasculature,[36] although recent evidence indicates that a chemical reaction to the suture material may also be a factor in inciting neuronal damage.[37,38] The model produces a partial, selective deafferentation injury. Histologically, demyelination and axonal degeneration are prominent, with loss of approximately 90% to 95% of myelinated and 75% of unmyelinated axons distal to the constriction site.[39] Residual myelinated fibers distal to the injury site are predominantly A delta (Aδ). At the constriction site, perineurium is disrupted and growth cones are abundant. In essence, this model produces a neuroma-in-continuity[39] with the periphery being innervated by a few abnormal large (Aβ) and small (Aδ) diameter myelinated fibers, and both abnormal and normal C fibers.[33]

The time course of electrophysiologic changes parallels that of histologic changes. From 1 to 3 days after the injury, myelinated fibers become unable to conduct impulses, then develop spontaneous activity (which may arise in the DRG)[40]; unmyelinated fibers continue to conduct impulses.[41] The DRG develops abnormal chemosensitivity and becomes a generator of abnormal ectopic activity.[40] Consistent with the increased spontaneous activity is an increase in metabolic activity in the spinal cord dorsal horn.[42] The time course of behavioral changes parallels that of electrophysiologic changes, and pain behaviors may be related, in part, to neuroma formation because the time course also parallels that of neuroma discharge.[39] Allodynia, hyperalgesia, and behavioral evidence of spontaneous pain or dysesthesia begin to develop within 2 to 3 days after the injury, reach peak severity in 10 to 14 days, and last about 2 months.[36,43]

The effects of CCI on central nervous system (CNS) structure and function are similar to those produced by the neuroma model in many respects, and these may represent the same abnormality in differing degrees.[40,41] Both produce spontaneous activity in myelinated fibers although the onset in CCI is earlier. C fibers become spontaneously active at a later time in both models. The typical discharge frequency and patterns of spontaneous activity in myelinated afferents in the constriction injury are nearly identical to those seen in the neuroma model. The underlying abnormalities that lead to spontaneous activity in the two injuries may be similar in that abnormal discharges can occur in the DRG, and the DRG is abnormally chemosensitive.[40]

The CCI model has been modified in an effort to mimic the effects of HIVD in causing human lumbar radiculopathy.[38,44,45] Specifically, chromic gut ligatures are placed around the root[38,44] or DRG,[45] common locations of nerve impingement by HIVD in humans,[1,2] to reproduce both the mechanical compression and possible chemical irritation that may lead to symptomatic HIVD in humans. This method has been used to study behavioral, histologic, and histochemical effects peripherally and within the spinal cord. It is the most direct attempt to simulate the pathophysiology of HIVD.

The Bennett and Xic model[36] represents partial injury to the whole nerve. In contrast is a model that causes a complete injury to a portion of the nerve, induced by ligation of one third to one half of the sciatic nerve.[35,46] The effects of this injury differ from that caused by whole nerve ligation in several regards. Behavioral changes are present in the immediate postoperative period, animals demonstrate hyperesthesia to repeated light touch (probably indicating sparing of the low threshold myelinated fibers), cold allodynia is not present, significant contralateral effects are present, and effects depend on sympathetic activity.

Partial injury may also be produced by threading a catgut suture through sciatic nerve, causing an inflammatory microgranuloma.[47] The histologic changes associated with this injury are similar to those caused by chromic suture ligation. Segmental demyelination, degeneration of large diameter fibers distal to the injury, and partial preservation of Aδ and C fibers are characteristic. Schwann cells and endoneurial connective tissue proliferate.[47,48] Conduction velocity across the lesion is reduced, particularly for large diameter fibers (Aα, Aβ), and behavioral evidence of hyperalgesia, allodynia, and spontaneous pain are present within 2 days.[47] This microgranuloma model has been applied to studies of the trigeminal nerve,[49] which permits study of lesion effects in a more physiologically and anatomically circumscribed setting.[32] The focal demyelination that is produced by the microgranuloma results in ectopic impulse generation with prolonged afterdischarges following orthodromic or antidromic stimulation.

The CCI models offer the ability to study partial injuries at peripheral and central locations of the nervous system. The models do not permit quantitative assessment of the compressive force, but the effect of the lesion appears similar regardless of the specific nature of ligation. CCI models may not simulate the mechanical effects of HIVD, but may provide a model of the inflammatory/chemical component of HIVD lacking in the acute compression models. The acute compression and CCI models may complement each other, particularly in view of the observation that acute compression does not induce hyperexcitabilty in dorsal root fibers, but induction of chronic injury by ligation constriction renders the fibers abnormally sensitive to acute mechanical compression.[4] The complementary nature of these models is emphasized in the CCI model using root or DRG ligation.[44] Compared to neuroma (transection) models, the CCI model may be more applicable to studies of HIVD by virtue of its axonotmetic rather than neurotmetic effects. However, the prominent hyperalgesia and allodynia that distinguish the CCI model from neuroma models is not a typical complaint of humans with HIVD.

281

Miscellaneous Models

Several other models have been proposed for studies of nerve dysfunction, but their general application has been limited and their applicability to HIVD is not known. Injection of lysophosphatidyl choline into rat saphenous nerve produces segmental demyelination. Axons that conduct through the lesion generate spontaneous ectopic impulses and the lesion site is abnormally sensitive to mechanical stimulation.[50] Injection of proteolytic agents into rat sciatic nerve[51] has been used to study pharmacologic responses to injury. Injection leads to depletion of neurotransmitter substances in the ipsilateral spinal cord dorsal horn, with partial recovery over 4 to 9 months, consistent with sprouting of primary afferent fibers.

A naturally occurring peripheral nerve lesion in pigs that resembles human carpal tunnel syndrome has been described.[52] Conduction velocity in the median nerve at the wrist is reduced in older animals compared to that of younger animals. Segmental demyelination within the median nerve occurs in animals with slowing of conduction, and complete fiber degeneration with loss of myelin and axons is present in animals with conduction block. The applicability of this natural lesion to studies of HIVD is uncertain, but it offers a method for in vivo evaluation of effects of compressive lesions, which could be studied at central as well as peripheral sites in the nervous system.

Central Effects of Peripheral Lesions

Peripheral nerve, root, and DRG lesions result in physiologic, anatomic, and pharmacologic changes within the spinal cord.[45,53-63] These central changes are of key importance in answering the question whether the stimulation of a nerve by HIVD can be "perceived" at the level of the spinal cord. Many of the models described above can be used to examine the central effects of peripheral nerve injury, but not every model has been used for this purpose. Few[44,59,60] have compared specifically the effects of different lesion types on central processes; consequently, we do not know whether the models are comparable in their effects. Some data reveal that the central responses to peripheral lesions vary with the nature of the injury (eg, transection versus chronic constriction).[44,58,59] Until more is known about the pathophysiologic changes occurring in human HIVD, we will not know which model is most accurate for use in determining whether the sensory effects of HIVD can be perceived at the spinal level.

Modulation of Pain

Modulation of pain associated with HIVD is typically pharmacologic, either by systemic drug administration (eg, analgesics) or administration into the spinal intrathecal or epidural space (eg, steroids). Less commonly, electrical stimulation in the brain or of the spinal cord (dorsal columns) is used to control pain. Most experimental work in nonhuman animals has focused on spinal cord mechanisms of pain control and has employed models described above. This work has been based on knowledge of (1) the transmitters and receptors in the spinal cord dorsal horn that mediate endogenous systems of inhibition descending from the brain stem (eg, norepinephrine acting at α_2-adrenoceptors), (2) local circuit control mechanisms that involve, principally, opiate receptors, and (3) spinal mechanisms that contribute to activity-dependent changes in excitability and lead to increased responses to both painful and nonpainful inputs.

When given systemically, opioids have direct effects in the periphery,[64] activate at supraspinal sites (eg, midbrain periaqueductal/ventricular gray systems) of descending inhibition, and act directly at the level of the spinal dorsal horn. The opiate receptor principally associated with analgesia is the μ receptor, which is present on nociceptor nerve terminals in the periphery and in the spinal dorsal horn and also at supraspinal sites, although peripheral κ (kappa) and central δ (delta) receptors likely also play a role in analgesia produced by opioids. Using a mononeuropathy model of incomplete sciatic nerve ligation similar to the CCI model, Yamamoto and Yaksh[58] reported that the receptor agonist morphine and the receptor agonist (D-Pen2, D-Pen5)-enkephalin (DPDPE) both attenuated responses to thermal stimulation of the affected (hyperalgesic) hind paw when these drugs were administered into the intrathecal space. Similarly, the α_2-adrenoceptor agonist ST-91 and the γ-aminobutyric acid (GABA) receptor agonist baclofen given intrathecally were effective in the same study. The latter outcomes are consistent with a recent report by Meyerson and associates[65] that spinal cord stimulation significantly increased the threshold for hindlimb withdrawal produced by innocuous mechanical stimuli in two CCI models[36,46] of sciatic nerve mononeuropathy. Spinal cord stimulation probably activates norepinephrine-containing axons descending the spinal cord from the pons and also increases the release of the inhibitory amino acid transmitter GABA in the dorsal horn.[66]

Because hyperalgesia is a characteristic feature of the mononeuropathy models described here, and hyperalgesia reflects activity-dependent increases in the excitability of central neurons, several studies have examined the role of the N-methyl-D-aspartic acid (NMDA) receptor in the initiation and maintenance of mononeuropathy-produced hyperalgesia. A cascade of events are initiated by persistent afferent input from the injured nerve.[67] The NMDA receptor is a cation channel that, when open, allows calcium (and other cations) to enter the neuron. The influx of calcium leads to translocation of protein kinase C, activation of nitric oxide synthase (NOS) and a host of other events. Meller and associates[68] reported that nitric oxide, the product of activation of NOS, mediated the thermal hyperalgesia produced by loose ligation of the sciatic nerve with chromic gut sutures. When given intrathecally, a blocker of NOS as well as a blocker of the production of cyclic guanosine 3,5′-monophosphate, which is stimulated by nitric oxide, both reversed the hyperalgesia in this model. Consistent with this report, Mao and associates[69] reported that the intrathecal administration of the NMDA channel blocker MK-801 similarly reduced nociceptive behaviors produced in the same mononeuropathy model. Further, they documented that local nerve anesthesia in conjunction with intrathecal MK-801 produced greater than additive effects (ie, were synergistic).

In a model of lumbar radiculopathy produced by placement of chromic gut sutures around the L4 and L5 dorsal roots in the rat,[38,44] Hayashi and associates[70] examined the efficacy of a more standard treatment for a variety of back related pains, epidural administration of a steroid. They found that betamethasone (Celestone®) given epidurally 3 days after loose ligation of the dorsal roots with chromic gut significantly attenuated the thermal hyperalgesia of the affected hindlimb when assessed 2 and 3 weeks postoperatively. Epidural injections of saline or bupivacaine 3 days postoperatively had no influence on the time course or magnitude of thermal hyperalgesia in this model. The efficacy of steroids in this model has been confirmed and extended by Lee, Weinstein, Spratt, and Gebhart (unpublished data, 1994), who found that dorsal root ligation with chromic gut sutures increased spinal cord activity of phospholipase A_2 (PLA$_2$), the enzyme inhibited by steroids. Epidural administration of steroids or PLA$_2$ inhibitors attenuated both the thermal hyperalgesia and the increase in PLA$_2$ activity.

References

1. Holt S, Yates PO: Cervical spondylosis and nerve root lesions: Incidence at routine necropsy. *J Bone Joint Surg* 1966;48B:407–423.
2. Lindblom K, Rexed B: Spinal nerve injury in dorso-lateral protrusions of lumbar disks. *J Neurosurg* 1948;5:413–432.
3. Smyth MJ, Wright V: Sciatica and the intervertebral disc: An experimental study. *J Bone Joint Surg* 1958;40A:1401–1418.
4. Howe JF, Loeser JD, Calvin WH: Mechanosensitivity of dorsal root ganglia and chronically injured axons: A physiological basis for the radicular pain of nerve root compression. *Pain* 1977;3:25–41.
5. Ochoa JL, Torebjork HE: Paraesthesiae from ectopic impulse generation in human sensory nerves. *Brain* 1980;103:835–853.
6. Parke W, Burchiel K, Rydevik B, et al: Nerve: Basic science perspectives, in Frymoyer JW, Gordon SL (eds): *New Perspectives on Low Back Pain*. Park Ridge, IL, American Academy of Orthopaedic Surgeons, 1989, pp 57–123.
7. Nordin M, Nystrom B, Wallin U, et al: Ectopic sensory discharges and paresthesiae in patients with disorders of peripheral nerves, dorsal roots, and dorsal columns. *Pain* 1984;20:231–245.
8. Nystrom B, Hagbarth K-E: Microelectrode recordings from transected nerves in amputees with phantom limb pain. *Neurosci Lett* 1981;27:211–216.
9. Loeser JD, Ward AA Jr, White LE Jr: Chronic deafferentation of human spinal cord neurons. *J Neurosurg* 1968;29:48–50.
10. Sweet WH: Animal models of chronic pain: Their possible validation from human experience with posterior rhizotomy and congenital analgesia. *Pain* 1981;10:275–295.
11. Granit R, Leksell L, Skoglund CR: Fibre interaction in injured or compressed region of nerve. *Brain* 1944;67:125–140.
12. Gelfan S, Tarlov IM: Physiology of spinal cord, nerve root, and peripheral nerve compression. *Am J Physiol* 1956;185:217–229.
13. Powell HC, Myers RR: Pathology of experimental nerve compression. *Lab Invest* 1986;55:91–100.
14. Dahlin LB, Nordborg C, Lundborg G: Morphologic changes in nerve cell bodies induced by experimental graded nerve compression. *Exp Neurol* 1987;95:611–621.
15. Gelberman RH, Hergenroeder PT, Hargens AR, et al: The carpal tunnel syndrome: A study of carpal canal pressures. *J Bone Joint Surg* 1981;63A:380–383.
16. Olmarker K, Rydevik B, Holm S, et al: Effects of experimental graded compression on blood flow in spinal nerve roots: A vital microscopic study on the porcine cauda equina. *J Orthop Res* 1989;7:817–823.
17. Weisl H, Osborne GV: The pathological changes in rats' nerves subject to moderate compression. *J Bone Joint Surg* 1964;46B:297–306.
18. Spencer DL, Miller JA, Bertolini JE: The effect of intervertebral disc space narrowing on the contact force between the nerve root and a simulated disc protrusion. *Spine* 1984;9:422–426.
19. Adrian ED: The effects of injury on mammalian nerve fibres. *Proc R Soc Lond B Biol Sci* 1930;106:596–618.

20. Wall PD, Waxman S, Basbaum AI: Ongoing activity in peripheral nerve: Injury discharge. *Exp Neurol* 1974;45:576–589.
21. Wiesenfeld Z, Lindblom U: Behavioral and electrophysiological effects of various types of peripheral nerve lesions in the rat: A comparison of possible models for chronic pain. *Pain* 1980;8:285–298.
22. Wall PD, Gutnick M: Properties of afferent nerve impulses originating from a neuroma. *Nature* 1974;248:740–743.
23. Wall PD, Gutnick M: Ongoing activity in peripheral nerves: The physiology and pharmacology of impulses originating from a neuroma. *Exp Neurol* 1974;43:580–593.
24. Devor M, Govrin-Lippmann R, Angelides K: Na⁺ channel immunolocalization in peripheral mammalian axons and changes following nerve injury and neuroma formation. *J Neurosci* 1993;13:1976–1992.
25. Matzner O, Devor M: Hyperexcitability at sites of nerve injury depends on voltage-sensitive Na⁺ channels. *J Neurophysiol* 1994;72:349–359.
26. Wall PD, Devor M: Sensory afferent impulses originate from dorsal root ganglia as well as from the periphery in normal and nerve injured rats. *Pain* 1983;17:321–339.
27. Govrin-Lippmann R, Devor M: Ongoing activity in severed nerves: Source and variation with time. *Brain Res* 1978;159:406–410.
28. Wall PD, Scadding JW, Tomkiewicz MM: The production and prevention of experimental anesthesia dolorosa. *Pain* 1979;6:175–182.
29. Scadding JW: Development of ongoing activity, mechanosensitivity, and adrenaline sensitivity in severed peripheral nerve axons. *Exp Neurol* 1981;73:345–364.
30. Loeser JD, Ward AA Jr: Some effects of deafferentation on neurons of the cat spinal cord. *Arch Neurol* 1967;17:629–636.
31. Brinkhus HB, Zimmermann M: Characteristics of spinal dorsal horn neurons after partial chronic deafferentation by dorsal root transection. *Pain* 1983;15:221–236.
32. Anderson LS, Black RG, Abraham J, et al: Neuronal hyperactivity in experimental trigeminal deafferentation. *J Neurosurg* 1971;35:444–452.
33. Bennett GJ: An animal model of neuropathic pain: A review. *Muscle Nerve* 1993;16:1040–1048.
34. Duncan D: Alterations in the structure of nerves caused by restricting their growth with ligatures. *J Neuropathol Exp Neurol* 1948;7:261–273.
35. Hylden JLK, Nahin RL, Humphrey E, et al: Abstract: An animal model of hyperalgesia: Partial sciatic nerve lesion. *Pain* 1987;29(suppl 4):S274.
36. Bennett GJ, Xie Y-K: A peripheral mononeuropathy in rat that produces disorders of pain sensation like those seen in man. *Pain* 1988;33:87–107.
37. Maves TJ, Pechman PS, Gebhart GF, et al: Possible chemical contribution from chromic gut sutures produces disorders of pain sensation like those seen in man. *Pain* 1993;54:57–69.
38. Kawakami M, Weinstein JN, Chatani K, et al: Experimental lumbar radiculopathy: Behavioral and histologic changes in a model of radicular pain after spinal nerve root irritation with chromic gut ligatures in the rat. *Spine* 1994;19:1795–1802.
39. Carlton SM, Dougherty PM, Pover CM, et al: Neuroma formation and numbers of axons in a rat model of experimental peripheral neuropathy. *Neurosci Lett* 1991;131:88–92.
40. Kajander KC, Wakisaka S, Bennett GJ: Spontaneous discharge originates in the dorsal root ganglion at the onset of a painful peripheral neuropathy in the rat. *Neurosci Lett* 1992;138:225–228.
41. Kajander KC, Bennett GJ: Onset of a painful peripheral neuropathy in rat: A partial and differential deafferentation and spontaneous discharge in A-beta and A-delta primary afferent neurons. *J Neurophysiol* 1992;68:734–744.
42. Price DD, Mao JR, Coghill RC, et al: Regional changes in spinal cord glucose metabolism in a rat model of painful neuropathy. *Brain Res* 1991;564:314–318
43. Attal N, Jazat F, Kayser V, et al: Further evidence for ''pain-related'' behaviours in a model of unilateral peripheral mononeuropathy. *Pain* 1990;41:235–251.

44. Kawakami M, Weinstein JN, Spratt KF, et al: Experimental lumbar radiculopathy: Immunohistochemical and quantitative demonstrations of pain induced by lumbar nerve root irritation of the rat. *Spine* 1994;19:1780–1794.
45. Chatani K, Kawakami, M, Weinstein JN, et al: Characterization of thermal hyperalgesia, c-fos expression, and alterations in neuropeptides after mechanical irritation of the dorsal root ganglion. *Spine* 1994;20:277–290.
46. Seltzer Z, Dubner R, Shir Y: A novel behavioral model of neuropathic pain disorders produced in rats by partial sciatic nerve injury. *Pain* 1990;43:205–218.
47. Lehmann HJ, Ule G: Electrophysiological findings and structural changes in circumscript inflammation of peripheral nerves, in Bargmann W, Schade JP (eds): *Topics in Basic Neurology*. Amsterdam, The Netherlands, Elsevier, 1964, pp 169–173.
48. Munger BL, Bennett GJ: Abstract: The peripheral axonal pathology in the constrictive model of peripheral neuropathy. *Anat Rec* 1990;226:70A.
49. Burchiel KJ: Ectopic impulse generation in focally demyelinated trigeminal nerve. *Exp Neurol* 1980;69:423–429.
50. Calvin WH, Devor M, Howe JF: Can neuralgias arise from minor demyelination? Spontaneous firing, mechanosensitivity, and afterdischarge from conducting axons. *Exp Neurol* 1982;75:755–763.
51. El-Bohy A, LaMotte CC: Deafferentation-induced changes in neuropeptides of the adult rat dorsal horn following pronase injection of the sciatic nerve. *J Comp Neurol* 1993;336:545–554.
52. Fullerton PM, Gilliatt RW: Median and ulnar neuropathy in the guinea-pig. *J Neurol Neurosurg Psychiatry* 1967;30:393–402.
53. Liu C-N, Chambers WW: Intraspinal sprouting of dorsal root axons: Development of new collaterals and preterminals following partial denervation of the spinal cord in the cat. *Arch Neurol Psychiat* 1958;79:46–61.
54. Devor M, Wall PD: Reorganisation of spinal cord sensory map after peripheral nerve injury. *Nature* 1978;276:75–76.
55. Kapadia SE, LaMotte CC: Deafferentation-induced alterations in the rat dorsal horn: I. Comparison of peripheral nerve injury vs. rhizotomy effects on presynaptic, postsynaptic, and glial processes. *J Comp Neurol* 1987;266:183–197.
56. Dubner R, Hylden JLK, Nahin RL, et al: Neuronal plasticity in the superficial dorsal horn following peripheral tissue inflammation and nerve injury, in Cervero F, Bennett GJ, Headley PM (eds): *Processing of Sensory Information in the Superficial Dorsal Horn of the Spinal Cord*. New York, NY, Plenum Press, 1989, pp 429–443.
57. Bennett GJ, Kajander KC, Sahara Y, et al: Neurochemical and anatomical changes in the dorsal horn of rats with an experimental painful peripheral neuropathy, in Cervero F, Bennett GJ, Headley PM (eds): *Processing of Sensory Information in the Superficial Dorsal Horn of the Spinal Cord*. New York, NY, Plenum Press, 1989, pp 463–471.
58. Yamamoto T, Yaksh TL: Spinal pharmacology of thermal hyperesthesia induced by incomplete ligation of sciatic nerve: Opioid and nonopiod receptors. *Anesthesiology* 1991;75:817–826.
59. Draisci G, Kajander KC, Dubner R, et al: Up-regulation of opioid gene expression in spinal cord evoked by experimental nerve injuries and inflammation. *Brain Res* 1991;560:186–192.
60. Garrison CJ, Dougherty PM, Kajander KC, et al: Staining of glial fibrillary acidic protein (GFAP) in lumbar spinal cord increases following a sciatic nerve constriction injury. *Brain Res* 1991;565:1–7.
61. Woolf CJ, Shortland P, Coggeshall RE: Peripheral nerve injury triggers central sprouting of myelinated afferents. *Nature* 1992;355:75–78.
62. Coderre TJ, Katz J, Vaccarino AL, et al: Contribution of central neuroplasticity to pathological pain: Review of clinical and experimental evidence. *Pain* 1993;52:259–285.

63. Chi S-I, Levine JD, Basbaum AI: Peripheral and central contributions to the persistent expression of spinal cord fos-like immunoreactivity produced by sciatic nerve transection in the rat. *Brain Res* 1993;617:225–237.
64. Stein C, Schafer M, Hassan AH: Peripheral opioid receptors. *Ann Med* 1995;27:219–221.
65. Meyerson BA, Ren B, Herregodts P, et al: Spinal cord stimulation in animal models of mononeuropathy: Effects on the withdrawal response and the flexor reflex. *Pain* 1995;61:229–243.
66. Linderoth B, Stiller C-O, Gunasekera L, et al: Gamma-aminobutyric acid is released in the dorsal horn by electrical spinal cord stimulation: An in vivo microdialysis study in the rat. *Neurosurgery* 1994;34:484–489.
67. Meller ST, Gebhart GF: Nitric oxide (NO) and nociceptive processing in the spinal cord. *Pain* 1993;52:127–136.
68. Meller ST, Pechman PS, Gebhart GF, et al: Nitric oxide mediates the thermal hyperalgesia produced in a model of neuropathic pain in the rat. *Neuroscience* 1992;50:7–10.
69. Mao J, Price DD, Mayer DJ, et al: Intrathecal MK-801 and local nerve anesthesia synergistically reduce nociceptive behaviors in rats with experimental peripheral mononeuropathy. *Brain Res* 1992;576:254–262.
70. Hayashi N, Weinstein JN, Kawakami M, et al: The effect of epidural steroid injection on the irritated nerve root: An animal model. *Orthop Trans* 1995;19:69.

Chapter 19

Biomechanics of Disk Herniation and Related Issues

Vijay K. Goel, PhD

Introduction

In a normal lumbar spinal segment, the disk and facets are the two main load-bearing components.[1] Both of these components show degenerative changes leading to disk herniations. Computed tomography and magnetic resonance imaging (MRI) techniques have been used to delineate changes in the disk (anulus and nucleus), facets, and adjacent vertebrae.[2,3] The physiologic events that occur in nonsurgical treatment of herniated lumbar disks as measured by MRI have also been documented.[4] Changes in the anulus include circumferential and radial tears, and rim lesions adjacent to end plates (laminae separation or delamination).[5,6]

With age, the gel-like nucleus pulposus changes into a granular structure, ultimately losing its incompressible nature, and the number of distinct layers in the anulus fibrosus decreases. Furthermore, the distinct region where anulus and nucleus meet becomes less evident,[7-9] and chemical composition of the disk changes. Hydration decreases, the collagen network of the anulus becomes less organized, and proteoglycan content may decrease.[10] These changes lead to disk resorption with loss of height and osteophyte formation in later stages. Changes in the facet progress from synovial reaction and cartilage destruction in early stages of capsular ligament laxity to subluxation with osteophyte formation in later stages. Other changes are annular bulging, calcification, stenosis, facet joint disease, and ligamentous hypertrophy. These degenerative changes occur more or less in parallel and can be grouped into three clinical stages.[11] In the second stage, instability is clearly present and the patient is symptomatic; herniation of disk material causing nerve root compression may occur, generally in persons between the ages of 30 and 50 years.

A herniated disk manifests itself in three different shapes (Fig. 1).[12] A protruded herniation causes eccentric bulging of an intact anulus fibrosus in comparison to the normal shape. An extrusion is characterized by disk material that extends beyond the anulus but is still in continuity with disk material within the disk space. In a sequestered herniation, disk material lies outside the anulus and is no longer in continuity with the disk material within the intervertebral space, presumably because healing of the defect in the anulus has occurred.

Posterior disk displacement/herniation is believed to be a cause of low back pain/sciatica, and the symptoms of sciatica have been related to nerve root

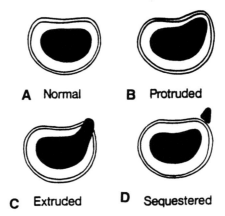

A Normal   **B** Protruded

C Extruded   **D** Sequestered

Fig. 1 *Classification of herniated disk shapes observed at operation. The shape of an intact "normal" disk is shown in A for the sake of comparison. (Adapted with permission from Frymoyer JW: Surgical indications for lumbar disc herniation, in Weinstein JN (ed): Clinical Efficacy and Outcome in the Diagnosis and Treatment of Low Back Pain. New York, NY, Raven Press, 1991, pp 117–124.)*

compression/irritation.[13] Entire surgical procedures and conservative treatment options are based on this tenet. There is no scientifically valid evidence that non-surgical treatment methods, such as braces, heat, ice, biofeedback, traction, manipulation, massage, steroids, acupuncture, and psychological support, improve the natural history of the problem.[12,13] Patients who do not respond to conservative treatment may be candidates for surgery. Surgical incision of a lumbar disk is the third most frequently performed orthopaedic surgical procedure, exceeded only by surgical fracture treatment and arthroscopy.[13] However, it is difficult to determine the beneficial effects of surgery as compared to conservative treatment after a few years, and it is virtually impossible after 10 years.[12,13] For most patients, the only real benefit from surgery is quicker relief from sciatic pain. The failure rate for primary surgical procedures, such as diskectomy and chemonucleolysis, varies from 15% to 40%,[13] and most failures are treated with repeat surgery. Reasons for failure include a new site of herniation, recurrent herniation at the same area, root scarring, missed herniations, migrated disk fragments, and postoperative diskitis.

Although the onset of low back pain and/or disk herniation is sometimes associated with a sudden injury, it is more often the result of cumulative damage to the spinal components induced by chronic loading of the spine.[1] Under chronic loading, the rate of damage may exceed the rate of repair by the cellular mechanisms of the body, thus weakening the structures to a point at which failure occurs under mildly abnormal loads. Chronic loading may occur under a variety of conditions. Lifting not only induces large axial compressive forces across the motion segment, but tends to be associated with twisting and bending of the trunk.[14-21] Persons with jobs requiring the lifting of objects of more than 11.3 kg more than 25 times per day have over three times the risk for acute prolapse of the lumbar intervertebral disk than people whose jobs do not involve lifting. If the body is twisted during lifting, the risk is even higher with less frequent lifting. An especially high risk for the prolapsed lumbar disk is associated with jobs involving the lifting of objects of more than 11.3 kg, with the body twisted and the knees unbent while lifting. Neither the lifting of objects of less than 11.3 kg nor twisting without lifting is associated with an increase in risk. Static loading influenced by posture during prolonged sitting and bending over also is associated with low back pain.[22,23] Vibration from such activities as driving a motor vehicle may compound the problems caused by prolonged sitting.[21] Kelsey and Hardy found that men who spend more than half of their workday in a car have a threefold increased risk of disk herniation.[24] Epidemiologic studies, however, do not indicate whether any load type (dynamic, heavy lifting, sedentary) is more harmful than the others.[22]

The repetitive loads experienced by the spine during daily living are complex (axial compressive load, flexion/extension, lateral bending, and axial twist)[1] and are shared by spinal muscles, facets, ligaments, and the disk of a motion segment. The loadsharing can be influenced by the type of loading, the geometry of the motion segment, and the stiffness of the participating structures. Because both the response of these structures to different load types and the resulting injury may differ, the effects of various load types, including complex loads on the disk, should be studied. The effects of quasistatic loads, dynamic (cyclic and impact) loads, and prolonged sitting (creep and viscoelasticity) should be included. Such studies will help determine the mechanism of injury leading to disk herniation, the biomechanical factors that may contribute to pain following herniation and prior to any treatment, and the biomechanical efficacy of conservative and surgical treatments. Both experimental and analytical approaches have been used to study the mechanics of the human spine in general and the disk in particular. Pertinent results from several studies are described next. At the end, a synthesis of the findings and their correlation to pain are presented.

Mechanism of Injury

Experimental Studies

Stokes and Greenapple[25,26] measured in situ strains in the disk fibers of a lumbar motion segment without posterior elements. The strains were of the order of 2% to 3% during normal load magnitudes; strains increased to about 6% to 10% for loads corresponding to extreme ranges of motion (eg, 8° of flexion and 6.5° of axial rotation). In torsional mode, there was a large difference in the strains in alternately aligned fiber directions. Larger strains were measured in fibers at posterolateral sites than in those at anterior sites. The authors also believed that the surface strain for intervertebral disks is very sensitive to disk height, diameter ratio, and fluid loss from the disk, but is less sensitive to the helix angle of the fibers themselves.

Axial forces experienced by a vertebra in vivo are of sufficient magnitude to induce fatigue fractures in the bony elements of the motion segment.[1] However, in vitro experiments, in which specimens were subjected to axial cyclic loads of varying magnitudes, have not indicated any damage to the disk per se.[27] Farfan[28] believes that compression failures of the vertebral end plates promote disk degeneration. The adult disk is avascular, and end plate microfractures can result in vascular ingrowth and concomitant formation of granular tissue or callus, which may lead to a decrease in the diffusion area for nutrition of the disk. As a result, the chemistry of the disk and the mechanical behavior of its constituents may be altered.

In response to cyclic axial twist (torsional loads), synovial fluid was discharged from the apophyseal joint capsules at some stage during testing.[29] When axial rotation exceeded +1.5°, bony failure of the facets and/or tearing of the capsular ligaments occurred. Cyclic torsional loads may lead to weakening and improper function of the apophyseal joints and disk. In the absence of synovial fluid, the facet joint may exhibit more bony contact and higher friction, which are likely to trigger degenerative changes in the facets and/or the disk. These results support the work of Farfan and associates[30] which reveals that cyclic torsional loads are detrimental to the spine and may lead to low back pain.

Cyclic flexion bending of a ligamentous spine subjected to "small" flexion bending moment led to a tangible increase in motion in the extension mode in comparison to the intact prefatigued spinal behavior.[31] This finding suggests that a partial loosening of the disk structure has occurred. The examination of dissected disks revealed fissures in the anulus of a few specimens; however, it was not possible to say whether these were caused by the cyclic bending test alone. These fissures become more relevant if the magnitude of the bending moment is large, which can happen in vivo when the muscle effectiveness in protecting the ligamentous spine decreases.

The testing of hyperflexed specimens in the axial compressive mode (flexion bending plus cyclic axial load) has resulted in disk prolapse in younger spinal specimens.[32] Wilder and associates[33] observed disk herniation in 75% of the calf segments tested. However, no herniations were found in the relatively older human specimens subjected to repetitive combined flexion, lateral bending and axial compression, and a constant axial torque. Combined repetitive loadings involving flexion bending, axial compression, and torque can produce radial cracks in the anulus and/or disk herniation. These findings, which support the epidemiologic findings,[19] suggest that disk herniations are related to age, and that many acute low back symptoms and frank disk herniations are part of the continuum of chronic, repetitive, low-grade trauma. From a biomechanical viewpoint, a prolonged sitting posture primarily induces a "constant" axial compressive load on the spine. As a result of this sustained loading, the viscoelastic (creep and relaxation) properties of the disk and, to some extent, those of the vertebra may be altered. It is very likely that, under chronic conditions, the degree of alteration may become so severe that any sudden activity undertaken by a subject after prolonged sitting (such as lifting a heavy load) may lead to a disk prolapse.

The disks are known to exhibit creep, relaxation, and hysteresis.[34-40] The nondegenerated disks creep slowly as compared to the degenerated or herniated disks, implying that a degenerated disk is less viscoelastic in nature. This characteristic may indicate a decrease in its ability to absorb the shocks of normal life. The magnitude of hysteresis increased with load and decreased with age.

Hansson and associates[34] monitored disk pressure across a motion segment and axial strains induced in the vertebral bodies of pigs subjected to sinusoidal vibration ranging from 1 to 12 Hz. A distinct resonance peak was observed at about 5 Hz. Disk pressure and strain data at resonance revealed a 2.5 times increase in load across the motion segment. This increase may explain the pathophysiology of seated whole-body vibrations.

Analytical Studies

The finite element (FE) technique has been used extensively to study the biomechanics of an intact lumbar spine motion segment. The results have not only delineated the roles of various elements in resisting the external loads but have revealed the roles of mechanical factors in initiating disk degeneration and herniation of the nucleus.[41]

Under axial compression, the intervertebral disk was predicted to bear most of the loads with a small contribution by the facets. At higher compressive loads, however, the inferior facet could also contact the lamina of the vertebra below, suggesting an increased role of the facets in resisting the loads.[42,43] The facets experience high loads in extension and also may impinge on the lamina at high extension. In the study of Kong and associates[44] on the effects of facet angle on the production of spondylolisthesis, the anteroposterior translation across the motion segment increased when the facet joints became more sagittally aligned, thereby suggesting that the disk experiences additional stresses. Under pure compression of the motion segment, intradiskal pressure (IDP) is proportional to the external load. In flexion, relatively large IDP is generated, whereas in pure extension, negative pressures of small magnitude have been predicted. The pressure rise in the nucleus due to torsion in the physiologic range of angular displacement ($< 3°$) is minimal compared to that accompanying axial compression.[41] In flexion, the ligaments are means of load transfer. The role of ligaments in torsion with a compressive preload was minimal for torsional angular displacement $< 3°$. Capsular ligaments experienced large strains in torsion for angular rotations $> 3°$.

Shirazi-Adl[45] has called attention to the vulnerability of the posterolateral portion of the disk. Under simulated loads representing heavy symmetric and nonsymmetric lifts, maximum anulus fiber strain occurred posterolaterally in the innermost annular layer. A progressive failure analysis was applied to a nonsymmetric lifting case with maximum loads of 4,000 N in compression and 400 N in anteriorly directed shear, and applied moments of 40, 25, and 50 N•m in flexion, lateral bending, and torsion, respectively. In the analysis, fiber elements with axial tensile strain exceeding an ultimate value of 16% were removed from the FE mesh to simulate the effects of fiber rupture.

Fiber rupture initiated posterolaterally in the innermost annular layer for compression and shear loads of 3,500 N and 350 N, respectively, at rotations of 10.0°, 6.2°, and 1.8°, respectively, in flexion, lateral bending, and axial rotation. The rupture progressed to the adjacent outer layer under forces and rotations of about 4,000 N, 400 N, 10.8°, 8.5°, and 3.7° in the specified directions. Further (radial) progression of the rupture toward the outer periphery was attained with increased loading up to the maximum loads used in the analysis.

Natarajan and associates[46] developed an iterative scheme to study the initiation and propagation of annular tears and end plate fractures in a three-dimensional (3-D) FE model of an L3–L4 body-disk-body unit. Analysis of the intact model under axial compression revealed that failure occurred first in the end plate (rather than anulus) at the junction of the anulus and end plate in the posterolateral region. Nearly twice the compressive load was required to initiate anulus failure, which then occurred on the inner surface of the anulus in the same region as the end plate failure. Sagittal plane bending moments (flexion and extension) in the presence of axial compressive preload similarly produced initial failure in the end plate.

The role of mechanical factors in producing laminae separation in disks with normal gel-like nucleus (the first sign of degeneration) is not fully understood. The role of interlaminar shear stresses (ILSS) in producing changes in the anulus, which have been overlooked so far in the literature, is crucial. The ILSS alone or in conjunction with other types of stresses, the initial fissures, and the loss of gel-like nucleus may cause delamination and further growth of cracks, hence leading to greater degeneration of the disk and disk herniation. This ILSS-based hypothesis is derived from the observation that high ILSS in a composite engineering structure can lead to failure by delamination.[6] Asymmetry in a composite structure, which may be due to the arrangement of the fibers in the layers or to structural damage, accelerates the delamination process by increasing the ILSS. Viewing the anulus as a composite structure, it is reasonable to expect that the ILSS, in conjunction with other types of stresses and chemical changes, may initiate cracks/laminae separation. Once the cracks appear, the entire disk structure becomes more asymmetric, leading to further degenerative changes due to an increase in ILSS. Goel and associates[6] used a fiber-reinforced concrete element to model the anulus of the detailed FE model of the L3–4 motion segment to predict the ILSS within the disk laminae. In response to a clinically relevant axial compressive load of 413 N, the maximum ILSS for an intact disk was 270 KPa in the posterolateral region; which is consistent with clinical observations that annular tears originate in the posterolateral region of the disk.

Furlong and Palazotto[47] formulated viscoelastic axisymmetric FE models of intact and denucleated disks. Radial stress along the anulus periphery increased with time (Fig. 2, *top*). In other regions, the stress magnitude decreased with time. This change suggests that a chronic, prolonged sitting posture may induce abnormally high stresses, especially if the individual engages in a relatively strenuous activity immediately after the sitting session. These stresses may lead to disk prolapse or to an injury to the soft tissue. In simulations of creep and impact using two-dimensional axisymmetric poroelastic FE models, Simon and associates[48] have shown the fluid phase to have a significant effect on the mechanical response of the disk-body unit. The authors speculated that the predicted relative fluid motion fields were possibly related to nutritional paths to the avascular interior of the disk.

The capability of poroelastic body-disk-body FE models of the disk has been extended to include the effects of osmotic pressure. Laible and associates[49] reasoned that the state of disk hydration depends on the balance between mechanical and osmotic pressures. In contrast to poroelastic-only formulations in which fluid pressure eventually goes to zero (relegating the load-bearing role entirely to the solid phase), the 3-D poroelastic-swelling models predicted that load-bearing by the fluid phase occurred even at equilibrium, with corresponding reductions in solid phase stresses. The analysis further revealed that swelling reduced disk height loss under compression, reversed inward bulging of the inner anulus, and modified disk fluid displacements.

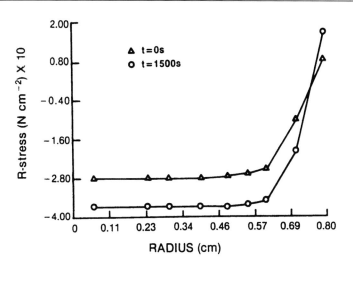

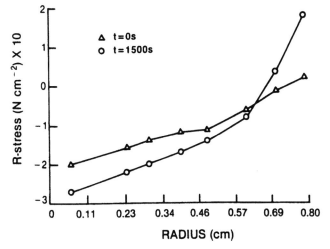

Fig. 2 *Radial stress versus radial distance in the disk of the healthy (**top**), and denucleated (**bottom**) specimen. The two curves in each are the variation in response with time t = 0 and 1,500 s. (Adapted with permission from Furlong DR, Palazotto AN: A finite element analysis of the influence of surgical herniation on the viscoelastic properties of the intervertebral disc. J Biomech 1983;16:785–795.)*

According to Goel and associates,[50] the response of the spine under dynamic loads is frequency dependent. Significant effects on the calculated biomechanical parameters (eg, displacement, disk bulge, intradiskal pressure, and loads transmitted through the facets) were predicted for a ligamentous two-motion segment model of L4–S1 when the frequency of external loading approached the natural frequency of the model in axial mode. Similar results were obtained by Kasra and associates.[51]

Cracks in the Anulus or Herniated Nucleus Pulposus

Experimental Studies

Disks of 20 cadaveric specimens, ranging in age between 14 and 63 years at time of death, were subjected to radial in–out injury, sparing only a peripheral layer 1 mm thick.[6,52] The specimens were subjected to axial loads, while disk contour measurements were taken using a 3-D profilometer. Contour differences between the intact specimens and the injured specimens were studied. In general, as load was increased, there was an increase in radial disk bulge. The creation of an in–out radial fissure also increased the radial disk bulge.

The 3-D motion behavior of intact and injured specimens in flexion, extension, lateral bending, and axial torsion was compared.[53] The experiment was repeated after simulating disk protrusion or herniation, an injury associated with low back pain prior to surgery. The disk herniation was created on the left side posterolaterally (within the vertebral canal) by cutting the left ligamentum flavum and the anulus horizontally. The nucleus pulposus was then gently teased out of the anulus. The teased nucleus was, therefore, not totally separated from its remaining part. The primary motion in flexion showed significant increases. The remaining five components of the motion did not show any significant changes with injury. There were no significant changes in extension. In lateral bending loads, the motion also increased, but at a reduced level of significance. Similar trends were exhibited in the right and left axial torsion modes. No significant increases were observed in the secondary motion components in any of the loading modes.

Analytical Studies

Natarajan and associates[46] studied how three different initial anulus injuries (radiating tear, circumferential tear, and rim lesion) modified the initiation and progression of failure. In the presence of each of these initial injuries, failure started first in the end plate posterolaterally, as it had in the intact case. These findings reinforced the concept that the end plates are the weak link in the body-disk-body unit. Despite some limitations (the posterior elements were not present and the model was linear), the study gave clinically relevant insights into the initiation and propagation of injuries that may lead to disk degeneration and herniation of the nucleus.

Shirazi-Adl,[54] using the FE model of a motion segment with a partially denucleated model (reduced intradiskal pressure as compared to the normal disk), predicted laminae separation following denucleation. Goel and associates[6] found that sequential removal of elements along one of the inner annular layers in the posterolateral region to simulate circumferential injury produced substantial increases in ILSS even for small tears. Elevated shear stresses (maximum: 360 KPa) were observed in the lateral aspect of the disk, on the same side as the injury. Introduction of a posterolateral radial crack increased ILSS beyond intact values, although significant increases did not occur until ≈70% of the annular depth had been compromised. Location of the maximum ILSS was again in the posterolateral region alongside the radial crack. Displacements, disk bulge, and coupled motions increased with injury as expected. Asymmetries in the disk structure brought about by injury (eg, cracks or tears) can produce large interlaminar shear stresses, which suggests that in the presence of the chemical and structural changes in the disk that accompany aging, ILSS may be an important cause of further degeneration through the mechanism of laminae separation. Similar results were obtained from the FE models that simulated disk protrusion phenomena described by Frymoyer[12] (Fig. 3 and Table 1). This change in stresses weakens the disk and will hasten the herniation of the nucleus.

After Surgery

Experimental Studies

Panjabi and associates[55] undertook a detailed 3-D investigation of the mechanical behavior of the lumbar motion segments affected by injuries to the two components of the disk. The sequential injuries considered were cutting a square window (5 × 5 mm) in the anulus on the right posterolateral side lateral to the neural foramen and total removal of the nucleus material. A significant increase in the primary, as well as secondary, coupled motion components with disk injuries was observed for almost all loading modes. However, the disk injuries simulated in the experiment were not realistic. Disk herniations usually occur within the vertebral canal. In this context, Goel and associates[53,56] undertook two clinically relevant biomechanical studies.

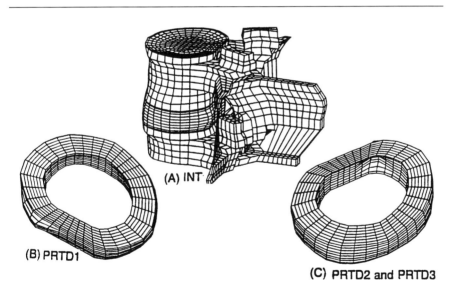

Fig. 3   *Finite element model simulations of the protruded disk shown in Figures 1B and C. In (**A**), the intact finite element model of a ligamentous motion segment–INT. In (**B**), the anulus of the intact model was modified to simulate disk protrusion–PRTD1. In (**C**), a small fissure of increasing depth was created in the protruded region of the anulus to create nucleus movement in posterolateral region–PRTD2 and PRTD3 models. For the sake of clarity the nucleus and other components of the models are not shown.*

Table 1 The predicted changes in biomechanical parameters in the three modified models described in Figure 3

Parameter	Model			
	INT*	PRTD1	PRTD2	PRTD3
Disk Bulge, mm (Posterior)	0.608	0.642	0.639	0.638
Intradiskal Pressure, MPa	0.360	0.358	0.358	0.358
Maximum Axial Interlaminar Shear Stress-ILSS, MPa	0.354	0.355	0.358	0.328

*The corresponding data for the intact model are provided for the sake of comparison; the data correspond to 400 N of axial compressive load

In the first study, they investigated the effects of disk protrusion or hernia-tion, an injury associated with low back pain prior to surgery, on the motion behavior of a spinal motion segment.[53] The second sequential injury was a partial diskectomy. The most significant increase in motion occurred in the flexion mode, followed by axial rotation and lateral bending, for specimens with partial diskectomy. These results, however, differed from those of Pan-jabi and associates[55] with respect to the effect of diskectomy on the second-ary, coupled motions. No significant increases were observed in these com-ponents after injury. This difference may be due to the unusual injury site chosen by Panjabi and associates and the large size of the anulus cut as well as the greater amount of nucleus material removed. In the second study, Goel and associates[56] used whole ligamentous lumbar spine specimens (T12-sacrum) for testing. This enabled them to study the effects of partial and total diskectomies across the involved and adjacent levels. Translational as well as rotational instabilities, although present, were less with partial diskectomy than with total diskectomy at the injury level. The instability above the injury level, however, was always observed, irrespective of the amount of nucleus re-moved.

Spencer and associates[57] used 122 lumbar intervertebral disks from 43 mon-grel dogs to study the effect of chemonucleolysis on the flexion, torsion, and lateral bending flexibilities of the disk (motion segments with posterior ele-ments removed). The dogs were killed 2, 4, 12, 26, and 52 weeks following in-jection with 0.1 to 0.15 ml of either crude collagenase, semipurified collage-nase, or chymopapain. Controls consisted of saline-injected and uninjected disks. Increases in disk flexibility ranging from 1.4 to 5.8-fold were found 2 weeks after injection with all three enzymes. The largest increase in flexion was noted in disks injected with chymopapain. By 3 months, all lateral bending flexibili-ties had returned to the control values. In general, however, flexion and torsion flexibilities did not return to the control values 6 months following chemonucle-olysis. The extent of the gross morphologic changes produced by each of the three enzyme preparations did not correlate with the acute increases in disk flex-ibility.

No explanations based on mechanical grounds could be offered to explain the efficacy of therapeutic intradiskal chymopapain injections. It is believed, how-ever, that the effectiveness of chymopapain injection in relieving pain comes from the decrease in disk bulge that results from the dissolution of the nucleus. The above studies did not document the effect of chymopapain on disk bulge per se.

The effects of the denucleation of a disk on the vibrational behavior of the lumbar spine were investigated in a study conducted on three 8- to 19-kg deeply anesthetized baboons.[58] The bioinstrumented animal was placed in a restraining chair and exposed to vibration in the 0 to 100 Hz range at 0.16 g root mean square acceleration. Once the data were recorded, the nucleus pulposi of the four disks were removed by suction and the experimental protocol was repeated. The removal of the nucleus pulposus increased transmissibility in the highest frequencies (doubled at 80 Hz). A shift toward higher values in the 10 to 30 Hz range was also observed. The acceleration data below 10 Hz were not reported by the authors. It is not yet known if these observations hold for humans.

Analytical Studies

The intact FE model of a lumbar motion segment was modified to investigate the effects of total denucleation of the disk with and without partial laminectomy and facetectomy to mimic an extreme effect of chymopapain injection or microsurgery in which spinal elements other than the disk are damaged the least (CHM) and total diskectomy (TDS) respectively on the kinetics of a ligamentous motion segment.[59-61]

For CHM and TDS models, the axial displacement and flexion–rotation angle were almost double the intact case. The increase in axial displacement was larger for the TDS model compared to the CHM model. The almost twofold decrease in stiffness computed for the injured models was compatible with the clinical observation of a decrease in disk space height following surgery.

In the intact model, the magnitude of bulging under 1,970 N of compressive load was maximum at the anterior location (2.13 mm), followed by the posterior (1.74 mm) and lateral (1.55 mm) locations. The inner wall of the anulus also bulged outward. The complete removal of the nucleus (CHM model) altered the bulging pattern. The posterior bulging (1.34 mm at 1,970 N) was less than the intact model (23% decrease). The innermost layer bulged inward due to the loss of nucleus pressure. The opposing directions of disk bulge for the innermost and outermost layers of the disk in the injured model may induce separation of the anulus layers with time. The disk bulge pattern for the TDS model was similar to that for the CHM model.

The load borne by the facets increased by 80% after denucleation compared to the intact model. The load-sharing mechanism thus was altered, and, as expected, altered the magnitude of other biomechanical parameters as well. The stresses in regions adjacent to the facets increased in comparison to the intact case. Due to the inclusion of posterior elements in the present model, a relatively less compressive load was transferred to the disk because of the increase in facet contact force in the CHM model. As a result, the changes in stresses within the vertebral body with denucleation were less drastic in comparison to the intact case. This finding differs from the published data. In the absence of posterior elements, especially the facets in the models developed by earlier investigators, applied loads were transferred to the disk; therefore, denucleation clearly increased the stress in the cortical bone due to the absence of nucleus pressure. The decrease in disk bulge following denucleation may help relieve pressure on the entrapped nerve roots and may be one of the mechanisms by which the beneficial effects of chymopapain therapy can be explained.

In the TDS model, the load borne by the facets is marginally less than in the intact model. The protective role of the facets thus has been reduced slightly. An expected increase in stress in the vertebral body is supported by the results. The local stresses in the regions adjacent to the facets also increased, although the load borne by the facets marginally decreased because of the decrease in facet contact area following partial excision of the facets. The decrease in the disk bulge in the posterior region may be sufficient to relieve pressure on the entrapped nerve roots.

Bone, as a living tissue, is known to change its shape and material properties with time (Wolff's Law/adaptive bone remodeling). To gain a better understanding of how chronic changes affect the spine (and to move a step closer toward more realistic models), the bone remodeling process recently has been incorporated into detailed FE models of the spine by Goel and associates.[62,63] The partial removal of the nucleus resulted in an extension of the bone margins resembling the osteophytes. Of course, the bone adaptive model prediction cannot explain the reasons why some patients get osteophytes following surgery and others do not.

Furlong and Palazotto[47] formulated viscoelastic axisymmetric finite element models of intact and denucleated disks. Radial stress along the anulus periphery increased with time. In other regions, the stress magnitude decreased with time. The increase in the stress levels, however, was greater for denucleated than healthy disks.

Kasra and associates[51] used the FE model to predict that the first natural frequency of the one motion segment ligamentous lumbar spine (L2–L3) decreased slightly following the removal of facet joints, but partial or complete removal of the disk nucleus significantly decreased the natural frequencies and the segmental stiffness. Under a step load, the stresses and strains throughout the segment increased approximately twofold in comparison with equivalent static values.

Conclusion

Modern imaging techniques and clinical observations have adequately delineated morphologic changes in the spinal structures that take place prior to disk herniation with sciatica/low back pain. Clinical outcomes of various conservative treatment options and surgery, although controversial, are well described in the literature. Mathematical models have provided reasonable estimates of the loads (magnitudes and types) experienced by the ligamentous spine during activities of daily living. The types of loads and activities linked with disk herniation have also been identified through epidemiologic studies. These observations have enabled bioengineers to undertake appropriate studies to address the role of mechanical factors in producing disk herniations and changes in the biomechanics following disk herniation and before and after treatment.

In vitro experimental studies have revealed that it is extremely difficult to produce disk herniations in intact ligamentous spinal segments subjected to loads of various types.[64] The repetitive complex loads (involving flexion, axial twist, lateral bending, and axial compression) can lead to loosening of spinal structures, annular tears, and frank disk herniations. Finite element models of the ligamentous spine, however, have predicted that quasistatic loads induce high stresses/strains in the posterolateral region even in the axial compression mode. Model predictions support end plate fractures. A decrease in the hydrostatic characteristics of the nucleus can lead to laminae separation. The delamination of the anulus layers can also occur in the posterolateral region due to high interlaminar shear stresses. The simulation of cracks in the posterolateral region of the anulus leads to an increase in disk bulge and interlaminar shear stresses. The predicted effects of cyclic loads on the motion segment are pronounced increases in stresses and strain in various structures and in the intradiskal pressure at the resonant frequencies. Simulation of prolonged sitting (creep and viscoelastic effects) through the finite element models reveals that the stresses in the posterolateral region of the disk increase with time. A person may increase chances of disk herniation if he/she attempts to undertake a strenuous activity (eg, lifting) immediately following prolonged sitting. Thus, the experimental and analytical models have been able to explain the role of mechanical factors in producing disk herniations.

From a biomechanical perspective, surgical procedures are effective in reducing pain due to a reduction in disk bulge following surgery. Both diskectomy and chemonucleolysis are effective procedures from a biomechanical point of view. The results also predict a decrease in disk height following surgery. This loss in disk height leads to an increase in the stresses/strains in the pars interarticularis regions, which can lead to spinal stenosis over time. Application of bone adaptive remodeling theories to spine also attest to the clinical observation that osteophytes can occur following disk herniation/surgery.

Acknowledgment

This work was supported in part by a grant from the National Institutes of Health (AR40166-4).

References

1. Goel VK, Weinstein JN (eds): *Biomechanics of the Spine: Clinical and Surgical Perspective*. Boca Raton, FL, CRC Press, 1989.
2. Modic MT, Ross JS: MRI, in Weinstein JN (ed): *Clinical Efficacy and Outcome in the Diagnosis and Treatment of Low Back Pain*. New York, NY, Raven Press, 1992, pp 57–66.
3. Herzog RJ: CT, in Weinstein JN (ed): *Clinical Efficacy and Outcome in the Diagnosis and Treatment of Low Back Pain*. New York, NY, Raven Press, 1992, pp 67–89.
4. Saal JA, Saal JS, Herzog RJ: The natural history of lumbar intervertebral disc extrusions treated nonoperatively. *Spine* 1990;15:683–686.
5. Garfin SR, Ozanne S: Spinal pedicle fixation, in Weinstein JN (ed): *Clinical Efficacy and Outcome in the Diagnosis and Treatment of Low Back Pain*. New York, NY, Raven Press, 1992, pp 137–174.
6. Goel VK, Monroe BT, Gilbertson LG, et al: Interlaminar shear stresses and laminae separation in a disc: Finite element analysis of the L3-L4 motion segment subjected to axial compressive loads. *Spine* 1995;20:689–698.
7. Andersson GBJ: Intervertebral disk: Clinical aspects, in Buckwalter JA, Goldberg VM, Woo SL-Y (eds): *Musculoskeletal Soft-Tissue Aging: Impact on Mobility*. Rosemont, IL, American Academy of Orthopaedic Surgeons, 1993, pp 331–347.

8. Marchand F, Ahmed AM: Investigation of the laminate structure of lumbar disc anulus fibrosus. *Spine* 1990;15:402–410.

9. Pearce RH: Morphologic and chemical aspects of aging, in Buckwalter JA, Goldberg VM, Woo SL-Y (eds): *Musculoskeletal Soft-Tissue Aging: Impact on Mobility.* Rosemont, IL, American Academy of Orthopaedic Surgeons, 1993, pp 363–379.

10. Urban JPG: The effect of physical factors on disk cell metabolism, in Buckwalter JA, Goldberg VM, Woo SL-Y (eds): *Musculoskeletal Soft-Tissue Aging: Impact on Mobility.* Rosemont, IL, American Academy of Orthopaedic Surgeons, 1993, pp 391–412.

11. Kirkaldy-Willis WH (ed): *Managing Low Back Pain,* ed 2. New York, NY, Churchill Livingstone, 1988.

12. Frymoyer JW: Surgical indications for lumbar disc herniation, in Weinstein JN (ed): *Clinical Efficacy and Outcome in the Diagnosis and Treatment of Low Back Pain.* New York, NY, Raven Press, 1992, pp 117–124.

13. Hanley EN Jr: The cost of surgical intervention for lumbar disc herniation, in Weinstein JN (ed): *Clinical Efficacy and Outcome in the Diagnosis and Treatment of Low Back Pain.* New York, NY, Raven Press, 1992, pp 125–133.

14. Andersson GB: Epidemiologic aspects on low-back pain in industry. *Spine* 1981;6:53–60.

15. Chaffin DB, Park KS: A longitudinal study of low-back pain as associated with occupational weight lifting factors. *Am Ind Hyg Assoc J* 1973;34:513– 525.

16. Damkot DK, Pope MH, Lord J, et al: The relationship between work history, work environment and low-back pain in men. *Spine* 1984;9:395–399.

17. Frymoyer JW, Pope MH, Clements JH, et al: Risk factors in low-back pain: An epidemiological survey. *J Bone Joint Surg* 1983;65A:213–218.

18. Kelsey JL, White AA III: Epidemiology and impact of low-back pain. *Spine* 1980;5:133–142.

19. Kelsey JL, Githens PB, White AA III, et al: An epidemiologic study of lifting and twisting on the job and risk for acute prolapsed lumbar intervertebral disc. *J Orthop Res* 1984;2:61–66.

20. Heliovaara M (ed): *Epidemiology of Sciatica and Herniated Lumbar Intervertebral Disc.* Helsinki, Finland, Social Insurance Institution, 1988.

21. Chaffin DB, Andersson G (eds): *Occupational Biomechanics.* New York, NY, John Wiley & Sons, 1984.

22. Wood PHN, Badley EM: Epidemiology of back pain, in Jayson MIV (ed): *The Lumbar Spine and Back Pain,* ed 3. Edinburgh, Scotland, Churchill Livingstone, 1987, pp 1–15.

23. Anderson JAD: Back pain and occupation, in Jayson MIV (ed): *The Lumbar Spine and Back Pain,* ed 3. Edinburgh, Scotland, Churchill Livingstone, 1987, pp 16–36.

24. Kelsey JL, Hardy RJ: Driving of motor vehicles as a risk factor for acute herniated lumbar intervertebral disc. *Am J Epidemiol* 1975;102:63–73.

25. Stokes I, Greenapple DM: Measurement of surface deformation of soft tissue. *J Biomech* 1985;18:1–7.

26. Stokes IA: Surface strain on human intervertebral discs. *J Orthop Res* 1987;5:348–355.

27. Liu YK, Njus G, Buckwalter J, et al: Fatigue response of lumbar intervertebral joints under axial cyclic loading. *Spine* 1983;8:857–865.

28. Farfan HF (ed): *Mechanical Disorders of the Low Back.* Philadelphia, PA, Lea & Febiger, 1973.

29. Liu YK, Goel VK, Dejong A, et al: Torsional fatigue of the lumbar intervertebral joints. *Spine* 1985;10:894–900.

30. Farfan HF, Cossette JW, Robertson GH, et al: The effects of torsion on the lumbar intervertebral joints: The role of torsion in the production of disc degeneration. *J Bone Joint Surg* 1970;52A:468–497.

31. Goel VK, Voo L-M, Weinstein JN, et al: Response of the ligamentous lumbar spine to cyclic bending loads. *Spine* 1988;13:294–300.

32. Adams MA, Hutton WC: Prolapsed intervertebral disc: A hyperflexion injury. *Spine* 1982;7:184–191.
33. Wilder DG, Pope MH, Frymoyer JW: The biomechanics of lumbar disc herniation and the effect of overload and instability. *J Spinal Disord* 1988;1:16–32.
34. Hansson T, Keller T, Holm S: The load on the porcine lumbar spine during seated whole body vibrations. *Orthop Trans* 1988;12:85.
35. Koeller W, Meier W, Hartmann F: Biomechanical properties of human intervertebral discs subjected to axial dynamic compression: A comparison of lumbar and thoracic discs. *Spine* 1984;9:725–733.
36. Kazarian LE: Creep characteristics of the human spinal column. *Orthop Clin North Am* 1975;6:3–18.
37. Hirsch C, Nachemson A: New observations on the mechanical behavior of lumbar discs. *Acta Orthop Scand* 1954;23:254–283.
38. Kazarian L: Dynamic response characteristics of the human vertebral column: An experimental study on human autopsy specimens. *Acta Orthop Scand* 1972;146(suppl):1–186.
39. Virgin WJ: Experimental investigations into the physical properties of the intervertebral disc. *J Bone Joint Surg* 1951;33B:607–611.
40. Twomey L, Taylor J: Flexion creep deformation and hysteresis in the lumbar vertebral column. *Spine* 1982;7:116–122.
41. Goel VK, Gilbertson LG: Applications of the finite element method to thoracolumbar spinal research: Past, present, and future. *Spine* 1995;20:1719–1727.
42. Yang KH, King AI: Mechanism of facet load transmission as a hypothesis for low-back pain. *Spine* 1984;9:557–565.
43. Shirazi-Adl A, Drouin G: Load-bearing role of facets in a lumbar segment under sagittal plane loadings. *J Biomech* 1987;20:601–613.
44. Kong WZ, Goel VK, Weinstein JN: Role of facet morphology in the etiology of degenerative spondylolisthesis in the presence of muscular activity. *Trans Orthop Res Soc* 1995;20:677.
45. Shirazi-Adl A: Strain in fibers of a lumbar disc: Analysis of the role of lifting in producing disc prolapse. *Spine* 1989;14:96–103.
46. Natarajan RN, Ke JH, Andersson GB: A model to study the disc degeneration process. *Spine* 1994;19:259–265.
47. Furlong DR, Palazotto AN: A finite element analysis of the influence of surgical herniation on the viscoelastic properties of the intervertebral disc. *J Biomech* 1983;16:785–795.
48. Simon BR, Wu JS, Carlton MW, et al: Poroelastic dynamic structural models of rhesus spinal motion segments. *Spine* 1985;10:494–507.
49. Laible JP, Pflaster DS, Krag MH, et al: A Poroelastic-swelling finite element model with application to the intervertebral disc. *Spine* 1993;18:659–670.
50. Goel VK, Park H, Kong W: Investigation of vibration characteristics of the ligamentous lumbar spine using the finite element approach. *J Biomech Eng* 1994;116:377–383.
51. Kasra M, Shirazi-Adl A, Drouin G: Dynamics of human lumbar intervertebral joints: Experimental and finite-element investigations. *Spine* 1992;17:93–102.
52. Brinckmann P, Porter RW: A laboratory model of lumbar disc protrusion: Fissure and fragment. *Spine* 1994;19:228–235.
53. Goel VK, Nishiyama K, Weinstein JN, et al: Mechanical properties of lumbar spinal motion segments as affected by partial disc removal. *Spine* 1986;11:1008–1012.
54. Shirazi-Adl A: Finite-element simulation of changes in the fluid content of human lumbar discs: Mechanical and clinical implications. *Spine* 1992;17:206–212.
55. Panjabi MM, Krag MH, Chung TQ: Effects of disc injury on mechanical behavior of the human spine. *Spine* 1984;9:707–713.
56. Goel VK, Goyal S, Clark C, et al: Kinematics of the whole lumbar spine: Effect of discectomy. *Spine* 1985;10:543–554.
57. Spencer DL, Miller JA, Schultz AB: The effects of chemonucleolysis on the mechanical properties of the canine lumbar disc. *Spine* 1985;10:555–561.

303

58. Quandieu P, Pellieux L, Lienhard F, et al: Effects of the Ablation of the nucleus pulposus on the vibrational behavior of the lumbosacral hinge. *J Biomech* 1983;16:777–784.
59. Kim YE, Goel VK, Weinstein J: The role of facets in denucleated discs: An analytical biomechanical study. *Trans Orthop Res Soc* 1988;13:330.
60. Kim YE: *An Analytical Investigation of Ligamentous Lumbar Spine Mechanics.* Iowa City, Iowa, University of Iowa, 1988. Dissertation.
61. Goel VK, Kim YE: Effects of injury on the spinal motion segment mechanics in the axial compression mode. *Clin Biomech* 1989;4:161–167.
62. Seenivasan G, Goel VK: Applying bone adaptive remodelling theory to ligamentous spine: Preliminary results of partial neucleotomy and stabilization. *IEEE Eng Med & Biol* 1994;13:508–516.
63. Goel VK, Weinstein JN, Gilbertson LG: Biomechanics of thoraco-lumbar spine stabilization, in Wiesel S (ed): *The Lumbar Spine*, ed 2. Philadelphia, PA, WB Saunders, 1996.
64. Adams MA, Dolan P: Recent advances in lumbar spinal mechanics and their clinical significance. *Clin Biomech* 1995;10:3–19.

Directions for Future Research

Differentiate between the anatomic, topographic, and temporal aspects of peripheral nerve, dorsal root ganglion, and dorsal root injuries.

To date, much of the nerve injury research has been performed using peripheral nerves. It is currently uncertain whether the data from this work can be extrapolated to the pathophysiologic mechanisms that underlie herniated nucleus pulposus (HNP) causing radiculopathy. The approach would be to apply the experimental procedures that were used with peripheral nerves to study dorsal root ganglion (DRG) and nerve roots. Methodologies should include electrophysiologic, biomechanical, biochemical, and histologic approaches.

Describe the biomechanics of the nerve root following herniation of the nucleus pulposus and the impact of herniation on sensory neurons.

Disk herniation usually occurs in the posterolateral direction and, therefore, is likely to impinge on the nerve root. Herniation displaces the nerve root, setting up compressive, tensile, and shear forces that ultimately impact on neurons (soma and/or axon).

It is possible to simulate force transmission based on realistic knowledge of the mechanical properties of the root, its geometry, and its anchoring. We need to know whether mechanical stresses act locally on axons (eg, at the site of herniation) or at a distance (in the DRG, or distal to it). This action can be predicted theoretically and confirmed by biopsy or pathology in appropriate models.

Also, we need to know if these stresses change with time after the herniation event, eg, due to viscoelastic properties of the tissues involved. What counts ultimately is the response of the neuron. Normal and/or shearing mechanical stresses and strains may impact at the level of the neuron in some of the following ways: by direct mechanical impact on the axon or soma; by direct impact on the Schwann cell/myelin sheath and only secondarily on the neuron; on the level of vascular flow, resulting in ischemic damage to the neuron or the myelin sheath; by stasis of endoneurial fluid; and on other nonneural cells or processes that release chemical mediators, which only secondarily affect the neuron. These possible mechanisms may require new, complex model systems.

To understand the mechanisms and their effect on the various forces and displacements on nerves, the following research would be valuable: (1) Determine how tissue displacement due to disk herniation results in increased forces (and stresses and strains) at the level of the nerve root and at the level of the individual axon. (2) Locate the stress and strain fields produced in the nerve root throughout its length, identifying the locations with the highest stress/strain. For example, determine whether longitudinal forces affect the DRG and spinal nerve. (3) Find how the stress and strain fields are altered over time as a result of the viscoelastic properties of the nerve root tissue. (4) Determine whether the axon, neuron, Schwann cell, and/or myelin sheath are affected directly by the altered stress/strain field, or only secondarily after direct mechanical impact on vascular flow, on the movement of endoneurial fluid, or on nonneural cells that release various mediator molecules involved in the production of inflammation/pain. Multidisciplinary studies are required to define the biomechanical state of the spinal tissues and the resulting biochemical and neurologic changes.

Study the pathologic effects of herniated nucleus pulposus in human nerve root, DRG, and spinal and peripheral nerves and their relation to pain.

The site of insult and pathologic effects of symptomatic HNP in humans is not established. The problem is due, in part, to the difficulty in obtaining human tissues, which generally are inaccessible premortem. This lack of human data impedes the ability to develop and validate models of HNP and impairs advances in treatment. Human necropsy studies can be used to correlate sites and magnitude of neural compression with presence or absence of premortem symptoms.

To define the structural changes associated with symptomatic injury to neural structures, it is suggested that autopsy specimens from individuals suffering radicular pain be evaluated histologically and correlated with the patient's history and premortem radiographic studies. These data, in turn, should be correlated with experimental models of neural injury and pain to aid in the development and validation of animal models. It is further suggested that premortem peripheral nerve biopsy, when feasible, may clarify the nature of the axonal injury induced by HNP. Human tissue samples may also be obtained at surgery to investigate possible pathologic changes at the interface between the HNP and the nerve root.

Further establish animal models that mimic the clinical phenomenon of disk herniation and radiculopathy.

Establishing the relevance of animal models to the human circumstance is critical to interpretation of results from animal experiments aimed at developing knowledge about mechanisms and treatment. This requires a better understanding of the consequences in humans of HNP whether or not it is followed by pain. Few, if any, psychophysical sensory studies in humans have been done. This lack of data is relevant to current animal models that, for the most part, are used to measure responses to thermal and/or mechanical stimuli to estimate the magnitude of hyperalgesia that develops after some experimental manipulation. Investigations should be undertaken to determine if there is evidence of either mechanical or thermal hyperalgesia in humans after HNP that is acutely associated with pain. If so, the hyperalgesia distribution should be studied in the affected root and outside of that area.

Determine the role of cytokines and other inflammatory mediators in animal models of radiculopathy.

Specific cytokines have been shown to be increased in both the peripheral nerve and spinal cord following pain-provoking peripheral nerve injury in animal models. Cytokines and other inflammatory mediators released from HNP can directly produce behaviors that are suggestive of neurogenic pain.

Future research should include use of immunohistochemical and in situ hybridization to localize various cytokines (eg, tumor necrosis factors, interleukins, transforming growth factors) in the DRG and spinal cord following dorsal root injuries. Furthermore, potential pharmacologic potentiation and/or attenuation of pain behaviors in nerve root injury animal models could be studied using specific cytokines or their inhibitors.

The technical difficulties inherent in producing nerve root injury animal models may be an obstacle to this research. Therefore, some basic experiments involving immunologic variables could be performed on the peripheral nervous system distal to the DRG. Results from these studies would then be compared with data obtained following dorsal root injuries. This type of comparison would provide a unique opportunity to address a fundamental basic science question as well as to gain a better understanding of pain following HNP.

Study the role of changes in the endoneurial environment in neuropathic pain.

The endoneurial environment influences the function of peripheral nerve fibers and is significantly altered in injured nerves associated with neuropathic pain states. It is suggested that a better understanding of the characteristics of the endoneurial environment in injured nerves will provide insights into the pathogenesis of neuropathic pain.

Edema, which is an early finding in nerve injuries, is associated with mast cell degranulation in which vasoactive compounds and cytokines are released. This release is followed by invasion of monocytes and other immune cells into the endoneurial environment. These cells further alter the environment through release of additional cytokines and other factors that lead to changes in the production of neurotrophins and their receptor concentrations in Schwann cells. Edema also increases the level of endoneurial fluid pressure, and this increase has been shown to cause nerve ischemia.

Future research might focus on determining the relationship of these variables to pain behaviors and exploring the role of therapies that influence the integrity of the endoneurial environment and the rate and quantity of demyelination and axonal degeneration and regeneration.

Characterize the changes triggered by HNP in the sensory cell body or its axon that render them electrically hyperexcitable.

Injured neurons may become hyperexcitable to mechanical, chemical, and metabolic events and substances normally present in the lower back, or generated following disk herniation. The resulting ectopic impulse discharge is probably an important substrate of back pain. To understand hyperexcitability, it is important to distinguish between the ability of neurons to be electrically excited, which depends on a single process (the Hodgkin-Huxley model), and events and substances capable of exciting already excitable neurons, of which there are very many (displacement, inflammatory mediators, peptides, etc). The electrical excitability process is the final common pathway for painful irritants and may be a good target for therapeutic intervention. Excitability depends on voltage, ligand, and mechanically gated ion channels in the neuronal membrane. We must learn how disk herniation causes the synthesis, local distribution and/or gating properties of these proteins to change, thereby rendering the neuron hyperexcitable. Prime targets for this investigation are sodium channels and mechanosensitive channels. Pharmacologic blockers of these channels should suppress the hyperexcitability and hence the neuronal firing and the pain.

Examine the changes in excitability of spinal neurons produced by manipulations of the DRG and dorsal root that contribute to radiculopathy.

All experimental models of peripheral nerve injury have been associated with changes in the excitability of spinal neurons, which is called "central sensitization." Central sensitization may be evoked by sustained nociceptor input (ie, is activity-dependent) and probably activates spinal N-methyl-D-aspartate glutamate receptors.

Study the contributions to central sensitization from DRG cells and afferent inputs from the spinal dorsal root. Electrophysiologic, pharmacologic, and molecular biological strategies currently available should be used to determine which DRG cells/axons contribute to activity-dependent changes in the spinal cord and to determine the neurotransmitter(s)/receptors involved.

Define the role of deafferentation in the pathogenesis of the radicular pain caused by HNP.

The mechanisms that underlie the radicular pain caused by HNP are not known. Compression of neural tissue by HNP may be associated with changes in neuronal structure and function outside the central neuroaxis that may give rise to pain. Central processes also may be involved in the pathogenesis of the radicular pain caused by HNP. Studies in animal models have demonstrated that neuronal injury at the level of the dorsal root, DRG, and peripheral nerve leads to anatomic, physiologic, and neurochemical changes within the spinal cord. Compression and disruption of dorsal root fibers by HNP, with subsequent deafferentation of the spinal cord dorsal horn, may contribute to the pathogenesis of pain of HNP by producing central deafferentation pain. Whether HNP causes deafferentation pain, and the role of deafferentation pain in the pathogenesis of the radicular pain of HNP, are not known, nor are the relative roles of central and peripheral processes in the production of radicular pain by HNP.

These issues need to be studied in animal models because the tissues and structures of interest are not readily accessible for studies in humans. Understanding the role of central mechanisms in the pathogenesis of pain caused by HNP is important because the management of deafferentation pain differs from management of other types of pain, and involvement of central nervous system processes raises the possibility of central modulation of pain caused by HNP.

Study the perception of lumbar radiculopathy or low back pain within the central nervous system.

An understanding of manifestations of low back pain and radiculopathy within the central nervous system would be useful. Because pain is a conscious perception, which has sensory-anatomic, affective, and cognitive components, it would seem important to consider the cerebral manifestations of pain in these conditions. A relatively new technology, positron emission tomography (PET), has potential use as a tool for further understanding of the pathogenesis of radicular pain and back pain within the central nervous system. This is especially important when considering that subjective pain is often the only clinical manifestation of these conditions.

Evaluate the cortical and thalamic representation of pain before and after surgery in a population experiencing lumbar radiculopathy and in an age-matched control population. Determine whether a radiculopathy group demonstrates increased blood flow in the area of the anterior cingulate gyrus when receiving the same painful stimulus as a normal group. Also evaluate a narcotic and a nonsteroidal anti-inflammatory agent for their effects on the normal population as well as the group experiencing radiculopathy.

The postoperative scan could conceivably be closer to the preoperative scan than to that of the normal control, possibly reflecting a residual emotion-based heightened awareness to pain. The effect of narcotics should be similar in both groups. A decrease in blood flow to the anterior cingulate gyrus would be expected because there are natural opioid receptors in this region. The subject group will probably still have a relative increase in blood flow to the anterior cingulate gyrus when compared to controls.

Evaluate the contribution of descending modulatory influences.

The altered behaviors (eg, hyperalgesia) that characterize animal models of radiculopathy can arise from a variety of influences, including alterations in the "tone" of modulatory symptoms descending from the brain stem, spinal cord influences on the excitability of spinal dorsal horn neurons, and spinal nociception.

Study the contributions of descending noradrenergic, serotonergic, GABAergic, and nonnociceptive reflexes. Electrophysiologic, pharmacologic, molecular, biologic, and behavioral methods should be used to determine the extent to which neuropathic pain input to the central nervous system alters bulbospinal modulatory pathways that, in turn, influence the activity and responsiveness of spinal neurons that initially receive the neuropathic input.

Section Three

Epidemiologic and Clinical Issues of Idiopathic Low Back Pain

Section Editor:
Edward N. Hanley, Jr, MD

Michele Crites Battié, PhD
Nikolai Bogduk, MD, PhD, BSc
Stephen L. Gordon, PhD
Harry N. Herkowitz, MD
Richard J. Herzog, MD
Richard L. Lieber, PhD
Manohar M. Panjabi, PhD
Malcolm H. Pope, Dr Med Sci, PhD

Jan K. Richardson, PT, PhD, OCS
Paul G. Shekelle, MD, PhD
Kanwaldeep S. Sidhu, MD
Tapio Videman, MD, Dr Med Sci

Overview

Low back pain of unknown etiology is extremely common in the adult population throughout the world. It has been suggested that this condition may be merely the consequence of normal aging of the spine and not a disease process or injury. Severity and disability vary greatly between different cultures and regions, although the incidence of back pain remains reasonably stable. Although three quarters of the adult population experience low back pain at some time, epidemiologic studies on this problem have been difficult to undertake because of difficulty in defining the amount of pain individuals have, the outcome of back pain episodes, the influence of various cultures and environments, and many other confounding factors. The underlying cause or causes of idiopathic low back pain remains an enigma. A major question is whether or not observed anatomic findings are pain-producing pathology or nonpain-producing degenerative change.

Some risk factors for the development of back pain have been defined. Most agree that evidence points to a multifactorial etiology. A history of prior low back pain is probably the most implicated risk factor for subsequent episodes of idiopathic low back pain. Physical loading may be a source of injury in primary back pain or it may exacerbate back pain or cause recurrent episodes in those individuals with a predisposition. Other factors that have been implicated are prolonged exposure to whole body vibration, impaired fibrinolysis, smoking, psychosocial problems, and job dissatisfaction.

Occupational practices and exposure may have some influence on back pain incidence and disability. It has been noted that individuals whose work involves heavy lifting have a higher incidence of back pain than sitting workers. Among individuals engaged in compensable work situations in the United States, 2% per year will file a claim for a low back pain incident. Of all injuries in the workplace, approximately 21% relate to the lumbar spine, and these account for 33% of costs. A small percentage (10% to 25%) of individuals affected account for the vast majority of cost. Of total cost, medical costs are approximately one third and disability payments an additional two thirds. There has been an attempt to develop preventive measures in the workplace by ergonomic studies and adaptation of workplace environments. These efforts have met with mixed success. It has been suggested that better efforts need to be undertaken by cooperation between the medical profession, workers, and management teams.

The role of skeletal muscle in the causation or exacerbation of low back pain remains controversial. Available evidence indicates that pain from the muscle is mediated through type III sensory nerves within the two major muscle groups of the spine: the erector spinae and the multifidi. Scientific studies indicate that pain of muscle origin originates from an injury and may be exacerbated by inflammation, ischemia, pressure, and persistent contraction. Whether or not muscle is a source of primary idiopathic low back pain remains controversial. The role of muscle in exacerbation of back pain caused by other noxious stimuli is yet to be defined.

Biomechanical issues in idiopathic low back pain are also a source of controversy. The role of "instability" or "insufficiency" in low back pain disorders remains to be confirmed. An untested definition of clinical instability has been proposed: "loss of ability of the spine under physiologic loads to maintain its pattern of displacement so that there is no neurologic deficit or pain." A "spine stabilizing system" has been proposed to explain the interactions between the spinal column and the muscles that surround and support it and are controlled through a central mechanism. This system may serve to explain compensatory mechanisms after injury or degeneration, with a breakdown in this system subjecting some individuals to more pain and disability.

Imaging studies have advanced greatly during the last decade. Magnetic resonance imaging appears to be the diagnostic imaging study of choice for disk degeneration, muscle changes, and neurologic problems within the lumbar spine. Most attention has been placed on the imaging patterns noted in aging and degenerated disks, with controversy over how to determine the difference between these two entities. Magnetic resonance imaging continues to be an evolving technology. Needs in this area are to determine what is normal and what is abnormal; to develop sensitivity, specificity, and accuracy data for use of these tests; and to correlate imaging findings with symptoms and outcomes of treatment.

Similar difficulties occur in the assessment of the clinical utility of various injection techniques for idiopathic back pain. It is generally agreed that these techniques can be useful to provoke or block pain, but the clinical implications of these tests and treatments remain difficult to define. It appears that injection techniques are useful for diagnosis and treatment of lumbar facet conditions, afflictions of the sacroiliac joint, and for isolated nerve root problems. Diskography remains controversial but is generally agreed upon as a reasonable test when morphologic abnormalities are correlated with pain provocation on injection. Radiofrequency neurotomy is controversial.

Exercises, patient education, and other means of physical therapy remain commonplace in the nonsurgical treatment of idiopathic low back pain conditions. Objective justification for their use, however, is difficult to find. There apparently is some evidence that thermal, electrical, and mechanical modalities may be of some benefit, but this benefit has been difficult to prove in a clinical setting due to the wide variety and overlap of treatments used for individuals with low back pain. Similar problems have been encountered with various exercise/conditioning programs. Although there is reasonable evidence that chronic low back pain is improved by physical therapy measures, data are lacking for the acute situation.

Spinal manipulation data indicate that it is helpful for acute low back pain but not proven efficacious for chronic low back pain conditions. Medications are frequently used for the treatment of low back pain conditions. There is reasonable evidence that nonnarcotic medication is helpful for pain control, but it is difficult to differentiate the beneficial effects of acetaminophen from those of nonsteroidal anti-inflammatory medications. Narcotics may be helpful in acute pain control but their use is associated with bothersome or serious side effects. Similar but less severe problems have been encountered with the use of "muscle relaxants."

Perhaps the most controversial area in the discussion of idiopathic low back pain is that of surgical intervention. Although it is commonly used, indications for spinal surgery (fusion) and the results of the procedure remain vague. A wide variety of outcomes has been reported, ranging from less than 30% success to 100% success. Most reports indicate surgical success in the 40% to 60% range, which is much less than that for herniated disk surgery or spinal stenosis surgery. Magnetic resonance imaging changes do not appear to be helpful in selecting patients for a procedure. Diskography may be more diagnostic of a "painful annular tear," but most individuals agree that the concept of an isolated "pain generator" is simplistic because many factors may be involved in the production of pain and its continuance. Additionally, it is difficult to compare the outcome of surgical interventions when the natural history of this problem is not delineated. Surgical treatment for this condition, when employed, consists of arthrodesis of the spine. Many argue this is a nonphysiologic treatment and most agree that the best technique is unknown. Should the surgery be anterior alone, posterior alone, or a combination of both? What is the role of instrumentation? If employed, surgery probably should be offered only to individuals with prolonged disability, true functional incapacity, and no confounding psychosocial problems.

Chapter 20

A Critical Review of the Epidemiology of Idiopathic Low Back Pain

Tapio Videman, MD, Dr Med Sci
Michele Crites Battié, PhD

Introduction

Whether it is measured in terms of related doctor visits,[1] industrial injury claims,[2] disability pensions,[3] or prevalence of symptom complaints in the general population, back pain is one of the most common and costly musculoskeletal problems facing the developed countries of the world. During a half century when medical advances have been made in understanding and managing many health problems, common back pain has continued to be an enigma of growing consequence.

The steady decrease in heavy physical work demands and the rise in leisure time exercise activities[4] might have been expected to have had beneficial effects on the problem. Yet back-related work absenteeism and disability awards have increased manyfold.[5] Concurrently, there appears to have been a dramatic shift in public perception of back pain as an "injury" or medical problem, and of its effect on work life in terms of disability.[6] The dramatic increase in back pain disability, despite the generally positive development in environmental exposures and no clear evidence of a concomitant increase in spinal morbidity, accentuates the puzzling development of this problem and the inadequacy of a biomedical model in formulating a solution. Although the role of the physical environment should not be ignored, the growing problem of disability from idiopathic low back pain suggests a need for a broadened perspective on underlying conditions and risk factors that goes beyond an examination of pathophysiologic conditions and includes the effects of sociocultural, legislative, and medical management factors.[3,5-9]

Epidemiologic studies have been conducted in an effort to identify risk factors and gain insights into the conditions underlying idiopathic low back pain. Although most of the studies have focused on individual physical factors and occupational physical demands, it is becoming common to consider a broader scope of potentially influential factors. Epidemiologic studies have faced significant challenges, however, that continue to limit their value. Among the greatest challenges are difficulties in defining the pain experience or outcome. As Miettinen[10] has cautioned, epidemiologic studies of ill-defined conditions are of limited value, and inferences to pathology can be misleading. Inadequate measures of environmental exposures and inadequate control of potentially confounding factors are problematic as well.

Defining Idiopathic Low Back Pain

Defining the problem is a critical yet muddy issue because of the myriad of symptom complaints that compose idiopathic low back pain. There is tremendous variability in how the presence and severity of back pain are identified and measured. Failure to distinguish between different back-related outcomes, such as acute and chronic back symptom complaints, industrial injury claims, back-related absenteeism, and disability pensions, all of which are predominantly related to idiopathic low back pain, may lead to further confusion and false conclusions.

Back pain is identified through numerous reporting systems, including population health surveys and symptom complaints recorded in clinical and workplace settings. The associated incidence rates vary considerably, depending on how back pain is defined.[11] Even in the case of fairly "hard" outcomes, such as industrial back injury claims and related absenteeism data, the figures result from such a complex chain of events that the occurrence of back pain incidents registered in the industrial setting cannot be equated to the occurrence of morbidity.[12] In other words, back-related absenteeism and disability pensions depend only in part on "morbidity" and back symptoms and depend to a major degree on social security legislation and cultural, psychosocial, and medical management factors.[13-23]

Idiopathic low back pain is identified by a complaint, which is an active behavior and can be influenced by a variety of factors other than pain and physical pathology. Although defining and quantifying pain will continue to be problematic, the development of standardized, validated outcome questionnaires has enhanced the investigation of idiopathic low back pain.[24]

Our limitation in understanding the condition is obvious by the inconsistencies in diagnoses for idiopathic low back pain. The diagnostic terms for such conditions are more closely associated with the specialty and training of the clinician than with the symptoms of the patients. Clear diagnoses are reserved for known diseases in which associated understanding of the underlying pathology provides information on prognosis and is a prerequisite for developing rationally based treatment. As long as common back pain remains a complaint in search of a disease, progress in prevention and medical management will be limited.

Although it is likely that there are several different conditions underlying it, in this chapter idiopathic low back pain is defined as all back symptoms for which the underlying pathophysiology is unknown.

Occurrence Rates

It is commonly concluded that approximately 75% of the population suffer from back problems at some time during their lives. In most studies the subjects have been asked if they have ever had back pain; the severity and the extent of the associated disability are often unknown. Reported lifetime incidences for back pain have varied in past decades from about 40% to more than 80%, with a trend toward higher percentages in the more recent studies than in studies from the fifties and sixties.[25-32] Lifetime incidences higher than 50% could be viewed as representing a "normal" phenomenon. Conversely, a lifetime incidence of 1% for a serious health condition is usually defined as a public health problem. Differentiating severe, disabling back pain conditions from transient feelings of discomfort could be important in investigating occurrence rates of idiopathic low back pain.

A few studies have demonstrated a decrease in the cumulative lifetime incidence of back pain around 60 years of age;[33] this decrease contradicts the definition of cumulative incidence. The causes for such findings are unclear, although it is possible to speculate. There is no obvious reason to believe that the decrease in the cumulative incidence is an age-cohort effect in which the earlier-born group would have less back pain than those born later. It is more likely that as people age they are more apt to forget back pain experiences, particularly when other morbidity becomes more dominant, and there is some evidence to support this theory.[34] In addition, selection may play a role: people with longer lifespans are healthier and may also have had less back pain, thereby decreasing the lifetime incidence in older age groups. Most likely, the explanation is a combination of increased forgetfulness of pain episodes with aging, selection, and decreased physical activity/loading, if we assume that physical loading during working years influences back pain experiences.

Natural History

Idiopathic low back pain is commonly believed to be a fairly benign, self-limited condition with recovery from symptoms occurring in several days or weeks from the time of onset in the vast majority of individuals.[35] Most can, however, expect to have a recurrent episode.[36-38] Recent studies of the natural history of back pain have suggested that in addition to its typically recurrent nature, persistent back pain occurs more often than previously believed.[39] The variations in the descriptions of the natural history may depend on the length of follow-up and the types of outcome measures used.

Suspected Risk Factors

In a review article, Hildebrandt[40] found 24 work-related and 55 individual factors that had been reported by at least one source as associated with low back pain (Table 1). Most of the work factors were variations of physical loading related to work tasks and the environment, as well as accident-related trauma (Table 2, Fig. 1).[41-55] Despite a few additions, such as impaired fibrinolysis, smoking, and job dissatisfaction, to the list of suspected risk factors over the past decade or so, few new ideas have surfaced to help explain the occurrence of back symptoms. Collectively, the work-related and individual factors studied explain little of the uncertainty in predicting back symptom reports and injury complaints. In a prospective, longitudinal study of back problems in more than 3,000 manufacturing workers in the United States, data on more than 50 commonly suspected risk factors explained less than 10% of the uncertainty in predicting who would or would not file industrial back pain complaints.[36]

Most studies of suspected risk factors have been retrospective or cross-sectional and are often prone to bias as well as presenting the ''chicken and egg''

Table 1 Back-related outcomes and their suspected risk factors

Outcome	Suspected Risk Factor
Degenerative changes in the disk and vertebra	Heavy physical loading, injuries, vibration, infections, smoking, and genetics
Reported symptoms	Personality and psychological stress*
Industrial injury claims	Work environment (job satisfaction)*
Disability due to low back pain	Neurologic and psychological (fear-avoidance) medical management factors
Absenteeism and pensions	Level of social security, employment/situation, and cultural factors*

*Besides all earlier (above) mentioned suspected risk factors

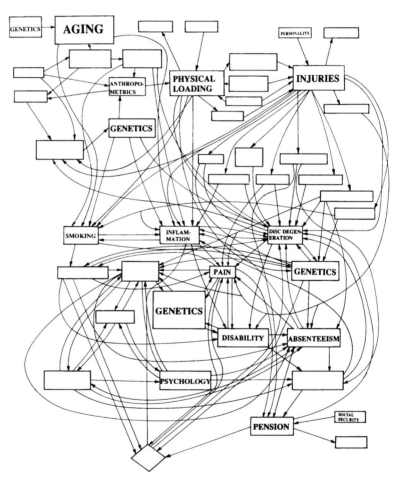

Fig. 1 *An abstract etiopathogenetic diagram of idiopathic low back pain that demonstrates the complexity of interrelationship of factors influencing back symptoms.*

dilemma. Prospective, longitudinal studies, which investigate factors measured at baseline as predictors of future back problems, typically provide a superior design with fewer difficulties in interpretation of results. More than a half dozen such studies have been conducted to identify predictors of back symptoms identified from health surveys.[16,25,26,55-59] The symptoms revealed from these surveys did not necessarily result in medical visits, filing of incident reports at the workplace, or time loss from work. These studies consistently find a history of back symptoms to be an indicator of future risk. Other clear risk indicators were comorbidities, particularly other types of symptoms/complaints, measures of psychological distress, and lower socioeconomic status, which is likely to be a marker for a variety of potential risk factors. Other factors associated to a lesser degree are greater age, smoking, chronic coughing, heavy occupational physical demands, and in nurses, poor patient handling skills. Although patient handling skill was associated with sudden-onset back pain in nurses, it was not associated with symptoms of gradual onset, which were more common.[55] Despite the number of associations identified, only small differences exist in risk of low back pain between various groups.[25] Therefore, it can be stated that everybody is at high risk, although some groups still have a risk above the high normal.

A number of prospective studies have been done to specifically investigate back pain reports and injury claims in the workplace.[11,17,36,41-44,46,52,55,60-63] These complaints are not solicited, as in the case of the survey studies; instead, they depend on persons actively coming forward to register a report of their problem. Most of the studies of work-related back pain reports focus on individual physical and workplace factors.[46,61,62] Higher fitness levels, defined as a composite score of aerobic capacity, strength, and flexibility measures, were associated with a lower incidence of back injury claims in firefighters.[61] Such an association was not found, however, in a large study of aircraft manufacturing workers who had less extreme occupational physical demands.[41-43] Other studies of lifting strength and general fitness parameters have found them to be poor predictors of subsequent back injury reports.[52,62,63] One exception is an early study by Chaffin and Park[46] in which a weak association was found between inadequate strength to meet specific job demands, as determined from isometric strength testing, and back pain reporting. However, strength in excess of job requirements did not appear to have an additional protective effect.[46]

A large study conducted among aircraft manufacturing workers was the first prospective, longitudinal study of work-related back pain reports to include psychosocial factors as possible predictors. Other than having current or recent back problems at the onset of the study, the strongest predictors of future reports were negative perceptions of the workplace, including low job task enjoyment and social support, and emotional distress.[17,36] These findings underline the complex nature of back pain reporting in industry. An extension of the same study of aircraft manufacturing workers investigated predictors of extended disability (work loss of greater than one month).[60] The only factors that were significantly associated with extended time loss and differed significantly between claims of short and long time loss were a low score on scale 10 of the Minnesota Multiphasic Personality Inventory (MMPI), indicating extroversion, and back pain elicited on straight leg raising, which was identified at the time of the baseline examination prior to filing the back injury claim. Although these factors were associated with subsequent back injury claims of extended time loss

Table 2 Back symptoms on health survey: Results of a prospective, longitudinal study

Study Subjects*

Factors Considered	Danish Male Employees Varied Occupations[25] (5,249/?)† 1 year	English Employees Varied Occupations[56] (2,891/?)† 1 year	Copenhagen Residents[16] (928/1,136)† 1 year		Finnish 1st-year Nurses[55] (255/255)† 1 year		Swedish Military Conscripts[26] (999/6,824)§ 2-3 years	Finnish Metal Industry Workers[37] (902/2,653)¶ 10 years	Newly Graduated Nurses[58] (179/?)** 1-1/2 years	French Commercial Travelers[59] (627/?)† 1 year
			1st episode	recurrent LBP	sudden onset	gradual onset				
Demographic										
Gender (female)	↑	↑††	↓	↑					↑	0
Age	↑		0	0				0	↑	0
Education	↓		0	0						
Living alone/divorced										
Social status	↓↑		↓	↓ (men)						0
Lifestyle										
Smoking	↓	↑ (women)	↑	↑			↑	0		
Alcohol consumption	0		0	0						
Leisure time physical activity	↓↑							↓ (men)		
Sport participation	↑									
"Psychic stress"/problems	↑									↑
Work Related										
Job classification			0	0				0		
Physical demands rating	↑↑		0	0	↑↑	0			0	0
Physical exertion					↓↓	0				
Patients' handling skill										
Patients' handling training									0	
Driving (10-12 hrs/wk)										↑
Uncomfortable car seat										↑
Social support/job satisfaction	↑		↓	0						
"Psychic stress" at work								↑ (women)		
Anthropometric										
Standing height	↑, > 181 cm	0	0	0	0	0	↑ (extremes)			
Obesity (relative weight)	0	0	0	0	0	0		0		

Leg length inequality			0		0
Scoliosis					0
Strength/endurance					
Isometric strength	0†	0 (men)	↓ (women)	0	0
Isometric back endurance		↓ (men)	0	0	0
Sit-up test	0†	0	↓ (women)	0	→
Psychophysical strength	0†				0
Aerobic capacity		0			
Flexibility					
Flexion/lateral bending	0†	↑ (men)	0	0	
Extension	0†	0		0	
Length of hamstrings		0	↓ (women)	0	
Psychometric					
Health locus of control				0	
Personality inventory (MHQ, MMPI)§§				0	
Anxiety				↑ 0	0
Hysteria				0 ↑↑	↑↑
IQ test				0	
Medical History					
Back pain history	↑↑	↑	↑↑		↑↑
Non-back symptom complaints			↑		↑↑
Health care utilization (for pain)	↑ (men)	↑ (men)			
Respiratory symptoms/↓ function	↑				↑↑

* ↑ = a positive association; ↓ = a negative association; ↑↑ = a strong positive association; ↓↓ = a strong negative association; 0 = not a predictor
† No. of volunteers/no. solicited, 1-year follow-up
§ No. of volunteers/no. solicited, 2- to 3-year follow-up
¶ No. of volunteers/no. solicited, 10-year follow-up
** No. of volunteers/no. solicited, 1.5-year follow-up
†† Troup and associates[56] found that the use of a test battery including all of these factors slightly enhanced the predictive value of subjects' history of low back pain
§§ MHQ = Middlesex Hospital Questionnaire; MMPI = Minnesota Multiphasic Personality Inventory

323

from work, they were poor predictors and are unlikely to be of any practical value in this regard.

Many epidemiologic studies have used statistics, such as *p*-values and risk ratios, to describe the effects of suspected risk factors. These statistics alone can be misleading in guiding prevention strategies. The *p*-values depend in part on the size of the study population, and a highly significant *p*-value can represent a very small effect that is of little or no practical significance. An additional strategy that has been used to put effect sizes in perspective is to estimate the variability in the outcome of interest that is explained by the suspected risk factor. For example, in the Boeing Study, job task enjoyment was a highly statistically significant predictor of industrial back injury claims; however, it explained less than 3% of the variability in whether someone would or would not file a back pain report.[17,36] This suggests that even if job task enjoyment, as defined in the study, was to be altered, it would be unlikely to have a major effect on industrial back pain reporting.

Associations of Loading, Spine Pathology, and Back Pain

Based on epidemiologic evidence, physical activity generally increases until the age of 20 to 30 years and thereafter decreases slowly. The curve for the incidence of back pain has a similar shape, except that it reaches its highest point 20 to 30 years later. The first signs of degenerative changes are visible before the age of 20 years, thereafter they increase steadily with age, although there is great variation between individuals (Fig. 2).[64,65] Many studies have shown that heavy physical loading and extreme positions are associated with a higher incidence of back symptoms,[27,28,30,32,54,55] but there are also studies in which this association has been unclear.[16,29,31,47,49] Linton[66] found an association between pain and general activity, but not between pain intensity and activity. Results from functional restoration rehabilitation programs have demonstrated little or no change in pain experienced with increased physical performance.[67] In an autopsy study, in which family members recalled severe back pain and workload histories, there was a linear association between severe back pain and heaviness

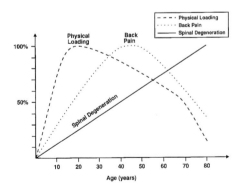

Fig. 2   *The lifetime changes of physical loading, back pain, and spine degeneration.*

of work after controlling for spine pathology.[68] Whether physical loading is important in the etiology of the conditions underlying back symptoms, or whether it primarily serves to exacerbate symptoms from an existing condition, is unclear.

Theoretical Considerations

Loading, stretching, or other irritation to pathologic structures usually produces pain, but it is likely that a feedback system exists between pain and loading, leading to the avoidance of loading (Fig. 3). Such a self-regulating system of minimizing pain by changes in physical loading is likely to dilute apparent associations between pain and pathology. Thus, even if spine pathology leads to back pain, which is modified by changes in physical activity/loading, the association between back pain and pathology may be obscured if simultaneous variations in physical loading are not controlled. It is also likely that the type of physical loading that exacerbates pain relates specifically to variations in underlying pathology. Such associations may be most clear in cases of severe back pathology, when even light loading can stimulate pain receptors.

In summary, physical loading is associated with back pain. Whether it is a causal factor, or simply modifies the effect of underlying pathology on symptoms, or both, is unclear. Self-regulation of physical loading to control pain may exist, thus confounding possible associations between pathology and symptoms, but evidence is lacking. The advancement and availability of imaging and other diagnostic tools may lead to more studies that simultaneously investigate the effects of spinal pathology and physical loading on back pain, and their interactions.

Epidemiologic Evidence of the Role of Pathophysiology

Clinicians and back pain researchers commonly state that intervertebral disk pathology is a likely culprit responsible for many back symptoms.[69-71] Except in the case of radicular symptoms, the importance of disk pathology has been increasingly questioned because the particular pathologic findings investigated have been poor predictors of the presence or absence of back pain. Yet, to date, no other conditions have captured more interest as primary suspects underlying symptoms. Although several studies have shown the importance of psychosocial parameters in pain expression, these factors may still be modifiers of pain;

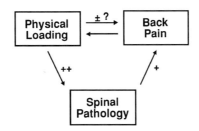

Fig. 3 *Theoretical concepts of the interactions between physical loading, back pain, and spinal pathology.*

325

in other words, mechanical or idiopathic low back pain is still likely to have a primary origin in pathology.[19,72-74]

Epidemiologic studies of the associations between spine pathology and back pain have yielded varying results. Frymoyer and associates[75] compared the radiographs of three groups of men between the ages of 18 and 55 years who had history of no back pain, of moderate back pain, or of severe back pain. The more prevalent radiographic findings in those with greater pain were traction spurs and/or L4-5 disk space narrowing. The frequency of Schmorl's nodes, claw spurs, disk heights at L3-4 and L5-S1 levels, the disk vacuum sign, and transitional vertebrae were similar in all three groups. In another study based on diskographic evaluations among back surgery candidates, annular ruptures were highly associated with patients' back pain reproduction, but "symmetric degeneration" without annular ruptures was not.[76] Such a finding is consistent with what is known about the innervation of disk structures.

In a study of former elite athletes, those with more spinal pathology, based on magnetic resonance imaging (MRI), had more reported back pain. However, overall, athletes, including former weight lifters and soccer players, reported less back-related pain than did referents with generally less pathology. These data emphasize the complexity of experiencing and reporting pain.[77] Several studies show a high frequency of abnormal findings among subjects without back pain. These findings are based on myelography, computed tomography (CT) scan,[78-81] and MRI studies.[82] For example, Jensen and associates[83] recently demonstrated that although 54% of subjects with a history of back pain had a disk protrusion identified on MRI, 27% of those without back pain had similar findings. In the same study, one of 98 subjects without pain and seven of 27 subjects with back pain had a disk extrusion. These findings show that such disk changes are common in the general population and frequently are not associated with the presence of symptoms; they emphasize that caution must be used when interpreting MRI findings in clinical studies. However, a higher prevalence of disk protrusions and extrusions among symptomatic subjects suggests that these findings may play a role in symptoms, although the number of severe findings was low. Similarly, in an autopsy study comparing lifetime back pain history recalled by subjects' family members, more problems were recalled among those with more pathology; however, degenerative changes also were common among those without a recalled pain history.[68,84]

In a recent study of 115 monozygotic twin pairs, the most commonly suspected risk factors for disk degeneration explained less than 10% of the variation in lumbar degenerative disk findings using MRI. Not surprisingly, age was associated with degenerative findings. However, the effects of age, ranging from 35 to 69 years, explained less than 10% of the variation. Conversely, familial aggregation, representing genetic influences and shared early environment, explained one to two thirds of the variation in lumbar disk degeneration. If disk degeneration and back pain are related, these results suggest that genetic influences may play a role in back symptoms.[65]

The Role of Pathophysiology

Tissue damage occurs when mechanical forces exceed the strength of a structure, or as a consequence of infection or other nonmechanical causes. In general, the pathophysiology of all tissue damage is similar: the acute phase is characterized by an "inflammatory reaction" including hyperemia, edema, and pain followed by proliferation of connective tissues and development of denser fibrotic tissue, including shrinkage of scar tissues. The inflammatory stage of any pathologic condition is most painful; however, most fibrotic structures have nerve endings and react to different stimuli, such that the shrinkage phenomenon could cause symptoms. Bone formation (osteophytes) at the tendon and ligament insertions is a common phenomenon associated with spinal degenerative processes. Most degenerative findings are irreversible; for example, scar tissue and bony formations do not disappear. The lack of innervation of some spine structures, eg, absence of nerve endings in cartilage or the inner part of the disk, means that only some spinal pathology can even in theory be related to pain. Simultaneously with pathogenetic processes, spine structures degenerate due to "pure aging," but these changes are not usually thought to be painful. Some new biochemical work gives hope that, in the future, we will be able to separate pathologic findings due to harmful environmental exposures from pure aging changes.

In summary, pathologic findings are not necessarily painful at the time of observation, although symptoms may have occurred in the early development of the pathologic process in innervated structures. Most pathologic findings are irreversible; therefore, when studying persons of any age, we see the accumulation of lifetime structural insults and degenerative changes (Fig. 4).

The Problems of Assessing Intervertebral Disk Pathology

Aside from gross pathology identified clinically, the reliability of using imaging techniques to assess degenerative changes has been and is still problematic. Possible effects are diluted by poor reliability and inaccuracy of parameters, which create uncertainty in interpreting the results of studies of the effects of disk degeneration on symptoms. The radiation risks of radiographs and CT

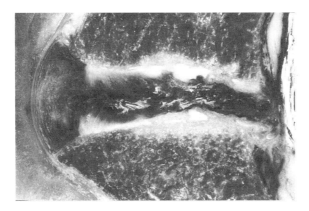

Fig. 4 *Cryomicrotomic section of severely degenerated presacral disk (the disk was injected with methylene blue before freezing, and the section was made by Dr. Wolfgang Rauschning).*

scans and, until recently, the costs and limited availability of MRI also have limited population-based studies. However, it currently is possible to use MRI safely to study disk degeneration in general populations. It is more informative in assessing the disk than is plain radiography, which allows indirect assessment based on disk height narrowing, osteophytes, and end plate irregularity. MRI does, however, have limitations in the types of changes that can be seen and the reliability with which they can be assessed.[85]

One methodologic problem with studying the associations of pain and MRI findings is that the most easily measured finding may not have any direct mechanism to produce pain, even in theory. The MRI image primarily describes the intervertebral disk's water content, which correlates well with degeneration. However, it is unclear how such changes, often judged through assessing disk signal intensity, correlate with pain producing pathology. The main suspected source of back pain is pathology in the outer layers of the anulus and around the nerve roots, but the reliability of detection by MRI is not clear. As with other assessments based on observation, the repeatability is suboptimal.[85] Some findings may eventually be assessed more reliably using the MRI digital data and quantitative methods. For example, certain dimensions, areas, and signal intensities can be assessed with such techniques, which provide continuous variables and improved repeatability, but there are many unresolved problems to evaluate, for example, annular pathology.[86]

In summary, the source of idiopathic low back pain is unclear. Although back pain is weakly associated with some structural changes in the spine, the specific pathologic findings commonly studied in the spine have a low specificity for back pain. One of the main obstacles to understanding common mechanical or idiopathic back symptoms is our inability to identify pain-producing pathology and to separate it from degeneration, which does not produce pain.[87]

Conclusion

Most of the adult population report experiencing back pain at some time, and the majority of these episodes are "idiopathic." To have experienced back pain would appear to be a more normal phenomenon than never to have done so. The severity of and resultant disability from these episodes, however, may vary substantially.

Most epidemiologic studies on idiopathic low back pain have focused on individual physical factors and occupational physical demands; however, consideration of a broader scope of potentially influential factors has become common. Because a back pain complaint is an active behavior, it can be influenced by a variety of factors other than physical pathology and pain.

Significant challenges, including difficulties in defining the pain experience or outcome, inadequate measures of environmental exposures, and inadequate control of potentially confounding factors, limit the value of epidemiologic studies of idiopathic low back pain. The difficulties in measuring both determinants and outcomes, along with problems with recall, tend to dilute associations. The highly variable course of back pain and its recurrent nature further complicate matters of classification.

Heavy physical loading parameters are to some degree associated with increased back pain, but the underlying mechanism is not fully understood.

Whether physical loading is important in the etiology of idiopathic low back pain, or whether it primarily exacerbates symptoms from an existing condition, or both, is unknown. Confusion about the effects of loading is exemplified by the common view that physical loading related to work is the main cause of idiopathic back pain and physical loading during leisure time is a preventive and therapeutic approach. However, there is little agreement regarding the types and amounts of exercise that are beneficial.[18] In addition to physical loading factors, such as heavy manual labor, bending, twisting, static work postures, vibration, and traumatic accidents, several other individual and psychosocial factors are suspected as determinants and modifiers of back pain. Collectively, the environmental and individual factors studied explain little of the uncertainty in predicting back symptoms and injury complaints. Despite a few additions, such as impaired fibrinolysis, smoking, and job dissatisfaction, to the list of suspected risk factors over the past decade or so, few new ideas have surfaced to help explain the occurrence of back symptoms.

The source of idiopathic low back pain is still unclear. We currently cannot differentiate pain producing pathology from simple aging changes. However, recent data suggest that we eventually may be able to use biochemical methods to detect differences in connective tissue related to pathology and aging. The value of imaging technology in revealing a structural cause for idiopathic low back pain is limited in part by the particular outcomes that are assessed and by less than optimal reading reliability. Given the resources that have been invested in MRI and other imaging, there have been relatively few comparisons of imaging findings to pathoanatomic and biochemical parameters.

Until understanding of the condition(s) underlying idiopathic low back pain and measures of this outcome and its suspected determinants are improved, epidemiologic studies will continue to be of limited value, and optimal prevention and treatment strategies are likely to remain elusive.

References

1. Cypress BK: Characteristics of physician visits for back symptoms: A national perspective. *Am J Public Health* 1983;73:389–395.
2. Spengler DM, Bigos SJ, Martin NA, et al: Back injuries in industry: A retrospective study. Overview and cost analysis: Injury factors. *Spine* 1986;11:241–251.
3. National Center for Health Statistics: *Prevalence of Selected Impairments, United States–1977*. Hyattsville, MD, Vital and Health Statistics: Series 10, No 134. US Department of Health and Human Services. (PHS) 81–1562, 1981.
4. Caspersen CJ, Merritt RK: Physical activity trends among 26 states, 1986–1990. *Med Sci Sports Exerc* 1995;27:713–720.
5. Nachemson AL: Problemets omfatting, in Ont i Ryggen: Orsaker, Diagnostik Och Behandling. Stockholm, Sweden, SBU, 1991, pp 8–28.
6. Allan DB, Waddell G: An historical perspective on low back pain and disability. *Acta Orthop Scand* 1989;234(suppl):1–23.
7. Andersson GBJ: The epidemiology of spinal disorders, in Frymoyer JW, Ducker TB, Hadler NM, et al (eds): *The Adult Spine: Principles and Practice*. New York, NY, Raven Press, 1991, vol 1, pp 107–146.
8. Hadler NM: To be a patient or a claimant with a musculoskeletal illness, in Hadler NM (ed): *Clinical Concepts in Regional Musculoskeletal Illness*. Orlando, FL, Grune & Stratton, 1987, pp 7–21.
9. *Social Security Statistical Supplement (1977-1979)*. HE 3.3/3:979, Washington, DC, Government Printing Office, 1979.

10. Miettinen OS (ed): *Theoretical Epidemiology: Principles of Occurrence Research in Medicine.* New York, NY, Wiley & Sons, 1985.
11. Rossignol M, Lortie M, Ledoux E: Comparison of spinal health indicators in predicting spinal status in a 1-year longitudinal study. *Spine* 1993;18:54–60.
12. Taylor PJ: International comparisons of sickness absence. *Proc Roy Soc Med* 1972;65:577–580.
13. Anderson RT: An orthopedic ethnography in rural Nepal. *Med Anthropol* 1984;8:46–59.
14. Andersson GB: Epidemiologic aspects of low-back pain in industry. *Spine* 1981;6:53–60.
15. Backenheimer MS: Demographic and job characteristics as variables in absences for illness. *Public Health Rep* 1968;83:1029–1032.
16. Biering-Sörensen F, Thomsen C: Medical, social and occupational history as risk indicators for low-back trouble in a general population. *Spine* 1986;11:720–725.
17. Bigos SJ, Battié MC, Spengler DM, et al: A prospective study of work perceptions and psychosocial factors affecting the report of back injury. *Spine* 1991;16:1–6.
18. Deyo RA, Cherkin D, Conrad D, et al: Cost, controversy, crisis: Low back pain and the health of the public. *Annu Rev Public Health* 1991;12:141–156.
19. Loeser J, Henderlite S, Condrad D: Incentive effects of workers compenstion benefits: A literature synthesis. *Med Care Res Rev* 1995;52:34–59.
20. Näyhä S, Videman T, Laakso M, et al: Prevalence of low back pain and other musculoskeletal symptoms and their association with work in Finnish reindeer herders. *Scan J Rheumatol* 1991;20:406–413.
21. Skovron ML, Szpalski M, Nordin M, et al: Sociocultural factors and back pain: A population-based study in Belgian adults. *Spine* 1994;19:129–137.
22. Volinn E, Van Koevering D, Loeser JD: Back sprain in industry: The role of socioeconomic factors in chronicity. *Spine* 1991;16:542–548.
23. Waddell G. A new clinical model for the treatment of low-back pain. *Spine* 1987;12:632–644.
24. Deyo RA, Andersson G, Bombardier C, et al: Outcome measures for studying patients with low back pain. *Spine* 1994;19(suppl 18):2032S–2036S.
25. Gyntelberg F: One year incidence of low back pain among male residents of Copenhagen aged 40–59. *Dan Med Bull* 1974;21:30–36.
26. Hellsing AL, Nordgren B, Schéle R, et al: Individual predictability of back trouble in 18-year-old men. *Manu Med* 1986;2:72–76.
27. Hult L: The Munkfors investigation. *Acta Orthop Scand* 1954;16(suppl):1–76.
28. Hult L: Cervical, dorsal and lumbar spinal syndromes. *Acta Orthop Scand* 1954:17(suppl):1–102.
29. Partridge RE, Duthie JJ: Rheumatism in dockers and civil servants: A comparison of heavy manual and sedentary workers. *Ann Rheum Dis* 1968;27:559–568.
30. Riihimäki H, Tola S, Videman T, et al: Low back pain and occupation: A cross-sectional questionnaire study of men in machine operating, dynamic physical work, and sedentary work. *Spine* 1989;14:204–209.
31. Sairanen E, Brushaber L, Kaskinen M: Felling work, low-back pain and osteoarthritis. *Scand J Work Environ Health* 1981;7:18–30.
32. Valkenburg HA, Haanen HCM: The epidemiology of low back pain, in White AA III, Gordon SL (eds): American Academy of Orthopaedic Surgeons *Symposium on Idiopathic Low Back Pain.* St. Louis, MO, CV Mosby, 1982, pp 9–22.
33. Videman T, Nurminen T, Tola S, et al: Low-back pain in nurses and some loading factors of work. *Spine* 1984;9:400–404.
34. Heikkilä JK, Koskenvuo M, Heliövaara M, et al: Genetic and environmental factors in sciatica: Evidence from a nationwide panel of 9365 adult twin pairs. *Ann Med* 1989;21:393–398.
35. Frymoyer JW, Nachemson A: Natural history of low back disorders, in Frymoyer JW, Ducker TB, Hadler NM, et al (eds): *The Adult Spine: Principles and Practice.* New York, NY, Raven Press, 1991, vol 2, pp 1537–1550.
36. Bigos SJ, Battié MC, Spengler DM, et al: A longitudinal, prospective study of industrial back injury reporting. *Clin Orthop* 1992;279:21–34.

37. Vallfors B: Acute, subacute and chronic low back pain: Clinical symptoms, absenteeism and working environment. *Scand J Rehabil Med* 1985;11(suppl):1–98.
38. Bergquist-Ullman M, Larsson U: Acute low back pain in industry: A controlled prospective study with special reference to therapy and confounding factors. *Acta Orthop Scand* 1977;170:1–117.
39. Von Korff M: Studying the natural history of back pain. *Spine* 1994;19(suppl 18):2041S–2046S.
40. Hildebrandt VH: A review of epidemiological research on risk factors of low back pain, in Buckle P (ed): *Musculoskeletal Disorders at Work*. London, England, Taylor & Francis, 1987, pp 9–16.
41. Battié MC, Bigos SJ, Fisher LD, et al: A prospective study of the role of cardiovascular risk factors and fitness in industrial back pain complaints. *Spine* 1989;14:141–147.
42. Battié MC, Bigos SJ, Fisher LD, et al: Isometric lifting strength as a predictor of industrial back pain reports. *Spine* 1989;14:851–856.
43. Battié MC, Bigos SJ, Fisher LD, et al: The role of spinal flexibility in back pain complaints within industry: A prospective study. *Spine* 1990;15:768–773.
44. Battié MC, Bigos SJ, Fisher LD, et al: Anthropometric and clinical measures as predictors of back pain complaints in industry: A prospective study. *J Spinal Disord* 1990;3:195–204.
45. Biering-Sörensen F: Physical measurements as risk indicators for low-back trouble over a one-year period. *Spine* 1984;9:106–119.
46. Chaffin DB, Park KS: A longitudinal study of low-back pain as associated with occupational weight lifting factors. *Am Ind Hyg Assoc J* 1973;34:513–525.
47. Damkot DK, Pope MH, Lord J, et al: The relationship between work history, work environment and low-back pain in men. *Spine* 1984;9:395–399.
48. Leavitt F: The physical exertion factor in compensable work injuries: A hidden flaw in previous research. *Spine* 1992;17:307–310.
49. Leino P: Physical loading and mental stress as determinants of musculoskeletal disorders. *Acta Universitatis Tamperensis* 1989;A282:56–60.
50. Linton SJ: Risk factors for neck and back pain in a working population in Sweden. *Work Stress* 1990;4:41–49.
51. Magora A: Investigation of the relation between low back pain and occupation. *IMS Industr Med Surg* 1970;39:504–510.
52. Ready AE, Boreskie SL, Law SA, et al: Fitness and lifestyle parameters fail to predict back injuries in nurses. *Can J Appl Physiol* 1993;18:80–90.
53. Riihimäki H: Low-back pain, its origin and risk indicators. *Scand J Work Environ Health* 1991;17:81–90.
54. Svensson H-O, Andersson GB: Low back pain in 40- to 47-year-old men: Work history and work environment factors. *Spine* 1983;8:272–276.
55. Videman T, Rauhala H, Asp S, et al: Patient-handling skill, back injuries, and back pain: An intervention study in nursing. *Spine* 1989;14:148–156.
56. Troup JD, Foreman TK, Baxter CE, et al: The perception of back pain and the role of psychophysical tests of lifting capacity. *Spine* 1987;12:645–657.
57. Leino P, Aro S, Hasan J: Trunk muscle function and low back disorders: A ten-year follow-up study. *J Chron Dis* 1987;40:289–296.
58. Harber P, Peña L, Hsu P, et al: Personal history, training and worksite as predictors of back pain in nurses. *Am J Ind Med* 1994;25:519–526.
59. Pietri F, Leclerc A, Boitel L, et al: Low-back pain in commercial travelers. *Scand J Work Environ Health* 1992;18:52–58.
60. Bigos SJ, Battié MC, Fisher LD, et al: Premorbid risk factors for back pain disability greater than one month. *Orthop Trans* 1993;17:285.
61. Cady LD, Bischoff DP, O'Connell ER, et al: Strength and fitness and subsequent back injuries in firefighters. *J Occup Med* 1979;21:269–272.
62. Mostardi RA, Noe DA, Kovacik MW, et al: Isokinetic lifting strength and occupational injury: A prospective study. *Spine* 1992;17:189–193.
63. Dueker JA, Ritchie SM, Knox TJ, et al: Isokinetic trunk testing and employment. *J Occup Med* 1994;36:42–48.

64. Heine J: Arthritis deformans. *Virch Arch Pathol Anat* 1926;260:521–663.
65. Battié MC, Videman T, Gibbons LE, et al: Determinants of lumbar disc degeneration: A study relating lifetime exposures and magnetic resonance imaging findings in identical twins. *Spine* 1995;20:2601–2612.
66. Linton SJ: The relationship between activity and chronic back pain. *Pain* 1985;21:289–294.
67. Rainville J, Ahern DK, Phalen L, et al: The association of pain with physical activities in chronic low back pain. *Spine* 1992;17:1060–1064.
68. Videman T, Nurminen M, Troup JD: Lumbar spinal pathology in cadaveric material in relation to history of back pain, occupation, and physical loading. *Spine* 1990;15:728–740.
69. Mooney V, Brown M, Modic M: Clinical perspectives, in Frymoyer JW, Gordon SL (eds): *New Perspectives on Low Back Pain.* Park Ridge, IL, American Academy of Orthopaedic Surgeons, 1989, pp 133–146.
70. Battié MC, Cherkin DC, Dunn R, et al: Managing low back pain: Attitudes and treatment preferences of physical therapists. *Phys Ther* 1994;74:219–226.
71. Cherkin DC, MacCornack FA, Berg AO: Managing low back pain: A comparison of the beliefs and behaviors of family physicians and chiropractors. *West J Med* 1988;149:475–480.
72. Greenough CG, Fraser RD: The effects of compensation on recovery from low-back injury. *Spine* 1989;14:947–955.
73. Linton SJ, Bradley LA, Jensen I, et al: The secondary prevention of low back pain: A controlled study with follow-up. *Pain* 1989;36:197–207.
74. Volinn E, Lai D, McKinney S, et al: When back pain becomes disabling: A regional analysis. *Pain* 1988;33:33–39.
75. Frymoyer JW, Newberg A, Pope MH, et al: Spine radiographs in patients with low-back pain: An epidemiological study in men. *J Bone Joint Surg* 1984;66A:1048–1055.
76. Moneta GB, Videman T, Kaivanto K, et al: Reported pain during lumbar discography as a function of anular ruptures and disc degeneration: A re-analysis of 833 discograms. *Spine* 1994:19:1968–1974.
77. Videman T, Sarna S, Battié MC, et al: The long-term effects of physical loading and exercise lifestyles on back-related symptoms, disability, and spinal pathology among men. *Spine* 1995;20:699–709.
78. Holt EP Jr: The question of lumbar discography. *J Bone Joint Surg* 1968;50A:720–726.
79. Hitselberger WE, Witten RM: Abnormal myelograms in asymptomatic patients. *J Neurosurg* 1968;28:204–206.
80. Rothman RH: A study of computer-assisted tomography. *Spine* 1984;9:548.
81. Wiesel SW, Tsourmas N, Feffer HL, et al: A study of computer-assisted tomography: I. The incidence of positive CAT scans in an asymptomatic group of patients. *Spine* 1984;9:549–551.
82. Boden SD, Davis DO, Dina TS, et al: Abnormal magnetic-resonance scans of the lumbar spine in asymptomatic subjects: A prospective investigation. *J Bone Joint Surg* 1990;72A:403–408.
83. Jensen MC, Brant-Zawadzki MN, Obuchowski N, et al: Magnetic resonance imaging of the lumbar spine in people without back pain. *N Engl J Med* 1994;331:69–73.
84. Kauppila LI, Videman T: Discographic findings and back pain history: An epidemiological study of 58 cadavers. *J Orthop Rheumatol* 1994;7:88–92.
85. Raininko R, Manninen H, Battié MC, et al: Observer variability in the assessment of disc degeneration on magnetic resonance images of the lumbar and thoracic spine. *Spine* 1995;20:1029–1035.
86. Videman T, Nummi P, Battié MC, et al: Digital assessment of MRI for lumbar disc dessication: A comparison of digital versus subjective assessments and digital intensity profiles versus discogram and macroanatomic findings. *Spine* 1994;19:192–198.
87. Saal JA: The pathophysiology of painful lumbar disorder symposium: Introduction. *Spine* 1995;20:1803.

Chapter 21

Occupational Hazards for Low Back Pain

Malcolm H. Pope, Dr Med Sci, PhD

Introduction

Low back pain (LBP) of occupational origin is at epidemic proportions, and its impact on industry and the medical community is great. LBP has been assessed epidemiologically, but this research has been hampered by problems with the definition, classification, and diagnosis of LBP and in quantifying physical exposures such as loads lifted and postures.

There are approximately 25 million workers with LBP in the United States; 1.2 million of these workers are disabled. In 10% of all patients with chronic health conditions, the diagnosis is LBP.[1,2] Rowe[3] studied workers in a single plant over a 10-year period and found that only upper respiratory illness exceeded LBP as a causative factor in work time lost. Thirty-five percent of the workers whose jobs require sitting and 47% of those indulging in physically demanding work made visits to the plant infirmary because of LBP during that time. Sick time used per worker averaged 4 hours a year, and 85% of these workers had recurrent episodes of LBP. Kelsey and White[2] estimate that approximately 2% of the workers in the United States sustain a compensable back injury each year, while Snook[4] found annual rates to range from 1% to 15%. The annual cost of LBP in the United States is currently estimated to be between $25 billion and $100 billion per year. LBP has become the most expensive health care problem in the United States in people aged 20 to 50 years. The total compensation cost for LBP is estimated at $4.6 billion and the cost per case is now well over $6,000 and is increasing.[5] However, only 25% of the cases account for this cost. As the duration of disability increases, the total cost increases. LBP is a factor in 21% of all compensable work injuries, but averages a third of the cost. Medical costs account for a third of the total cost, and disability payments account for the remainder.[6]

This chapter will present some methods for primary and secondary prevention of LBP. The epidemiologic relationships between LBP and physical loading of the spine will be examined first.

Occupational Biomechanics

Lifting

There are many studies in which it has been determined that LBP is associated with heavy lifting.[7-15] In addition, Snook[4] found that a worker was three times more likely to have a compensable LBP injury if the job involved heavy lifting. Magora[11] found that LBP also occurred in workers whose jobs required sitting, because sitting itself is a plausible cause for LBP. The National Institutes for Occupational Safety and Health (NIOSH) have stated that: (1) one third of the United States workforce is currently required to exert significant strength as part of their jobs; (2) overexertion was claimed as the cause of LBP by over 60% of workers; (3) 500,000 overexertion injuries occur in the United States per year (in 5% of workers per year); (4) overexertion injuries account for one fourth of all occupational injuries although some industries report that over half of these injuries are caused by overexertion; (5) approximately two thirds of overexertion injuries involved lifting loads; (6) less than one third of patients with LBP returned to their previous job.

The estimation of stresses on various parts of the musculoskeletal system during lifting activities will require a complex model that accounts for such factors as: (1) instantaneous positions and accelerations of the extremities, head, and trunk; (2) changes in spinal geometry; and (3) strength variations in different muscle groups and people.

Recent efforts have been made to extend a biomechanical model to include: (1) an estimate of the stresses on the lumbosacral disk; (2) the addition of external loads on the hands (for example, when handling materials); and (3) an evaluation of the effects of various muscle group strengths on the performance of the person being studied.

Abdominal pressure has been proposed as a major source of column support. Data obtained by Asmussen and Poulsen[16] suggest that the general effectiveness of this reflex mechanism is limited, however. A maximum pressure of 150 mm Hg appears to be possible with physically fit individuals, although 90 mm Hg is probably a more reasonable limit for those who are less physically fit. It should be noted, though, that this spinal relief may not be possible when a person is carrying a load for a sustained period. If assumed to be a well-developed reflex in an individual, abdominal pressurization probably can relieve approximately 10% to 20% of lumbar spinal column compression.

The back-stooped posture, when lifting a heavy or bulky load, actually reduces the compressive loading on the L5-S1 disk below that predicted when lifting with a more erect back. The reasons for the larger compression forces when lifting with the back near vertical in this example are that (1) the load moment arm is increased; and (2) the vertical component of both the body weight and hand forces add more directly to the compressive forces on the more vertical spine. Of course, the shearing forces are greater when lifting with the back flexed. Also, depending on the precise curvature of the lumbar spine during the lift, the articular facet capsules and the posterior ligaments may be overstrained, especially with the more flexed torso posture required when performing a stoop type of lift.

It appears that people often lift loads with their backs rather than their legs. In so doing, the energy necessary to move the body-load-mass combination is minimized. Although it was commonly believed that ''back lifting'' was more stressful than ''leg lifting,'' this theory does not appear to be true in regard to compression loading of the column, especially when lifting loads that are larger than can be brought between the knees or loads that are located horizontally away from the feet. Disk pressure measurements have shown the pressure to be similar when ''back lift'' and ''leg lift'' methods were compared, provided the moment arm to the load was kept constant.

If a person can maintain the torso in a completely erect position while lifting, then the compressive force on the L5-S1 disk is minimized. Because of limited shoulder strength and arm reach, this minimization can only be accomplished by lifting a small object held in close to the body. The most important principle when lifting loads is to minimize the distance of the load from the L5-S1 disk, especially if the load is heavy.

Pulling and Pushing

There is much less information on pushing and pulling activities and their role in work-related LBP. Magora[11] found increased LBP in those whose jobs involved reaching and pulling, and the NIOSH[17] reported that 20% of injury claims for LBP involved pushing or pulling loads. Damkot and associates[18] measured pushing exposure by multiplying the weight of pushed objects by the number of pushing efforts required each day. The controls averaged 326 weightday units, and the group with severe LBP averaged 1,612 weightday units. There was a tendency for increased severity of LBP in those with increased pulling requirements. White and Panjabi[19] have shown theoretically that high loads on disks and other structures result from pulling activities. Because body posture plays an important role in the force capability in both pushing and pulling, posture is probably very important in the etiology of LBP resulting from pulling/pushing activities.

Twisting

Twisting was found to be related to LBP in several studies.[11,20] Basmajian[21] reported antagonistic activity of the deep trunk muscles, and Morris and associates[22] found antagonistic activity of the multifidus rotators muscles, during axial rotation. My colleagues and I[23] found high levels of antagonistic activity in both abdominal and posterior back muscles. These levels were justified because of the apparent need to maintain posture during twisting activities. Thus, the high levels of antagonistic muscle activities and the resultant spinal loads in reaction to those contractions may be the reason for the apparent relationship between twisting and LBP.

Slipping

Slipping, tripping, and falling are common factors attributed to causing LBP. Troup and associates[24] reported that 36% of accidents resulting in LBP were falls. Manning and Shannon[25] found that slipping, tripping, or falling were factors in 70% of accidents resulting in LBP. Andersson and Legerlof[26] found that a high percentage of occupational accidents were caused by falls, of which 42% were initiated by slipping and 14% by tripping. Grieve[27] has pointed out that manual exertion often causes workers to slip because the exertions often result in tangential forces at the foot interface. Magora[11] showed that the most expensive injuries for industry are those for which there is a traumatic event, such as a slip or fall, associated with the onset.

335

Sitting Postures

There is increased risk of LBP in workers with jobs that require sitting.[9,28-30] Results of these studies show an increase in back pain symptomatology in subjects with LBP who are required to sit for prolonged periods. Kelsey[31] found that the risk of disk herniation increased threefold in men who spend more than half their workday in a car. It is unclear whether this increase is caused by the sitting posture, vibration, or by a combination of both. Nachemson and Elfstrom[32] and Andersson and Ortengren[33] have evaluated the sitting posture by electromyographic and intradiskal pressure measurements and have found that disk pressure can be very high in the worker bending forward at 20° and the worker sitting unsupported. However, it should be noted that there are other studies in which sitting was not determined to be a substantial risk factor for LBP.[34,35] These findings may be because jobs that require sitting are often less physically demanding. However, there are physiologic reasons to change working posture to improve both disk nutrition and soft tissue tone: posture-related fatigue and sickness/work absence decrease.[29,30,36]

Sitting is a position in which the weight of the body is transferred to the supporting area mainly by the ischial tuberosities of the pelvis and their surrounding soft tissues. Depending on the chair and posture, some proportion of the total body weight will also be transferred through the legs to the floor, as well as to the backrest and armrests.

Three different types of sitting postures can be distinguished and will be referred to as anterior, middle, or posterior. In the middle posture, the center of mass of the trunk is directly above the ischial tuberosities. This posture is quite unstable because the ischial tuberosities act as a pivot. In the middle posture, the lumbar spine is either straight or in slight kyphosis. The anterior (forward leaning) posture is adopted most often when desk work is performed. The center of mass is in front of the ischial tuberosities, whereas in the posterior (backward leaning) posture, the center of mass is behind the ischial tuberosities. The latter posture is obtained by a backward rotation of the pelvis, resulting in kyphosis of the lumbar spine. It is a posture typically assumed in chairs with reclining backrests, such as lounge chairs.

In general, the posture of a seated person depends not only on the design of the chair, but on the person's sitting habits and the task to be performed. The height and inclination of the seat of the chair, the position, shape, and inclination of the backrest, and the presence of other types of support all influence the resulting posture. The chair should also permit regular and easy alterations in posture, because continuous sitting in one position is a risk factor for LBP.

Information on the biomechanics of sitting comes from radiographic and electromyographic studies of muscles, disk pressure measurements, and from studies of seat pan pressure. Radiographic studies show that the pelvis rotates backward and the lumbar spine flattens when sitting. Andersson and Troup[37] found that changes in pelvic rotation influenced the shape of the lumbar spine because the sacral-horizontal angle changed, that is, the foundation of the lumbar spine changed. There must be compensation for this change in angle in order to maintain the trunk's upright position.

In vivo pressures measured within a lumbar disk when a patient sits without a lumbar support have been found to be about 35% higher than those obtained when the patient is standing. To study the influence of supports, disk pressures have also been measured in patients seated in different chairs with different back supports. Results of these studies confirmed that the disk pressure is considerably lower in standing than in unsupported sitting. Of different unsupported sitting postures, the lowest pressure was found when sitting with the back straight. The reasons for this increased pressure in sitting postures are: (1) an increase in the trunk load moment when the pelvis is rotated backward and the lumbar spine and torso are rotated forward; and (2) the deformation of the disk itself caused by flattening of the lumbar spine.

Inclination of the backrest backward from vertical and an increase in lumbar support resulted in a decrease in disk pressure. The disk pressure measurements can be interpreted as follows: (1) when backrests are used, part of the body weight is transferred to them when a person leans back, reducing the load on the lumbar spine caused by the upper body weight; (2) an increase in backrest inclination (leaning the backrest more backward) means an increase in load transfer to the backrest and results in a reduced disk pressure; (3) the use of armrests supports the weight of the arms, reducing the disk pressure; and (4) the use of a lumbar support changes the posture of the lumbar spine toward lordosis and hence reduces the deformation of the lumbar spine and corresponding disk pressure.

Typical seated office work has also been studied. Compared to the performance of other tasks, writing at a desk resulted in a decrease in disk pressure. This decrease was expected, because the arms can be well supported by the desk. Other office activities, such as typing and lifting a phone at arm's length, increased the pressure because of larger external load moments imparted to the spine during such tasks.

Electromyography (EMG) has also been used to study the activity of back muscles when sitting. High EMG activity levels indicate muscle contractions. Generally, similar activity levels have been recorded when standing and sitting without a back support. There is general agreement that the myoelectric activity decreases during sitting when (1) the back is slumped forward in full flexion; (2) the arms are supported; or (3) a backrest is used.

Standing Postures

Muscle activity is required to maintain an upright posture, but as long as the body is well aligned, with respect to the center of gravity, the activity is minimal. Any shift in the center of gravity of the trunk requires active counterbalancing by muscle force to maintain equilibrium. Muscle forces are also required to counterbalance the moment caused by an outstretched arm, an external weight or any other force applied to the trunk, head, and upper extremities. The combined effect of all these forces on the lumbar spine produces a moment that must be counterbalanced by the spinal muscles to maintain equilibrium. This moment is referred to in this chapter as the load moment. A much more complex situation occurs when asymmetry prevails. In such postures as lateral flexion, rotation, and combinations thereof, other appropriate muscles will contract. In rotation and lateral bending, high levels of activity occur contralateral to the direction of postural asymmetries, while the activities on the ipsilateral side are minimal. This asymmetry in muscle activity can lead to unequal stress concentrations on the different component structures of the spine. To maintain low muscle forces and consequently low stresses on the spine structures when standing, an upright symmetric posture should always be advocated, and all material should be handled as close to the body as possible.

Postural Fixity

The problem of postural fixity, that is, of remaining in the same posture for long periods of time, is that static loading of muscles and joint tissues will occur, which can often lead to discomfort. This problem is often exaggerated in offices, and electronic and small parts assembly workplaces, where movements are limited or stereotyped. Sitting work is often physically less demanding than production-line work. However, it is important to change work posture often. Postural fatigue and resultant absence from work have been found to decrease when postural changes are frequent.

Cyclic Loading

Cyclic loading, or vibration, has been shown to have many, and quite varied, effects on the human body. An extensive description is given by Dupuis and Zerlett.[38] Of concern to the spine is the fatigue life of the tissues. Fatigue, which is defined as a loss of strength resulting from intermittent stresses over time, can lead to material failure. This can occur with relatively small stresses compared to those required for a static stress failure. A material's fatigue life (the number of loading cycles it can withstand) depends on the range of stress imposed. For most materials, there is a stress below which the material's fatigue life can be considered infinite. Even a small increase in that stress, over that limit, can cause a significant decrease in the material's fatigue life.

There is a strong relationship between vehicular vibration and LBP.[39] Kelsey[31] found that truck drivers were four times more likely than others to have had a disk herniation. In addition, those driving more than 20 miles a day have four times as much LBP and twice the incidence of herniated nucleus pulposus. If the transmission of vibration through the human body is measured in the laboratory, the natural frequency will be accompanied by enhanced transmission and a greater absorption of energy. Damkot and associates[18] suggested that exposure to vehicular vibration, lifting, pulling, and pushing combine as important risk factors for LBP.

Mechanical studies have also been performed to evaluate the effect of vibration with various postures, in single or multiple directions. With mounting epidemiologic evidence associating LBP with vibration environments, there has been an increasing focus on the mechanical effect of occupational vibrations on the low back. Most of this work has been related to the study of seating and motor vehicles.

Dupuis and Zerlett[38] looked at the seated environment as a design problem. They suggested it was necessary to record the three-dimensional motions, analyze the data with human tolerances in mind, and finally, design a seat to protect the vehicle operator. If possible, measures should be taken to reduce vibration transmission. Unfortunately, good vibration tolerance data has yet to be determined for all people. The most serious consequence of providing a seat in a vehicle is that man's most effective isolation mechanism, the legs, is lost, yet the alternative (to drive the vehicle while standing) is clearly unacceptable.

Basic studies of vibration have focused on the following mechanical parameters; resonant frequency, transmissibility, impedance, spinal muscle activity, and effects on the materials comprising the spine.

The natural frequency is that at which an object, such as a bell, will freely vibrate after it has been struck mechanically. The frequency at which a simple spring-mass system will freely vibrate is proportional to the square root of the stiffness divided by the mass in a single degree of freedom system. For a given mass, natural frequency depends on stiffness. When a structure having a particular natural frequency is moved by some periodic oscillating force at the structure's natural frequency, a condition called resonance occurs, which has major mechanical consequences. In this situation it takes very little additional energy to keep the structure vibrating at its natural frequency, and the associated stress can lead to the structure's mechanical failure. Failure occurs because the structure oscillates at its maximum capacity, thus creating the greatest possible strains on the components. As a result, the structure is at its greatest susceptibility for fatigue failure.

The primary source of vibration in a vehicle is its interaction with the ground surface, but any component of the vehicle—engine, wheels, or drive shaft, for example—can be a source. In some cars, driving 50 to 60 mph on the expressway and the joints in the concrete slabs, which are placed at 15-feet intervals, are factors that can lead to a 6 Hz continuous vibration. In helicopters the rotor and wind buffeting also have vibration effects, and in semitrailers interaction between the trailer and the tractor may be an important source of vibration. Under some conditions the natural frequency of the vehicle suspension is approached, resulting in a violent response of the vehicle. Over very smooth ground the vehicle component (tires, for example) may excite the chassis and again the vibration may be excessive.

The natural frequency of a single degree of freedom structure can be determined by acceleration transmissibility and driving point impedance. Acceleration transmissibility is used to determine the output acceleration in the simple structure caused by a given input or driving acceleration. At resonance the transmissibility exceeds 1. In mechanical driving point impedance studies the driving force is divided by the structure's resultant velocity. Resonance occurs when both the driving force and resultant velocity are in phase and the impedance/frequency curve reaches a maximum.

Vibrational transmission can also be characterized by transfer functions describing the relationship of input acceleration, and measured output acceleration, at a point in the body. In frequency ranges where attenuation is low, resonances occur, causing increases in the transfer function magnitude. In a standing subject the first resonance occurs at the hip, shoulder, and head at about 5 Hz. In sitting subjects, resonance occurs at the shoulders at 5 Hz and to some degree also at the head. Further, a significant resonance from shoulder to head occurs at about 30 Hz.

Mechanical studies of seated vehicle operators subjected to vertical vibration in order to determine the resonant frequency have been summarized by Dupuis and Zerlett.[38] They found resonant frequencies of 4 to 6 Hz when the upper torso vibrates vertically with respect to the pelvis, and 10 to 14 Hz when there is a bending vibration of the upper torso with respect to the lumbar spine. Resonant frequencies of standing and supine subjects, and resonant frequencies of seated subjects as affected by side to side or fore-aft vibrations have also been reported.

Using accelerometers implanted in the lumbar region, Pope and associates[40] showed that the resonant frequency in the lumbar region of the vertically vibrated, seated operator was 4.5 Hz, indicating that maximum strain was occurring in the seated operator's lumbar region at resonances of 4.5 Hz. Much of the dynamic response is caused by the combined rotation and vertical compression of the pelvis-buttocks system.

The muscular effort of driving is considerable. This effort involves the forces necessary to maintain posture, control the vehicle, and resist its movements. The components of vibration and shock may not be enough to cause acute injury, but lateral thrusts may add to the spinal stress. Thus, there may be a symbiotic effect of vibration and posture.

Assessing the Workplace

Worksite Sampling

Worksite sampling should be carried out by a trained ergonomic evaluation team to document potentially harmful exposures or loads. The approach is successful for nonrepetitive or unstructured work but can also be helpful for routine, repetitive work that has not been previously analyzed. The evaluation team can observe the tasks and record the physically stressful exposures on a checklist or, more commonly, the tasks are video recorded. Later analysis will identify all tasks that are required of the workers, identify potentially hazardous job postures, measure the actual loads being handled, and record postural extremes. Often a job analyst will observe the worker and "check" the activities performed from a list. These lists of common manual tasks have been used in one study to improve job placement procedures for individuals with physical impairments.[41] Slipping is an important cause of injury that results in LBP. Measurement of slip resistance is not difficult. Strandberg,[42] for example, listed more than 60 different meters to measure the slip resistance. The meters measure the frictional characteristics of the floor. If the slip resistance is greater, then a worker is less likely to slip.

Worksite Simulation

In complex loadings, it has been helpful to simulate the task in the laboratory. The worker can stand on a load cell and motions can be quantified by an automated computer-based motion analysis system. This enables the team to analyze all the intrinsic and extrinsic factors and make appropriate recommendations.

Posture Analysis

Corlett and associates[43] have developed a method to record potentially stressful postures, called posture targeting. This procedure requires the job analyst to observe a worker at random during the workday, and to record the configuration of various body segments. The method is quite tedious and human observation errors are common, however.

A three-axis electrogoniometer (BT, Isotechnologies, Hillsborough, NC) is used in the workplace to determine the flexion-extension, axial rotation, and lateral bending of the trunk. These data are recorded on a portable data logger and subsequently analyzed by computer (Fig. 1).

Analysis of Strength Demands

Quite often the forces applied by the worker are unknown. To obviate this problem, a handheld load cell that quantifies the force applied in different directions by the worker has been developed. The technique is applicable to pulling and pushing activities as well as lifting. If necessary, these data can be used in a computer model such as that of Garg and Chaffin[44] to predict disk loads.

Vibration Measurement

The United States standard for vibration measurement is given by the Society of Automotive Engineers (SAE J1013). Accelerations are measured by a disk 250 mm in diameter made of molded rubber with an accelerometer inset. The disk is designed to sit comfortably between the ischial tuberosities, and the acceleration results are usually analyzed with a ride meter. Most ride meters compute and assign weighting factors to the overall root mean squared acceleration based on tolerance curves. Thus, it is possible for a person to perform normal driving tasks while the loads to the spine are directly measured.

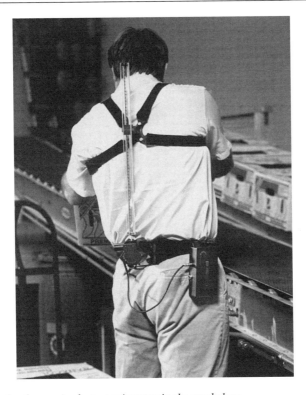

Fig. 1 *Use of a three-axis electrogoniometer in the workplace.*

Prevention

Several alternative prevention models exist but, unfortunately, none of these has been properly evaluated. The three main preventive approaches are: (1) selecting the right worker for the right job; (2) training the worker to use correct work techniques; and (3) (most desirable) designing the job to the worker. The first approach has legal limitations, but the others will be discussed in the following paragraphs.

Education

Fifty percent of compensable LBP is associated with lifting, but instructions on the ''proper'' lifting technique have been a matter of some controversy. The principle of safe lifting that has the greatest basis in biomechanics is to hold the object as close to the body as possible. This is more important than keeping a ''straight back.'' It is important that the worker use a smooth lifting technique, without jerking, in order to minimize the effect of dynamic loads on the spine. When performing those critical tasks involving twisting, it is important that the worker turn with the feet instead of twisting the trunk to reduce the torsional loads on the intervertebral disks.[45]

Back schools are a relatively recent innovation. Topics such as physical health, general back education, lifting techniques, and the importance of psychosocial factors are discussed. Most back schools stress that there is a responsibility for recovery that rests with the patient, and that there may not be complete absence of pain. Results of controlled studies indicate that the back school is better than a placebo and may be economically superior to physical therapy and other forms of treatment.[46] It is probable that the back school is much less effective for those with chronic LBP. Preventive schools may very well by helpful but controlled studies are lacking.

Workplace Design

To design a workplace that minimizes the stresses on the back is a difficult task. Measurement and optimization of posture, external load, trunk motion, and vibration is worthwhile. In lifting, the weight is not the only important factor, and the dimensions of the load should be kept compact so that the spine load moment can be minimized by keeping the load close to the center of gravity of the body. As stated earlier, the best prevention of back stress is to avoid lifting the load at all, but if this is not possible the load must be kept at a level such that the load moment does not exceed that recommended by NIOSH.[17]

The NIOSH Workpractices Guide for Manual Lifting gives the permissible load for a given posture for a person of a certain size. The guide clearly indicates the disadvantages of lifting loads above the shoulder, with the suggested limits being as much as 50% lower than in lifting loads knuckle height. The guide specifically calls for the measurement of object weight, horizontal location of the hands, vertical travel distance, frequency of lifting, and duration of the period with which lifting has occurred. All of these factors should be taken into account to minimize the total stress on the spine during a workday. As important as this guide is, it specifically does not include a number of important variables. The guide is only applicable to smooth lifting, two-handed symmetrical lifting in the sagittal plane, and the lifting of moderate width objects. In addition, the standing postures should be unrestricted, there should be suitable handles on the object, favorable environmental conditions, and the worker should not be performing any other activities simultaneously. If any of these other provisions do apply, then the load should be reduced even further. When the object is large and heavy, a hoist or crane to assist in its movement should be available. This crane must be conveniently placed, otherwise the worker will not use it. Pushing or pulling force requirements, which are often ignored, should be made low, certainly below 225 N, and the hands should be placed around the hip to waist level when making a maximum exertion so as to minimize spine load moments. The floor surfaces and areas where pushing and pulling activities occur must be kept clean and dry and workers should be instructed to wear shoes with traction.

Sitting is a common posture in the workplace, and has become even more prevalent. Although sitting offers certain advantages, the seat design must be carefully thought out to avoid muscle fatigue or excessive spine loads. Available chairs vary considerably because there are many different opinions on user requirements. Regardless of usage, it is important to adjust the chair to fit the worker. Andersson and associates[47] showed that spinal stress could be minimized if the backrest angle was designed to be 110° or more, and the seat pan angle was 6°, and if there were additional curved support for the lumbar spine. The depth of the seat is important because it should make use of the backrest possible. This means that the seat pan should not be too deep. Interactions with the work surface must also be considered in seating. Tilting the work surface toward the worker is a good way to prevent unnecessary forward flexion of the neck and back. A semiseated posture can also be an advantage in certain jobs.

Seat vibration should be minimized. Cyclic loading should not exceed the International Standards Organization requirements. Vibration isolation seats should be used where possible, and firm cushions with lumbar support should be employed. If possible, the arms and the feet should be supported. The posture should permit the backrest to be used where possible. One method of reducing whole body vibration is to reduce the vibration input. This can only be done by the choice of vehicles and by training drivers to choose the vehicle they drive, and to reduce vibration by changing their driving speed and style. Many of these factors are within the control of the operator and can be influenced by training.

Conclusion

Occupational LBP is of major importance both economically and in terms of disability. The incidence of LBP increases each year, and major steps should be taken toward prevention. Although it is often problematic, prevention is by far the most advantageous option. Epidemiologic studies clearly indicate the role of mechnical loads on the etiology of occupational LBP, therefore, it is essential that the basic occupational biomechanics be understood. Methods for measuring the mechanical environment of the worker have been developed. This information can be used to adapt the workplace to prevent injuries. It is probable that most mechanical risk factors, along with psychosocial factors, combine for total risk for LBP. The combined efforts of the medical community along with labor and management are required in order to promote prevention of LBP.

References

1. Kelsey JL, Pastides H, Bisbee GE Jr, et al (eds): *Musculo-skeletal Disorders: Their Frequency of Occurrence and Their Impact on the Population of the United States.* New York, NY, Prodist, 1978.
2. Kelsey JL, White AA III: Epidemiology and impact of low-back pain. *Spine* 1980;5:133–142.
3. Rowe ML: Low back pain in industry: A position paper. *J Occup Med* 1969;11:161–169.
4. Snook SH: Low back pain in industry, in White AA III, Gordon SL (eds): American Academy of Orthopaedic Surgeons *Symposium on Idiopathic Low Back Pain.* St. Louis, MO, CV Mosby, 1982, pp 23–38.
5. Andersson GBJ, Pope MH, Frymoyer JW, et al: Epidemiology and cost, in Pope MH, Andersson GBJ, Frymoyer JW, et al (eds): *Occupational Low Back Pain: Assessment, Treatment and Prevention.* St. Louis, MO, Mosby-Year Book, 1991, pp 95–113.
6. Social Security Statistical Supplement, Suppl Doc No HE 3.3/3:979. Washington, DC, Government Printing Office, pp 1977–1979.
7. Brown JR: Lifting as an industrial hazard. *Am Ind Hyg Assoc J* 1973;34:292–297.
8. Chaffin DB: Human strength capability and low-back pain. *J Occup Med* 1974;16:248–254.
9. Hult L: Cervical, dorsal and lumbar spinal syndromes. *Acta Orthop Scand* 1954;17(suppl):1–102.
10. Magora A: Investigation of the relation between low back pain and occupation: IV. Physical requirements: Bending, rotation, reaching and sudden maximal effort. *Scand J Rehabil Med* 1973;5:186–190.
11. Magora A: Investigation of the relation between low back pain and occupation: VI. Medical history and symptoms. *Scand J Rehabil Med* 1974;6:81–88.
12. Rowe ML: Preliminary statistical study of low back pain. *J Occup Med* 1963;5:336–341.
13. Snook SH, Campanelli RA, Hart JW: A study of three preventive approaches to low back injury. *J Occup Med* 1978;20:478–481.
14. Andersson GBJ, Ortengren R, Nachemson A: Quantitative studies of back loads in lifting. *Spine* 1976;1:178–185.
15. Svensson HO, Andersson GB: Low-back pain in 40- to 47-year-old men: Work history and work environment factors. *Spine* 1983;8:272–276.
16. Asmussen E, Poulsen E: On the role of the intraabdominal pressure in relieving the back muscles while holding weights in a forward inclined position. *Commun Dan Natl Assoc Infant Paral* 1968;28:3.
17. National Institute for Occupational Safety and Health: *Work Practices Guide for Manual Lifting.* Cincinnati, OH, Division of Biomedical and Behavioral Science, 1981, (DHHS Publication No 81–122).
18. Damkot DK, Pope MH, Lord J, et al: The relationship between work history, work environment and low-back pain in men. *Spine* 1984;9:395–399.
19. White AA III, Panjabi MM (eds): *Clinical Biomechanics of the Spine.* Philadelphia, PA, JB Lippincott, 1978.
20. Frymoyer JW, Pope MH, Costanza MC, et al: Epidemiologic studies of low-back pain. *Spine* 1980;5:419–423.
21. Basmajian JV (ed): *Muscles Alive: Their Functions Revealed by Electromyography,* ed 4. Baltimore, MD, Williams & Wilkins, 1978.
22. Morris JM, Benner G, Lucas DB: An electromyographic study of the intrinsic muscles of the back in man. *J Anat* 1962;96:509–520.
23. Pope MH, Andersson GB, Broman H, et al: Electromyographic studies of the lumbar trunk musculature during the development of axial torques. *J Orthop Res* 1986;4:288–297.
24. Troup JD, Martin JW, Lloyd DC: Back pain in industry: A prospective survey. *Spine* 1981;6:61–69.
25. Manning DP, Shannon HS: Slipping accidents causing low-back pain in a gearbox factory. *Spine* 1981;6:70–72.

26. Andersson R, Lagerlof E: Accident data in the new Swedish information system on occupational injuries. *Ergonomics* 1983;26:33–42.
27. Grieve DW: Slipping due to manual exertion. *Ergonomics* 1983;26:61–72.
28. Lawrence JS: Rheumatism in coal miners: Occupational factors. *Brit J Industr Med* 1955;12:249–261.
29. Kroemer KH, Robinette JC: Ergonomics in the design of office furniture. *Industr Med Surg* 1969;38:115–125.
30. Magora A: Investigation of the relation between low back pain and occupation: Physical requirements. Sitting, standing and weight lifting. *Industr Med Surg* 1972;41:5–9.
31. Kelsey JL: An epidemiological study of acute herniated lumbar intervertebral discs. *Rheum Rehabil* 1975;14:144–159.
32. Nachemson A, Elfstrom G: Intravital dynamic pressure measurements in lumbar discs: A study of common movements, maneuvers and exercises. *Scand J Rehabil Med* 1970;(suppl 1):1–40.
33. Andersson BJ, Ortengren R: Myoelectric back muscle activity during sitting. *Scand J Rehabil Med* 1974;(suppl 3):73–90.
34. Westrin CG: Low back sick-listing: A nosological and medical insurance investigation. *Scand J Soc Med* 1973;(suppl 7):1–116.
35. Bergquist-Ullman M, Larsson U: Acute low back pain in industry: A controlled prospective study with special reference to therapy and confounding factors. *Acta Orthop Scand* 1977;170(suppl):1–117.
36. Griffing JP: The occupational back, in Fleming AJ, D'Alonzo CA (eds): *Modern Occupational Medicine*, ed 2. Philadelphia, PA, Lea & Febiger, 1960, pp 219–227.
37. Andersson GBJ, Troup JDG: Worker selection, in Pope MH, Andersson GBJ, Frymoyer JW, et al (eds): *Occupational Low Back Pain: Assessment, Treatment, and Prevention*. St. Louis, MO, Mosby-Year Book, 1991, pp 239–250.
38. Dupuis H, Zerlett G (eds): *The Effects of Whole-Body Vibration*. Berlin, Germany, Springer-Verlag, 1986.
39. Frymoyer JW, Pope MH, Clements JH, et al: Risk factors in low-back pain: An epidemiological survey. *J Bone Joint Surg* 1983;65A:213–218.
40. Pope MH, Wilder DG, Jorneus L, et al: The response of the seated human to sinusoidal vibration and impact. *J Biomech Eng* 1987;109:279–284.
41. Smith P, Armstrong TJ, Liza GD: IECSs can play crucial role in enabling handicapped employees to work safely, productively. *Indus Eng* 1982;13:98–105.
42. Strandberg L: Ergonomics applied to slipping accidents, in Kvalseth TO (ed): *Applied Ergonomics: Selected Cases and Practical Issue*. London, England, IPC Science and Technology Press, 1982.
43. Corlett EN, Madeley SJ, Manenica I: Posture targetting: A technique for recording working postures. *Ergonomics* 1979;22:357–366.
44. Garg A, Chaffin DB: A biomechanical computerized simulation of human strength. *AJIE Tr* 1975;7:1–15.
45. Hickey DS, Hukins DW: Relation between the structure of the annulus fibrosus and the function and failure of the intervertebral disc. *Spine* 1980;5:106–116.
46. Bergquist-Ullman M, Larsson U: Acute low back pain in industry: A controlled prospective study with special reference to therapy and confounding factors. *Acta Orthop Scand* 1977;170(suppl):1–117.
47. Andersson BJ, Örtengren R, Nachemson AL, et al: The sitting posture: An electromyographic and discometric study. *Orthop Clin North Am* 1975;6:105–120.

Chapter 22
Skeletal Muscle Pathophysiology in Low Back Pain

Richard L. Lieber, PhD

Introduction

As detailed elsewhere in this volume, low back pain is responsible for a great deal of suffering and loss of work throughout the world. Because most individuals have experienced soreness associated with exercise of specific muscle groups, it is reasonable to investigate the lumbar musculature as a source of pain in patients suffering from low back pain. In this chapter, the relevant anatomy of the lumbar musculature will first be reviewed. Next, the eccentric contraction model of muscle injury will be presented to provide insights into muscle injury damage mechanisms and subjective symptoms. This type of injury occurs in most individuals with intense exercise training. Finally, neurophysiologic studies of muscle pain will be reviewed because they may relate to low back pain. Much of the work described in this chapter has been performed on limb musculature; therefore, I will extrapolate to possible implications in low back pain.

Lumbar Extensor Musculature

Anatomy

The muscles of the back often have been portrayed in anatomy texts as a single bulky mass that extends between the sacrum and iliac crest and the thorax. However, recent anatomic dissections have demonstrated that the back muscles are clearly divided into two major groups—the erector spinae and multifidus muscles (Outline 1). These two distinct functional units have large differences in innervation that probably indicate significant functional differences,[1] although the detailed biomechanical function of these groups remains only partially elucidated.[2] The erector spinae muscles are further subdivided into medial and lateral divisions known as the longissimus thoracis and iliocostalis lumborum, respectively. Both of these divisions are further subdivided into thoracic and lumbar portions.[1,3] In addition to these major muscle groups, several smaller muscles exist that form direct connections between analogous portions of adjacent vertebrae. These muscles are the interspinales, which connect the spines of adja-

Outline 1 Back muscle anatomic components

Multifidus muscles (medial)
Erector spinae muscles (lateral)
    Lateral division
        Iliocostalis lumborum
            Thoracic
            Lumbar
    Medial division
        Longissimus thoracis
            Thoracic
            Lumbar

cent vertebrae, and the intertransversarii, which connect the transverse processes of adjacent vertebrae.

Multifidus Muscles The multifidus muscles represent the deepest muscle group in the lumbar region (Fig. 1, *top*) and consist of multiple separate bands arising from each vertebral lamina and inserting from two to four segments below the level of origin (Fig. 1, *bottom*). The shortest fascicle of each muscle inserts onto the mamillary process of the vertebra located two segments caudally; longer, more superficial fascicles insert sequentially onto subsequent vertebrae three or more segments lower (Fig. 1). Thus, the shortest band of the multifidus arising from L1 inserts on L3, and subsequent bands insert sequentially on L4, L5, and the sacrum. Obviously, multifidus muscles arising from lower regions will consist of fewer fascicles as the number of vertebrae caudal to the origin decreases. All multifidus muscles that arise from a given level are innervated by the medial branch of the primary dorsal rami of the spinal nerves from a single segment, that is, each band of multifidus muscle is innervated from a single dorsal ramus. The principal action of the multifidus is sagittal rotation; however, the multisegmental nature of the muscle as well as its complex three-dimensional (3-D) orientation in the cranial-caudal and medial-lateral directions make this description a gross oversimplification.[4]

Longissimus Thoracis This muscle is the medial division of the erector spinae. The lumbar fascicles of the longissimus thoracis are composed of five bands that arise from the lumbar transverse processes and attach caudally onto the iliac crest (Fig. 2, *top left*). Each band arising from vertebrae L1 to L4 is actually a small fusiform muscle that has an elongated and flattened caudal tendon of insertion. The juxtaposition of many of these caudally located tendons forms the lumbar intermuscular aponeurosis, which easily is recognized intraoperatively or in cadaveric specimens. The thoracic component of the longissimus thoracis is composed of long slender muscles with pronounced caudal tendons that juxtapose to form the strong erector spinae aponeurosis (Fig. 2, *top right*). It is this aponeurosis that forms the boundary of the lumbar paraspinal muscles dorsally.

Iliocostalis Lumborum This muscle is the lateral division of the erector spinae. The iliocostalis lumborum muscles lie laterally to the longissimus thoracis muscles and arise from the tip of the transverse processes of vertebrae L1 to L4 in the lumbar region and thus are composed of four small, broad bands

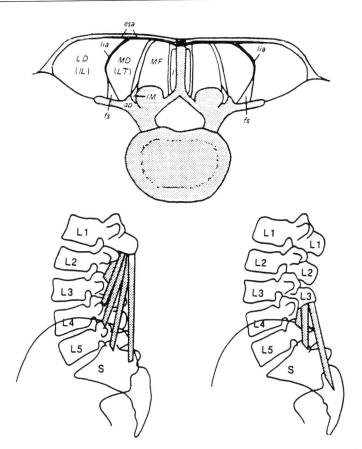

Fig. 1   *Schematic arrangement of multifidus muscle in cross-section (**top**) (Reproduced with permission from Bogduk N: A reappraisal of the anatomy of the human lumbar erector spinae. J Anat 1980;131:525–540.) and longitudinal section (**bottom**) (Reproduced with permission from Kalimo H, Rantanen J, Viljanen T, et al: Lumbar muscles: Structure and function. Ann Med 1989;21:353–359.). esa = erector spinae aponeurosis; lia = lumbar intermuscular aponeurosis; LD = lateral division; IL = iliocostalis lumborum; MD = medial division; LT = longissimus thoracis; MF = multifidus; I = interspinalis; fs = fat-filled space; ap = accessory process; IM = intertransversarii mediales.*

(Fig. 2, *bottom left*). In contrast to the more medially located musculature, there are no prominent caudal tendons, thereby giving the iliocostalis lumborum a much more fleshy appearance.

The mechanical properties of the lumbar muscles have not been measured directly. It is not clear, based on the description provided in the literature, whether the individual muscles that make up the spine extensors are very strong pennate muscles that generate large forces with a relatively small excursion or whether they contain relatively long muscle fibers and generate smaller forces. This difference is important because these architectural features are the major determinant of muscle function, but they can be determined only from microdissection of fixed tissue.[5] Microdissection of fixed tissue from the upper extremities of

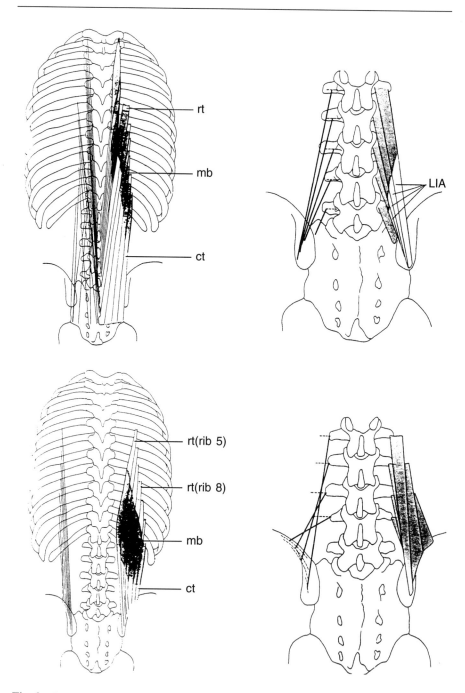

Fig. 2 *Longissimus thoracis (medial division of erector spinae) schematic of lumbar (**top left**) and thoracic (**top right**) regions and iliocostalis lumborum (lateral division of the erector spinae) schematic of lumbar (**bottom left**) and thoracic (**bottom right**) regions. rt = rostral tendon; mb = muscle belly; ct = caudal tendon; LIA = lumbar intermuscular aponeurosis. (Reproduced with permission from Macintosh JE, Bogduk N: The morphology of the lumbar erector spinae. Spine 1987;12:658–668.)*

humans has provided such insights.[6-8] It has been demonstrated, using other animals, that antigravity extensors (for example, the vastus lateralis and medial gastrocnemius) often have an architectural design that suits them for high force production; that is, they have a large number of relatively short fibers.[9-11] Analogous studies are required to define the architecture of the back muscles more completely.

Muscle Fiber Type Distribution

The distribution of fiber types within muscles provides insights into muscle function. For example, those muscles that are frequently activated in a postural role often contain a predominance of type 1 or "slow" muscle fibers.[12] In humans, type 1 fibers predominate in the vastus intermedius and soleus muscles. These muscle fibers are characterized by their slow contraction speed and extremely high endurance, which clearly suit their function. The few studies on the back extensor muscles are compromised somewhat by the lack of detail provided by the authors as to the actual sampling site of the biopsy among the five major components of back musculature. Given this limitation, there is general agreement that there is a slight predominance of type 1 fibers, with reported percentages of these fibers ranging from 49% to 67% (Table 1). Because, in many limb muscles, the deeper musculature tends to have a greater proportion of highly oxidative and slow muscle fibers,[13] it might be reasonable to guess that the deeper portions of the back extensor muscles would have the greatest proportion of type 1 fibers.

Highly oxidative type 1 fibers often are contrasted with low oxidative capacity type 2 fibers. In humans and other species, type 2 fibers exist as two subtypes, types 2A and 2B (or 2X), both of which have fast contraction times but also have quite different oxidative capacities. Type 2A fibers have, in many cases, as high an oxidative capacity as type 1 fibers (Fig. 3), whereas type 2B fibers have a much lower oxidative capacity altogether. In summary, it is not appropriate to measure the percentage of type 2 fibers and then discuss a muscle's fatigability without a knowledge of the percentage of each subtype present.

Skeletal Muscle Injury

Injury to muscle fibers can occur as a result of direct trauma, disease, application of myotoxic agents (such as local anesthetics), inflammatory processes,

Table 1 Back muscle fiber type percentages

Muscle Reported	Sample Studied	Type 1 Percentage
"Superficial" erector spinae	6 normal young men	58%
"Deep" erector spinae	6 normal young men	55%
Deep part of the multifidus	45 herniated disk patients	62% (females) 58% (males)
Deep part of the multifidus	12 control cadaver samples	63% (females) 61% (males)
Multifidus	17 patients with lumbar derangement	67%

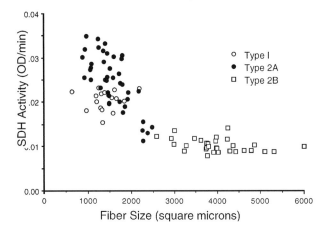

Fig. 3 *Oxidative capacity of individual muscle fibers of different types. Fibers were identified using the monoclonal antibody panel provided by Stefano Schiaffino (Padova, Italy). Note that it is a misconception that type 1 fibers must have higher oxidative capacities than type 2 fibers. In fact, type 2A fast fibers can have a higher oxidative capacity than type 1 fibers.*

or intense exercise. The degree to which muscle injury relates to low back pain is not currently known. However, injury and the pain that accompanies it have been studied using a number of experimental models. Results from these studies shed light on the mechanism of muscle fiber injury and on factors that influence the pain associated with it.

Muscle Injury Due to Eccentric Contractions

One of the surest methods for inducing skeletal muscle injury and soreness is to lengthen a muscle while it is activated. This active lengthening has been termed "eccentric contraction," where contraction simply denotes that the muscle is actively generating force during the lengthening maneuver. This muscle injury model has been studied in animals and humans for over 20 years. Most of the results discussed in the following paragraphs have been reported for a number of species and specific movements and, thus, probably are generally representative of changes that occur in all muscles.

Creatine Kinase as an Indicator of Muscle Damage

It has been reported that eccentric exercise results in a significant increase in serum creatine kinase (CK) levels 24 to 48 hours after the exercise bout,[14,15] an increase that may persist for 3 to 6 days, depending on the precise nature of the exercise (Fig. 4, open circles). CK is an intramuscular enzyme responsible for maintaining adequate adenosine triphosphate (ATP) levels during muscle contraction. Its appearance in the serum is interpreted as an increased permeability or breakdown of the membrane surrounding the muscle cell. Increased CK levels resolve in 7 to 14 days. In a similar delayed fashion, muscle pain accompanying eccentric exercise peaks 24 to 48 hours after the exercise bout, but it resolves more rapidly than CK levels. Peak CK levels are not strongly cor-

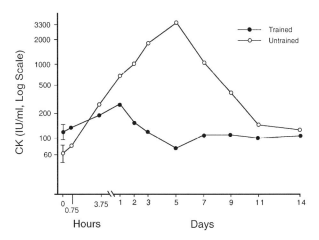

Fig. 4 *Time course of serum creatine kinase (CK) levels after a bout of eccentric exercise in untrained (open circles) or trained (filled circles) young men. Note the delayed and prolonged increase in CK levels in untrained individuals is attenuated after training. (Reproduced with permission from Lieber RL: Skeletal muscle response to injury, in Butler JP (ed): Skeletal Muscle Structure and Function. Baltimore, MD, Williams & Wilkins, 1992.)*

related with either the timing of increased muscle pain or the magnitude of tissue injury. This has been demonstrated quantitatively in both animal and human models of eccentric exercise.[16]

Another widely agreed upon finding is that training prevents or at least attenuates the magnitude of muscle injury that occurs after eccentric exercise (Fig. 4, solid circles). This training effect is produced only after eccentric training of the specific muscle group being tested. Thus, there is a very high degree of specificity regarding the protective effect of exercise. General increased fitness neither prevents nor attenuates eccentric contraction-induced muscle injury.

Mechanisms of Muscle Fiber Injury

Based on results of experimental studies of skeletal muscles directly subjected to eccentric exercise, it is widely thought that the very early events that cause muscle injury are mechanical in nature.[17,18] For example, during cyclic eccentric exercise of the rabbit tibialis anterior, significant mechanical changes were observed in the first 5 to 7 minutes of exercise.[19] After this time period, histologic examination revealed that a small fraction of muscle fibers appeared larger, more rounded, and more lightly staining than surrounding normal muscle fibers. Recent immunohistochemical studies have revealed structural disruption of the cytoskeleton within the fibers at these very earlier time periods.[20,21] This disruption may provide further insight into the damage mechanism.

Fiber Type Specific Damage

Both animal and human studies have provided evidence for selective damage of fast fiber types after eccentric exercise.[22-24] In human studies, this damage was confined to the type 2 muscle fibers in general, but in animal studies, damage has been further localized to the type FG (fast-glycolytic; often equated to type 2B) fast fiber subtype. Because FG fibers are the most highly fatigable muscle fibers,[25] it has been speculated that their high degree of fatigability may predispose them to injury. In fact, authors of several clinical studies have proposed that the fatigability of back muscles may be a predisposing factor to injury. However, it is difficult to test this idea directly because there are many other differences between type FG fibers and other muscle fibers. Further studies are required to elucidate the basis for fiber type specific injury to skeletal muscle and to document whether this is a predisposing factor to low back pain.

Inflammation After Muscle Injury

Direct evidence of inflammatory cells within skeletal muscle in both animals and humans after eccentric exercise has been presented.[26,27] Armstrong and associates[26] and McCully and Faulkner[27] documented that the early events are followed by infiltration of circulating monocytes that become macrophages after entering the tissue. My coworkers and I measured the time course of torque generation in rabbit dorsiflexors after a single eccentric exercise bout and found a progressive decline in force that was delayed and occurred over a 2- to 3-day period (Fig. 5). We hypothesized that the mechanism for the progressive decline in force was the infiltration of inflammatory cells and the associated proteolytic degradation of muscle tissue. In our model, the progressive force de-

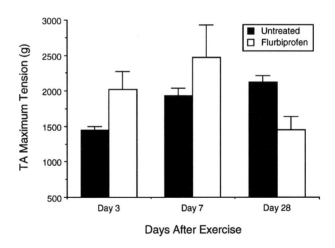

Fig. 5 *Time course of torque change for flurbiprofen-treated (unfilled bars) and untreated (filled bars) muscles. Isometric torque was measured noninvasively with the servomotor holding the ankle fixed in about 10° of plantarflexion and activating the peroneal nerve. The untreated muscles experience a transient decrease in torque, which returns to normal around 15 days. In contrast, the flurbiprofen-treated muscles generated a significantly higher torque early in the treatment period (3 and 7 days) and a significantly lower torque later in the experimental period (28 days). (Reproduced with permission from Mishra DK, Fridén J, Schmitz MC, et al: Anti-inflammatory medication after muscle injury: A treatment resulting in short-term improvement but subsequent loss of muscle function. J Bone Joint Surg 1995;77A:1510–1519.)*

cline was about the same order of magnitude as the force decline that occurred due to the mechanical injury itself. Cellular infiltration was uniquely associated with the eccentric exercise itself; isometrically-exercised muscles were devoid of infiltrating cells, and the same force decrement was not observed after isometric exercise of the same duration. A similar scenario has been proposed in human exercise studies.[28]

Because the inflammatory process itself can cause damage in excess of that originally experienced by the tissue, it is possible that prevention of inflammation would improve muscle status following injury. Based on this assumption, nonsteroidal anti-inflammatory drugs (NSAIDs) are commonly prescribed to provide analgesia and improve performance. The specific objective effects of the NSAID on muscle function are, however, poorly understood. Moreover, it is difficult to test muscle function in humans because the analgesic effect of NSAIDs may themselves permit improved performance. My coworkers and I tested the anti-inflammatory medication, flurbiprofen, in the rabbit muscle injury described above. Muscles were exercised with a single eccentric exercise bout after which the anti-inflammatory medication was given for 7 days. Muscle contractile properties were measured for the 28 days following the exercise, and a most interesting result was obtained. Muscles treated with the NSAID demonstrated a significant short-term improvement in contractile function, but a subsequent loss in function (Fig. 5). The inflammation process itself, which occurred secondary to the initial muscle injury, also resulted in additional delayed ''injury'' to the muscle, and we suggested that the eventual functional recovery of the muscle was dependent on the inflammatory process (Fig. 6). By suppressing the initial inflammatory reaction, the NSAID permits improved performance in early time periods, but appears to suppress the stimulus that may be needed for cellular remodeling in longer time periods.[29] These data may have implications in the use of NSAIDs for pain treatment associated with neuromuscular injury.

Skeletal Muscle Pain

Source of Pain in Skeletal Muscle

Whether low back pain directly results from events within the paraspinal muscles is not known. Numerous investigators have documented the existence of pain in skeletal muscles resulting from a number of different situations, including blunt trauma, eccentric exercise, injection of noxious agents, and peripheral nerve disease. However, none of these studies have been performed explicitly on back muscles. For that reason, I have extrapolated from studies of limb muscles to the situation that might occur in back muscles.

It is clear that muscle fiber damage does not necessarily cause pain. This statement is based on the observation that muscle biopsies obtained from patients with primary muscle diseases, such as Duchenne muscular dystrophy, reveal major disruptions of the myofibrillar and sarcotubular apparatus and, yet, the patients themselves remain pain-free. Thus, pain within muscle that occurs after

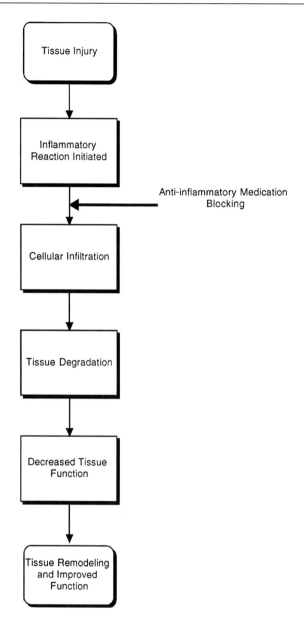

Fig. 6 *Hypothetical effect of anti-inflammatory medication on the normal progress of tissue injury and healing. In the absence of medication, tissue injury results in an inflammatory reaction, which further degrades tissue prior to healing. If the inflammatory reaction is blocked, complete tissue remodeling does not occur, resulting in decreased remodeling.*[29]

fiber injury is a result of secondary events that take place after the damage itself. For this reason, and based on experimental data obtained from investigations of muscles, tendons, and joints, muscle pain is thought to result from stimulation of nociceptors within the muscle itself.

Skeletal Muscle Innervation

Muscles are supplied by a rich and extensive network of receptors that are innervated by small myelinated (group III) and unmyelinated (group IV) afferent nerve fibers. These fibers conduct much more slowly (Table 2) than either the α-motoneurons that project to the muscle fibers (extrafusal muscle fibers), the γ-motoneurons that project to the muscle spindles (intrafusal muscle fibers), or even the Ia afferents that feed back from muscle spindles to the spinal cord.

Cutaneous Receptors Encode Specific Sensations

Much of the understanding of the neurophysiologic basis of sensation is based on studies of cutaneous receptors. Using the technique of intraneural microstimulation and microrecording (Fig. 7), Torebjörk and Ochoa[30,31] have generated a large experimental base that has improved understanding of the anatomic and physiologic basis of pain. With their method, electric activity of single afferent axons can be measured in awake human volunteers in such a way that electrophysiologic events can be associated with subjective reports of sensation and localization.[30] In a typical experiment, a microelectrode (200 μm diameter) was inserted through the skin into an underlying nerve trunk and identified as impaling digital cutaneous afferents either by recording afferent activity while stroking the skin or by evoking sensations projected to the skin while stimulating electrically through the electrode. A second recording electrode was placed more proximally on the forearm (Fig. 7). The receptive field was then mapped using von Frey hairs and the conduction velocity calculated from measurement of the latency and conduction distance between stimulating and recording sites. Once the single unit was characterized, stimulation was applied and the elementary characteristics resulting were documented.

These investigators matched the receptive field of a recorded single unit that was defined by cutaneous stimulation with a painter's brush with the field to which a "pure" sensation was projected during microstimulation. They also matched the sensory unit type with the subjective interpretation of the sensation (for example, tickle, pressure, pain) to yield confidence that the evoked sensations were indeed the result of the isolated activity of a single unit (Table 3). This study allowed correlation between the subjective sensation and the afferent unit type.[31]

The numerous experiments revealed several sensations subjectively agreed upon between subjects: tapping or vibration, pressure, and tickling. When the stimulation frequency was changed, the intensity of the sensations increased, but the basic nature of the sensation did not change. This result suggested that the afferent activity actually encoded the elementary sensation and was not coded

Table 2 Properties of afferent fibers in peripheral nerve

Fiber Group	Myelinated?	Axon Diameter (μm)	Average Conduction Velocity (m/s)
I	Yes	15	90-100
II	Yes	10	40-50
III	Yes	5	20-30
IV	No	< 1	1

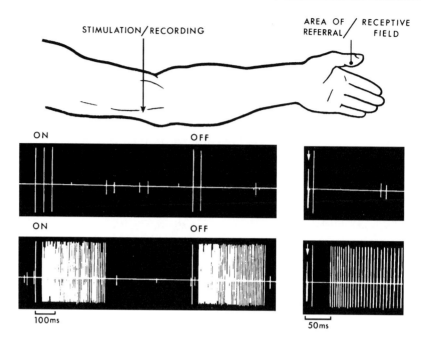

Fig. 7 *Method for intraneural identification of sensory units. A microelectrode is placed within a nerve and stimulated to elicit a sensation. This sensation can be emulated for cutaneous afferents by gently stroking receptive fields on the skin. (Reproduced with permission from Torebjörk HE, Ochoa JL: Specific sensations evoked by activity in single identified sensory units in man. Acta Physiol Scand 1980;110:445–447.)*

Table 3 Sensations associated with intraneural stimulation of mechanoreceptors in the human hand[31]

Unit Type	Sensation
Rapidly adapting (RA)	Intermittent tapping
Pacinian corpuscles (PC)	Vibration or tickle
Slowly adapting I (SA I)	Pressure
Slowly adapting II (SA II)	No sensation

by the frequency of the action potentials. In addition, the size of the receptive field was not influenced by stimulus frequency. Correlation between the elementary sensations and single unit electrophysiology revealed that the rapidly adapting (RA) units (Table 3) encoded the tapping-flutter sensation (but never pressure or tickling), the pacinian corpuscles (PC) units encoded vibration, the slowly adapting (SA) I units were associated with the sensation of pressure, and the SA II units were not associated with any particular sensation at all. These data indicate that afferent activity by specific receptors within the skin encodes specific sensations.

Nociception in Skeletal Muscle

Although the bulk of the data on the neurophysiology of pain has been obtained from similar studies of cutaneous receptors, muscle and visceral pain are much more clinically relevant. It was estimated, in a 1990 survey, that 14% of the United States population suffers from chronic pain related to muscles and joints.[32]

The extensive studies by Mense and associates[33-35] provide a wealth of understanding regarding these nociceptive mechanisms in muscle and viscera. They delineated several important differences between muscle (and visceral) pain compared to cutaneous pain: (1) whereas cutaneous pain is localized with great accuracy, muscle pain is difficult to localize; (2) although increasing activation intensity of cutaneous receptors does not change the size of the receptive field, increasing muscular pain intensity results in referral to remote sites, such as other muscles, fascia, tendons, joints, or ligaments; and (3) muscle pain is associated with symptoms mediated through the autonomic nervous system, such as decreased blood pressure, nausea, and sweating, whereas cutaneous pain is not.

Unlike analogous studies of the skin, repetitive electrical stimulation of muscle afferents results only in painful sensations. Increasing the intensity does not modify the subjective nature of the pain and only serves to elicit the description of a ''cramp'' as well as a decreased ability to localize the site of the pain source.[36] Additionally, the magnitude of referred pain is positively correlated to the stimulation frequency of deep nociceptive fibers.

Factors That Modulate Nociception in Skeletal Muscle

The type III and type IV nociceptors in skeletal muscle have been studied primarily in the cat hindlimb preparation. The relative percentage of motor and sensory nerves innervating the lateral gastrocnemius-soleus muscles has been shown to be approximately 60% motor and 40% sensory (Table 4). Of the sensory nerves, about 40% of them can be classified as nociceptive, suggesting an overall high sensibility within these muscles (15% to 20% of the innervating axons).

Factors affecting nociception are demonstrated by recording from single nociceptive afferents from anesthetized cats and experimentally perturbing the system. For example, Mense and Meyer[33] measured the discharge activity of these group III afferents and saw almost no activity on light touch with a painter's brush (Fig. 8), some activity on moderate touch, and high activity with noxious touch (pinching the muscle with forceps). No activity was observed on passive stretch of the muscle within the physiologic range (6 mm in this case), but if the muscle was stretched 9 or 12 mm, a moderate level of activity was recorded. This made teleologic sense because nociceptors are designed to not only signal tissue damage but to prevent it as well.

Inflammatory Factors Other causes of increased output from nociceptors were injection of factors presumed to be involved in the inflammatory response, such as bradykinin (BK, cleaved from precursor plasma proteins), 5-hydroxytryptamine (5HT, released from platelets following vascular damage), and prostaglandins (PG, a by-product of the cylooxygenase pathway). All receptors studied showed clear signs of BK-induced sensitization characterized

359

Table 4 Fiber composition of the nerve to the lateral gastrocnemius-soleus cat muscle[43]

Nerves	Number	Percentage
Myelinated (1200)		
Motor	720	60%
Aα Skeletomotor	382	53%
Aβ Skeleto- and fusimotor	14	2%
Aγ Fusimotor	324	45%
Sensory	480	40%
I Spindle primary sensory endings (Ia)	144	30%
Golgi tendon organs (Ib)	72	15%
II Spindle secondary endings	144	30%
III "Free" nerve endings	110	23%
Unmyelinated (2000)		
Motor		
C Vasomotor	1000	50%
Sensory		
IV Sensory	1000	50%

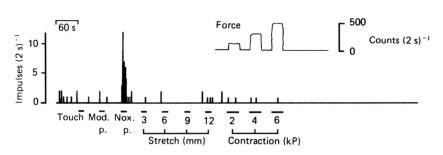

Fig. 8 *Recording from intramuscular type III afferents with pressure of different levels (left) and with stretch above and beyond the physiologic range (6 mm in this case). (Reproduced with permission from Mense S, Meyer H: Different types of slowly conducting afferent units in cat skeletal muscle and tendon. J Physiol 1985;363:403–417.)*

by a lowered threshold to local pressure stimulation (Fig. 9). Because BK is known to release PGE2 from cells, it can actually potentiate its own action. This finding led to the idea that compounds that block the effect of PG synthesis (for example, acetylsalicylic acid, ASA) might reduce or abolish the stimulatory action of BK. This was, in fact, the case. There was a complete lack of effect of BK within 15 minutes of injection of ASA, thereby demonstrating the peripheral effect of ASA because connections with the central nervous system were cut in this experiment.

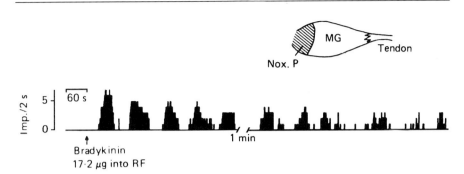

Fig. 9   *Demonstration of increased type III afferent activity in cat soleus muscle nociceptors with application of bradykinin. (Reproduced with permission from Mense S, Meyer H: Bradykinin-induced modulation of the response behaviour of different types of feline group III and IV muscle receptors.* J Physiol *1988;398:49–63.)*

Ischemia Ischemia for prolonged periods (up to about 15 minutes) is not painful and does not evoke sympathetic reflexes.[37] However, if a muscle contracts under ischemic conditions, pain rapidly develops. BK probably is involved in this response because kinin is released from plasma proteins during ischemia.[38] Mense and Stahnke[34] demonstrated activation of group IV muscle receptors during ischemic contractions. Muscle contraction alone did not elicit the response, but afferent activity increased fourfold when the same contraction was performed while occluding the nutrient artery.

Reflex-Mediated Pain In some of the older clinical literature, there are reports suggesting that increased activity or excitability of the γ motor system causes the painful spasms that sometime appear in skeletal muscle. Increased activity of the γ motor system would then lead to increased discharge frequency in muscle spindle afferent fibers. The increased discharge frequency would, in turn, lead to increased activation of α motoneurons. By this mechanism, a vicious cycle could result that would be so strong it could lead to ischemic contractions and pain by any one of a number of mechanisms described above. Unfortunately, experimental evidence supporting this concept is lacking.[35] The main finding of these studies was that resting activity of the γ-motoneurons was reduced significantly by inflammation and that the reflex excitability of the neurons also was inhibited. These results demonstrated that nociceptive muscle afferents actually inhibit homonymous γ motoneurons. The inhibition may represent an advantage to the muscle because it could reduce potential damaging forces on it that would result from an increase in γ motoneuron activity.

Development of Chronic Pain It is conceivable that some of the mechanisms just described could be relevant to development of chronic muscle pain in the lower back musculature. Obviously, objective, prospective clinical data are not available, and these ideas mostly represent an educated guess based on synthesis of available literature. Nevertheless, a plausible scenario may be as follows.[39] Due to some peripheral injury (trauma, ischemia, pressure, and so forth), endogenous sensitizing substances and pain-producing substances (for example, kinins and prostaglandins) are released. The main action of these sub-

361

stances is vasodilatation and increased permeability of the microcirculation (Fig. 10), which results in increased interstitial fluid pressure. Further deposition of vasoactive substances and venous occlusion could result in tissue ischemia that itself would result in release of more vasoactive substances. Within the muscle, lack of oxygen could lead to a reduced adenylate charge within the fiber, loss of calcium homeostasis, and tissue damage similar to that seen during intense exercise. Muscle contracture and structural disruption could result in further exacerbating ischemic damage. Of course, these ideas are speculative and further experiments are required to determine the extent to which such mechanisms operate in low back pain.

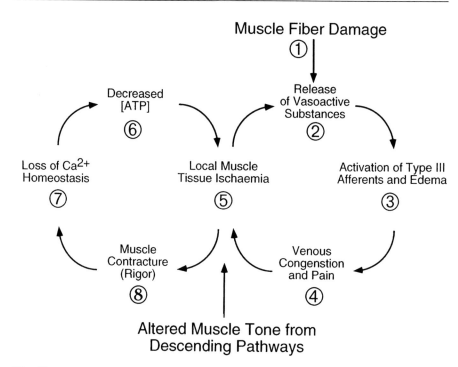

Fig. 10 *Putative peripheral mechanism for development and maintenance of chronic pain. The self-sustaining cycle begins (right portion of panel) with a lesion to muscular or nervous tissue (1). This results in release of vasoneuroactive substances such as kinins, potassium, and prostaglandins (2). Increased capillary permeability and direct activation of type III afferent fibers result in pain and swelling (3). Increased interstitial fluid flow provides an inhibition of venous outflow (4) that also causes some degree of local tissue ischemia (5). Low tissue oxygenation due to ischemia exacerbates pain- and edema-producing mechanisms. Within the muscle itself, decreased tissue perfusion results in decreased levels of ATP within the cell (6), especially in muscle fibers with low oxidative capacity (the type 2B or type FG muscle fibers). Loss of adenylate charge results in loss of muscle cell Ca2+ homeostasis that can activate endogenous proteases and allow permanent myofilament activation (rigor, 7). Increased tissue activation exacerbates both the ischemic condition of the tissue (8) and tissue injury exacerbates pain producing release of neuroactive substances (2).[44]*

Prediction of Low Back Pain Unfortunately, there is little agreement among investigators as to specific muscular sources of low back pain or interventions that relieve the pain. Most published studies represent anecdotal summaries of relatively specific patient populations. As expected, it has been postulated that low back pain results from excessive fatigue of back musculature. A number of straightforward methods have been developed to quantify fatigue,[40-42] and investigators generally have reported that individuals with greater lumbar muscle fatigability are at greater risk for development of low back pain. It would be a mistake to interpret these results directly in terms of fatigability of muscles themselves because a major factor affecting such functional fatigue tests is the neural activation pattern, which is very difficult to control. In fact, in one of the few studies of this type, careful measurement of back muscle function via isometric testing and of erector spinae structure via magnetic resonance imaging revealed that patients with chronic low back pain had less extensor strength and endurance and lower density in their erector spinae muscles compared to healthy subjects.[43] However, it is not clear whether this was the cause or the result of the pain (or neither). The largest prospective study of low back pain to date followed 3,020 Boeing Corporation workers over a 4-year period and, unfortunately, demonstrated that there were no useful morphologic or performance predictors of low back pain. Parameters measured included the traditional anthropometric measures as well as reflex asymmetry, toe extensor and calf muscle girth asymmetry, and the presence of back pain on straight leg raise.[44] No estimates of back muscle fatigue were attempted. Based on an average follow-up of over 3 years, no useful predictors for the development of low back pain were obtained.

Summary

Although a great deal is known regarding the gross anatomy of back muscles and their innervation, relationships between anatomic structure, muscle fiber recruitment, and movement are lacking. Such studies are relatively rare in the extemity literature; therefore, it is not surprising that detailed kinematic analysis of the lumbar spine during locomotion is not available. It is also difficult to study this problem in detail in the absense of an adequate animal model. It would be important to describe the microscopic architectural and histochemical properties of the muscles described above in order to gain insights into their function. The recruitment pattern of the various muscles during normal movements must also be understood in order to compare patients with painful symptoms to those without such symptoms. Finally, it is desirable to develop noninvasive diagnostic methods to identify factors contributing to low back pain and to perform a prospective, large scale study on which (if any) of these factors have useful predictive value.

References

1. Kalimo H, Rantanen J, Viljanen T, et al: Lumbar muscles: Structure and function. *Ann Med* 1989;21:353–359.
2. Macintosh JE, Bogduk N: The morphology of the lumbar erector spinae. *Spine* 1987;12:658–668.

3. Bogduk N: A reappraisal of the anatomy of the human lumbar erector spinae. *J Anat* 1980;131:525–540.

4. Macintosh JE, Bogduk N: The biomechanics of the lumbar multifidus. *Clin Biomech* 1986;1:205–213.

5. Sacks RD, Roy RR: Architecture of the hind limb muscles of cats: Functional significance. *J Morphol* 1982;173:185–195.

6. Lieber RL, Jacobson MD, Fazeli BM, et al: Architecture of selected muscles of the arm and forearm: Anatomy and implications for tendon transfer. *J Hand Surg* 1992;17A:787–798.

7. Lieber RL, Fazeli BM, Botte MJ: Architecture of selected wrist flexor and extensor muscles. *J Hand Surg* 1990;15A:244–250.

8. Jacobson MD, Raab R, Fazeli BM, et al: Architectural design of the human intrinsic hand muscles. *J Hand Surg* 1992;17A:804–809.

9. Lieber RL, Blevins FT: Skeletal muscle architecture of the rabbit hindlimb: Functional implications of muscle design. *J Morphol* 1989;199:93–101.

10. Wickiewicz TL, Roy RR, Powell PL, et al: Muscle architecture of the human lower limb. *Clin Orthop* 1983;179:275–283.

11. Friederich JA, Brand RA: Muscle fiber architecture in the human lower limb. *J Biomech* 1990;23:91–95.

12. Edgerton VR, Smith JL, Simpson DR: Muscle fibre type populations of human leg muscles. *Histochem J* 1975;7:259–266.

13. Lexell J, Downham D, Sjostrom M: Distribution of different fibre types in human skeletal muscles: A statistical and computational study of the fibre type arrangement in m. vastus lateralis of young, healthy males. *J Neurol Sci* 1984;65:353–365.

14. Evans WJ, Meredith CN, Cannon JG, et al: Metabolic changes following eccentric exercise in trained and untrained men. *J Appl Physiol* 1986;61:1864–1868.

15. Clarkson PM, Johnson J, Dextradeur D, et al: The relationships among isokinetic endurance, initial strength level, and fiber type. *Res Q Exerc Sport* 1982;53:15–19.

16. Newham DJ: The consequences of eccentric contractions and their relationship to delayed onset muscle pain. *Eur J Appl Physiol* 1988;57:353–359.

17. Lieber RL, Fridén J: Muscle damage is not a function of muscle force but active muscle strain. *J Appl Physiol* 1993;74:520–526.

18. Warren GL, Hayes DA, Lowe DA, et al: Mechanical factors in the initiation of eccentric contraction-induced injury in rat soleus muscle. *J Physiol* 1993;464:457–475.

19. Lieber RL, Woodburn TM, Fridén J: Muscle damage induced by eccentric contractions of 25% strain. *J Appl Physiol* 1991;70:2498–2507.

20. Lieber RL, Schmitz MC, Mishra DK, et al: Contractile and cellular remodeling in rabbit skeletal muscle after cyclic eccentric contractions. *J Appl Physiol* 1994;77:1926–1934.

21. Lieber RL, Thornell L-E, Fridén J: Muscle cytoskeletal disruption occurs within the first 15 minutes of cyclic eccentric contraction. *J Appl Physiol* 1996;80:278–284.

22. Lieber RL, Fridén J: Selective damage of fast glycolytic muscle fibres with eccentric contraction of the rabbit tibialis anterior. *Acta Physiol Scand* 1988;133:587–588.

23. Fridén J, Sjöström M, Ekblom B: Myofibrillar damage following intense eccentric exercise in man. *Int J Sports Med* 1983;4:170–176.

24. Fridén J: Changes in human skeletal muscle induced by long-term eccentric exercise. *Cell Tissue Res* 1984;236:365–372.

25. Burke RE, Levine DN, Tsairis P, et al: Physiological types and histochemical profiles in motor units of the cat gastrocnemius. *J Physiol* 1973;234:723–748.

26. Armstrong RB, Ogilvie RW, Schwane JA: Eccentric exercise-induced injury to rat skeletal muscle. *J Appl Physiol* 1983;54:80–93.

27. McCully KK, Faulkner JA: Injury to skeletal muscle fibers of mice following lengthening contractions. *J Appl Physiol* 1985;59:119–126.

28. Cannon JG, Orencole SF, Fielding RA, et al: Acute phase response in exercise: Interaction of age and vitamin E on neutrophils and muscle enzyme release. *Am J Physiol* 1990;259:R1214–R1219.

29. Mishra DK, Fridén J, Schmitz MC, et al: Anti-inflammatory medication after muscle injury: A treatment resulting in short-term improvement but subsequent loss of muscle function. *J Bone Joint Surg* 1995;77A:1510–1519.

30. Torebjörk HE, Ochoa JL: Specific sensations evoked by activity in single identified sensory units in man. *Acta Physiol Scand* 1980;110:445–447.

31. Ochoa J, Torebjörk E: Sensations evoked by intraneural microstimulation of single mechanoreceptor units innervating the human hand. *J Physiol* 1983;342:633–654.

32. Magni G, Caldieron C, Rigatti-Luchini S, et al: Chronic musculoskeletal pain and depressive symptoms in the general population: An analysis of the 1st National Health and Nutrition Examination Survey data. *Pain* 1990;43:299–307.

33. Mense S, Meyer H: Different types of slowly conducting afferent units in cat skeletal muscle and tendon. *J Physiol* 1985;363:403–417.

34. Mense S, Stahnke M: Responses in muscle afferent fibres of slow conduction velocity to contractions and ischaemia in the cat. *J Physiol* 1983;342:383–397.

35. Mense S, Skeppar P: Discharge behaviour of feline gamma-motoneurones following induction of an artificial myositis. *Pain* 1991;46:201–210.

36. Torebjörk HE, Ochoa JL, Schady W: Referred pain from intraneural stimulation of muscle fascicles in the median nerve. *Pain* 1984;18:145–156.

37. Lewis T, Pickering GW, Rothschild P: Observations upon muscular pain in intermittent claudication. *Heart* 1931;15:359–383.

38. Mitchell JH, Schmidt RF: Cardiovascular reflex control by afferent fibers from skeletal muscle receptors, in Shepherd JT, Abboud FM, Geiger SR (eds): *The Cardiovascular System: Vol 3. Peripheral Circulation and Organ Blood Flow: Part 2.* Bethesda, MD, The American Physiological Society, 1983, pp 623–658.

39. Mense S: Considerations concerning the neurobiological basis of muscle pain. *Can J Physiol Pharmacol* 1991;69:610–616.

40. Roy SH, De Luca CJ, Casavant DA: Lumbar muscle fatigue and chronic lower back pain. *Spine* 1989;14:992–1001.

41. Biering-Sorensen F: A prospective study of low back pain in a general population: I. Occurrence, recurrence and aetiology. *Scand J Rehabil Med* 1983;15:71–79.

42. Frymoyer JW, Pope MH, Costanza MC, et al: Epidemiologic studies of low-back pain. *Spine* 1980;5:419–423.

43. Hultman G, Nordin M, Saraste H, et al: Body composition, endurance, strength, cross-sectional area, and density of MM erector spinae in men with and without low back pain. *J Spinal Disord* 1993;6:114–123.

44. Battie MC, Bigos SJ, Fisher LD, et al: Anthropometric and clinical measures as predictors of back pain complaints in industry: A prospective study. *J Spinal Disord* 1990;3:195–204.

Chapter 23
Low Back Pain and Spinal Instability

Manohar M. Panjabi, PhD

Low back pain is a significant problem of the industrialized societies, costing an estimated \$15 to \$50 billion per year in the United States.[1-4] There is a 50% to 70% chance of a person having low back pain during his or her lifetime,[5] with a prevalence of about 18%.[6] Thus, more than 30 million people in the United States may have low back pain at any time, and 10 million of them have chronic symptoms.[2] Specific causes for most of the low back pain problems are unknown. Although negative social interaction (for example, dissatisfaction at work) has been found to relate to low back pain, a significant portion of the problem is of mechanical origin; this portion is often referred to as spinal instability.[7]

The problem of clinical instability is controversial and not well understood. Clinical instability of the spine has been defined as the loss of the spine's ability to maintain its patterns of displacement under physiologic loads so there is no initial or additional neurologic deficit, no major deformity, and no incapacitating pain.[8] Clinical studies of patients with spine pain would be ideal for testing this hypothesis. However, carrying out such studies has not been easy and the results have not been encouraging.

Clinical instability of the spine has been studied in vivo since 1944 when Knutsson, using functional radiographs, attempted to relate low back pain to retrodisplacement of a vertebra during flexion.[9] There have been several similar studies over the past 50 years, but the results have been unclear. In association with back or neck pain, some investigators found increased motion,[10-13] whereas others found decreased motion.[14-16] Some reasons for the uncertainties have been the variability in the voluntary efforts of the subjects to produce spinal motion, the presence of muscle spasm and pain during the radiographic examination, lack of appropriate control subjects matched in age and gender, and the limited accuracy of in vivo methods for measuring motion. These problems, although not insurmountable, are difficult to resolve in a clinical setting.

Clinical Assessment of Spinal Instability

The first systematic approach to the analysis of clinical stability of the spine was undertaken in a biomechanical study of the cervical spine. Fresh cadaveric functional spinal units or motion segments (two adjacent vertebrae with interconnecting disk, ligaments, and facet joints, but devoid of musculature)[17,18] were

367

loaded either in flexion or extension, and the anatomic elements (disk, ligaments, and facet joints) were transected either from anterior to posterior or from posterior to anterior. This process resulted in the development of a checklist for the diagnosis of instability in the cervical spine.[8] A similar biomechanical experiment was performed for the lumbar spine, and results of this study led to the development of a checklist for lumbar spine instability.[8,19]

The lumbar spine checklist uses several elements, such as biomechanical parameters, neurologic damage, and anticipated loading on the spine (Table 1). A point value system is used to determine stability or instability. The anterior elements include the posterior longitudinal ligament and all anatomic structures anterior to it (two points). The posterior elements are all anatomic structures posterior to the posterior longitudinal ligament (two points). The intervertebral translation (two points) is measured either on flexion-extension or resting radiographs (Fig. 1). The rotation (two points) is measured either on flexion-extension radiographs (Fig. 2, *top*) or on resting radiographs (Fig. 2, *bottom*). Damage to the cauda equina is given three points, and the anticipated high loading on the spine is given one point.

If the sum of the points is five or more, then the spine is considered clinically unstable. This systematic approach to the assessment of clinical instability is an important tool for the clinician, and a prospective controlled study to validate the predictions of the checklist would be beneficial.

The Spinal Stabilizing System

In addition to the spinal column, the surrounding muscles and their controlled and precise activation play important roles in the mechanical stability of

Table 1 Checklist for the diagnosis of clinical instability in the lumbar spine

Element	Point Value[*]
Anterior elements destroyed or unable to function	2
Posterior elements destroyed or unable to function	2
Radiographic criteria[†]	4
Flexion-extension radiographs	
Sagittal plane translation > 4.5 mm or 15%	2
Sagittal plane rotation	
> 15° at L1-2, L2-3, and L3-4	2
> 20° at L4-5	2
> 25° at L5-S1	2
Resting radiographs[†]	
Sagittal plane displacement > 4.5 mm or 15%	2
Relative sagittal plane angulation > 22°	2
Cauda equina damage	3
Dangerous loading anticipated	1

[*]A point value total of 5 or more indicates clinical instability
[†]*See Figures 9, 10A & 10B for measurement techniques*
(Reproduced with permission from White AA, Panjabi MM (eds): *Clinical Biomechanics of the Spine*, ed 2. Philadelphia, PA, JB Lippincott, 1990.)

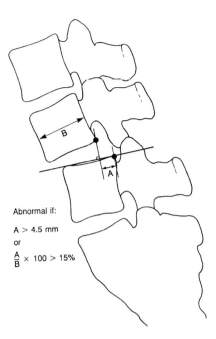

Abnormal if:

A > 4.5 mm

or

$\frac{A}{B} \times 100 > 15\%$

Fig. 1 *Measurement of vertebral translation or displacement in the lumbar spine. A method for measuring sagittal plane translation or displacement. If the translation or displacement is as much as 4.5 mm or 15% of the sagittal diameter of the adjacent vertebra, it is considered abnormal. These measurements are to be used in conjunction with the checklist in Table 1. (Reproduced with permission from White AA, Panjabi MM (eds):* Clinical Biomechanics of the Spine, *ed 2. Philadelphia, PA, JB Lippincott, 1990, p 354.)*

the spinal column, especially in dynamic conditions and under heavy loads. As a result, the spinal stabilizing system of the spine can be divided into three subsystems: spinal column, spinal muscles surrounding the spinal column, and control unit (Fig. 3).[20] Under normal conditions, the three subsystems work in harmony and provide mechanical stability. The spinal column provides information, such as position, loads, and motions of each vertebra, in a dynamic fashion. The control unit computes the needed stability and appropriately activates the muscles. Experimental data concerning each of the three subsystems and how the various components contribute to the overall stability of the spine will be discussed next.

The Spinal Column

Biomechanical studies under controlled laboratory conditions have provided some insight into the role of spinal column components (disk, ligaments, and facets) in providing spinal stability. Details of some of these studies are provided below. The load displacement curve was used as a measure of physical properties of the spine. The curve may be linear or nonlinear. In man-made structures, such as a steel spring, in which the load displacement curve is linear, the ratio of the load applied, and the displacement produced is constant. Such a curve

369

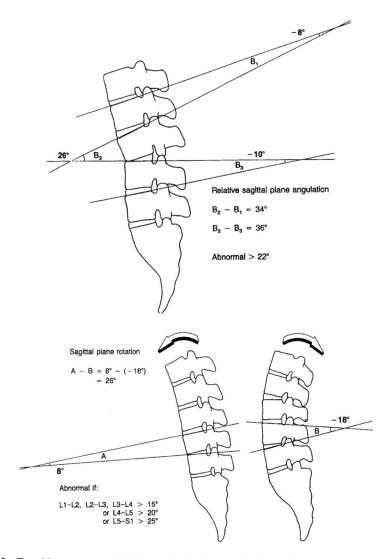

Fig. 2   Top, *Measurement of relative sagittal plane angulation in the lumbar spine. A method of measuring relative sagittal plane angulation of the L4-5 functional spinal unit on a static (resting) lateral radiograph. Relative sagittal plane angulation greater than 22° is abnormal and potentially unstable in the lumbar spine. Note that this means 22° greater than the amount of angulation above or below the functional spinal unit. By convention, negative values denote lordosis, and positive values kyphosis.* **Bottom**, *Measurement of sagittal plane rotation in the lumbar spine. A method of measuring sagittal plane rotation of the L4-5 functional spinal unit on dynamic (flexion-extension) lateral radiographs. The sagittal plane rotation is the difference between the Cobb measurements taken in flexion (A degree) and extension (B degree). Sagittal plane rotation greater than 15° at L1-2, L2-3, and L3-4, greater than 20° at L4-5, or greater than 25° at L5-S1 is abnormal and potentially unstable. These measurements are to be used in conjunction with the checklist in Table 1. (Reproduced with permission from White AA, Panjabi MM (eds):* Clinical Biomechanics of the Spine, *ed 2. Philadelphia, PA, JB Lippincott, 1990, p 355.)*

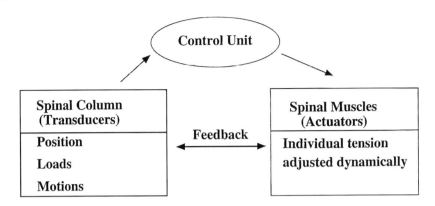

Fig. 3   *The spinal stabilizing system can be thought of as consisting of three subsystems: spinal column; muscles surrounding the spine; and motor control unit. The spinal column carries the loads and provides information about the position, motion, and loads of the spinal column. This information is transformed into action by the control unit. The action is provided by the muscles which must take into consideration the spinal column, but also the dynamic changes in spinal posture and loads. (Reproduced with permission from Panjabi MM: The stabilizing system of the spine. Part I. Function, dysfunction, adaptation, and enhancement.* J Spinal Disord *1992;5:383–389.)*

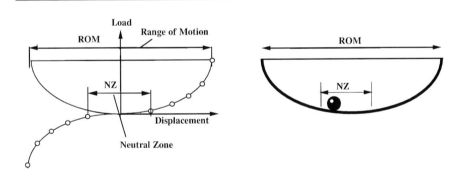

Fig. 4   **Left**, *Spine segment exhibits a nonlinear load displacement curve, indicating a changing relationship between the applied load and the displacements produced. Addition of neutral zone parameter, representing laxity of the spine segment around neutral position, to the range of motion parameter better describes the nonlinearity of the spinal characteristics.* **Right**, *A ball in a bowl is a graphic analogy of the load displacement curve.*

can be represented by a single value, namely the slope of the line, or stiffness. In contrast, the load displacement curve of the spine is nonlinear. A typical load displacement curve of a spinal segment for flexion-extension is shown in Figure 4, *left*. The spine is flexible at low loads and stiffens with increasing loads. The slope of the line (stiffness of the spine) varies with load. This behavior is not adequately represented by a single stiffness value. It has been suggested that two parameters be used: neutral zone, and range of motion. The neutral zone is that part of the range of motion within which there is minimal resistance to intervertebral motion.[21,22] For the purpose of visualization, the load displacement curve can be described using the analogy of a ball in a bowl. The load displacement curve is transformed into a bowl by flipping the extension curve around the displacement axis. In this bowl, we place a ball. The ball moves easily within the neutral zone but requires greater effort to move it along the sloping sides of the bowl (Fig. 4, *right*). The shape of the bowl indicates the spinal stability. A deeper bowl, such as a wine glass, is a representation of a more stable spine while a more shallow bowl, such as a soup plate, represents a less stable spine. This "ball in a bowl" analogy will be used later to explain a new hypothesis of low back pain.

Markolf and Morris[23] performed experiments using functional spinal units to show that an injury to the disk did not alter its mechanical properties under axial compressive load. However, in two later studies,[24,25] the opposite was found to be true. The differences lie in the directions of loading. Markolf and Morris applied only compression load. In the study by my colleagues and me,[25] the response of the intact functional spinal unit before and after the disk injuries was measured under the action of six forces of compression, tension, anterior and posterior shear, and left and right shear; and six moments of flexion, extension, left and right rotations, and left and right bendings. For each of these load types, complete three-dimensional (3-D) motion was measured. Results of the two studies are shown in Figure 5. As can be seen, there are significant changes in the spinal behavior after both the annular and nucleus injuries. The magnitude of the changes is greater after the removal of the nucleus than when the anulus defect is created. These findings have been independently confirmed by Goel and associates.[24]

Posner and associates[19] studied the effect of cutting spinal ligaments on stability. Eighteen functional spinal units from L1-2, L3-4, and L5-S1 were used. The specimen was loaded in either flexion or extension, while the ligaments were transected sequentially either from posterior to anterior or anterior to posterior. The effect of each ligament transection was documented using the intervertebral motion measurement. Under flexion loading and posterior to anterior cutting, there were incremental motion increases with significant residual motion after facet joint transection. In extension loading and anterior to posterior cutting, a significant residual deformation was found after the anterior half of the disk was cut. Results of this study formed the basis for development of the checklist for the diagnosis of clinical instability in the lumbar spine, which was discussed earlier.[8]

The facet joints are important components of the spinal column. They carry axial load and limit the axial rotation at any level in the lumbar spine to about 2° to either side. This small movement is the result of highly congruent joint surfaces of the mating inferior and superior facets. It has been shown in several experiments, beginning with those of Farfan and associates,[26] that transection of the facets significantly increases axial rotation. However, the role of injury to the facets on the coupled motions of the lumbar spine and the effect of partial transections of the facets on the spinal motion are factors that have not been studied extensively.

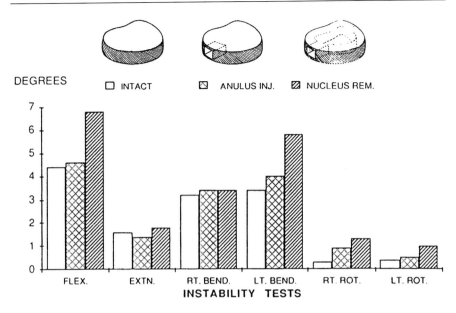

Fig. 5 *Effects of disk injury on the mechanical properties of a lumbar functional spinal unit. Three states of the disk were investigated: intact, with anulus injury on left side, and after removal of the nucleus. Instability tests were conducted using pure moments of flexion, extension, right lateral bending, left lateral bending, left rotation, and right rotation. The bar graph shows the main motions for the intact and two injuries due to each of the six physiologic loads. Anulus injury with nucleus removal produced greater changes than the anulus injury alone. The maximum absolute changes were seen in flexion and left lateral bending. On the percentage changes, it was the axial rotation that exhibited the greatest effect of the disk injury. (Reproduced with permission from Panjabi MM, Krag MH, Chung TQ: Effects of disc injury on mechanical behavior of the human spine. Spine 1984;9:707–713.)*

Using fresh human cadaveric two-vertebra lumbar spine specimens, Abumi and associates[27] studied the effects of graded facetectomy on the motions of the spine. Using the techniques of noninjurious multidirectional flexibility testing, they studied normal behavior and motion increases after each injury. The study was 3-D, thus providing complete documentation of the kinematic changes caused by the injuries. Besides the uninjured specimen, five injuries were studied: (1) Transection of supraspinous and intraspinous ligaments; (2) Left unilateral medial facetectomy; (3) Bilateral medial facetectomy; (4) Left unilateral total facetectomy; and (5) Bilateral total facetectomy. Changes in the range of motion and the statistical significance are given in Table 2. The major conclusions were that transection of the supraspinous and intraspinous ligaments did not affect lumbar spine motion in any way. However, unilateral medial facetectomy increased flexion. Total facetectomy of one side increased the axial rotation to the opposite side. Complete facetectomy increased the axial rotation to both sides. The extension and lateral bending movements were not increased by any of the injuries.

Table 2   Average ranges of motion (standard deviations) in degrees at 8 Nm for each of the six moment types for the intact and injured functional spinal unit*

Moment Type	INT Mean (SD)	SSL & ISL Mean (SD)	Left UMF Mean (SD)	BMF Mean (SD)	Left UTF Mean (SD)	BTF Mean (SD)
Flexion	8.22 (2.57)	9.99 (3.58)	11.32 (3.67)[†]	11.86 (3.88)[†]	12.44 (3.62)[†]	13.61 (2.69)[†]
Extension	4.00 (1.40)	3.71 (1.54)	4.41 (1.80)	4.56 (2.19)	5.30 (2.28)	5.76 (2.47)
Left axial rotation	3.31 (1.36)	3.34 (1.56)	3.55 (1.04)	3.64 (1.21)	3.74 (1.08)	7.85 (3.04)[†]
Right axial rotation	3.68 (1.78)	3.75 (1.87)	3.81 (1.51)	4.07 (1.25)	5.49 (1.68)[†]	7.58 (2.92)[†]
Right lateral bending	5.53 (2.01)	6.46 (2.21)	7.13 (2.53)	7.39 (2.73)	7.31 (2.35)	7.66 (2.60)
Left lateral bending	5.78 (2.94)	6.42 (2.74)	6.37 (2.45)	6.65 (2.73)	6.75 (3.07)	7.31 (3.37)

*INT = intact; SSL & ISL = transection supraspinous and intraspinous; UMF = unilateral medial facetectomy; BMF = bilateral medial facetectomy; UTF = unilateral total facetectomy; BTF = bilateral total facetectomy
[†]$p < 0.05$
(Reproduced with permission from Abumi K, Panjabi MM, Kramer KM, et al: Biomechanical evaluation of lumbar spinal stability after graded facetectomies. *Spine* 1990;15:1142–1147.)

It is not difficult to appreciate that all cutting studies of the spinal column, as previously described, are artificial in the sense that in a real-life situation an individual spinal component is seldom injured alone. In a real injury, several anatomic components of the spinal column are injured, but to varying degrees. To simulate these injuries, Perey[28] used a drop-mass trauma model. However, the resulting spinal instability was not studied. Willen and associates[29] studied changes in spinal posture due to trauma. Actual trauma may result in multidirectional instability. This aspect was evaluated for the first time by my colleagues and me,[30] using porcine spine specimens from the cervical region. The onset and progression of instability as a result of increasing trauma without gross fractures has also been studied.[31] Multidirectional instability caused by high-speed spinal trauma in human thoracolumbar specimens has been investigated recently.[32] The main findings of these in vitro trauma studies have been that even simple trauma, such as axial compression, affects multidirectional instability of the spinal column. In addition, the neutral zone (a measure of the low load response or spinal laxity) was found to be affected by trauma to a greater extent than range of motion.

In summary, the stabilizing role of the various components of the spinal column has been studied by simulating injuries and trauma and determining the effect on the stiffness and ranges of motion of the spinal specimen. The reason for the abundance of this experimental work is not necessarily because of the greater importance of the spinal column in low back pain problems, but more likely because of the difficulties in studying the other two components of the spinal stabilizing system.

The Muscles

The importance of muscles in stabilizing the spinal column is quite obvious when a cross-section of the human body is viewed at the lumbar level. Not only is the area of the total cross-section of the numerous muscles surrounding the spinal column much bigger than that of the spinal column, but the muscles have significantly larger lever arms and thus have a relatively large mechanical advantage, compared to the spinal column, in stabilizing the spine. There is a lack of experimental work relating the muscular forces to spinal stability. Euler, a Swiss scientist, developed his mathematical theories for buckling of upright slender columns in 1744, as described by Timoshenko and Gere.[33] Critical load of a column was defined as that weight on the top of the column that would cause it to begin to buckle (Fig. 6, *left*). In other words, if an actual column was stiffer than the critical load column, then the column would stand and remain stable (Fig. 6, *left center*). On the other hand, if the column was more flexible than the critical load column, then the column would buckle and be unstable (Fig. 6, *right center*). When fresh cadaveric lumbar spine specimens (L1-sacrum) are used, the critical load for the lumbar spine has been determined to be about 90 N.[34] This is much smaller than the in vivo load of 1500 N found on the spine in 20 degrees of flexion.[35] This difference between the in vitro and in vivo loads can be explained on the basis that the muscles act as guy wires in stabilizing the spine (Fig. 6, *right*).

There are some interesting clinical observations concerning the role of muscles in stabilizing the spine. For example, patients with low back pain have muscle spasm. Although it is uncertain whether the muscle spasm occurs before the low back pain, its presence in patients with low back pain does not negate the hypothesis that the muscle spasm represents additional forces that are attempting to stabilize an unstable spinal column. In patients with polio and inadequate muscle function, there is a collapse of the spinal column. There has also been a study of firefighters, in whom better conditioning of muscles by physical exer-

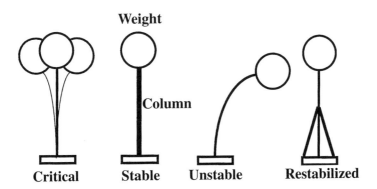

Fig. 6 *Buckling of a column carrying a load:* **Left**, *A column with a critical load is at the brink of buckling or instability.* **Left center**, *A stiffer column is stable.* **Right center**, *A more flexible column is unstable.* **Right**, *The weaker column can be restabilized by adding guy wires.*

cise (increased muscle strength and better coordination of muscle forces) resulted in a lower frequency of low back pain.[36]

Because of the insurmountable difficulties with measuring muscle forces in vivo, my colleagues and I[37] developed an in vitro model to simulate the effect of muscle forces. Fresh cadaveric human lumbar spine specimens were used. Multidirectional instabilities were measured before injury and after several injuries of increasing severity. After each injury, muscle forces (maximum 60 N) were applied to the spinous process, directed anteriorly and inferiorly. The main findings of the study were that, under flexion loading, there were increasing neutral zones and ranges of motion with increasing severity of the injury. However, when muscle forces were applied there was a difference in the changes seen in neutral zone and range of motion. For the most severe injury, the application of the 60 N muscle force brought the neutral zone to its near-normal value while the range of motion was significantly larger than normal. We hypothesize that this differential behavior of the neutral zone and range of motion parameters probably indicates that the role of the muscle forces in stabilizing the spinal column is, first and foremost, to decrease the neutral zone. This hypothesis needs to be validated by other in vitro and, especially, in vivo experiments.

The Control Unit

The etiology of low back pain in most patients is not known. It can be hypothesized that a certain percentage of these patients may have suboptimal muscle control, especially under dynamic conditions. There are only two studies that have specifically concentrated on this aspect of low back pain. In the first study, the sway of the center of gravity of the body in patients with spinal canal stenosis was determined.[38] The patients were challenged to exercise until claudication occurred, and were tested before and after claudication. There were differences in the sway measurements in the patients with stenosis and compared to controls as well after the claudication. In a second study, the variations in balance were quantified by body sway in middle-aged adults.[39] There were two groups of subjects: those with low back dysfunction and those who had no history of low back pain. A direct comparison was made between the two groups. Each group was tested for eight tasks. The tasks were of increasing difficulty, from the simplest: to stand on both feet on a stable surface with eyes open; to the most difficult: to stand on one foot on an unstable surface with eyes closed. In performing the most difficult task, the measurement of body sway was significantly greater in the patients with low back pain compared to the normal controls (Fig. 7). In both these studies, larger body sway indicates suboptimal muscle control. Presently, etiology for this type of muscle control dysfunction is not known.

Pain, Motion, and Fusion

Based on the definition of spinal instability presented earlier, the instability hypothesis assumes a relationship between abnormal intervertebral motion and low back pain. The corollary to this hypothesis is that a decrease in the intervertebral motion in a patient with low back pain would reduce the pain. My

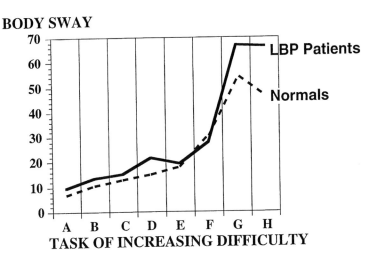

Fig. 7 *Two groups of subjects, low back pain patients and normal control patients, were studied for their body sway while performing tasks (A-H) of increasing difficulty.[39] See text for details. The low back pain patients had significantly greater sway compared to the normals at the two most difficult tasks.*

colleagues and I have conducted a biomechanical experiment to test this hypothesis.[40]

About 10 years ago, Magerl[41] developed an external fixator for the lumbar spine, with the intent to stabilize a spinal fracture in a patient using an external fixator. Olerud and associates[42] used this fixation device to produce instantaneous fusion; the purpose was to use the external fixator for the diagnosis of spinal instability in patients with low back pain. The hypothesis was that the decrease in motion caused by the application of the external fixator would lead to a decrease in pain and, therefore, identify the spinal level causing the pain. This idea of identifying pain location was adopted by Grob and associates,[43] who developed a cervical spine fixator constructed of Kirschner (K-) wires to be used for the same purpose. The pain was significantly reduced by the application of this external fixator. My colleagues and I used this fixator and designed an in vitro biomechanical study, using fresh cadaveric cervical spine specimens, to simulate the mechanical aspects of the use of the external fixator in the clinical situation.[40] The purpose of our study was to answer several interesting questions. Does the application of the fixator reduce intervertebral motion? If this occurred, was it direction-specific? Which parameter reduced the most, neutral zone or range of motion? Results of the study showed that ranges of motion for flexion, extension, lateral bending, and axial rotation decreased by 40%, 27%, 32%, and 58%, respectively, when the external fixator was applied. All neutral zones decreased to a greater extent: 76%, 76%, 54%, and 69%, respectively (Fig. 8). Thus, on average, the range of motion decreased by 39.3% while the neutral zone decreased by 68.8% following application of the external fixator.

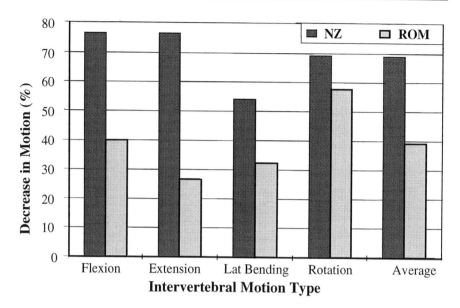

Fig. 8   *Decreases in motion at a cervical spine segment due to the application of an external fixator at the same level to a fresh cadaveric human cervical spine specimen. (Reproduced with permission from Panjabi MM, Lydon C, Vasavada A, et al: On the understanding of clinical instability.* Spine *1994;19:2642–2650.)*

How can the findings of the in vivo clinical study,[43] in which the application of the external fixator decreased neck pain, and the in vitro biomechanical study,[40] in which the application of the same fixator to a cadaveric cervical spine specimen produced results as described, be combined? These findings are interpreted in the following discussion, with the help of an innovative use of the load displacement curve.

A Hypothesis to Relate Pain to Motion

Using the "ball in a bowl" analogy of the load displacement curve (Fig. 4, *right*), stable and unstable situations can be represented, and the hypothesis of the motion-pain relationship can be interpreted in the following manner. For each person without spine pain there is a normal neutral zone and range of motion (Fig. 9, *top*). When an injury occurs, an anatomic structure, such as the capsular ligament, is injured. The neutral zone is bigger, and the ball moves freely over a larger distance (Fig. 9, *center*). This combination of injury to an anatomic structure, which may thus become more sensitive, and the spinal column, which develops a larger neutral zone, may cause pain. The spinal stabilizing system may react by actively limiting the neutral zone via activation of the muscles or by formation of osteophytes and surgical fusion (Fig. 9, *bottom*). In the analogy, the ball is anchored, and the spine is again pain-free. Please note that these interactions between the neutral zone, pain, and spinal state (injury and resta-

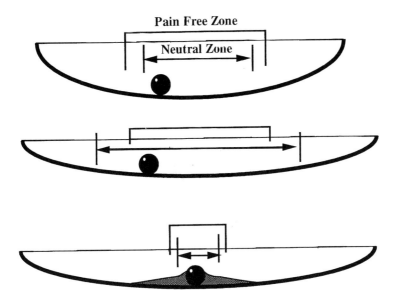

Fig. 9   *A graphic interpretation of the motion-pain hypothesis.* **Top**, *Normal spine.* **Center**, *Painful spine has greater neutral zone.* **Bottom**, *Spine is made pain-free, indicated by decreased neutral zone.*

bilization) constitute an as-yet unproven hypothesis that must be tested and validated by future clinical studies.

A Mathematical Model of Spinal Stabilization

Recently, a mathematical model was developed to estimate the mechanical stability of the human lumbar spine in vivo,[44] taking into consideration all of the three stabilizing subsystems: the spinal column, muscles, and the motor control unit. The model consisted of five rigid vertebrate, the rib cage, pelvis, and 90 muscle fascicles. Each intervertebral joint had three rotational degrees of freedom with nonlinear load-displacement characteristics. The insight into the motor control strategy of muscle recruitment patterns was achieved with surface electromyographic recordings. Young, healthy subjects were tested while performing a variety of tasks involving trunk flexion, extension lateral bending, and twisting. The spine stability index, a measure of relative stability, was computed. Coincidentally, the depth of the bowl (Fig. 4), may be equated to the spinal stability index. Spinal instability is represented by a shallow bowl and a lower spinal stability index. On the other hand, a more stable spine is represented by a deeper bowl and a higher stability index.

The results of the mathematical model indicated that there was an ample stability safety margin (higher stability index) in the tasks that required large muscular effort, such as lifting weights (Fig. 10). However, the tasks that demanded

379

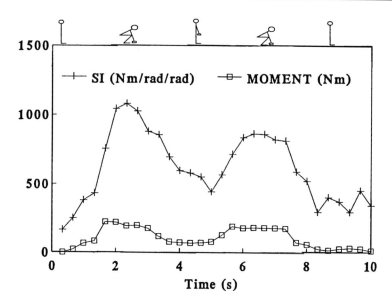

Fig. 10 *Stability index (SI) of the in vivo lumbar spine during the lifting task. The SI followed the pattern of a lumbar moment: spine stability was high during the periods when the moment demands were high and the spine stability was low when the moment diminished. The negative value of SI would indicate spine instability. (Reproduced with permission from Cholewicki J, McGill SM: Mechanical stability of the in vivo lumbar spine: Implications for injury and chronic low back pain.* Clin Biomech *1996;11:1–15.)*

very little muscle activity, such as upright standing with no external loads, were characterized by a smaller stability index that described the whole system as being just on the verge of spine buckling. For example, the stability index during lifting a load from the floor follows the same pattern as the bending moment in the lumbar spine. The greater the muscular effort needed during the lifting task, the higher the stability index. This theory is evidenced by the bending moment demands about the L4-5 joint. The opposite is true for lighter tasks with very low bending moment, seen at the beginning and end of the lifting task in Figure 10.

This study supports the hypothesis of neutral zone and low back pain. It seems that tasks that challenge spine stability the most are the ones in which spine posture is maintained within its neutral zone and there are very few muscles activated to stabilize the spine. While healthy individuals may rely on the passive, osteoligamentous structures to maintain spine stability in such tasks, the injured or degenerated spine must be compensated with the additional muscle activation to prevent spine collapse. This scenario may lead to the prolonged static muscle activity during standing or sitting, chronic muscle fatigue, and weakness. In turn, these muscles will be inadequate in providing stability to the spinal column during other, more challenging tasks. Conversely, injury to the spine can occur during performance of very light tasks, when the stability index is low and errors in motor control can occur.

Recent In Vivo Experimental Studies

In all of the clinical studies presented here, range of motion was used to indicate the degree of spinal instability because this parameter is relatively easy to measure radiographically. In some of the recent studies, other parameters have been suggested as indicators of back problems. In one study, the subjects were asked to perform sagittal plane motion. More out-of-sagittal-plane motions were observed in subjects with low back pain than were seen in the control subjects.[15] Similarly, out-of-sagittal-plane torques were observed in patients with low back pain performing flexion-extension against resistance in a strength testing machine.[45] Neutral zone has been suggested as an indicator of clinical spinal instability.[21] The neutral zone, being a much smaller parameter than the range of motion, is difficult to measure directly using traditional methods of radiography. However, changes in the neutral zone may alter the pattern of motion. Such pattern changes have been observed in a recent in vivo porcine study. In vivo motions were measured using an intervertebral motion measurement device that is attached to the K-wires threaded into the spinous processes.[46] Injury to the facets resulted in significant changes in the motion pattern, especially in the neutral region. Muscle activation stabilized the spine, smoothing the erratic motion pattern. There have also been attempts to measure alterations in the motion, presumably caused by altered neutral zone, in subjects performing axial rotation.[47] This noninvasive technique has yet to be tested in patients with low back pain. In conclusion, the new modes of in vivo testing for clinical instability have evolved because the traditional parameter, range of motion, has been used for the past 50 years without providing clear answers. The new methods attempt to focus on the pattern of motion throughout the range of motion, and subtle changes in it around the neutral position. It will be interesting to see how these new modalities fare when they are used in well-designed, controlled clinical trials.

Summary

Clinical instability is an important cause of low back pain. Although there is some controversy concerning the definition of low back pain, it is most widely agreed that loss of the normal pattern of spinal motion (more motion or different motion pattern) is what causes pain and/or neurologic dysfunction. Based on biomechanical experiments, a checklist has been developed for a systematic diagnosis of clinical instability. The stabilizing system of the spine may be divided into three subsystems: (1) the spinal column and (2) the surrounding muscles, well coordinated by (3) the motor control unit. A large number of biomechanical studies of the spinal column have provided insight into the role of the various anatomic structures of the spinal column. On the other hand, there have not been many studies on the role of muscles, or dynamic muscle control, in spinal stability. The neutral zone was found to be a more sensitive parameter than range of motion in documenting the effect of mechanical destabilization of the spine caused by injury. In another study, the neutral zone was again found to be the more sensitive parameter, but this time in restabilizing the spine by simulated muscle forces. Regarding neuromuscular control, increased body sway was found in patients with low back pain, indicating the importance of a muscle control system. Results of an experiment relating spinal fixation to decreased neck pain concluded that the neutral zone was the parameter most increased by injury and decreased by the fixation and, therefore, possibly a measure of clinical instability. A hypothesis relating the neutral zone to pain has been presented, and a mathematical model has been constructed that can predict the degree of stability or instability associated with a given task. It supports the neutral zone hypothesis, and predicted the potential for injuries during light lifting tasks. Some recent studies have attempted to look at the changes in the patterns of motion, instead of the range of motion, as the indicators of spinal instability.

References

1. Andersson GBJ, Pope MH, Frymoyer JW: Epidemiology, in Pope MH, Frymoyer JW, Andersson G (eds): *Occupational Low Back Pain.* New York, NY, Praeger, 1984, pp 101–114.
2. Frymoyer JW, Pope MH, Clements JH, et al: Risk factors in low-back pain: An epidemiological survey. *J Bone Joint Surg* 1983;65A:213–218.
3. Morris A: Identifying workers at risk to back injury is not guesswork. *Occup Health Saf* 1985;54:16–20.
4. Spengler DM, Bigos SJ, Martin NA, et al: Back injuries in industry: A retrospective study. I. Overview and cost analysis. *Spine* 1986;11:241–245.
5. Biering-Sorensen F: Low back trouble in a general population of 30-, 40-, 50-, and 60-year-old men and women: Study design, representativeness and basic results. *Dan Med Bull* 1982;29:289–299.
6. Nagi SZ, Riley LE, Newby LG: A social epidemiology of back pain in a general population. *J Chron Dis* 1973;26:769–779.
7. Nachemson AL: Advances in low-back pain. *Clin Orthop* 1985;200:266–278.
8. White AA, Panjabi MM (eds): *Clinical Biomechanics of the Spine*, ed 2. Philadelphia, PA, JB Lippincott, 1990.
9. Knutsson F: The instability associated with disk degeneration in the lumbar spine. *Acta Radiol* 1944;25:593–609.
10. Dvorak J, Antinnes JA Panjabi M, et al: Age and gender related normal motion of the cervical spine. *Spine* 1992;17(suppl 10):S393–S398.
11. Dvorak J, Panjabi MM, Grob D, et al: Clinical validation of functional flexion/extension radiographs of the cervical spine. *Spine* 1993;18:120–127.
12. Friberg O: Lumbar instability: A dynamic approach by traction-compression radiography. *Spine* 1987;12:119–129.
13. Lehmann TR, Brand RA: Instability of the lower lumbar spine. *Orthop Trans* 1983;7:97.
14. Dvorak J, Panjabi MM, Novotny JE, et al: Clinical validation of functional flexion-extension roentgenograms of the lumbar spine. *Spine* 1991;16:943–950.
15. Pearcy M, Portek I, Shepherd J: The effect of low-back pain on lumbar spinal movements measured by three-dimensional X-ray analysis. *Spine* 1985;10:150–153.
16. Pearcy M, Shepherd J: Is there instability in spondylolisthesis? *Spine* 1985;10:175–177.
17. Panjabi MM, White AA III, Johnson RM: Cervical spine mechanics as a function of transection of components. *J Biomech* 1975;8:327–336.
18. White AA III, Johnson RM, Panjabi MM, et al: Biomechanical analysis of clinical stability in the cervical spine. *Clin Orthop* 1975;109:85–96.
19. Posner I, White AA III, Edwards WT, et al: A biomechanical analysis of the clinical stability of the lumbar and lumbosacral spine. *Spine* 1982;7:374–389.
20. Panjabi MM: The stabilizing system of the spine. Part I. Function, dysfunction, adaptation, and enhancement. *J Spinal Disord* 1992;5:383–389.
21. Panjabi MM: The stabilizing system of the spine: Part II. Neutral zone and instability hypothesis. *J Spinal Disord* 1992;5:390–397.

22. Panjabi MM, Goel VK, Takata K: Physiologic strains in lumbar spinal ligaments: An in vitro biomechanical study. *Spine* 1982;7:192–203.

23. Markolf KL, Morris JM: The structural components of the intervertebral disc: A study of their contributions to the ability of the disc to withstand compressive forces. *J Bone Joint Surg* 1974;56A:675–687.

24. Goel VK, Goyal S, Clark C, et al: Kinematics of the whole lumbar spine: Effect of discectomy. *Spine* 1985;10:543–554.

25. Panjabi MM, Krag MH, Chung TQ: Effects of disc injury on mechanical behavior of the human spine. *Spine* 1984;9:707–713.

26. Farfan HF, Cossette JW, Robertson GH, et al: The effects of torsion on the lumbar intervertebral joints: The role of torsion in the production of disc degeneration. *J Bone Joint Surg* 1970;52A:468–497.

27. Abumi K, Panjabi MM, Kramer KM, et al: Biomechanical evaluation of lumbar spinal stability after graded facetectomies. *Spine* 1990;15:1142–1147.

28. Perey O: Fracture of the vertebral end-plate in the lumbar spine: An experimental biomechanical investigation. *Acta Orthop Scand* 1957;25(suppl):1–101.

29. Willen J, Lindahl S, Irstam L, et al: The thoracolumbar crush fracture: An experimental study on instant axial dynamic loading. The resulting fracture type and its stability. *Spine* 1984;9:624–631.

30. Panjabi MM, Duranceau JS, Oxland TR, et al: Multidirectional instabilities of traumatic cervical spine injuries in a porcine model. *Spine* 1989;14:1111–1115.

31. Oxland TR, Panjabi MM: The onset and progression of spinal injury: A demonstration of neutral zone sensitivity. *J Biomech* 1992;25:1165–1172.

32. Panjabi MM, Oxland TR, Lin RM, et al: Thoracolumbar burst fracture: A biomechanical investigation of its multidirectional flexibility. *Spine* 1994;19:578–585.

33. Timoshenko SP, Gere JM (eds): *Mechanics of Materials*. New York, NY, Van Nostrand Reinhold, 1972.

34. Crisco JJ: *The Biomechanical Stability of the Human Lumbar Spine: Experimental and Theoretical Investigations*. New Haven, CT, Yale University, 1989. Dissertation.

35. Nachemson A, Morris JM: In vivo measurements of intradiscal pressure: Discometry, a method for the determination of pressure in the lower lumbar discs. *J Bone Joint Surg* 1964;46A:1077–1092.

36. Cady LD, Bischoff DP, O'Connell ER, et al: Strength and fitness and subsequent back injuries in firefighters. *Occup Med* 1979;21:269–272.

37. Panjabi M, Abumi K, Duranceau J, et al: Spinal stability and intersegmental muscle forces: A biomechanical model. *Spine* 1989;14:194–200.

38. Hanai K, Ishii K, Nojiri H: Sway of the center of gravity in patients with spinal canal stenosis. *Spine* 1988;13:1303–1307.

39. Nies N, Sinnott PL: Variations in balance and body sway in middle-aged adults: Subjects with healthy backs compared with subjects with low-back dysfunction. *Spine* 1991;16:325–330.

40. Panjabi MM, Lydon C, Vasavada A, et al: On the understanding of clinical instability. *Spine* 1994;19:2642–2650.

41. Magerl F: External skeletal fixation of the lower thoracic and the lumbar spine, in Uhthoff HK, Stahl E (eds): *Current Concepts of External Fixation of Fractures*. Berlin, Germany, Springer-Verlag, 1982, pp 353–366.

42. Olerud S, Sjöström L, Karlstrom G, et al: Spontaneous effect of increased stability of the lower lumbar spine in cases of severe chronic back pain: The answer to an external transpeduncular fixation test. *Clin Orthop* 1986;203:67–74.

43. Grob D, Dvorak J, Panjabi MM, et al: External fixator of the cervical spine: A new diagnostic tool. *Unfallchirurg* 1993;96:416–421.

44. Cholewicki J, McGill SM: Mechanical stability of the in vivo lumbar spine: Implications for injury and chronic low back pain. *Clin Biomech* 1996;11:1–15.

383

45. Parnianpour M, Nordin M, Kahanovitz N, et al: The triaxial coupling of torque generation of trunk muscles during isometric exertions and the effect of fatiguing isoinertial movements on the motor output and movement patterns. *Spine* 1988;13:982–992.
46. Kaigle AM, Holm SH, Hansson TH: Experimental instability in the lumbar spine. *Spine* 1995;20:421–430.
47. Kumar S, Panjabi MM: In vivo axial rotations and neutral zones of the thoracolumbar spine. *J Spinal Disord* 1995;8:253–263.

Chapter 24

The Role of Magnetic Resonance Imaging in the Assessment of Disk Degeneration and Diskogenic Pain

Richard J. Herzog, MD

Introduction

With the development and implementation of magnetic resonance imaging (MRI) both the clinician and the investigator of spinal disease were provided with a new diagnostic tool to noninvasively study the normal and pathologic conditions of the human lumbar intervertebral disk. MRI provides a means to evaluate both the structural and the biochemical status of a disk. It creates images or topographic maps based on the location, concentration, and relaxation times of mobile hydrogen ions. High resolution imaging can be performed directly in any plane to optimally evaluate each component of the spinal motion segment. Currently, there are no known biologic risks of MRI. Absolute contraindications for undergoing an MRI examination include cardiac pacemakers or other implanted electric devices, which may dysfunction in a strong magnetic field and whose failure would be an immediate threat to patient health; metallic foreign bodies in the orbit or central spinal column; brain aneurysm clips; metallic cochlear implants; and some heart valves and vascular stents. Other metallic objects in the body, for example, posterior spinal instrumentation or hip prostheses, may generate significant artifacts and degrade the MR images, but their presence does not preclude performing an MRI examination.

Although MRI may provide unique information concerning the biochemical and morphologic status of a disk, its precise role in patient care remains to be clarified. Some of the questions that must be addressed include: (1) Is it possible with MRI to determine if a patient's pain is originating from the disk or peridiskal tissue? (2) What is the clinical significance of a normal or abnormal MRI study? (3) Do all MRI equipment and imaging protocols provide similar information? (4) What are the reliability and precision of MRI interpretations? (5) How does MRI compare to other diagnostic modalities in diagnosing the source of a patient's symptoms and affecting patient outcome? (6) How may MRI, in the future, provide new insights into understanding the natural history of degenerative disk disease? Several of these issues will be addressed in this chapter, because its purpose is to clarify the value of MRI in the evaluation of annular tears, disk disruption, and diskogenic pain.

Terminology

Before discussing these questions, it is necessary to define some of the terminology used in this chapter. One area of persistent debate and disagreement among spinal clinicians and investigators is the difference, if any, between normal disk aging and disk degeneration. Little has changed since Pritzker[1] stated almost two decades ago, ''The term 'degeneration' as commonly applied to the intervertebral disc covers such a wide variety of clinical, radiologic, and pathologic manifestations that the word is really only a symbol of our ignorance about disc disease.'' By combining the results of present and past spinal investigators, it appears that normal aging of the disk is related predominantly to the transformation of the nucleus pulposus (NP) from a turgid gel of proteoglycans, which is enmeshed in a random network of collagen filaments and morphologically distinct from the inner anulus, into a more desiccated fibrocartilaginous structure, which appears morphologically and biochemically similar to the inner anulus.

With aging, there is a gradual transformation of the biochemical composition and organization of a disk.[2] The greatest changes occur in the NP. Beginning in the second decade of life, the nucleus becomes more fibrous, begins to lose its hydrostatic swelling capacity, and manifests cellular metaplasia. While it may contain small clefts, it still maintains an organized structure. With aging, there is a gradual change in the annular collagen structure, with separation and possible infolding of inner annular fibers,[3,4] but no complete fiber disruption. In addition, annular hydration decreases slightly. Disks with this morphologic appearance are present in individuals beyond the age of 70 years and demonstrate normal signal intensity on T2-weighted MR images,[5] even though the degree of hydration of the disk has decreased with aging. The signal intensity of a disk on a T2-weighted MR image represents more than just the state of disk hydration, it also depends on the disk's macromolecular composition and organization.[6,7] Whether biochemical changes without structural alterations of the disk are sufficient to affect T2-weighted signal intensity requires further investigation.[8] It is possible that a mild reduction in disk T2 signal may be a manifestation of disk aging, whereas a marked reduction in disk signal may reflect disk disruption.

Should these age-related changes be classified as degeneration? Buckwalter[2] states that ''In the sense that these age-related changes result in progressive loss of normal tissue structure, composition, and biologic and mechanical function they are a form of degeneration.'' To me, degeneration of the disk implies, mechanical failure of the disk, which precipitates progressive macroscopic disorganization of the NP and the anulus fibrosus. This disorganization may be secondary to fatigue failure of the disk matrix[2] and concomitant development of complete annular tears, or to acute annular disruption that may be secondary to trauma or surgery. It appears from pathologic studies[9-11] and experimental animal models[12] that the necessary condition for the progressive deterioration of a disk depends on the development of a complete radial annular tear. This condition results in the disruption of the structural integrity of the nucleus and anulus; loss of nuclear fibrocartilage; and the possibility of nuclear, annular, or end plate herniation. It is this condition of the disk that manifests reduced T2-weighted signal intensity on an MR image.[10] Perhaps this state of disk failure should be referred to as advanced disk degeneration or disk disruption to distinguish it from an aging disk that has not failed. Although both aging and advanced degeneration of a disk will alter its material and structural properties, it is usually a disk with a complete annular tear or marked degeneration that precipitates a patient's symptoms.[13] Whether this pain is related to biochemical mediators, mechanical deformation of nociceptive fibers, an immunologic response to disk material, or possibly to an end plate microcompartment syndrome requires further investigation. When aged disks are injected at diskography and they have no evidence of major macroscopic disruption, they typically elicit no pain.[14]

Detectable Annular Abnormalities

Before discussing the use of MRI to predict whether a fissured or degenerated disk is the source of a patient's pain, it is important to describe the annular abnormalities that may be detected by MRI and which may precipitate a patient's pain and/or predispose a disk to failure. A radial annular tear represents disruption of contiguous annular lamellae, with the cleft oriented perpendicular or obliquely to the lamellar fibers. A complete radial tear, that is, a disk rupture, extends from the NP to the surface of the disk, whereas an incomplete radial tear originates from the NP and extends into the inner or outer annular fibers, leaving some peripheral annular fibers intact. The use of MRI for detection of these tears depends on the type of tissue within a tear (for example, extracellular matrix, chondroid material, or fibrovascular tissue, the tissue adjacent to a tear that provides tissue contrast) and the resolution of the MRI equipment. On T2-weighted images, a normal outer anulus demonstrates low signal intensity (Fig. 1). Because the material in an annular fissure is more hydrated than the normal anulus, it should be detected as a focus of increased signal intensity within, or at the margin, of the dark outer annular fibers. An annular fissure may also be detected in a disk with advanced degeneration (Fig. 2). In addition, if annular tears contain neovascularity,[15] they should be possible to detect by the administration of an intravenous contrast agent (for example, gadolinium-

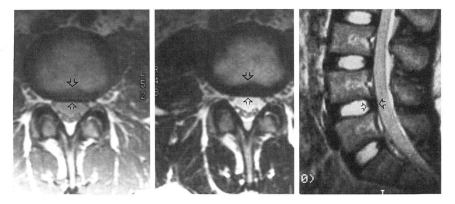

Fig. 1 *The outer anulus (arrows) demonstrates low signal intensity on the axial proton density and T2-weighted images (**left and center**), and on the sagittal T2-weighted image (**right**).*

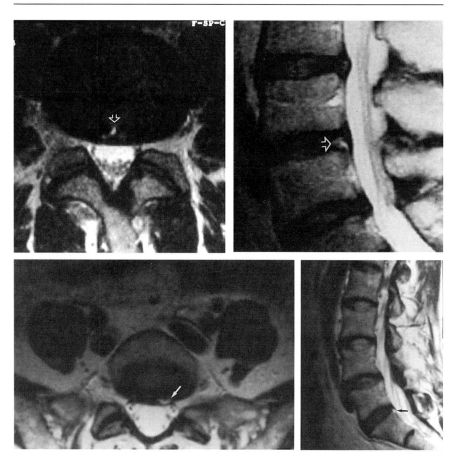

Fig. 2 *An annular fissure (arrow) is present in the central segment of the posterior anulus on the axial (**top left**) and sagittal (**top right**) T2-weighted images at the L4-5 disk level. On another patient, at the L5-S1 disk level, there is a peripheral annular fissure located at the posterolateral margin of the disk at its insertion into the ring apophysis. The fissure is delineated on the axial (**bottom left**) and sagittal (**bottom right**) T2-weighted images.*

diethylenetriamine pentaacetic acid; Gd-DTPA), if there is adequate vascularity in the annular tear, contrast diffusion out of the vessels, and an adequate extracellular space to accumulate contrast (Fig. 3). Optimal scanning techniques, that is, thin sections, small matrix size, limited field of view, and fat-suppressed T1-weighted images, should also be used.

Concentric and peripheral rim tears of the anulus have also been described.[16,17] With a concentric tear, the annular cleft is located in a vertical plane between annular lamellae. With a peripheral rim tear, the cleft is oriented in a horizontal transverse plane and is located at the site of attachment of the outer annular fibers into the vertebral ring apophysis. Horizontal tears may also be located at the disk/end plate interface or within the anulus. Concentric and peripheral annular tears have been detected pathologically in otherwise normal disks. It has been hypothesized that these tears may be due to a traumatic event

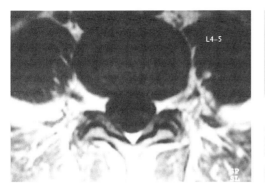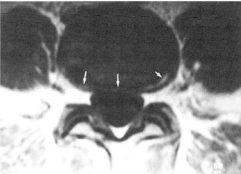

Fig. 3 *On the precontrast T1-weighted axial image* (**left**), *there is no evidence of a fissure in the posterior outer anulus. After the intravenous injection of gadolinium-diethylenetriamine pentaacetic acid, a circumferential annular fissure is identified in the posterior outer annular fibers (arrows) on the T1-weighted axial image* (**right**).

and are independent from disk aging or degeneration.[16] In order to image these tears, it is necessary to optimize both the spatial and contrast resolution of the MR images.

Detection of Annular Tears

Yu and associates[10] have demonstrated that with MRI it is possible not only to detect the normal changes of disk aging, but also to define when a disk becomes ruptured and degenerated. They evaluated 134 disks in 28 cadavers, from those of neonates to those of adults beyond the age of 70 years. They correlated high resolution MRI studies performed on cadaveric specimens to the same specimens after cryomicrotoming. Although the results of this study provide important information concerning the maturation and degeneration of a disk, the study is limited by the number and age distribution of the cadavers studied, most of whom were older than 50 years of age at the time of death. The authors classify the normal maturation of a human intervertebral disk into three stages: neonatal, transitional, and adult. In the neonatal disk, the NP is a gelatinous structure containing notochordal remnants. The margins of the nucleus are easily differentiated from the inner anulus. In the transitional disk, the NP becomes more turgid but it is still clearly separate from the anulus fibrosus. Organized fibrous tissue is detected in the equator of the disk. The transitional disk represents the most common type in the first three decades of life. With the transformation of the transitional disk into an adult disk, there is no longer a sharp demarcation between the NP and the inner anulus fibrosus. These disks contain some nuclear discoloration and nuclear clefts, but the anulus is intact.

The authors[10] first found an adult disk in a cadaver that was 19 years old at the time of death. This was the predominant type of disk in cadavers that were older than 30 years at death. On the T2-weighted MR images, the central portion of these disks, including the NP and the inner anulus fibrosus, demonstrated high signal intensity, and the outer annular collagenous fibers demonstrated low signal intensity. Only one of 60 of these disks demonstrated low signal intensity on MR T2-weighted images. Adult disks were present in most cadavers up to the age of 70 years at death. In the pathologic literature, this type of disk has been referred to as an early degenerated disk even though it may not progress to a ruptured disorganized disk.[18] In 20 of the disks, the authors[10] detected radial annular tears that extended from the nucleus to the surface of the disk. Although these disks had more discoloration and narrower disk spaces than the normal adult disk, there was no disorganization of the disk fibrocartilage. Seven of these disks demonstrated low signal intensity on the T2-weighted images. The radial tear was demonstrated on the MRI in five of the seven disks.

The authors[10] designated a disk as degenerated if there was disintegration of the fibrocartilage of the nucleus and a torn or totally disrupted anulus. Endplate osteophytes and sclerosis were also associated with this type of a disk. A degenerated disk was present in 17% of the adult cadavers and not present in cadavers younger than 40 years at death. These disks had either low T2-weighted signal intensity when dense fibrous tissue was present in the nucleus or increased signal intensity when there were fluid-filled fissures in the nucleus. T2-weighted images were optimal in differentiating between the different disk types. Yu and associates[10] hypothesized that the development of a radial tear was a critical factor in the development of disk degeneration, even when no herniation was present. With a radial tear, there was replacement of the nuclear fibrocartilage with disorganized collagen and fluid-filled fissures. Although the majority of the disks in cadavers that were older than 70 years at death had radial tears, normal adult disks were also present.

The sensitivity of MRI to detect annular tears has been studied both in cadaveric specimens and in patients. Yu and associates[17] compared the findings of high resolution MRI performed on cadaveric spines to pathologic analysis. Only radial and transverse tears were detected with MRI. Transverse tears were most frequently detected pathologically. They occurred at all levels but were most frequently located in the anterior anulus at the L1-2, L2-3, and L3-4 disk levels. The transverse tears appeared on MRI T2-weighted images as areas of increased signal intensity and corresponded to the shape and location of the fissures detected on the pathologic sections. MRI is the only imaging modality that can be used to detect concentric and peripheral rim annular tears that do not communicate with the NP. Radial tears were found in 21% to 35% of the disks in cadavers older than 40 years at death, and were rare in younger specimens. Radial tears were detected on MRI images as areas of high signal intensity on T2-weighted images. In order to test the sensitivity of MRI to detect radial tears, Yu and associates[19] compared diskography and high resolution MRI to histopathologic analysis of cadaveric lumbar spines. Diskography indicated the presence of 15 radial tears in 36 cadaveric disks. Disk degeneration was present on histopathology in all disks containing radial tears. With T2-weighted images, only ten of 15 radial tears were detected. There was decreased nuclear signal intensity in 13 of 15 degenerated disks, and the tears were detected as areas of high signal intensity. All diskographically normal disks had high signal intensity on T2-weighted images.

Gunzburg and associates[20] also compared diskography, MRI, and histology in human cadaveric disks. All three studies were not performed on all specimens. No data were presented on the reliability of the observations, which is important considering the small number of cases and the number that were classified as mild. Of all the disks with a normal appearance on MRI, 25% had abnormal diskograms (eight of 11 had only grade 1 changes). Of all disks with normal diskograms, 8% had abnormal MRI findings (3 of 4 disks had grade 1 changes). It is difficult to draw any conclusions from these observations because all the disks, including 43% of those with a normal diskogram and 48% of those with a normal MRI, showed histopathologic evidence of disk degeneration. No annular tears were detected on their MRI studies.

Annular tears created in animal models and detected in human pathologic specimens may contain granulation tissue. Nguyen and associates,[21] using a dog model, studied contrast enhancement of the intervertebral disk after surgically disrupting the anulus. Contrast enhancement of the disk was first seen 2 weeks postoperatively. T2-weighted nuclear signal intensity was normal in the disks at this time. Histology demonstrated small vessels penetrating the vertebral end plate and posterior anulus. There was no evidence of inflammatory cells.

For MRI to have an impact on elucidating the possible importance of annular tears as a cause of back pain, it must be able to detect these tears in living subjects. Ross and associates[15] performed MRI examinations on 30 patients who had not undergone surgery and who had symptoms suggesting disk disruption or herniation. An annular tear was defined as a linear or globular focus of increased signal intensity in the outer anulus on T2-weighted or postcontrast T1-weighted images. In the lumbar spine, they[15] detected 12 annular tears with contrast-enhanced images. Only four of the 12 tears were detected on the standard T2-weighted nonenhanced images. Ross and associates[15] subdivided the annular tears into central tears that extended towards the nucleus and tears adjacent to the vertebral body end plate. The central tears were much more common in this selected group of patients. A surgical biopsy performed on one of the disks with an annular tear demonstrated vascularized granulation tissue within the outer anulus and no disk herniation. Krodel and associates[22] recently reported on the histologic analysis of disks from 15 patients who demonstrated MRI disk enhancement and then underwent anterior interbody fusion. Pathologic vessels were detected in all 15 disks that had enhanced on the MRI study.

Modic and associates[23] used contrast-enhanced MRI to evaluate 25 patients with acute lumbar radiculopathy, that is, pain below the knee and positive root tension signs. These patients were imaged within 2 weeks of the onset of their symptoms and at 6 weeks and 6 months after their presentation. Although there was strong presumptive clinical diagnosis of a disk herniation, only 18 of the 25 patients had a herniated nucleus pulposus (HNP) on their imaging study. Two patients had synovial cysts associated with central canal stenosis, and of the remaining five patients, one had only an annular tear, two had a disk bulge, two had facet arthrosis, and one was normal. The authors defined annular tears on the MRI images as linear areas of enhancement on contrast-enhanced images or increased signal intensity in the anulus on T2-weighted images. Fifteen patients had annular tears; 11 enhanced and four did not. All disks with annular tears were degenerated; that is, they demonstrated low signal intensity on the T2-weighted images. The presence of annular tears was highest in the older patients. The authors[23] attempted to identify abnormalities, such as the size of a disk herniation, the presence of enhancement of the margins of a herniation, nerve root enhancement, or the presence of annular tears, that may provide re-

liable prognostic indicators of patient outcome. At 6 weeks, patients with annular tears were more than twice as likely to show no clinical improvement compared to patients without tears, but this finding was not predictive of eventual
patient outcome. At 6 months, patients with enhancing annular tears tended to
be more symptomatic than patients with nonenhancing tears. The statistical
power of this study was limited due to the small number of patients.

Although these studies have documented that it is possible to detect annular
tears with nonenhanced and contrast-enhanced MRI, they do not address the sensitivity or specificity of MRI in detection of annular tears in patients or whether
detection of an annular tear on an MRI study has clinical significance. In order
to determine the significance of an annular tear detected on an MRI study performed on symptomatic patients, it is important to know the prevalence of annular tears in asymptomatic patients. This problem is similar to that of determining the significance of detecting a disk bulge, herniation, or degeneration on
an MRI study.

Findings in Asymptomatic Subjects

Considering the well-documented pathologic evidence of disk degeneration
and herniation in the early decades of life, and their increased incidence with
advancing age,[18] it is not surprising that diskal abnormalities are frequently detected on MRI scans performed on asymptomatic patients. One important finding in the MRI studies performed on asymptomatic patients is the age at which
different types of abnormalities are first detected. This information becomes relevant when a symptomatic patient presents with a similar finding. The report by
Boden and associates[24] probably is the most frequently referenced report on the
MRI appearance of the lumbar spine in asymptomatic patients. The criteria for
consideration as an asymptomatic patient are quite different in the various MRI
studies. Boden and associates[24] studied 67 subjects with no history of back pain,
radicular pain, or neurogenic claudication. No history of back pain was defined
as no episode of pain that lasted more than 24 hours or required time off from
work. A subject who experienced recurrent episodes of back pain could still be
included in this study. The youngest group of asymptomatic subjects were aged
20 to 39 years. In this group, an HNP was present in 21%, a disk bulge in 56%,
disk degeneration (defined as decreased T2 signal intensity and decreased disk
height) in 34%, and stenosis in 1%. Evidence of disk degeneration increased
with increasing age of the patients. Stenosis was rare below the age of 60 years.
In the 60- to 80-year-old group, stenosis was present in 21%, HNP in 36%, disk
degeneration in 93%, and disk bulge in 79%. In this study, there was no assessment of the presence of annular tears. It cannot be assumed that because they
were not mentioned, they were not present.

Jensen and associates[25] reported on the MRI appearance of the lumbar spine
in people without back pain. They studied 98 subjects, mean age 48 years, who
were pain-free at the time of imaging and who had no history of back pain lasting more than 48 hours or of radiculopathy. In this asymptomatic population,
52% had a disk bulge, 27% a disk protrusion, and 1% a disk extrusion. In the
20- to 29-year-old group, 20% demonstrated a disk bulge and 15% a disk protrusion. The prevalence of disk bulge increased with increasing age up to the
50- to 59-year-old group and the prevalence of disk protrusion increased up to

the 40- to 49-year-old group. Annular tears were also detected in 14% of the asymptomatic patients. All disks with annular tears had abnormal nuclear signal intensity and all but one were associated with a disk bulge or protrusion. The authors[25] did not provide the criteria employed to diagnose an annular tear or the location of these tears.

There have been only a limited number of reports concerning MRI findings of the lumbar spine in asymptomatic subjects younger than 20 years of age. Gibson and associates[26] reported on 20 asymptomatic adolescents in whom four "minor central disc protrusions" were detected. Two of these subjects reported a history of prior mild back pain. Paajanen and associates[27] also reported on the MRI findings of the lumbar spine in young patients with low back pain. They evaluated 75 patients aged 20 ± 1 year and 34 controls aged 20 ± 0.6 years. Disk degeneration was defined as decreased disk T2-weighted signal intensity. This was detected in 57% of the symptomatic subjects and 35% of the asymptomatic subjects.

It is evident from these studies that the full spectrum of disk pathology is present at an early age and can be detected by MRI in asymptomatic individuals. Even though these findings are common, they still may have prognostic significance when present in a patient with back or radicular symptoms. Sward and associates[28] evaluated the MRI appearance of the lumbar spine for evidence of disk degeneration in 24 elite male gymnasts, median age 23 years, and 16 nonathlete controls, median age 26 years. Disk degeneration defined as reduced T2-weighted disk signal intensity was present in 75% of the athletes and 31% of the controls. When the two groups were pooled, there was a significant correlation between reduced disk signal intensity and back pain. A history of back pain was present in 79% of the athletes and 38% of the nonathletes who had evidence of disk degeneration on the MRI examination. At the time of the MRI, only 38% of the athletes and 0% of the nonathletes were experiencing back pain; therefore, it does not appear that the presence of low disk signal was predictive of current pain.

Findings in Symptomatic Patients

Magnetic Resonance Imaging Versus Diskography

If an abnormality is detected on an imaging study performed on a symptomatic patient, the clinician who ordered the study must decide whether it is the cause of a patient's symptoms, although it generally is accepted that an HNP, which correlates to a patient's symptoms and physical examination, detected on an MRI study is a clinically significant finding. Because annular tears and disk degeneration are omnipresent in the adult population, it is more difficult to prove that they are the cause of a patient's symptoms. Moreover, because diskogenic pain has a somatotopic rather than a dermatomal pattern of pain projection, it also may be difficult to clinically localize the symptomatic level.

Currently, diskography offers the only objective means to evaluate the morphologic status of a disk and to determine if a disk is the source of a patient's pain. It is easy to validate with cadaveric studies that diskography accurately depicts the morphologic condition of a disk.[29] It is more difficult to determine the significance of the pain provoked in patients at the time of disk injection. In the clinical assessment of other joints in the body, a patient's description of his or her pain is critical for the examining clinician to arrive at an accurate diagnosis. Unfortunately, because of the psychosocial issues that frequently cloud the assessment of a patient with acute or chronic back pain, the veracity of a patient's symptoms may be questioned. The fact that the treatment of diskogenic pain is difficult does not negate the importance of the disk as a potential pain generator. The work of Fernstrom[30] indicates that diskogenic pain may explain both local and referred symptoms. The pain he elicited at diskography could be reproduced at the time of surgery by stimulating the posterior surface of the disk in patients who experienced local pain at diskography, or by stimulating a nerve root in the patients who complained of referred pain with the disk injection.

If it is accepted that annular fissures and/or advanced disk degeneration are a potential etiology of back or referred pain, and that exact pain provocation when injecting a morphologically abnormal disk is presumptive evidence that a specific disk is the source of pain, then an important question arises. Can any noninvasive examination provide the same information as diskography? It was hoped that with its biochemical and morphologic assessment of the disk, MRI might provide information similar to that obtained by diskography. Two questions needed to be answered: (1) What is the significance of demonstrating a normal or abnormal disk on an MRI? (2) Are there any specific pathologic changes in the disk that can be detected on an MRI study that may indicate whether a disk is the source of a patient's pain? To answer these questions it is necessary to compare MRI scans to diskography performed on the same patient, with minimal time elapsing between the two.

Schneiderman and associates[31] compared MRI to diskography in the evaluation of 36 patients being considered for lumbar fusion for back pain. They demonstrated a 99% accuracy with MRI in predicting detection of morphologic degeneration of the disk using diskography. Diskography was considered abnormal if there were changes of disk degeneration or herniation and MRI was considered abnormal if there was decrease in T2-weighted disk signal intensity. The exact pattern of abnormal morphology detected on the diskogram could not be predicted from the MRI findings. Although the authors[31] concluded that changes in disk signal intensity accurately reflected the morphologic conditions of the disk, and that diskography was not indicated when an MRI demonstrated normal disk signal intensity, they also concluded that diskography may still be needed with an abnormal MRI in order to evaluate a patient's pain response. The authors[31] reported that normal MRI disk signal intensity indicated normal disk morphology on the diskogram in all patients with symptoms of greater than 2 months duration. Linson and Crowe[32] compared MRI to diskography in a prospective study of 50 patients. Using decreased T2-weighted disk signal as the criterion to diagnose disk degeneration, there was a 94% correlation between MRI and diskographic morphologic changes. Five percent of the MRI normal disks were abnormal on diskography. There was no discussion concerning the blinding of the MRI readers or assessing reader variation in these studies.

After initial optimistic reports on the ability of MRI to accurately define disk morphology,[31-33] there were several reports of disks that were normal on MRI but degenerated or disrupted on diskography. Zucherman and associates[34] reported on a group of 18 patents in whom MRI did not accurately reflect disk architecture or predict pain response. There was a mean of 2.5 months between the MRI and diskograms. No MRI protocols were presented in the report. It also is not stated whether the MRI reader was blinded to the patient status at the time of the retrospective analysis of the MRI images. In the discussion section, the authors[34] state that on T2-weighted sequences in several patients, an area of high signal intensity was identified extending through the posterior anulus. Even with the presence of this abnormality, these patients were classified as having normal MRI studies.

Although loss of T2-weighted signal in a disk may indicate disk degeneration, an important question is whether it has prognostic value in determining whether a degenerative disk is the source of a patient's pain. Collins and associates[35] reported on a prospective evaluation of 29 patients with chronic low back pain who were being considered for surgery. All symptomatic disks were found to be degenerated on MRI, as manifested by decreased T2 signal, and on diskography. The morphologic findings at diskography correlated with the MRI findings in 90%. Of the 57 degenerated disks detected on diskography, only 23% were symptomatic. Annular disruption was present with diskography in 10 of 13 symptomatic disks and 9 of 44 asymptomatic disks. MRI could not be used to identify the symptomatic level, particularly when multilevel disease was present. The severity of disk degeneration detected on MRI had no predictive value in determining which disks were symptomatic. The presence of a bulging anulus associated with disk degeneration on the MRI had some predictive value, with 10 of 13 symptomatic disks demonstrating annular bulges. Even though 7% of disks had a normal MRI appearance and an abnormal diskogram, the authors concluded that if a disk was normal on an MRI, it need not be injected when performing diskography. This conclusion appears to based on the fact that the diskographic abnormal and MRI normal disks were asymptomatic.

Simmons and associates[36] compared MRI to diskography in 164 patients who had low back pain with or without radiculopathy. The MRIs were performed on a variety of scanners, and the scanning protocols were not presented. Any mention in the radiology report of decreased disk signal intensity or a disk bulge was considered abnormal. Diskography and MRI correlated at disk levels in 80% of the disks. Thirteen percent of disks that were abnormal on MRI had normal diskograms. Of the MRI abnormal disks, 37% were asymptomatic. Thirty-four disks had a normal MRI and abnormal diskogram; 21 of these produced exact symptoms on diskography. It is difficult to evaluate the results of this study because of its methodology.

Buirski[37] prospectively evaluated 892 patients with chronic low back pain. He classified the appearance of a disk on MRI into six patterns and was able to show that changes in disk signal intensity patterns reflected the progression of disk degeneration demonstrated with diskography. In this group of patients, he did not assess whether these changes had predictive value in determining whether a degenerated disk was the pain generator. Using the same MRI criteria, Buirski and Silberstein[38] compared the appearance of 184 disks in 115 patients with chronic low back pain who were being considered for spinal fusion to 63 symptom-free controls who had no history of pain requiring analgesics, bed rest, or hospitalization. They detected 1.6 abnormal disks per symptomatic patient and 1.2 abnormal disks per control. There was no statistically significant difference in the distribution of abnormal signal intensity patterns in the two groups. In the symptomatic patients, the more degenerated the disk appeared in their MRI classification scheme, the more likely it was to be painful at diskography. No abnormal lumbar disk signal intensity pattern specifically indicated whether a disk would be painful with diskography. The authors[38] concluded that MRI is accurate in the assessment of disk morphology but diskography is the only technique able to assess whether a specific disk is the source of a patient's symptoms. Because they injected only disks that demonstrated an abnormal pattern on MRI, it is not possible to determine from their data the significance of a disk with a normal MRI pattern.

Horton and Daftari[39] used MRI and diskography to study 25 patients who were diagnosed as having chronic diskogenic pain, had not responded to conservative therapy, and were being considered for spinal fusion. On T2-weighted sagittal images, 63 disks were classified according to signal intensity and appearance of the posterior anulus (flat, bulged, or torn). Disk morphology on diskography was classified as normal or degenerated. A positive diskogram required both a positive pain response and a degenerated morphology. There were 19 positive diskograms in the 25 patients. Abnormal disk morphology was present in 71% of the disks at diskography but only 55% of these abnormal disks elicited a positive pain response. Some of the MRI disk patterns correlated to the morphologic changes detected on diskography. Only 1 of 18 disks that had normal MRI signal intensity had a positive diskogram with concordant pain. This disk had a posterior intra-annular cleft on its diskogram. The highest rate of positive diskography correlated to disks that demonstrated no signal on the T2-weighted images. All nine disks demonstrating a tear in the anulus and the posterior longitudinal ligament on the MRI had abnormal morphology on diskography, but only five of these disks had a positive pain response. The authors concluded that diskography may be obviated in a patient with diskogenic pain, who demonstrates a torn outer anulus-associated absent T2-weighted signal intensity.

A study comparing MRI and diskography for the evaluation of annular tears and lumbar disk degeneration was reported by Osti and Fraser.[40] They evaluated 108 disks in 33 consecutive patients with low back pain. MRI signal intensity was graded as normal, reduced, or absent on T2-weighted images. The following morphologic classification of the disk was employed on diskography: type 1, normal; type 2, normal NP associated with an inner or outer annular fissure without contrast extravasation; type 3, normal NP associated with an annular fissure and contrast extravasation; and type 4, disorganization of the NP and contrast extension throughout the disk space, with or without contrast extravasation. Comparison of the MRI appearance of the disks and the diskographic findings is presented in Table 1. The patient's pain provocation is compared with the MRI and diskographic morphologic types in Table 2. Of the 60 disks with normal MRI signal intensity, 25% showed type 2, 20% type 3, and 10% type 4, diskographic changes. In addition, 20% of the disks with normal MRI signal intensity elicited typical pain with diskography. From these findings, it appears that a normal MRI would not be sufficient to exclude a painful disk containing annular tears. Of the 15 disks with absent MRI signal, 40% showed type 3 and 60% type 4 diskographic changes. Although all disks with absent MRI signal had abnormal morphology at diskography, only 60% pro-

Table 1 Comparison of the results of magnetic resonance imaging (MRI) and diskography

MRI Signal Intensity	No. of Disks	Diskography Type*			
		1	2	3	4
Normal	60	27	15	12	6
Decreased	39	0	9	15	15
Absent	15	0	0	6	9

*Type 1, normal; type 2, normal nucleus pulposus (NP) associated with an inner or outer annular fissure without contrast extravasation; type 3, normal NP associated with an annular fissure and contrast extravasation; type 4, disorganization of the NP and contrast extension through the disk space with or without contrast extravasation

Table 2 Comparison of the type of diskographic degeneration and magnetic resonance imaging (MRI) signal pattern to patient's pain response at diskography

Pain at Diskography	No. of Disks	Diskography Type*				MRI Signal		
		1	2	3	4	Normal	Decreased	Absent
None	39	24	6	0	9	33	3	3
Atypical	36	3	15	6	12	15	18	3
Typical	39	0	3	27	9	12	18	9

*Type 1, normal; type 2, normal nucleus pulposus (NP) associated with an inner or outer annular fissure without contrast extravasation; type 3, normal NP associated with an annular fissure and contrast extravasation; type 4, disorganization of the NP and contrast extension through the disk space with or without contrast extravasation

voked typical pain when they were injected. It was not possible to use the MRI signal characteristics of the disk to predict the patient's pain response. Of the patients reporting typical pain with diskographic injection, 69% had abnormal MRI signals, all had degenerated patterns on diskography, and 92% had contrast extending to the outer anulus.

Osti and Fraser[40] concluded that MRI is a useful screening modality for patients with disabling disk disease. If a patient has pain and an abnormal MRI, it can be assumed that the abnormal disk on the MRI is the source of a patient's pain. If the MRI is negative, or if definitive proof is needed to demonstrate that a specific disk is the cause of a patient's pain, then diskography is needed. A potential source of bias in this study is that the interpretation of the MRI images and diskograms was performed by the same observer. There was no mention of observer blinding or assessment of intraobserver reader variation. One possible reason for the normal MRI signal intensity in disks containing annular fissures may be explained by results from the authors' previous animal experiments.[12] In an animal model of disk degeneration, T2-weighted images failed to demonstrate abnormal signal intensity in disks until 12 months after diskal injury. It is possible that patients with recent annular tears may still demonstrate normal MRI T2-weighted signal. Currently, it is unknown how long it takes for a normal human disk to lose its signal intensity after developing an

397

annular tear. It is also possible that there was a decrease in the disk signal intensity that was not detected visually.

Videman and associates,[41] using T1- and proton density-weighted images, compared visual assessment of disk signal intensity in human disks to digital intensity profiles of regions of interest in the disk. The digital method showed differences between disks that were not shown by the visual method, particularly in younger subjects. The authors[41] concluded that digital assessments of disk signal intensity offer more precise and detailed information about disk desiccation than do subjective readings. Even though the digital method showed more variation than the visual method, it does not necessarily mean that the digital method is more accurate. In addition, quantitative evaluation of disk signal intensity is very dependent on scanning techniques,[42] and its reliability and precision are unproven.[43] Sether and associates[44] also demonstrated the difficulty of visually detecting subtle differences in MRI disk signal intensity. When evaluating the signal intensity changes of aging disks, they were able to detect differences in MRI signal intensity by direct measurement from the monitor, but not by visual inspection.

Diskography and the High Intensity Zone

Results from several studies have indicated that decreased or absent T2-weighted disk signal intensity has a poor predictive value in determining whether a fissured or degenerated disk is painful. However, Aprill and Bogduk[45] reported on an abnormal high intensity zone (HIZ) in the disk that was highly correlated to disk degeneration and positive pain provocation at diskography. They evaluated the MRI scans of 500 patients who had a history of intractable back pain, with or without leg pain, and at least 3 months of symptoms. A HIZ represented a focus of increased signal within the anulus that was separate from the signal intensity of the nucleus. The fact that the HIZ did not appear to contact the nucleus may be a function of image resolution or an oblique orientation of the abnormality with respect to the MRI scan plane. The authors did not report on the appearance of the T2-weighted signal intensity of the nucleus in the disks containing a HIZ.

A HIZ was present in 143 of the 500 patients. Forty-one of these 143 patients also had a diskogram combined with a computed tomographic (CT) study, that is, disko-CT. In all patients with a HIZ, either a grade 3 (four patients) or a grade 4 (37 patients) annular disruption was present on the disko-CT. Grade 3 disruption represented contrast extending into the outer third of the disk, and grade 4 represented contrast extending into the outer third of the disk associated with circumferential extension of contrast between the outer annular lamellae. Of the 68 patients who had a grade 4 annular disruption on disko-CT, 37 had a HIZ on MRI, and of the seven disks with a grade 3 annular disruption, four had a HIZ. Three of seven disks with grade 3 annular disruption had exact pain reproduction. Of the 68 disks with a grade 4 annular disruption, 35 had exact pain reproduction, 16 had similar pain reproduction, and 17 had no pain. In patients with a HIZ disk, pain provocation was exact in 31, similar in seven, and none in two. In disks without a HIZ, pain provocation was exact in seven, similar in 15, and none in 56. Exact pain reproduction occurred only with injection of grade 3 (3 disks) and grade 4 (35 disks) annular abnormalities. Reproduction of symptoms was related to the degree of disk degeneration. The sensitivity of HIZ in detecting exact pain reproduction was 82% and the specificity, 89%.

The results of this study demonstrate that in this subset of patients, it is highly likely that a disk containing a HIZ represents a degenerated painful disk. The authors postulate that a HIZ represents inflamed nuclear material trapped between annular fibers. It is also possible that the HIZ represents granulation tissue in the outer anulus secondary to an annular tear. The fact that the healing potential of the disk appears limited to the outer annular fibers, at least in animal models,[46] may explain why the HIZ is limited to the outer margin of the disk. Although it is tempting to hypothesize that a HIZ represents a torn, painful, and possibly inflamed anulus, it will not be possible to determine the significance of this finding until the prevalence of a HIZ is determined in a larger set of patients with low back pain and in asymptomatic patients. Future analysis of the histopathology of a HIZ should provide insight into explaining its MRI appearance and, perhaps, its role in the causation of back pain.

In all of the previous studies comparing MRI to diskography, diskography was used as the standard for diagnosing the presence of diskogenic disease. However, the accuracy of diskography has been questioned. Holt[47] found diskography to be positive in up to 37% of asymptomatic subjects. Hudgins[48] reported a 22% false-positive and 17% false-negative rate, and Yasuma and associates[49] reported a 32% to 56% false-negative rate for diskography. Whereas Hudgins[48] and Yasuma and associates[49] assessed the limitations of diskography in depiction of accurate disk morphology related to disk herniations, Holt[47] reported on the pain response to injection. Walsh and associates[50] demonstrated a 0% false-positive rate for diskography in a small number of asymptomatic patients when both an abnormal image and substantial pain were considered criteria for a positive test. Proponents of diskography state that if provocation diskography is not painful in a normal subject, then exact pain reproduction with disk injection is indicative that the disk is the source of a patient's symptoms.

It may not be possible to use MRI to predict whether a fissured or degenerated disk is the cause of a patient's symptoms; however, it may be possible to detect evidence of incipient disk failure that could be retarded or prevented with appropriate therapeutic regimens. Infolding of the inner annular fibers appears to be an early event in the development of disk degeneration (Fig. 4).[3,4] The infolding may reflect matrix failure due to increased compressive load on the anulus as the nucleus loses its hydrostatic capacity with aging. Schiebler and associates[51] reported on in vivo and ex vivo MRI of early disk degeneration. They performed high resolution MRI imaging, with a pixel size of 0.18 mm and slice thickness of 3 mm, of cadaveric spines and compared the images to histopathologic findings. Using this technique, it was possible to detect on the MRI infolding of the annular fibers, annular tears, and separation of the NP and the inner anulus from the hyaline end plates. They[51] described a central dot in the disk, best seen on a proton density-weighted image, which they believed represented the infolded fibers. They also demonstrated that disks with evidence of early degeneration but not herniation had normal T2-weighted MRI signal intensity.

Schiebler and associates[51] also evaluated routine MRI scans performed on patients to determine if changes of altered annular morphology could be detected.

399

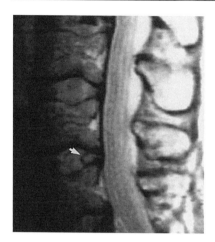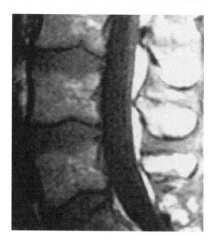

Fig. 4 *There appears to be infolding of the inner annular fibers (arrow) at the L4-5 disk level on the proton density-weighted image (***left***). This is not identified on the T1-weighted image (***right***).*

Infolding of the anulus could be detected even on clinical studies in which high resolution techniques were not used. Although these observations indicate that it may be possible to detect altered annular morphology prior to failure, further experimental and clinical validation is needed, particularly the assessment of observer accuracy and reliability, before it will be possible to determine the significance of these findings. It is tempting to try to improve the MRI spatial resolution by using thinner sections or a smaller field of view, but this may adversely affect image resolution due to a decrease in MRI signal.[52] With the implementation of the new high field strength 4-Tesla MRI systems, it may be possible to achieve image resolution in patients that equals the resolution currently achieved only in ex vivo specimens.

Biochemical Composition of the Disk

It has been hypothesized that altered disk nutrition due to changes in the diffusion properties of the vertebral end plates may be the initiating event in transformation of the composition and structure of the disk. With Gd-DTPA enhanced imaging, it may be possible to noninvasively study the diffusion properties of a disk. Ibrahim and associates[53] recently reported on the assessment of contrast enhancement of rabbit disks. Contrast enhancement of the disk was detected by observation and measurement in animals receiving a minimum dose of 0.3 mmol/kg of contrast. Enhancement was first detected near the vertebral end plates and later in the center of the disk. It progressively increased with time and with the amount of contrast. With the administration of 0.1 mmol/kg of contrast, which is the standard clinical dose, there was less than 10% enhancement of the disk, and this was not detected visually. Only when enhancement exceeded 25% was it evident on visual inspection. It is not stated in the study whether the observers were blinded to the contrast dosage when they were analyzing the images. Considering that new gadolinium contrast agents have been approved for clinical use at dosages of 0.3 mmol/kg, it may be possible to evaluate the diffusion properties of the disk end plate complex. Although the size and charge of the gadolinium chelates is quite different from those of the normal solutes that diffuse into the disk, studying the diffusion of the gadolinium chelates may still provide useful information on the diffusion capacity of the disk and end plate.

Another early age-related change detected in the human intervertebral disk is decreased aggregation and amount of diskal proteoglycans and decreased hydration of the nucleus pulposus. Because routine MR images are based on the concentration of mobile hydrogen ions, along with their T1 and T2 relaxation times, it would seem that MRI would provide an excellent means to assess the biochemical status of a disk.[8,54,55] Unfortunately, the signal intensity generated depends not only on the hydration level of the disk, but also is intimately related to the hydrogen atoms' biochemical environment, which is in a constant state of flux in healthy and degenerated disks. In addition, the acquisition of this information is extremely dependent on imaging methodologies and the equipment used.[7] Realizing these difficulties, it still may be possible with MRI to create topographic maps of disk relaxation parameters and possibly pH.

Chatani and associates[56] evaluated the topographic differences of relaxation times in the normal adult bovine disk and compared their relationships to water content. They demonstrated a positive linear relationship between T1 and water content. There was a decrease in T2 with decreased water content only when water content was at least 75% of diskal weight, but no marked change when water content was below 75%. T1 and T2 were affected differently by changes in water content; therefore, it is possible that T2-weighted images, which are used clinically to assess the degree of disk hydration, may not be the optimal means to obtain this information. The T1 and T2 values were also different in different parts of the disk as a result of the differences in the composition and structure of the macromolecular constituents.

Another potential application of MRI, the detection of alterations in disk relaxation values as a means of diagnosing disk degeneration, was reported by Boos and associates.[42] They compared the diurnal variation of the relaxation times of the hydrogen ions in normal and degenerated disks. When comparing the morning and evening values, they detected less of a decrease in the T1 of degenerated disks when compared to normal disks.

Magnetization transfer (MT) is a new technique that also offers promise as a means of studying the biochemical status of a disk.[57] It has been used in clinical MRI to improve image contrast. With MT, it is possible to measure the cross-relaxation between free and macromolecular bound protons of tissue water. MT may provide new insights into the changing biochemical environment of the disk associated with disk degeneration.

It also is possible that studying the changes of disk contour with MRI may give insight into incipient biomechanical failure of the disk. Beattie and associates[58] studied the effect of lordosis on disk contour in supine patients. By performing ''dynamic'' MRI studies they were able to demonstrate small changes in the posterior margin of normal disks with changes in spinal posture. Some manufacturers have attempted to construct an MRI scanner in which the patient may be imaged while seated or standing. If image quality could be maintained, this may be the optimal method to evaluate patients with diskogenic pain, radicular symptoms, or claudication.

As a result of the noninvasiveness and absent biologic risk of MRI, it may be possible with repeated studies to follow any structural or biochemical markers that are proven to be indicative of disk deterioration and to assess the effect of different therapeutic regimens on the progression of the degenerative process. Although the MRI detection of diskal pathology may not be useful for diagnosing whether a disk is painful, it may have some predictive value in guiding patient therapy. The preliminary results reported by Modic and associates[23] suggest that the presence of an annular fissure in a symptomatic patient may be indicative of a poorer outcome with conservative care. If this is true, earlier surgical intervention may be indicated in these patients. An expanded prospective clinical study may answer this question.

Reliability of MRI

The purpose of this chapter has been to provide insight into the potential strengths and limitations of MRI as an experimental tool to expand the understanding of disk degeneration and as a diagnostic tool in assessing patients with suspected diskogenic pain. Although this chapter has focused on the precision of MRI, it is also necessary to discuss its reliability. In the studies reported by Jensen and associates[25] and Brant-Zawadzki and associates,[59] the MRI examinations were interpreted by two expert neuroradiologists from the same institution. Interobserver agreement for a limited number of diagnoses (normal, disk bulge, disk protrusion, or disk extrusion) was only 80% ($\kappa = 0.59$). Raininko and associates[60] reported on observer variability in the assessment of disk degeneration on MRI studies of the lumbar and thoracic spine. Three independent readers—an orthopaedic surgeon, a general radiologist, and a spinal radiologist—evaluated MR images of the lumbar spine in 122 subjects, 17% of whom had back symptoms at the time of the MRI. Twenty cases were reevaluated to test for intraobserver variation. Each observer graded 12 different findings related to disk degeneration. Intraobserver agreement in the assessment of lumbar spine images was generally greater than 0.70 but interobserver agreement was poorer. The interobserver agreement between the orthopaedist and the general radiologist and between the general radiologist and the spinal radiologist was 0.50 and that between the orthopaedist and the spinal radiologist was 0.40. The authors concluded that the substantial interobserver disagreement limits comparisons of evaluations by different readers. This study did not address the accuracy of the interpretations or the effect of the different diagnoses on therapeutic decisions. The findings in these studies are relevant when trying to assess the imaging results generated in a single or multicenter clinical study in which the results of two or more readers are combined. Inter- and intraobserver variability along with observer accuracy must be critically assessed for all current and future applications of MRI.

The value of MRI in assessing patients with back and radicular pain is still evolving. Its efficacy and cost effectiveness must be demonstrated to justify its continued use. Conjecture and speculation will no longer be accepted by the United States health care system as the basis for ordering a diagnostic imaging study. Only by performing and completing large prospective outcome studies will it be possible to determine the value of diagnostic tests. Unfortunately, such studies will require a large investment of time and resources, which at this moment are in limited supply.

References

1. Pritzker KP: Aging and degeneration in the lumbar intervertebral disc. *Orthop Clin North Am* 1977;8:66–77.
2. Buckwalter JA: Aging and degeneration of the human intervertebral disc. *Spine* 1995;20:1307–1314.
3. Yasuma T, Arai K, Yamauchi Y: The histology of lumbar intervertebral disc herniation: The significance of small blood vessels in the extruded tissue. *Spine* 1993;18:1761–1765.
4. Yasuma T, Koh S, Okamura T, et al: Histological changes in aging lumbar intervertebral discs: Their role in protusions and prolapses. *J Bone Joint Surg* 1990;72A:220–229.
5. DeCandido P, Reinig JW, Dwyer AJ, et al: Magnetic resonance assessment of the distribution of lumbar spine disc degenerative changes. *J Spinal Disord* 1988;1:9–15.
6. Modic MT, Masaryk TJ, Ross JS, et al: Imaging of degenerative disk disease. *Radiology* 1988;168:177–186.
7. Weidenbaum M, Foster RJ, Best BA, et al: Correlating magnetic resonance imaging with the biochemical content of the normal human intervertebral disc. *J Orthop Res* 1992;10:552–561.
8. Tertti M, Paajanen H, Laato M, et al: Disc degeneration in magnetic resonance imaging: A comparative biochemical, histologic, and radiologic study in cadaver spines. *Spine* 1991;16:629–634.
9. Friberg S, Hirsch C: Anatomical and clinical studies on lumbar disc degeneration. *Acta Orthop Scand* 1949;19:222–242.
10. Yu SW, Haughton VM, Ho PS, et al: Progressive and regressive changes in the nucleus pulposus: Part II. The adult. *Radiology* 1988;169:93–97.
11. Yu S, Haughton VM, Sether LA, et al: Criteria for classifying normal and degenerated lumbar intervertebral disks. *Radiology* 1989;170:523–526.
12. Osti OL, Vernon-Roberts B, Fraser RD: Anulus tears and intervertebral disc degeneration: An experimental study using an animal model. *Spine* 1990;15:762–767.
13. Moneta GB, Videman T, Kaivanto K, et al: Reported pain during lumbar discography as a function of anular ruptures and disc degeneration: A re-analysis of 833 discograms. *Spine* 1994;19:1968–1974.
14. Vanharanta H, Sachs BL, Ohnmeiss DD, et al: Pain provocation and disc deterioration by age: A CT/discography study in a low-back pain population. *Spine* 1989;14:420–423.
15. Ross JS, Modic MT, Masaryk TJ: Tears of the anulus fibrosus: Assessment with Gd-DTPA-enhanced MR imaging. *Am J Roentgenol* 1990;154:159–162.
16. Osti OL, Vernon-Roberts B, Moore R, et al: Annular tears and disc degeneration in the lumbar spine: A post-mortem study of 135 discs. *J Bone Joint Surg* 1992;74B:678–682.
17. Yu SW, Sether LA, Ho PS, et al: Tears of the anulus fibrosus: Correlation between MR and pathologic findings in cadavers. *Am J Neuroradiol* 1988;9:367–370.
18. Miller JA, Schmatz C, Schultz AB. Lumbar disc degeneration: Correlation with age, sex, and spine level in 600 autopsy specimens. *Spine* 1988;13:173–178.
19. Yu SW, Haughton VM, Sether LA, et al: Comparison of MR and diskography in detecting radial tears of the anulus: A postmortem study. *Am J Neuroradiol* 1989;10:1077–1081.
20. Gunzburg R, Parkinson R, Moore R, et al: A cadaveric study comparing discography, magnetic resonance imaging, histology, and mechanical behavior of the human lumbar disc. *Spine* 1992;17:417–426.

21. Nguyen CM, Ho K-C, Yu SW, et al: An experimental model to study contrast enhancement in MR imaging of the intervertebral disk. *Am J Neuroradiol* 1989;10:811–814.
22. Krödel A, Reinhard P, Stäbler S, et al: Abstract: Pathological disc vascularization: MRI and histological findings. *J Bone Joint Surg* 1995;77B:14.
23. Modic MT, Ross JS, Obuchowski NA, et al: Contrast-enhanced MR imaging in acute lumbar radiculopathy: A pilot study of the natural history. *Radiology* 1995;195:429–435.
24. Boden SD, Davis DO, Dina TS, et al: Abnormal magnetic-resonance scans of the lumbar spine in asymptomatic subjects: A prospective investigation. *J Bone Joint Surg* 1990;72A:403–408.
25. Jensen MC, Brant-Zawadzki MN, Obuchowski N, et al: Magnetic resonance imaging of the lumbar spine in people without back pain. *N Engl J Med* 1994;331:69–73.
26. Gibson MJ, Szypryt EP, Buckley JH, et al: Magnetic resonance imaging of adolescent disc herniation. *J Bone Joint Surg* 1987;69B:699–703.
27. Paajanen H, Erkintalo M, Kuusela T, et al: Magnetic resonance study of disc degeneration in young low-back pain patients. *Spine* 1989;14:982–985.
28. Sward L, Hellstrom M, Jacobsson B, et al: Disc degeneration and associated abnormalities of the spine in elite gymnasts: A magnetic resonance imaging study. *Spine* 1991;16:437–443.
29. Adams MA, Dolan P, Hutton WC: The stages of disc degeneration as revealed by discograms. *J Bone Joint Surg* 1986;68B:36–41.
30. Fernstrom U: A discographical study of ruptured lumbar intervertebral discs. *Acta Chir Scand* 1960;258(suppl):1–60.
31. Schneiderman G, Flannigan B, Kingston S, et al: Magnetic resonance imaging in the diagnosis of disc degeneration: Correlation with discography. *Spine* 1987;12:276–281.
32. Linson MA, Crowe CH: Comparison of magnetic resonance imaging and lumbar discography in the diagnosis of disc degeneration. *Clin Orthop* 1990;250:160–163.
33. Gibson MJ, Buckley J, Mawhinney R, et al: Magnetic resonance imaging and discography in the diagnosis of disc degeneration: A comparative study of 50 discs. *J Bone Joint Surg* 1986;68B:369–373.
34. Zucherman J, Derby R, Hsu K, et al: Normal magnetic resonance imaging with abnormal discography. *Spine* 1988;13:1355–1359.
35. Collins CD, Stack JP, O'Connell DJ, et al: The role of discography in lumbar disc disease: A comparative study of magnetic resonance imaging and discography. *Clin Radiol* 1990;42:252–257.
36. Simmons JW, Emery SF, McMillin JN, et al: Awake discography: A comparison study with magnetic resonance imaging. *Spine* 1991;16(suppl 6):S216–221.
37. Buirski G: Magnetic resonance signal patterns of lumbar discs in patients with low back pain: A prospective study with discographic correlation. *Spine* 1992;17:1199–1204.
38. Buirski G, Silberstein M: The symptomatic lumbar disc in patients with low-back pain: Magnetic resonance imaging appearances in both a symptomatic and control population. *Spine* 1993;18:1808–1811.
39. Horton WC, Daftari TK: Which disc as visualized by magnetic resonance imaging is actually a source of pain? A correlation between magnetic resonance imaging and discography. *Spine* 1992;17(suppl 6):S164–S171.
40. Osti OL, Fraser RD: MRI and discography of annular tears and intervertebral disc degeneration: A prospective clinical comparison. *J Bone Joint Surg* 1992;74B:431–435.
41. Videman T, Nummi P, Battié MC, et al: Digital assessment of MRI for lumbar disc desiccation: A comparison of digital versus subjective assessments and digital intensity profiles versus discogram and macroanatomic findings. *Spine* 1994;19:192–198.

42. Boos N, Wallin A, Gbedegbegnon T, et al: Quantitative MR imaging of lumbar intervertebral disks and vertebral bodies: Influence of diurnal water content variations. *Radiology* 1993;188:351–354.
43. Modic MT, Herfkens RJ: Intervertebral disk: Normal age-related changes in MR signal intensity. *Radiology* 1990;177:332–334.
44. Sether LA, Yu S, Haughton VM, et al: Intervertebral disk: Normal age-related changes in MR signal intensity. *Radiology* 1990;177:385–388.
45. Aprill C, Bogduk N: High-intensity zone: A diagnostic sign of painful lumbar disc on magnetic resonance imaging. *Br J Radiol* 1992;65:361–369.
46. Hampton D, Laros G, McCarron R, et al: Healing potential of the anulus fibrosus. *Spine* 1989;14:398–401.
47. Holt EP Jr: The question of lumbar discography. *J Bone Joint Surg* 1968;50A:720–726.
48. Hudgins WR: Diagnostic accuracy of lumbar discography. *Spine* 1977;2:305–309.
49. Yasuma T, Ohno R, Yamauchi Y: False-negative lumbar discograms: Correlation of discographic and histological findings in postmortem and surgical specimens. *J Bone Joint Surg* 1988;70A:1279–1290.
50. Walsh TR, Weinstein JN, Spratt KF, et al: Lumbar discography in normal subjects: A controlled prospective study. *J Bone Joint Surg* 1990;72A:1081–1088.
51. Schiebler ML, Camerino VJ, Fallon MD, et al: In vivo and ex vivo magnetic resonance imaging evaluation of early disc degeneration with histopathologic correlation. *Spine* 1991;16:635–640.
52. Constable RT, Henkelman RM: Contrast, resolution, and detectability in MR imaging. *J Comput Assist Tomogr* 1991;15:297–303.
53. Ibrahim MA, Jesmanowicz A, Hyde JS, et al: Contrast enhancement of normal intervertebral disks: Time and dose dependence. *Am J Neuroradiol* 1994;15:419–423.
54. Hickey DS, Aspden RM, Hukins DW, et al: Analysis of magnetic resonance images from normal and degenerate lumbar intervertebral discs. *Spine* 1986;11:702–708.
55. Jenkins JP, Hickey DS, Zhu XP, et al: MR imaging of the intervertebral disc: A quantitative study. *Br J Radiol* 1985;58:705–709.
56. Chatani K, Kusaka Y, Mifune T, et al: Topographic differences of 1H-NMR relaxation times (T1, T2) in the normal intervertebral disc and its relationship to water content. *Spine* 1993;18:2271–2275.
57. Paajanen H, Komu M, Lehto I, et al: Magnetization transfer imaging of lumbar disc degeneration: Correlation of relaxation parameters with biochemistry. *Spine* 1994;19:2833–2837.
58. Beattie PF, Brooks WM, Rothstein JM, et al: Effect of lordosis on the position of the nucleus pulposus in supine subjects: A study using magnetic resonance imaging. *Spine* 1994;19:2096–2102.
59. Brant-Zawadzki MN, Jensen MC, Obuchowski N, et al: Interobserver and intraobserver variability in interpretation of lumbar disc abnormalities: A comparison of two nomenclatures. *Spine* 1995;20:1257–1264.
60. Raininko R, Manninen H, Battie MC, et al: Observer variability in the assessment of disc degeneration on magnetic resonance images of the lumbar and thoracic spine. *Spine* 1995;20:1029–1035.

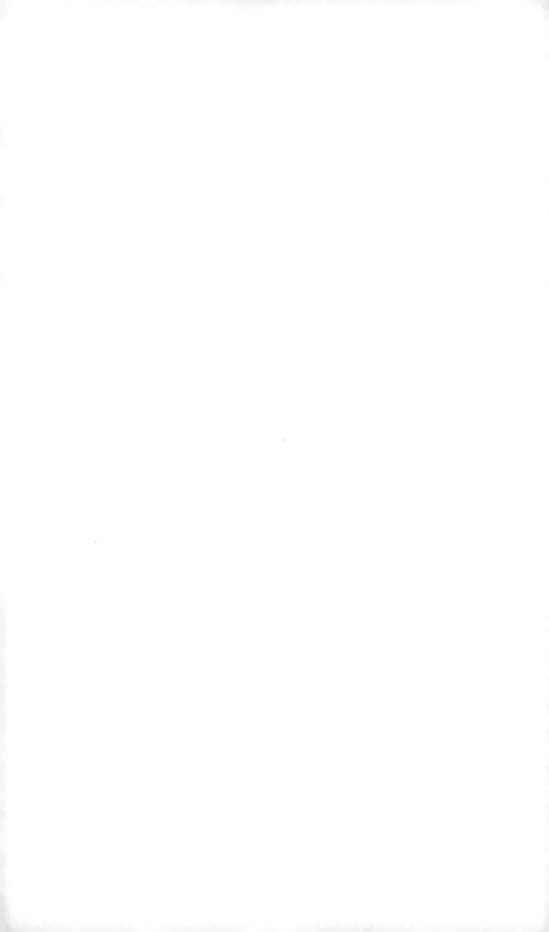

Chapter 25

Needle Techniques in the Diagnosis of Low Back Pain

Nikolai Bogduk MD, PhD, BSc

Introduction

In the assessment of patients with low back pain there will be instances where, after clinical examination and conventional investigations, no diagnosis is evident. The patient has back pain, perhaps with referred pain in the lower limb, but neurologic examination is normal. Spinal movements may be restricted, the back may be tender; plain radiographs, computed tomography (CT) scans, and even magnetic resonance imaging (MRI) are normal or equivocal. There is no evidence of disk herniation. This scenario is not uncommon and, indeed, may be typical of the majority of presentations of lumbar spinal pain.

The physician has two options. One is to call a halt to investigations and offer a diagnosis of *lumbar spinal pain of unknown origin*, as prescribed by the International Association for the Study of Pain (IASP).[1] But without an anatomic diagnosis, treatment cannot be targeted. At best, the patient will undergo whatever is the currently popular program of management, be it manipulation, physiotherapy, work-hardening, or behavioral therapy, or even surgery, as a last resort.

The other option is to pursue a diagnosis. The objective is to pinpoint the source of pain in order to institute therapy that is specific to the source. But medical imaging is notoriously useless in pinpointing the source of idiopathic back pain. Once tumors, fractures, and disk herniation have been excluded, there is nothing to be seen on radiograph or CT that legitimately and reliably correlates with a source of pain.

The only means available of finding a source of pain are needle procedures designed to provoke or anesthetize putatively painful structures. Needles provide access to structures that are not accessible to manual examination, and a particular structure can be incriminated if selectively provoking that structure reproduces the patient's pain. It is more compelling if anesthetizing a particular structure totally relieves the patient's pain. However, caveats apply. With respect to provocation, it must be shown that provoking other structures fails to reproduce the patient's pain. With respect to anesthesia, it must be shown that the response is real and physiologic, and that it is not confounded by a placebo response.

The Techniques

Techniques have been developed whereby access can be gained to the lumbar zygapophyseal joints, the sacroiliac joints, the lumbar disks, and the nerve-root sleeves (Table 1). Although the back muscles have been deemed to be a potent source of back pain, no selective needle procedures have been developed to test if a particular muscle or group of muscles is the primary source of pain. Techniques such as trigger point injections for low back pain have not been subjected to scientific scrutiny.

Zygapophyseal joint blocks were developed because there are no other means of diagnosing pain from these joints. There are no diagnostic clinical features of lumbar zygapophyseal joint pain,[2-5] nor are painful joints reliably evident on CT.[6]

Diskogenic pain cannot be diagnosed clinically,[7] or by plain radiography or CT. In this context, diskogenic pain means pain stemming from the disk itself, as opposed to radicular pain caused by disk prolapse. In some instances, diskogenic pain can be diagnosed by MRI. Some disks exhibit a distinctive high intensity zone in the posterior anulus fibrosus, and this sign correlates strongly with the presence of a painful grade 4 fissure in that disk. This sign has high specificity and a high positive predictive value.[8] However, the sign has a low prevalence and only a modest sensitivity; there are patients with diskogenic pain who do not exhibit the sign. Disk stimulation (also called diskography) is the only available means of determining whether or not a patient has diskogenic pain.

There are no clinical features diagnostic of sacroiliac joint pain[9] or of pain stemming from the dural sleeves of the lumbar nerve roots. Diagnostic blocks constitute the only means of identifying these sources of pain.

Zygapophyseal Joint Blocks

The lumbar zygapophyseal joints can be provoked with injections of contrast medium that distend the joint capsule or by injections of hypertonic saline that ostensibly irritate the joint. As a diagnostic technique, however, joint provocation is unreliable. It has been formally shown that the results of provocation cor-

Table 1 The needle procedures available for the diagnosis of low back pain and the conditions that they identify

Condition	Procedure[*]
Zygapophyseal joint pain	Intra-articular blocks
	Medial branch blocks
Sacroiliac joint pain	Intra-articular blocks
Diskogenic pain	Disk stimulation
	± Diskography
	± CT diskography
Radicular pain	Root sleeve blocks

*CT = computed tomography

relate poorly with relief of pain following controlled diagnostic blocks of these joints.[10]

Diagnostic blocks are the only reliable means of identifying lumbar zygapophyseal joint pain. To prove that a zygapophyseal joint is the source of a patient's pain, that pain must be abolished by selectively anesthetizing that joint.

Zygapophyseal joints may be blocked by intra-articular injections of local anesthetic or by blocking the nerves that innervate them: the medial branches of the lumbar dorsal rami[11] (Fig. 1). With either technique, the injections must be discrete.

The lumbar zygapophyseal joints admit less than 2 ml and usually not more than 1 ml of solution. If greater volumes are used to infiltrate these joints, the solution will rupture the joint capsule and spread to adjacent structures.[12,13] Such spread not only destroys the specificity of the block, it also risks complications resulting from epidural or even intrathecal spread of local anesthetic.[14,15]

Similar considerations pertain to medial branch blocks. A volume of 0.5 ml is sufficient to infiltrate one of these nerves (Fig. 2); larger volumes are unnecessary and risk spread of the local anesthetic to distant sites and structures.

The technical aspects of zygapophyseal joint blocks have been detailed in other sources.[2-4,11] The critical feature is that they must be performed under fluoroscopic control in order to ensure accuracy and safety.

Controls

Controls are the most critical aspect of zygapophyseal joint blocks. It has been shown that the placebo response rate of lumbar zygapophyseal joint blocks can be as high as 32%,[4] and the false-positive rate for lumbar zygapophyseal joint blocks is 38%.[16]

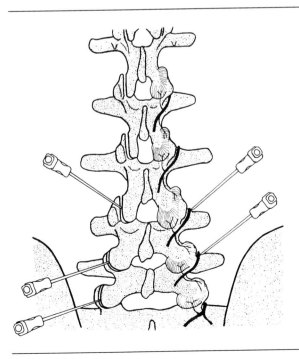

Fig. 1   *A sketch illustrating the procedures for blocking lumbar zygapophyseal joints. On the left, needles are shown as they would appear during intra-articular blocks. On the right, needles are shown in place to block the medial branches of the L3 and L4 dorsal rami, which innervate the L4-5 zygapophyseal joint. (Courtesy of Dr. Nikolai Bogduk, Callaghan, NSW, Australia.)*

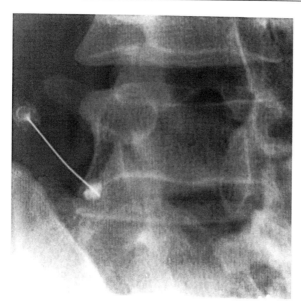

Fig. 2 *A posteroanterior radiograph of a lumbar spine showing a needle in position to block the left L5 dorsal ramus. Contrast medium (0.5 ml) has been injected to indicate that the target point is well infiltrated and that the injectate does not spread to other sites. (Courtesy of Dr. Charles Aprill, New Orleans, LA.)*

A single diagnostic block is liable to error; patients may respond for reasons other than the pharmacologic effect of the agent injected. Indeed, because of the relatively low prevalence of lumbar zygapophyseal joint pain, it transpires that for every three apparently positive diagnostic blocks, two will be wrong.[16] The only way to circumvent this problem is to perform control blocks in each and every patient. Otherwise, the operator is simply guessing which block is truly positive, with the odds being 2:1 against guessing correctly.

Unfortunately, performance of control blocks has not been standard practice in the past. As a result, none of the earlier literature on the prevalence of zygapophyseal joint pain or its treatment is reliable. All studies were potentially polluted by inordinate numbers of false-positive responders. This lack of reliability, however, does not detract from the legitimacy of the diagnosis of zygapophyseal joint pain. The condition occurs, and it can be diagnosed only by diagnostic blocks; but those blocks must be controlled.

Two types of control are available. Under research conditions, patients could undergo a series of diagnostic blocks among which placebo agents, such as normal saline, would be used. At least three blocks, however, would be required: one using local anesthetic in the first instance in order to establish prima facie that the joint in question is putatively a source of pain; and then, at least two others. The second injection could not simply be placebo because in that situation, patients would come to know that "the first one works and the second one never does." The placebo and an active agent must be assigned randomly. For the second block, the patient gets saline or a local anesthetic, and for the third block the patient receives the reciprocal agent. This protocol will screen out placebo responders, but it is onerous for both the patient and the physician. Furthermore, health care providers are not likely to be disposed to paying for placebo blocks, regardless of their scientific propriety.

The alternative is comparative local anesthetic blocks, in which on two separate occasions, different local anesthetic agents are used to block the target joint. A true-positive response is one in which the patient obtains complete relief on both occasions, but longer-lasting relief when the longer-acting agent is used.[17] This protocol is expedient because it requires only two blocks each with active agents. There are no ethical issues about performing sham procedures. Furthermore, in a recent study that compared comparative blocks to placebo, comparative blocks were found to be highly specific.[18]

Physicians and insurers may be reluctant to seemingly double the work and cost of diagnostic blocks by adding controls. However, they must recognize that double blocks are the only way of ensuring reliable results. Single blocks may be cheaper but they are scientifically unreliable and clinically useless. Moreover, they are a financial waste because for every positive responder there will be two false-positive responders who risk being committed to unjustified subsequent therapy. The waste lies not in the second block but in the consumption of unjustified therapy.

Prevalence

Using controlled blocks, the prevalence of lumbar zygapophyseal joint pain has been established. It differs in different populations. In a U.S. population, using comparative local anesthetic blocks, the prevalence of lumbar zygapophyseal joint pain was found to be 15% with a 95% confidence interval (CI) of 10% to 20%.[2] In an Australian population of rheumatology patients under single-blind, placebo-controlled conditions, the prevalence was found to be 40% (95% CI: 27% to 53%).[4]

The differences in prevalence might be ascribed to the fact that the Australian patients were older, suffered pain of spontaneous onset, and had been referred to rheumatologists; whereas the American patients were largely younger, injured individuals under the care of surgeons, and had been referred to specialized spine centers. Perhaps odious is the possibility that Australian and American patients respond differently to their pain and its investigation.

Of concern is the fact that generous diagnostic criteria were applied in these studies. Patients were considered positive if they reported greater than 50% relief of their pain. A cynical observer rightly might require 100% relief to be convinced. Very few of the American patients obtained complete relief; but it was not uncommon among the Australians, 32% of whom had complete or virtually complete abolition of their pain.

Lumbar zygapophyseal joint pain is not a rare entity. Using controlled blocks, its prevalence proves to be greater than some nihilistic estimates,[19] but less than previous, uncontrolled enthusiastic estimates.[20,21]

Reliability

Zygapophyseal joint blocks have face validity and construct validity. Face validity is ensured because these blocks are performed under fluoroscopic control. Radiography demonstrates that the needles go where they are supposed to go. Contrast medium can be used to prove that other structures are not infiltrated.

Construct validity relies on controls being exercised in each and every case. Blocks make sense and provide compelling diagnostic data only if placebo responses are reduced or eliminated. Repeat blocks with different local anesthetic

411

agents or challenge with normal saline are required to ensure that the patient has responded physiologically in accordance with the pharmacology of the agents used. The high false-positive rate of single diagnostic blocks and the low prevalence of zygapophyseal joint pain make control blocks mandatory in each and every case. Without controls, zygapophyseal joint blocks will be falsely positive in two out of every three positive cases.

Sacroiliac Joint Blocks

Opinions on the sacroiliac joint as a source of back pain have ranged from denial to almost religious enthusiasm, but the controversy has been fought with little evidence. Aficionados of manual medicine claim that a variety of signs are indicative of sacroiliac joint pain,[22,23] but none have ever been validated. There are no diagnostic features of sacroiliac pain on conventional clinical examination.[9] Imaging studies may be positive in inflammatory disorders of this joint,[24] but there are no diagnostic signs of so-called mechanical disorders.

Of importance is the distinction between sacroiliac joint blocks and infiltration of the interosseous sacroiliac ligament. The ligament is accessible to needles introduced from behind and may be infiltrated as an office procedure; the joint is not. The sacroiliac joint lies deeply anterior and cannot be entered from behind or without radiographic control.

Techniques for anesthetizing the sacroiliac joint have only recently been developed.[9,22,25] Stressing this joint in normal volunteers with intra-articular injections of contrast medium produces a characteristic pattern of pain centered over the sacral sulcus and radiating into the lower limb.[26] Blocking the joint with local anesthetic relieves similar patterns of pain in some patients.[9]

Population studies indicate that sacroiliac joint pain is not rare among patients with low back pain. Its prevalence is about 12%,[9] but this may be an underestimate because patients were preselected from a random sample on the basis of clinical signs.

The face validity of sacroiliac joint blocks is self evident because the blocks must be performed under fluoroscopic control (Fig. 3), and the injection of contrast medium to obtain an arthrogram confirms intra-articular placement of the needle (Fig. 4). With respect to construct validity, remarks pertain that are identical to those pertaining to zygapophyseal joint blocks. Controls are essential to exclude false-positive responses.

Strictly controlled studies of sacroiliac joint blocks have been performed but results have not yet been published. They stand to confirm that the prevalence of sacroiliac joint pain is about 15% among patients with pain primarily over the sacral sulcus.

Disk Stimulation

Diskography is perhaps the most vehemently contested controversy in the field of back pain.[27-30] However, no other technique has been devised to establish the diagnosis of diskogenic pain. Much of the controversy about diskography stems from confusion about the purpose of this diagnostic test. Although origi-

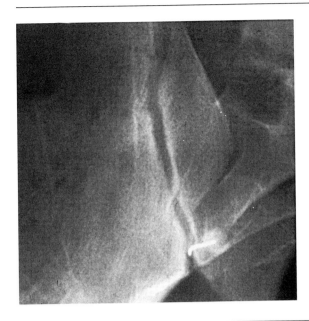

Fig. 3 *A close-up posterior view of a left sacroiliac joint with a needle introduced into its cavity at its lower pole. (Courtesy of Dr. Charles Aprill, New Orleans, LA.)*

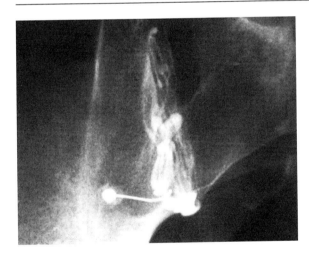

Fig. 4 *A close-up posterior view of a left sacroiliac joint following the injection of 1.0 ml of contrast medium into the joint. (Courtesy of Dr. Charles Aprill, New Orleans, LA.)*

nally introduced to pursue disk herniation, it is no longer used in this regard. Nor is the test used to evaluate disk morphology as a diagnostic criterion.

The purpose of diskography is to determine if a disk is the source of a patient's pain. For this purpose, the critical phase of diskography is disk stimulation. A needle introduced into the nucleus pulposus is used to distend the disk in an effort to stretch the anulus fibrosus and evoke the patient's accustomed pain (Fig. 5). The injection of contrast medium confirms accurate placement of the needle into the nucleus pulposus. The procedure is analogous to palpating for tenderness, save that a needle is used instead of a palpating finger.

413

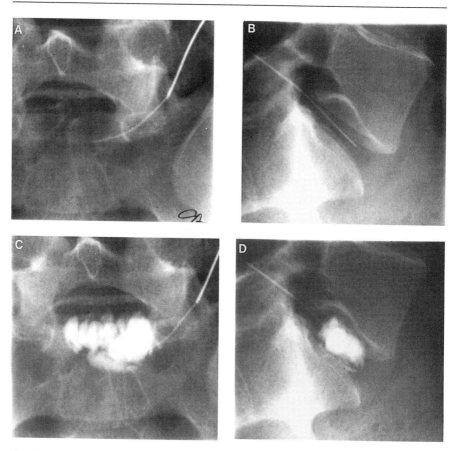

Fig. 5 *Stages in the conduct of disk stimulation. Posterior (**A**) and lateral (**C**) views of a needle passed into the nucleus pulposus of the L5-S1 disk.* **B** *and* **D**, *Similar views of the same disk after injection of contrast medium into the nucleus. (Courtesy of Dr. Nikolai Bogduk, Callaghan, NSW, Australia.)*

Disk stimulation is highly specific. Previous studies of diskography in normal volunteers[31] have been repudiated on methodological grounds.[32] Stringent, modern studies have shown that disk stimulation in normal volunteers does not evoke pain.[33] Painful disks occur only in patients with back pain.

Disk stimulation looks for a distinctive entity, which is not disk degeneration nor disk herniation. It is a condition in which the external appearance of the disk is essentially normal, and the disk looks normal on CT. The condition is one in which the pain stems from the disk itself, ostensibly from the anulus fibrosus. It is not pain due to compression of nerve roots.

The condition in question is internal disk disruption, which is characterized by the presence of radial fissures extending into the outer third of the anulus fibrosus but not breaching the perimeter of the disk. This pathology can be visualized by CT diskography.[34]

Early studies demonstrated a strong correlation between grade 3 fissures of the anulus fibrosus and reproduction of the patient's pain by disk stimulation.[35]

More recent studies have shown that this correlation is independent of disk de-generation[36] (Table 2). Radial tears are a distinctive, separate entity.
The etiology of painful radial tears remains conjectural,[30-37] but once present and symptomatic, they can be demonstrated by CT diskography. However, what is critical is the rigor and discipline required to perform and interpret disk stimulation correctly.

Controls

Simply stimulating a disk to reproduce a patient's pain is an inadequate di-agnostic test, for it does not show that stimulating another disk (or any struc-ture) in the patient's back does not have the same effect. For this reason, con-trols are required in each and every case.

Guidelines for the conduct and interpretation of disk stimulation have been laid down by the IASP[1] and by the International Spinal Injection Society.[38,39] They stipulate that, for a diagnosis of diskogenic pain to be made, not only must stimulation of a given disk reproduce the patient's accustomed pain, but also stimulation of adjacent disks must not reproduce their pain. These criteria guard against nonspecific and false-positive responses. It also means that single-level disk stimulation is unreliable and that triple-level positive disk stimulation can-not be interpreted as positive.[29,30]

Prevalence

The diagnostic criteria for internal disk disruption laid down by the IASP[1] are that not only must disk stimulation be positive, but the disk must also exhibit a grade 3 fissure on CT diskography. A formal study, adhering to these criteria, explored the prevalence of internal disk disruption in a population of patients with chronic low back pain.[7]

Of 92 consecutive patients who completed investigations, 39% satisfied the diagnostic criteria for internal disk disruption.[7] Of all conditions that have been sought among patients with chronic low back pain of unknown origin, under scientific conditions, internal disk disruption has the highest prevalence. It is three times more common than sacroiliac joint pain, and nearly three times more common than zygapophyseal joint pain. Furthermore, it has been shown to be an independent disorder.

When disk stimulation, zygapophyseal joint blocks, and sacroiliac joint blocks are all performed on the same patients, few patients emerge with multiple dis-orders. Patients may be positive to one or another investigation, but typically

Table 2 Correlation between annular disruption and reproduction of pain by disk stimulation[36]

Pain Reproduction	Annular Disruption			
	Grade 3	Grade 2	Grade 1	Grade 0
Exact	43	29	6	4
Similar	32	36	21	8
Dissimilar	9	11	6	2
None	16	24	67	86

$\chi^2 = 148$; $p < 0.001$

are negative to the others. A tiny minority of patients are positive to both disk stimulation and to zygapophyseal joint blocks.[40] Otherwise, internal disk disruption and zygapophyseal joint pain occur as separate entities.

Reliability

The face validity of disk stimulation is obvious. Radiography is used to prove that the needle has entered the nucleus pulposus. The injection of contrast medium will indicate that the injection is contained within the disk.

The construct validity of disk stimulation depends critically on obtaining control observations. An adjacent disk must be stimulated and found not to reproduce the patient's pain. Unless this is done, the procedure is not valid, for a nonspecific effect will not have been excluded.

Critical as well is the fidelity with which the patient's pain is reproduced. The accustomed pain should be exactly reproduced. "Any pain" does not constitute a positive response. It is in this respect that disk stimulation is open to abuse. The technique is reliable but its execution and interpretation are not necessarily so. Only adherence to the strict guidelines guards against false-positive interpretations. An emerging development in this regard is disk-manometry, in which injection pressures are calibrated and monitored.[41] Once refined, manometry may serve to standardize the stress applied to the disk and reduce false-positive interpretations of responses.

Nerve Root Blocks

Nerve root blocks were devised as a means of determining which segmental nerve mediates a patient's pain. They can be applied in cases of radicular pain when imaging studies are equivocal, or when zygapophyseal joint blocks and disk stimulation fail to pinpoint the source of pain.

Root blocks are performed under fluoroscopic control. Along a posterolateral approach, a needle is passed into the intervertebral foramen so that its tip lies at the bottom of the pedicle.[42] From this point, local anesthetic can be injected to infiltrate the spinal nerve, its roots, and their dural sleeve (Fig. 6). A positive response occurs when the patient's pain is totally abolished.

Utility

The primary utility of needle procedures is that they provide information; they enable the source of the patient's pain to be specified. This alone can be of benefit for it allays patient anxiety about being labeled a malingerer or being told that the pain is imaginary. It is also practical in that it protects patients from undergoing therapy inappropriate to the source of pain. If nothing else, needle procedures can serve to prevent patients being assigned to therapies that, in principle, are destined to fail.

Ideally, however, needle procedures should have therapeutic utility. A diagnosis having been established, therapy should target the offending structure. However, few options are available in this regard.

Intra-articular steroids were heralded as a treatment for zygapophyseal joint pain,[11] but a controlled trial has shown that they are no more effective than nor-

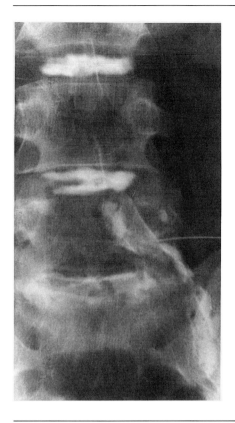

Fig. 6 *Posterior radiograph of a lumbar spine following the injection of contrast medium to outline the right L5 nerve-root sleeve, prior to blocking the root with local anesthetic. (Courtesy of Dr. Charles Aprill, New Orleans, LA.)*

mal saline.[43] The only other therapeutic option for zygapophyseal joint pain is percutaneous radiofrequency neurotomy. This procedure has had a checkered history. Introduced as "facet denervation," the original procedure was shown to be based on inaccurate surgical anatomy.[11] Subsequent revisions were shown to be technically inadequate.[44] Nevertheless, the procedure is sound in principle.

Radiofrequency neurotomy is designed to coagulate the medial branches of the lumbar dorsal rami and thereby interrupt nociception from a painful zyga- pophyseal joint. The procedure is not trivial. Care must be taken to ensure ac- curate placement of the electrodes and to achieve adequate coagulation of the target nerves.[44]

North and associates[45] have recently shown a strong correlation between re- sponse to diagnostic blocks and success with radiofrequency neurotomy. Pa- tients who respond to blocks are likely to benefit from neurotomy. Few patients who are not positive to blocks benefit from the procedure. This argues against a placebo effect. However, no studies have yet formally compared radiofre- quency neurotomy with strict placebo.

With respect to sacroiliac joint pain, there is no valid therapeutic option. No injection procedures have been claimed, let alone proven, to be of benefit for sacroiliac joint pain. Theoretically, surgery, perhaps in the form of anterior plat- ing of the joint, might be an option; this has not been formally explored in pa- tients with proven sacroiliac joint pain.

With respect to disk stimulation, there are two putative benefits, one positive and one negative. The positive use is that treatment can be directed at the offending disk. At present, surgery is the only available option, in the form of disk excision and arthrodesis. However, reports of the efficacy of this treatment are mixed. Some claim good results with anterior interbody fusion of segments that are abnormal on MRI and positive to disk stimulation,[46,47] but others report dismal results.[48] This is clearly an area that requires clarification.

The negative use of disk stimulation lies in its potential to prevent unnecessary surgery. Spinal fusions are sometimes, if not often, undertaken on the basis of ''clinical features'' and ''imaging studies,'' neither of which has any diagnostic or prognostic validity. Multilevel positive disk stimulation should warn a surgeon against operating. If everything in the patient hurts, what guarantee can the surgeon offer that the operation will relieve the patient's pain?

Nerve root blocks are not a diagnostic tool in the conventional sense, for they do not pinpoint sources of pain. Rather, they are a discriminating test to determine which nerve is mediating the patient's pain. In cases of radicular pain they are used to assist surgeons in deciding which segmental level, if any, should be surgically explored. There is no point decompressing a level that is not related to the patient's symptoms.

Root blocks can have prognostic value. Some investigators have explored what is known as ''the steroid response.'' At the time of investigation, an aliquot of corticosteroid is injected along with the local anesthetic, and the patient's response is monitored. If the patient obtains sustained relief of pain lasting 2 weeks or more, the relief is ascribed to the steroid, for the effect of the local anesthetic should have worn off within a matter of hours. This ''steroid effect'' correlates with the outcome of surgery, but only in a negative predictive sense. Patients who have had radicular pain longer than 1 year in duration who fail to obtain a steroid response are most unlikely to respond to surgery.[49]

Discussion

The two cardinal advantages of needle procedures are that they can target specific structures and that they can be controlled. No other diagnostic technique offers the same advantages in the assessment of back pain.

Dissidents abound, but it is not clear what the grounds for dissent are. They cannot be intellectual, because the validity of the procedures has been established, and the prevalence of the entities diagnosed is too great to be ignored (Table 3). The orthopaedist cannot, in all honesty, refuse to look for conditions that constitute 15%, 13%, and 39% (a total of 67%) of the causes of chronic low back pain, conditions that cannot otherwise be identified.

Table 3 The prevalence of various sources of low back pain as determined using needle procedures under controlled conditions

Diagnostic Entity	Prevalence	95% Confidence Limits
Zygapophyseal joint pain	15%	10% to 20%
Sacroiliac joint pain	13%	6% to 20%
Internal disk disruption	39%	29% to 49%

The resistance may be practical. Individuals who cannot perform diagnostic blocks or disk stimulation, or who do not have access to these procedures, will be unwilling or unable to implement them. However, under these circumstances, it is the patient who is denied the benefit.

Utility is the one arena in which proponents of needle procedures still lack evidence. It has not been shown that finding a painful disk leads to better outcome. It has not been shown that finding multiple disks prevents needless surgery. There is tentative evidence that radiofrequency neurotomy is worthwhile for proven zygapophyseal joint pain, but the evidence is insufficiently compelling to justify an overhaul of the management of back pain. The treatment of sacroiliac joint pain is still on the drawing board.

References

1. Merskey H, Bogduk N (eds): *Classification of Chronic Pain: Descriptions of Chronic Pain Syndromes and Definition of Pain Terms*, ed 2. Seattle, WA, IASP Press, 1994, p 178.
2. Schwarzer AC, Aprill CN, Derby R, et al: Clinical features of patients with pain stemming from the lumbar zygapophysial joints: Is the lumbar facet syndrome a clinical entity? *Spine* 1994;19:1132–1137.
3. Schwarzer AC, Derby R, Aprill CN, et al: Pain from the lumbar zygapophysial joints: A test of two models. *J Spinal Disord* 1994;7:331–336.
4. Schwarzer AC, Wang SC, Bogduk N, et al: Prevalence and clinical features of lumbar zygapophysial joint pain: A study in an Australian population with chronic low back pain. *Ann Rheum Disord* 1995;54:100–106.
5. Revel ME, Listrat VM, Chevalier XJ, et al: Facet joint block for low back pain: Identifying predictors of a good response. *Arch Phys Med Rehabil* 1992;73:824–828.
6. Schwarzer AC, Wang SC, O'Driscoll D, et al: The ability of computed tomography to identify a painful zygapophysial joint in patients with chronic low back pain. *Spine* 1995;20:907–912.
7. Schwarzer AC, Aprill CN, Derby R, et al: The prevalence and clinical features of internal disc disruption in patients with chronic low back pain. *Spine* 1995;20:1878–1883.
8. Aprill C, Bogduk N: High-intensity zone: A diagnostic sign of painful lumbar disc on magnetic resonance imaging. *Br J Radiol* 1992;65:361–369.
9. Schwarzer AC, Aprill CN, Bogduk N: The sacroiliac joint in chronic low back pain. *Spine* 1995;20:31–37.
10. Schwarzer AC, Derby R, Aprill CN, et al: The value of the provocation response in lumbar zygapophyseal joint injections. *Clin J Pain* 1994;10:309–313.
11. Bogduk N, Aprill C, Derby R: Diagnostic blocks of synovial joints, in White AH (ed): *Spine Care: Diagnosis and Conservative Treatment*. St. Louis, MO, CV Mosby, 1995, pp 298–321.
12. Dory MA: Arthrography of the lumbar facet joints. *Radiology* 1981;140:23–27.
13. Moran R, O'Connell D, Walsh MG: The diagnostic value of facet joint injections. *Spine* 1988;13:1407–1410.
14. Goldstone JC, Pennant JH: Spinal anaesthesia following facet joint injection: A report of two cases. *Anaesthesia* 1987;42:754–756.
15. Thomson SJ, Lomax DM, Collett BJ: Chemical meningism after lumbar facet joint block with local anaesthetic and steroids. *Anaesthesia* 1991;46:563–564.
16. Schwarzer AC, Aprill CN, Derby R, et al: The false-positive rate of uncontrolled diagnostic blocks of the lumbar zygapophysial joints. *Pain* 1994;58:195–200.
17. Barnsley L, Lord S, Bogduk N: Comparative local anaesthetic blocks in the diagnosis of cervical zygapophysial joint pain. *Pain* 1993;55:99–106.

18. Lord SM, Barnsley L, Bogduk N: The utility of comparative local anesthetic blocks versus placebo-controlled blocks for the diagnosis of cervical zygapophysial joint pain. *Clin J Pain* 1995;11:208–213.

19. Jackson RP: The facet syndrome: Myth or reality? *Clin Orthop* 1992;279:110–121.

20. Lewinnek GE, Warfield CA: Facet joint degeneration as a cause of low back pain. *Clin Orthop* 1986;213:216–222.

21. Destouet JM, Gilula LA, Murphy WA, et al: Lumbar facet joint injection: Indication, technique, clinical correlation, and preliminary results. *Radiology* 1982;145:321–325.

22. Fortin JD: Sacroiliac joint dysfunction: Biomechanics, diagnosis, and rehabilitation, in Vleeming A, Mooney V, Snijders C, et al (eds): *First Interdisciplinary World Conference on Low Back Pain and its Relation to the Sacroiliac Joint.* San Diego, CA, University of California, 1992, pp 383–399.

23. Hesch J, Aisenbrey JA, Guarino J: Manual therapy evaluation of the pelvic joints using palpatory and articular spring tests, in Vleeming A, Mooney V, Snijders C, et al (eds): *First Interdisciplinary World Conference on Low Back Pain and its Relation to the Sacroiliac Joint.* San Diego, CA, University of California, 1992, pp 435–459.

24. Bellamy N, Park W, Rooney PJ: What do we know about the sacroiliac joint? *Semin Arthritis Rheum* 1983;12:282–313.

25. Aprill CN: The role of anatomically specific injections into the sacroiliac joint, in Vleeming A, Mooney V, Snijders C, et al (eds): *First Interdisciplinary World Conference on Low Back Pain and its Relation to the Sacroiliac Joint.* San Diego, CA, University of California, 1992, pp 373–380.

26. Fortin JD, Dwyer AP, West S, et al: Sacroiliac joint: Pain referral maps upon applying a new injection/arthrography technique. Part I: Asymptomatic volunteers. *Spine* 1994;19:1475–1482.

27. Nachemson A: Lumbar discography: Where are we today? *Spine* 1989;14:555–557.

28. Executive Committee of the North American Spine Society: Position statement on discography. *Spine* 1988;13:1343.

29. Bogduk N: Diskography. *Am Pain Soc J* 1994;3:149–154.

30. Bogduk N, Aprill C, Derby R: Discography, in White AH (ed): *Spine Care: Diagnosis and Conservative Treatment.* St. Louis, MO, CV Mosby, 1995, pp 219–238.

31. Holt EP Jr: The question of lumbar discography. *J Bone Joint Surg* 1968;50A:720–726.

32. Simmons JW, Aprill CN, Dwyer AP, et al: A reassessment of Holt's data on "the question of lumbar discography." *Clin Orthop* 1988;237:120–124.

33. Walsh TR, Weinstein JN, Spratt KF, et al: Lumbar discography in normal subjects: A controlled, prospective study. *J Bone Joint Surg* 1990;72A:1081–1088.

34. Sachs BL, Vanharanta H, Spivey MA, et al: Dallas discogram description: A new classification of CT/discography in low-back disorders. *Spine* 1987;12:287–294.

35. Vanharanta H, Sachs BL, Spivey MA, et al: The relationship of pain provocation to lumbar disc deterioration as seen by CT/discography. *Spine* 1987;12:295–298.

36. Moneta GB, Videman T, Kaivanto K, et al: Reported pain during lumbar discography as a function of anular ruptures and disc degeneration: A re-analysis of 833 discograms. *Spine* 1994;17:1968–1974.

37. Bogduk N: The lumbar disc and low back pain. *Neurosurg Clin N Am* 1991;2:791–806.

38. Bogduk B: Proposed discography standards, in *ISIS Newsletter.* Daly City, California, International Spinal Injection Society, 1994, vol 2, pp 10–13.

39. Derby R: A second proposal for discography standards, in *ISIS Newsletter.* Daly City, California, International Spinal Injection Society, 1994, vol 2, pp 108–122.

40. Schwarzer AC, Aprill CN, Derby R, et al: The relative contributions of the disc and zygapophyseal joint in chronic low back pain. *Spine* 1994;19:801–806.

41. Derby R: Lumbar discometry, in *ISIS Newsletter.* Daly City, California, International Spinal Injection Society, 1993, vol 2.

42. Bogduk N, Aprill C, Derby R: Selective nerve root blocks, in Wilson DJ (ed): *Interventional Radiology of the Musculoskeletal System.* London, England, Edward Arnold, 1995, pp 121–132.
43. Carette S, Marcoux S, Truchon R, et al: A controlled trial of corticosteroid injections into facet joints for chronic low back pain. *N Engl J Med* 1991;325:1002–1007.
44. Bogduk N, Macintosh J, Marsland A: Technical limitations to the efficacy of radiofrequency neurotomy for spinal pain. *Neurosurgery* 1987;20:529–535.
45. North RB, Han M, Zahurak M, et al: Radiofrequency lumbar facet denervation: Analysis of prognostic factors. *Pain* 1994;57:77–83.
46. Newman MH, Grirstead GL: Anterior lumbar interbody fusion for internal disc disruption. *Spine* 1992;17:831–833.
47. Gill K, Blumenthal SL: Functional results after anterior lumbar fusion at L5-S1 in patients with normal and abnormal MRI scans. *Spine* 1992;17:940–942.
48. Knox BD, Chapman TM: Anterior lumbar interbody fusion for discogram concordant pain. *J Spinal Disord* 1993;6:242–244.
49. Derby R, Kine G, Saal JA, et al: Response to steroid and duration of radicular pain as predictors of surgical outcome. *Spine* 1992;17(suppl 6):S176–S183.

Chapter 26

Physical Agents and Exercise in Low Back Pain

Jan K. Richardson, PT, PhD, OCS
Stephen L. Gordon, PhD

Low back pain is a common medical problem that reportedly occurs in 60% to 80% of the population;[1] individuals in their fourth decade of life are at the greatest risk.[2] Waddell[3] defines low back pain as being a benign, self-limiting condition that is so commonly experienced that it could almost be interpreted as a normal occurrence in life. Most patients with acute low back pain categorized as sciatica or nonspecific back pain will recover within 30 days;[4] however, early intervention can reduce time to recovery and decrease the potential for an acute episode to become chronic (Table 1). Early intervention is usually comprehensive, and includes exercises to enhance mobility and strength, patient education, and pain management, and often includes a component of physical agents (also known as physical modalities). However, the precise role of these interventions needs further study. Physical agents can be broadly categorized into thermal, electrical, and mechanical techniques. The overall goal of physical therapy intervention is to optimize functional outcome and performance. Exercise programs often are included in a complete rehabilitation plan for acute and chronic low back pain. Paradigms of intervention should be selected based on examination to enhance each patient's optimal performance and functional outcome.

Table 1 Prevalence of back pain and sciatica in the adult population of the United States

Group	Percentage
Any LBP	60-80
Ever had LBP persisting 2 weeks	14
Point prevalence of LBP for 2 weeks	7
LBP with sciatica (2 weeks' duration)	1.6
Undergo lumbar spine surgery	1-2

LBP = low back pain
(Adapted with permission from Deyo RA, Loeser JD, Bigos SJ: Herniated lumbar intervertebral disk. *Ann Intern Med* 1990;112:598–603.)

This chapter will address the management of patients by means of surgical and nonsurgical care, identify major physical agents and exercise study results, and forecast the new horizons for the physical therapist's intervention in the management of patients with low back pain. Study designs in future trials must be improved by separating physical methods and mobility exercises rather than clustering treatment nonspecifically with generalized patient groups. Physical agents will be discussed first, followed by exercise.

Physical Agents in Low Back Pain

Physical agents have been used to promote tissue healing and reduce pain. Whether thermal, electrical, or mechanical, these physical methods are most commonly used by physical therapists in conjunction with procedures such as exercise, manipulation, and mobilization techniques.

To date, researchers have grouped physical agents in clinical trials. It has been difficult to demonstrate a significant improvement with one type of therapeutic intervention compared to another or compared to a control group when the therapeutic interventions used have included a clustering of physical agents or of physical agents with exercises.

Acute low back pain has been defined in the Agency for Health Care Policy and Research (AHCPR) Clinical Practice Guidelines as involving symptoms lasting for less than 3 months.[4] Therefore, the transitional phase between acute and chronic can be termed subacute. The operational definitions of these terms as used in this discussion will be as follows: acute, 7 days or less; subacute, more than 7 days but not longer than 7 weeks; and chronic, pain lasting 7 weeks or longer. It is important to define pain duration and to identify the neurophysiologic and psychosocial changes that occur with each phase, in order to treat each phase accordingly.

Establishing a differential diagnosis in patients with low back pain is sometimes difficult. However, Nachemson[5] has stated that a pathoanatomic cause of symptoms was identified in only 15% of all patients with low back pain of more than 3 months' duration. The etiology of low back pain is unclear partly because of a lack of good models to study its cause and effect relationships.

DeRosa and Porterfield[6] discussed the history of the development of treatment strategies based on the pathophysiologic hypotheses related to tissue dysfunction and differential diagnosis. They reviewed treatment interventions based on the disk diagnosis model of Mixter and Barr, and Cyriax, the joint model of Maitland, and the myofascial diagnosis syndromes of Travell. They argue that these models, which have prescribed methods of treatment, are based on pathology of specified tissue, and that identifying with even minimal certainty the exact tissues involved in most instances of low back pain is virtually impossible. Therefore, they conclude that in the case of activity-related spinal disorders, attention should be focused not on the identification of faulty tissue, but on determining the mechanical stress or combination of stresses that provoke familiar symptoms.

A scientific approach to the assessment and management of activity-related spinal disorders was established by the Quebec Task Force on Spinal Disorders.[7] DeRosa and Porterfield[6] modified the Quebec Task Force classification system from 11 categories to only seven, with the compelling argument that a universally accepted classification scheme for activity-related low back pain would allow for improved communications regarding appropriateness and efficacy of physical therapy and would permit scientific investigation of treatment methods. Table 2 outlines the modified physical therapy diagnosis classification by DeRosa and Porterfield.[6] It should be noted that these categories are not mutually exclusive. Although these classifications are functionally related, further refinement and study are needed because they are not universally accepted or used and to date have not been proved valid or reliable.

Thermal Agents

Of the three categories of physical agents, thermal agents are the best known, dating back to the historic use of heat and cold for healing purposes. The effective use and generalized acceptance of heat and cold in the reduction of pain, increase in circulation, and decrease in inflammation has already been established[8] and will not be discussed here. However, this broad acceptance in practice may account for the lack of current scientific trials designed to assess the isolated effects of ice or heat, utilizing hydrocollator packs, on low back pain. In several current studies, thermal agents were used either in combination with other thermal agents or combined with electrical and mechanical agents and exercise, massage, or mobilization.[9-12]

Koes and associates[9] studied 256 patients from the Netherlands who had nonspecific back and neck complaints of at least 6 weeks' duration. Subjects who had not received manual therapy or physiotherapy within the last 2 years were randomized into four groups: those receiving physiotherapy (including physical agents of heat, electrotherapy, ultrasound, shortwave diathermy, and/or exercise and massage); those receiving manual therapy, consisting of manipulation and mobilization of the spine (as per directives of the Dutch Society for Manual Therapy); those receiving continued physician-directed treatment (with analgesics and nonsteroidal anti-inflammatory drugs, plus advice regarding posture, exercises, sports, and bed rest); and those receiving placebo treatment (a physical examination, with subsequent sessions of detuned shortwave diathermy for 10 minutes and detuned ultrasound for 10 minutes). All practitioners were permitted to choose their usual therapeutic intervention except the physiotherapists who were restricted from using manipulative techniques. Each group was analyzed

Table 2 Modified physical therapy diagnosis classification*

Category	Definition
1	Back pain without radiation
2	Back pain with referral to extremity, proximally
3	Back pain with referral to extremity, distally
4	Extremity pain greater than back pain
5	Back pain with radiation and neurologic signs
6	Postsurgical status (< 6 months or > 6 months)
7	Chronic pain syndrome

*Based on Quebec Task Force on Spinal Disorders classification system
(Reproduced with permission from DeRosa CP, Porterfield JA: A physical therapy model for the treatment of low back pain. *Phys Ther* 1992;72:261–269.)

to determine the severity of the main complaint, the global perceived effect, and physical function.

Of the 256 patients, 65 received manual therapy, and 66, physical therapy. Compared to the other groups, the patients receiving manual therapy showed a faster and larger improvement in physical function. However, Koes and associates[10] concluded that the differences in effectiveness between physiotherapy and manual therapy could not be shown. In a 1-year follow-up study of the same 256 patients with nonspecific back and neck complaints, Koes and associates[11] determined that the manual therapy group showed consistently better results for physical functioning than the physiotherapy group at all follow-up measurements except for global perceived effect (patients' assessment of overall benefit). Criticism has been raised as to the different conclusions in each of the articles by Koes and associates, in light of the fact that they all report on the same set of data.[13] This issue, in addition to the restrictions imposed upon the physical therapists from employing manipulation or manual techniques which might have otherwise been employed for this diagnostic group, renders the comparative results of minimal benefit.

Several recent studies have considered the effectiveness of combined components of physical therapy intervention. Hansen and associates[12] compared intensive back muscle exercises to conventional physiotherapy, including heat and ice, massage and exercise, and a control group. Among 150 patients, conventional physical therapy was the best treatment for the males, and intensive back exercises, which include typical extension exercises used by physical therapists, appeared to be most effective for the females. Also of interest was the conclusion that patients with physically demanding occupations tended to respond better to conventional physical therapy, whereas patients with less physically strenuous job functions responded most effectively to intensive back exercises. This study showed that patients with chronic or subchronic low back pain were successfully treated with both physical therapy and intensive dynamic back exercises, but not with the placebo-control treatment. In one study,[14] the pain-relieving effects of moist heat and shortwave diathermy on tender joints were objectively measured with a pressure algometer. Both treatments were effective in relieving pain; shortwave diathermy was more effective at decreasing the sensitivity of both moderate and sensitive trigger points. In another study,[15] ten patients showed an immediate but short-term analgesic effect in over a 24-hour period with the combined use of high voltage galvanic stimulation and ultrasound in the treatment of low back pain.

There are several well-documented thermal effects of ultrasound, such as enhancement of wound healing, increased tendon extensibility, increased blood flow, increased range of motion, and reduction of scar tissue.[16,17] Draper and associates[18] studied 16 subjects divided into two groups: ultrasound treatment on precooled tissue, or ultrasound with no preceding treatment. Both treatment groups received 10 minutes of continuous ultrasound delivered topically at 1.5 watts/cm^2. Tissue temperature was measured with a 23-gauge hypodermic needle microprobe inserted 5 cm deep into the subjects' anesthetized triceps sural muscles. A significant difference between the two treatment methods was measured, with ultrasound alone increasing tissue temperature an average of 4.0 ± 0.83°C, whereas ultrasound preceded by ice increased tissue temperature by only 1.8 ± 1.0°C above pretreatment baseline levels. These trials, which were not performed on low back patients, should be reproduced in the spine to demonstrate that similar temperature changes occur in deep low back muscles and can have similar benefits to patients with low back pain.

Electrical Agents

The use of electrical physical agents, such as transcutaneous electrical nerve stimulation (TENS) and electrical muscle stimulation (EMS), for patients with low back pain has been the topic of several studies.

Pope and associates[19] studied 164 patients who were attending the health center of a chiropractic college, with additional subjects recruited by advertisement. Seventy patients were randomly assigned to a manipulation group. There were three comparison groups: transcutaneous muscle stimulation (TMS) (28 patients), soft-tissue massage (37 patients), and corset (29 patients). Patients in the manipulation group were seen three or more times weekly by a chiropractor, and the massage group was seen by a massage therapist for 15 minutes, three times weekly. Patients in the TMS group were instructed in the use and application of the unit with self-control of amplitude based on patient tolerance. Compliance was defined as 7 hours' use per day on average as measured by an internal compliance meter. Each patient in the TMS group was scheduled to return once a week for 3 weeks. A trained technician checked if the patient used the unit correctly and printed out the compliance report. Patients in the corset group were measured and fitted for a soft Freeman lumbosacral corset. Patients were instructed to wear the corset during waking hours but could remove the corset for up to 10 minutes, three times daily. Patients were scheduled to be seen once a week during the 3 weeks, at which time a technician checked for proper application and recorded compliance as reported by the subject's diary. During the 3 weeks, the dropout rate was highest in the corset, TMS, and massage groups and lowest in the manipulation group.

At the conclusion of the study, there were no significant differences among treatment methods in any of the objective ratings of spinal function and pain scores. However, the measure of patient confidence in their treatment was highest in the group that received manipulation. This could be attributed to the fact that the patients in the manipulation group were treated by doctors of chiropractic versus a trained technician and additionally could be seen more than three times weekly, resulting in the potential for a ''halo effect,'' compared to the other three groups. Other design flaws included differences in length of sessions; differences in frequency of sessions per week; and administration of massage and TMS by technicians rather than by a chiropractor or another health professional. These factors may have produced differences within the groups, eliminated the issue of patient confidence, and controlled for intergroup reliability. One also needs to question the fact that subjects were attending the clinic for treatment from the onset, which would make them more confident in manipulation as a viable treatment.

In another study[20] with a similar design, it was concluded that manipulation had a greater short-term benefit compared to stroking massage and TMS in patients with subacute low back pain, and there was a significant difference between the manipulation and corset groups. This study had several limitations, including the dropout rate and the use of stroking massage in contrast to deep massage. Hot packs were also used for 10 minutes prior to both the manipulation and massage treatments. However, a chiropractor assisted in the management of both the corset and TMS groups.

A case study by Starring[21] described the use of electrical stimulation in conjunction with exercise for the muscles of the lumbar spinal region to a patient with pain and hypermobility at L5-S1. The patient's treatment consisted of electrical stimulation to the paraspinal muscles and exercise with the use of moist heat, ice, and ultrasound for pain relief. The patient who had been seen by a chiropractor for approximately 9 weeks, with failed results, was then treated by a physical therapist. After eight sessions during a 2-week period, the patient had full range of trunk motion in all planes, no low back or radicular pain on returning to erect posture from forward bend, and improved stability of L5-S1 with segmental mobility testing. At the conclusion of treatment, the patient returned to full function and even began a running program. This case study needs to be substantiated in a well-designed study with larger numbers of patients.

McQuain and associates[22] studied 40 healthy, sedentary, premenopausal women in a single-blind controlled study to determine the effects of capacitively coupled electrical stimulation on the strength of the lumbar paraspinal muscles and bone mineral in the lumbar spine. The study was based on the hypothesis that isometric back extensor strength could be augmented by electrical stimulation. Research studies[23] have shown that muscle strength and bone mass are correlated and that bone mass and muscle mass can be increased with exercise or diminished with inactivity. Therefore, bone mineral was measured with an absorptiometer to evaluate whether electrical stimulation had a measurable effect on bone mass. It was concluded that isometric back extensor strength could be significantly increased with low frequency electrical stimulation and maintained with continued stimulation for up to a year, but that there was no effect on bone density in the lumbar spine. It still remains to be seen whether this strength change in any way serves to prevent low back pain or is potentially effective for strengthening in a patient with acute or subacute back pain.

Several clinical studies are identified in the AHCPR guidelines[4] that address the use of TENS in patients with low back pain. Few of the investigations deal with acute low back pain. In general, there does not appear to be a significant difference between active and placebo treatment. In a more recent study, Marchand and associates[24] studied 42 subjects experiencing chronic low back pain for more than 6 months. Subjects were randomly assigned to three groups: those receiving TENS twice weekly for 10 weeks; placebo-TENS, using a standard unit that was short circuited so that current did not reach the electrode; and a control, whose subjects were informed they would receive treatment in 6 months. Visual analog scale (VAS) pain ratings were taken before and after each treatment session to measure the short-term effect of TENS, and additionally, long-term effects were measured by patient rating at home every 2 hours for a 3-day period before, and 1 week, 3 months, and 6 months after treatment sessions. When comparing the subject pain evaluations made immediately before and after the treatment sessions, intensity and unpleasantness of chronic low back pain were decreased in both the TENS and placebo-TENS group. TENS was evaluated as significantly more efficient than placebo-TENS in reducing pain intensity, but not pain unpleasantness. In addition, TENS produced a significant additive effect over repeated treatment sessions for intensity and relative unpleasantness, in contrast to placebo-TENS.

At this time, the benefits of TENS are not clearly documented; however, risks to the patient are low and the costs are considered low to moderate. When treating patients with chronic low back pain, TENS may be considered as a possible short-term analgesic intervention in a comprehensive approach to pain management rather than as an isolated or sole long-term treatment technique; however, further research is required.

Mechanical Agents

Mechanical physical agents produce a compression or distraction force when applied to a patient. These agents can include intermittent compression devices, auto traction or passive mechanical traction, and massage.

The AHCPR Guidelines[4] describe the lack of well-designed clinical studies of traction applied to low back pain. Most of the traction is applied by mechanical or manual means (ie, a harness pulling on the pelvis). In short, traction has not proved to be significantly beneficial to warrant a general recommendation.

Tesio and Merlo[25] studied 44 patients with unremitting low back pain with or without radiation, in whom one or more conservative approaches had failed. Pain duration was 1 month or longer. The design randomly allocated the patients to either autotraction (AT) or passive traction (PT). The AT device supports the body under the axilla with gravity providing the spinal distraction. The study design allowed for a crossover (Fig. 1) if the first physical agent failed. Patients' responses were assessed following the third session for AT and the fifth session for PT, and patient responders were identified. "Responders" were those subjects who reported full recovery or improvement. Responders to AT were treated with three more sessions and responders to PT were treated with five more sessions. Nonresponders were crossed over to the other physical agent following a 4- to 5-day delay to lessen carryover effects. Both groups were treated by the same physical therapist. After the initial treatments, 17 of 22 pa-

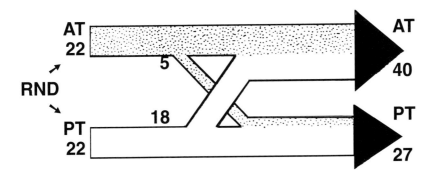

Fig. 1 *The trial design. Forty-four patients were randomly (RND) allocated to autotraction (AT, 22 subjects) or to conventional passive traction (PT, 22 subjects). Nonresponders to either treatment (5 AT patients, 18 PT patients) were "crossed-over" to the other treatment. (Reproduced with permission from Tesio L, Merlo A: Autotraction versus passive traction: An open controlled study in lumbar disc herniation.* Arch Phys Med Rehabil *1993;74:871.)*

tients were responders to AT with the remaining five crossing over to PT, in comparison to 18 of 22 PT crossing over to AT. A limitation of the study was the possible placebo effect that was associated with the AT because of the complexity of equipment, thereby possibly giving the perception that AT was more modern.

However, the response to AT did not appear to be solely a placebo effect, with the rate of response to AT (75%) being greater than three times that of PT (22%). Three months following treatment, 63% of AT responders still reported relief from pain. Although the scientific basis and mechanism of AT is not currently explained, it appears that there is sufficient evidence to encourage further studies of AT so that, in the future, it may be recommended to a broader range of patients with low back pain.

In a recent review, Reitman and Esses[26] define massage as systematic maneuvers of body tissue for which the intent is to improve circulation, encourage relaxation, decrease pain through interaction with the nervous system, promote nutritive exchange, and increase soft-tissue mobility. Massage appears to effect short-term relief in many conditions including low back pain; however, it may not necessarily produce long-term pain management. Even though there have been no prospective, controlled trials that demonstrate the efficacy of massage, the rationale for its use is sound. Physical therapists have long used hand massages, versus those with mechanical appliances, as a component of therapeutic intervention, to facilitate exercise, mobility, and functional movement rather than as an isolated treatment physical agent. Again, further research is required to document the value of specific inteventions for specific classifications of low back pain.

Exercise and Low Back Pain

Exercise is often a recommended component of nonsurgical programs to relieve existing low back pain and prevent its recurrence, and its use may be considered cost-effective. Results of several studies[1,27,28] and the AHCPR guidelines[4] suggest that exercise may have a positive effect on chronic low back pain in particular. The review recommendations in this chapter are based on a broad weighting of the overall evidence rather than on the critical scientific assessment of statistical or design/implementation flaws in specific studies.

There appear to be many technical flaws within the current literature, eg, vague descriptions of exercise programs, nonuniform and unblinded outcome measures, clinical trial design shortcomings, and variable results even within a single study. Koes and associates[29] described in great detail some of the methodologic flaws in existing exercise studies and studies with other therapeutic interventions.

This section is intended as an overview assessment of major exercise study results, but is not an in-depth critique of the investigative design, methodology, and implementation of each investigation. Clearly, improved study designs in future trials will improve credibility of and help generalize exercise recommendations for specific patient groups. The review of studies on exercise are separated into three classifications: acute low back pain, chronic low back pain, and prevention of low back pain.

Acute Low Back Pain

Acute low back pain, defined as pain lasting for 7 weeks or less,[7] may be further categorized into subacute phases. Episodes of acute low back pain may resolve within 1 to 2 months[1] using a variety of treatments, or, in some cases, without treatment. Therefore, it may be difficult to demonstrate a significant improvement of one form of intervention, compared to a different intervention or a control group, with no intervention.

Lindstrom and associates[30,31] studied 103 factory workers with subacute low back pain (6 weeks' duration) for a period of 3 years. Subjects were randomized into a custom, graded exercise program or a control group. All subjects received continuous medical care from the primary care physician. There was a significant improvement in early return to work, reduced sick leave used, and many strength parameters in the exercise group compared to the control group. Individual graded exercise programs emphasized working to a quota instead of to a moderate pain threshold. The exercise patients seemed to learn that it was safe to initiate mobility early, while regaining function. In another study,[32] McKenzie extension exercises were compared to a 45-minute "mini back school" without exercises. In the 100 patients randomized into these two groups and evaluated at 1 year, there was a significant improvement in the exercise group for outcome measures, including return to work, decrease in pain recurrence, and the amount of pain and degree of mobility at the time of evaluation.

The results of several studies suggest that there may be no significant benefit to adding an exercise program during the acute phase of low back pain. Four treatment combinations—traction, exercises, manipulation, and corset—and no treatment were compared during a randomized trial of 322 outpatients.[33] At 4 weeks, the treatment groups showed small, generally nonsignificant benefits over spontaneous improvement with no treatment. Even the small benefits disappeared at 4 and 16 months. In a smaller study,[34] 28 patients with acute low back pain were randomized to lumbar flexion, manipulation, or home care. There was no statistical difference among groups in terms of pain, spinal flexion, or functional activity. In addition, bed rest and/or exercise proved to be of no benefit in acute low back pain.[35] It is a generally accepted fact based on scientific trials that bed rest longer than 48 hours is not beneficial in the relief of low back pain.

Faas and associates[36] studied 473 acute low back pain cases randomized to a usual care, exercise, or placebo group. For most outcome variables there was no significant difference between groups. These results continued for up to 12 months. In the early time periods, the exercise group fared worse for such variables as fatigue and emotional problems. Accordingly, Faas and associates did not recommend exercise in the acute period. In a separate study of the same patient population,[37] it is reported that sickness absence was increased during the first 3 months in the exercise group. It was to be expected that the exercise group may have expressed some additional early pain and/or fatigue from their additional exertions. However, Faas and associates'[36] earlier study generated several letters to the editor[38] that specifically criticized the nature of the exercise program used. The general consensus of these comments was that the exercises were incomplete and, therefore, unlikely by design to be of any benefit.

431

In a recent trial,[39] 186 patients with acute, nonspecific low back pain, were randomized to one of three groups: bed rest, back mobilizing (exercise), or continuation of ordinary activities (control). The exercise program was a single visit to the physical therapist and an instruction sheet on extension and lateral bending movements to be repeated ten times a day. The exercise program was very limited in scope and not individualized for each patient. At 3 and 12 weeks, the control group had better results in several important variables, such as measures of pain duration, pain intensity, and days absent from work. The bed rest group fared worse than the exercise group. At the 3-week evaluation, the exercise group averaged 61 sets of the brief program prescribed. If exercising patients did little else, it is not surprising that their recovery was diminished.

To date, there is a lack of scientifically rigorous trials on the effects of a well-designed exercise program for acute low back pain. Several studies (not described in this review) clearly recommend that extensive bed rest is detrimental to recovery. Thus, early mobility and activity is valuable. The recent AHCPR guidelines on acute low back pain[4] recommend, but with weak evidence, that exercise may be valuable. If exercise is to be recommended, then a complete and specified program is likely to be more beneficial than an abbreviated and general program.

Chronic Low Back Pain

Most episodes of acute low back pain resolve before becoming a debilitating and chronic condition. However, there are still millions of patients with chronic low back pain who represent the majority of the large public health cost of this condition.

Risch and associates[40] compared the effects of an extension exercise training program with the results of other patients with chronic pain who were placed on a wait list (placebo) before beginning to exercise. The treated group increased lumbar strength, reported less pain, and decreased psychosocial dysfunction; however, there was no statistical difference in self-reported daily activities. Physiologic examination[41] of integrated electromyographies in patients with chronic low back pain showed significant decreases in endurance and strength of the spinal muscles, indicating an underlying need to restore these muscles to normal functional levels. Deyo and associates[42] studied the effect of a flexibility exercise program as part of a study of TENS. A sham TENS group served as the control. After 4 weeks of exercise, the exercise group showed improvement in pain measures and self-rated activity. The effects disappeared 2 months after the exercise was stopped, supporting the need for continuation of exercises and patient compliance. In a study of three classes of radiographically identified spinal instability, it was determined that a program with education, extension exercises, and an extension brace produced significant reductions in a pain interference scale (improved wellness) that could be recommended for most classifications of low back pain.[43] The importance of patient education and the need for patient compliance in a home environment was also emphasized.

Several studies have considered different levels of exercise intensity and supervision. Jarvikoski and associates[44] compared two thorough exercise programs: one guided by pain, the other with more intensive training with the rationale of "no pain, no gain." The intensive program yielded better long-term results in pain and daily function. There was no statistical gain in return to work in either group. The authors claim socioeconomic factors may dominate in determining return to work. In another study,[45] highly intensive, less intensive (one-fifth the intensity), and placebo-treated patients with chronic low back pain were compared. The two treatment exercise programs were given for 3 months. The high-intensity training fared significantly better for most of the outcome measures at time periods up to 1 year. The duration of exercise may partially explain the strongly positive results. In yet another study,[46] demographic differences between patients with chronic low back pain were analyzed. Intensive, dynamic exercises were recommended for females and those with sedentary jobs. Conventional physical therapy and isometric exercises produced a better response in males and those with demanding physical occupations.

Frost and associates[47] compared patients in a twice-weekly for 4 weeks exercise program to a control group in moderately disabled chronic low back pain patients. Both groups received brief training and an instruction sheet for home exercises. The supervised exercise group responded significantly better on many pain and function measures during the 6-month study period. Based on this study, education and advice alone (without follow-up) may not be sufficient to produce changes in patient results. Reilly and associates,[48] using a similar design, showed that supervised patients exercised about three times as much as those with instruction sheets only. Again, outcome measures were significantly better for the supervised group. Supervised, formal intervention by a physical therapist teaching individualized patient exercises based on diagnosis and lifestyle will be the most beneficial to patients and their functional outcome.

Several studies have considered the issue of the effectiveness of complete programs (behavior, education, and exercise components) in the care of chronic low back pain. Turner and associates[49] compared aerobic exercise, behavioral training, and a combination of these to a wait-listed group for moderately disabled patients with low back pain. The combination treatment produced the best results in the immediate posttreatment period. At 6- and 12-month follow-ups, all treatment groups had similar positive results. Klaber Moffett and associates[50] compared a complete back school program with an exercise only program; the complete program had the longer-lasting effect. Mayer and associates[51] demonstrated that 87% of chronic patients in a functional restoration program returned to work compared to 41% in a group of historic controls with no treatment. The nontreatment group also had twice as many subsequent surgeries. In a long-term study[52] (average 3 years) after completion of a multidisciplinary back program, telephone interviews documented a generally good outcome. Overall, 68% had returned to work but only 49% retained their original jobs. There was a strong relationship between length of follow-up and successful outcome. In a retrospective cohort study,[53] it was shown that a complete back care program produced results similar to previously published surgical studies in patients with herniated disks and radiculopathy at an average follow-up time of 31 months.

Exercise, alone or in combination with other education or training programs, appears to be an important element in the rehabilitation of the patient with chronic low back pain in terms of both functional measures and return to work. It has yet to be established, however, which exercise regimens would be most beneficial for specific groups of patients.

Prevention of Low Back Pain

Some of the studies discussed here focused on the issue of preventing further episodes of low back pain. There is some overlap among designs and outcomes of articles reviewed in the section on chronic low back pain. Most of the prevention articles include discussions of epidemiologic studies to determine if healthy and physically fit individuals experience more or less low back pain than their counterparts. While the majority of these data seem to define a role for fitness in the prevention of low back pain, some studies do not support that association. Epidemiologic studies are not covered in depth in this current review.

Grundewall and associates[54] studied hospital workers grouped into a complete exercise program and a control group. The exercise group had reduced days lost from low back complaints and less low back pain. The authors demonstrated the cost effectiveness of this ''on the job'' exercise program in terms of a 10:1 cost benefit ratio. In another study of hospital workers, Donchin and associates[55] showed that a calisthenics group experienced fewer painful months than back school or control groups. There was a correlation between large increases in flexibility and abdominal strength. This demonstrates the relevance of mobility, strength, and function in a pain management program. Kellett and associates[56] showed that an exercise group, which included aerobic components, had a significantly reduced incidence of sick days attributable to low back pain compared to a control group. However, there was no accompanying change in aerobic fitness of the worker. Recently, Lahad and associates[57] reviewed much of the prevention literature and concluded that intervention studies uniformly showed positive effects from exercise and that longer time periods of exercise and greater numbers of subjects are required so as to define specific recommendations.

It appears that exercise programs are successful in reducing the future occurrence of low back pain. However, precise programs and classification of subjects have not been defined, encouraging the continuation of further studies in this area.

Discussion of Exercise for Low Back Pain

The underlying physiologic rationale for exercise and the positive and negative issues related to flexion, extension, and aerobic exercises have been discussed.[28,58,59] Jackson and Brown[58] discuss the underlying evidence to support indications for exercise in patients with low back pain, and they conclude that a complete exercise program (flexion, extension, and aerobic) may be beneficial to: (1) decrease pain; (2) strengthen weak muscles (strength and endurance gains are valuable); (3) decrease mechanical stress (stretching tight muscles); (4) improve fitness (a well-substantiated fact); (5) stabilize hypermobile segments; (6) improve posture; (7) improve trunk mobility (empirically valid); and (8) use when other approaches fail (valid in terms of the general physiological benefits of conditioning).

Outline 1 contains general exercise guidelines that are based on summaries provided by Jackson and Brown[59] and Jenkins and Borenstein.[27]

In summary, exercise is a commonly recommended and helpful component of a well-designed program for the complete rehabilitation and secondary prevention of low back pain. In the acute phase it is difficult to provide rigorous

Outline 1 General guidelines for the use of exercise in low back patients

Indications for Flexion Exercises	Indications for Extension Exercises
Mechanical LBP/painful extension	Postural LBP in flexion
Osteoarthritis in lumbar spine	Mechanical LBP/painful flexion
Spondylolisthesis	Disk prolapse, after acute phase
Spinal stenosis	Ankylosing spondylitis
Contraindications for Flexion Exercises	**Contraindications for Extension Exercises**
Acute disk prolapse	Acute disk prolapse
Immediately after long rest (hyperhydrated)	Multioperated back/disruption of muscles
Postural low back	Scarring with limited flexion
Presence of lateral trunk shift/list	Spinal stenosis/spondylolisthesis

LBP = low back pain
(Adapted with permission from Jackson CR, Brown MD: Analysis of current approaches and a practical guide to prescription of exercise. *Clin Orthop* 1983;179:46–54 and Jenkins EM, Borenstein DG: Exercise for the low back pain patient. *Baillieres Clin Rheumatol* 1994;8:191–197.)

proof of benefit, except to substantiate the need for early mobility as is now recognized for joint rehabilitation in the extremities, especially with postsurgical care. Clearly, long-term bed rest is not indicated in any situation. Rapid, progressive return to normal function is best with or without prescribed exercise. In chronic and preventive research studies, there is strong evidence to support exercise, both alone and in combination with other interventions, such as physical methods, as an important factor in improved patient outcomes.

Conclusion

Few well-designed physical agent and/or exercise studies exist, especially for acute low back pain. Therefore, it is difficult to prove or disprove in a fully rigorous manner the potential benefit of any single physical agent or specific exercise program. The absence of prospective controlled studies should not be misconstrued as meaning there is no efficacious benefit to the use of exercise, mobilization, and physical methods.

Some recommendations or guidelines advocate no intervention because of concern for cost containment and lack of scientific trials that prove efficacy. In many other clinical circumstances, medical and health care providers are under a similar state of lack of knowledge as to the exact diagnostic interpretation or treatment plan for individual patients. Practitioners who treat patients with low back pain must use their best clinical judgment based on knowledge and experience to reduce pain in a practical and effective way. A lack of professional intervention may result in patients' improper use of bed rest or over-the-counter medicines.

Scientific support exists for some aspects of physical methods and exercise as components of a well-designed patient management plan. Anecdotal information supports the general improvement of most patients with low risk and at low to moderate cost. Well-designed clinical studies are needed to determine the value of specific interventions for well-defined classes of patients.

References

1. Deyo RA: Nonsurgical care of low back pain. *Neurosurg Clin N Am* 1991;2:851–862.
2. Griffiths HJ (ed): *Imaging of the Lumbar Spine.* Gaithersburg, MD, Aspen Publishers, 1991, pp 1–5.
3. Waddell G: A new clinical model for the treatment of low-back pain. *Spine* 1987;12:632–644.
4. Bigos SJ, Bowyer O, Braen GR: *Acute Low Back Problems in Adults.* Rockville, MD, US Department of Health and Human Services (AHCPR Pub No 95–0642), 1994.
5. Nachemson AL: The natural course of low back pain, in White AA III, Gordon SL (eds): American Academy of Orthopaedic Surgeons *Symposium on Idiopathic Low Back Pain.* St. Louis, MO, CV Mosby, 1982, pp 46–51.
6. DeRosa CP, Porterfield JA: A physical therapy model for the treatment of low back pain. *Phys Ther* 1992;72:261–272.
7. Spitzer WO: Report of the Quebec Task Force on Spinal Disorders: Scientific approach to the assessment and management of activity-related spinal disorders. A monograph for clinicians. *Spine* 1987;12:S1–S59.
8. Knight KL: Cold as a modifier of sports-induced inflammation, in Leadbetter WB, Buckwalter JA, Gordon SL (eds): *Sports-Induced Inflammation.* Park Ridge, IL, American Academy of Orthopaedic Surgeons, 1990, pp 463–477.
9. Koes BW, Bouter LM, van Mameren H, et al: A randomized clinical trial of manual therapy and physiotherapy for persistent back and neck complaints: Subgroup analysis and relationship between outcome measures. *J Manipulative Physiol Ther* 1993;16:211–219.
10. Koes BW, Bouter LM, van Mameren H: The effectiveness of manual therapy, physiotherapy, and treatment by the general practitioner for nonspecific back and neck complaints: A randomized clinical trial. *Spine* 1992;17:28–35.
11. Koes BW, Bouter LM, van Mameren H, et al: Randomised clinical trial of manipulative therapy and physiotherapy for persistent back and neck complaints: Results of one year follow-up. *Br Med J* 1992;304:601–605.
12. Hansen FR, Bendix T, Skov P, et al: Intensive, dynamic back-muscle exercises, conventional physiotherapy, or placebo-control treatment of low-back pain: A randomized, observer-blind trial. *Spine* 1993;18:98–108.
13. Miglis MF: Shades of straight: Diversity among purists. *J Manipulative Physiol Ther* 1992;18:406–407.
14. McCray RE, Patton NJ: Pain relief at trigger points: A comparison of moist heat and shortwave diathermy. *J Orthop Sports Phys Ther* 1984;5:175–178.
15. Quirion-De Girardi C, Seaborne D, Savard-Goulet F, et al: The analgesic effect of high voltage galvanic stimulation combined with ultrasound in the treatment of low back pain: A one-group pretest/post-test study. *Physiother Canada* 1984;36:327–333.
16. Ziskin MC, Michlovitz SL: Therapeutic ultrasound, in Michlovitz SL, Wolf SL (eds): *Thermal Agents in Rehabilitation.* Philadelphia, PA, FA Davis, 1986, pp 141–176.
17. Spiker JC: Ultrasound, in Prentice WE (ed): *Therapeutic Modalities in Sports Medicine,* ed 2. St. Louis, MO, Times Mirror/Mosby College Publishing, 1990, pp 129–147.
18. Draper DO, Schulthies S, Sorvisto P, et al: Temperature changes in deep muscles of humans during ice and ultrasound therapies: An in vivo study. *J Orthop Sports Phys Ther* 1995;21:153–157.

19. Pope MH, Phillips RB, Haugh LD, et al: A prospective randomized three-week trial of spinal manipulation, transcutaneous muscle stimulation, massage and corset in the treatment of subacute low back pain. *Spine* 1994;19:2571–2577.
20. Hsieh CY, Phillips RB, Adams AH, et al: Functional outcomes of low back pain: Comparison of four treatment groups in a randomized controlled trial. *J Manipulative Physiol Ther* 1992;15:4–9.
21. Starring DT: The use of electrical stimulation and exercise for strengthening lumbar musculature: A case study. *J Orthop Sports Phys Ther* 1991;14:61–64.
22. McQuain MT, Sinaki M, Shibley LD, et al: Effect of electrical stimulation on lumbar paraspinal muscles. *Spine* 1993;18:1787–1792.
23. Sinaki M, McPhee MC, Hodgson SF: Relationship between bone mineral density of spine and strength of back extensors in healthy postmenopausal women. *Mayo Clin Proc* 1986;61:116–122.
24. Marchand S, Charest J, Li J, et al: Is TENS purely a placebo effect? A controlled study on chronic low back pain. *Pain* 1993;54:99–106.
25. Tesio L, Merlo A: Autotraction versus passive traction: An open controlled study in lumbar disc herniation. *Arch Phys Med Rehabil* 1993;74:871–876.
26. Reitman C, Esses SI: Conservative options in the management of spinal disorders: Part II. Exercise, education, and manual therapies. *Am J Orthop* 1995;24:241–250.
27. Jenkins EM, Borenstein DG: Exercise for the low back pain patient. *Baillieres Clin Rheumatol* 1994;8:191–197.
28. Wheeler AH, Hanley EN Jr: Nonoperative treatment for low back pain: Rest to restoration. *Spine* 1995;20:375–378.
29. Koes BW, Bouter LM, van der Heijden GJ: Methodological quality of randomized clinical trials on treatment efficacy in low back pain. *Spine* 1995;20:228–235.
30. Lindstrom I, Ohlund C, Eek C, et al: Mobility, strength, and fitness after a graded activity program for patients with subacute low back pain: A randomized prospective clinical study with a behavioral therapy approach. *Spine* 1992;17:641–652.
31. Lindstrom I, Ohlund C, Eek C, et al: The effect of graded activity on patients with subacute low back pain: A randomized prospective clinical study with an operant-conditioning behavioral approach. *Phys Ther* 1992;72:279–293.
32. Stankovic R, Johnell O: Conservative treatment of acute low-back pain: A prospective randomized trial. McKenzie method of treatment versus patient education in "mini back school." *Spine* 1990;15:120–123.
33. Coxhead CE, Inskip H, Meade TW, et al: Multicentre trial of physiotherapy in the management of sciatic symptoms. *Lancet* 1981;1:1065–1068.
34. Zylbergold RS, Piper MC: Lumbar disc disease: Comparative analysis of physical therapy treatments. *Arch Phys Med Rehabil* 1981;62:176–179.
35. Gilbert JR, Taylor DW, Hildebrand A, et al: Clinical trial of common treatments for low back pain in family practice. *Br Med J* 1985;291:791–794.
36. Faas A, Chavannes AW, van Eijk JT, et al: A randomized, placebo-controlled trial of exercise therapy in patients with acute low back pain. *Spine* 1993;18:1388–1395.
37. Faas A, van Eijk JT, Chavannes AW, et al: A randomized trial of exercise therapy in patients with acute low back pain: Efficacy on sickness absence. *Spine* 1995;20:941–947.
38. Bunch RW: Letter: A randomized, placebo-controlled trial of exercise therapy in patients with acute low back pain. *Spine* 1994;19:1101–1104.
39. Malmivaara A, Hakkinen U, Aro T, et al: The treatment of acute low back pain: Bed rest, exercises, or ordinary activity? *N Engl J Med* 1995;332:351–335.
40. Risch SV, Norvell NK, Pollock ML, et al: Lumbar strengthening in chronic low back pain patients: Physiologic and psychological benefits. *Spine* 1993;18:232–238.
41. Robinson ME, Cassisi JE, O'Connor PD, et al: Lumbar iEMG during isotonic exercise: Chronic low back pain patients versus controls. *J Spinal Disord* 1992;5:8–15.
42. Deyo RA, Walsh NE, Martin DC, et al: A controlled trial of transcutaneous electrical nerve stimulation (TENS) and exercise for chronic low back pain. *N Engl J Med* 1990;322:1627–1634.

43. Spratt KF, Weinstein JN, Lehmann TR, et al: Efficacy of flexion and extension treatments incorporating braces for low back pain patients with retrodisplacement, spondylolisthesis, or normal sagittal translation. *Spine* 1993;18:1839–1849.

44. Jarvikoski A, Mellin G, Estlander AM, et al: Outcome of two multimodal back treatment programs with and without intensive physical training. *J Spinal Disord* 1993;6:93–98.

45. Manniche C, Hesselsoe G, Bentzen L, et al: Clinical trial of intensive muscle training for chronic low back pain. *Lancet* 1988;2:1473–1476.

46. Hansen FR, Bendix T, Skov P, et al: Intensive, dynamic back-muscle exercises, conventional physiotherapy, or placebo-control treatment of low-back pain: A randomized observer-blind trial. *Spine* 1993;18:98–108.

47. Frost H, Klaber Moffett JA, Moser JS, et al: Randomised controlled trial for evaluation of fitness programme for patients with chronic low back pain. *Br Med J* 1995;310:151–154.

48. Reilly K, Lovejoy B, Williams R, et al: Differences between a supervised and independent strength and conditioning program with chronic low back syndromes. *J Occup Med* 1989;31:547–550.

49. Turner JA, Clancy S, McQuade KJ, et al: Effectiveness of behavioral therapy for chronic low back pain: A component analysis. *J Consult Clin Psychol* 1990;58:573–579.

50. Klaber Moffett JA, Chase SM, Portek I, et al: A controlled, prospective study to evaluate the effectiveness of a back school in the relief of chronic low back pain. *Spine* 1986;11:120–122.

51. Mayer TG, Gatchel RJ, Mayer H, et al: A prospective two-year study of functional restoration in industrial low back injury: An objective assessment procedure. *JAMA* 1987;258:1763–1767.

52. Lanes TC, Gauron EF, Spratt KF, et al: Long-term follow-up of patients with chronic back pain treated in a multidisciplinary rehabilitation program. *Spine* 1995;20:801–806.

53. Saal JA, Saal JS: Nonoperative treatment of herniated lumbar intervertebral disc with radiculopathy: An outcome study. *Spine* 1989;14:431–437.

54. Gundewall B, Liljeqvist M, Hansson T: Primary prevention of back symptoms and absence from work: A prospective randomized study among hospital employees. *Spine* 1993;18:587–594.

55. Donchin M, Woolf O, Kaplan L, et al: Secondary prevention of low-back pain: A clinical trial. *Spine* 1990;15:1317–1320.

56. Kellett KM, Kellett DA, Nordholm LA: Effects of an exercise program on sick leave due to back pain. *Phys Ther* 1991;71:283–293.

57. Lahad A, Malter AD, Berg AO, et al: The effectiveness of four interventions for the prevention of low back pain. *JAMA* 1994;272:1286–1291.

58. Jackson CP, Brown MD: Is there a role for exercise in the treatment of patients with low back pain? *Clin Orthop* 1983;179:39–45.

59. Jackson CP, Brown MD: Analysis of current approaches and a practical guide to prescription of exercise. *Clin Orthop* 1983;179:46–54.

Chapter 27

A Critical Appraisal of the Use of Medications and Spinal Manipulation for Idiopathic Low Back Pain

Paul G. Shekelle, MD, PhD

Introduction

The choice of symptom relief measures for patients with idiopathic low back pain often includes medications and/or spinal manipulation. In this chapter, I will discuss the scientific evidence for the use of common medications and spinal manipulation for patients with idiopathic low back pain.

Medications

Analgesics are medications that relieve pain. Acetaminophen, nonsteroidal anti-inflammatory drugs (NSAIDs), such as aspirin, ibuprofen, and naproxen, and narcotics are all analgesics that have been used to treat low back pain. They provide pain relief for patients with low back pain in exactly the same manner they provide pain relief for patients with a headache or twisted ankle, ie, there is nothing specific about their mechanism of action with respect to patients with low back pain. Although there have been relatively few randomized controlled trials in which analgesics are compared with placebos as treatment for patients with low back pain, those that have been performed have generally shown that pain relief is greater in groups treated with analgesics.[1-4] Data from a recent systematic overview of the efficacy of NSAIDs for low back pain reported a pooled odds ratio for improvement at 1 week of 0.53 (95% confidence interval 0.32-0.89) favoring NSAIDs.[5] Narcotic analgesics may be more chemically potent pain relievers than acetaminophen or NSAIDs for patients with low back pain, but in two of three clinical trials, narcotic analgesics were found to be no more effective than NSAIDs or acetaminophen in relieving pain.[6-8] These data, combined with the potential for abuse, habituation, and addiction that exist with use of narcotics, may mean that their regular use by the patient with low back pain should not be recommended. Acetaminophen or NSAIDs should be the first medication options for pain relief in patients with idiopathic low back pain. No conclusive evidence exists that suggests there is a therapeutic difference between either acetaminophen or NSAIDs or between any of the various types of NSAIDs. The choice of medication should be made on the basis of cost, poten-

Table 1 Efficacy of muscle relaxants for low back pain

Reference	Type of Pain	Treatment Comparisons and Results

Arbus et al[10] — Subacute or chronic

Pain severity (scale of 1 to 5): Improvement at day 14 ($p < 0.02$)

Tetrazepam	2.09
Placebo	0.98

Baratta[11] — Acute

Global evaluation by physician ($p < 0.05$):

	Cyclobenzaprine	Placebo
Patients with marked improvement	23	2
Patients with moderate improvement	18	13

Basmajian[12] — Subacute or chronic

Effect on muscle spasm (change from pretreatment on a scale of 1 to 5, absent to severe, p = NS):

Cyclobenzaprine	-1.0
Diazepam	-1.0
Placebo	-1.1

Basmajian[4] — Acute neck + back

Patients with marked or moderate improvement at 4 days (p = 0.006):

Cyclobenzaprine	Diflunisal	Cyclobenzaprine + Diflunisal	Placebo
26	24	32	21

Borenstein et al[13] — Acute

Days to resolution of pain ($0.05 < p < 0.10$):

	Naproxen	Naproxen + Cyclobenzaprine
Patient rating	12.5	8.5
Physician rating	14	7

Boyles[14] — Acute

Patients with marked to complete relief at 7 days (p = NS):

Carisoprodol	70%
Diazepam	45%

Physician assessment of overall improvement at 7 days (p = 0.059):

Carisoprodol	74%
Diazepam	49%

Casale[15] — Chronic in acute phase

Patients with improvement in pain behavior at 4 days ($p < 0.001$):

Dantrolene	100%
Placebo	40%

Improvement on Visual Analog Scale pain ($p < 0.001$):

Dantrolene	50%
Placebo	9%

Dapas[16] — Acute

Patient's rating of pain severity (scale of 1 to 5, p < NS):

	Day 1	Day 10
Baclofen	4.0	1.75
Placebo	4.0	2.3

Reference	Type of Pain	Treatment Comparisons and Results
Gold[17]	Acute	Number of patients reporting overall symptomatology improved at 48 hours ($p < 0.01$ versus placebo; $p = $ NS between treatments): Orphenadrine 7/20 Phenobarbital 3/20 Placebo 0/20 Number of patients reporting pain intensity reduced at 48 hours ($p < 0.01$ favoring orphenadrine): Orphenadrine 9/20 Phenobarbital 3/20 Placebo 4/20
Hindle[18]	Acute	Overall response at 7 days ($p < 0.01$): *Carisoprodol* *Butalbital* *Placebo* Excellent 7 0 0 Good 5 2 2 All others 2 13 12
Hingorani[19]	Acute in hospital	Subjective improvement in pain and tenderness at 5 days ($p = $ NS): Diazepam 76% Placebo 72%
Klinger et al[20]	Low back strain	Patient assessment of post-treatment pain ($p < 0.001$): % pain relief Orphenadrine 92.5 Placebo 12.5
Middleton[21]	Acute	Patient symptoms at 7 days: *Methocarbanol* *Chlormezanone* Absent 27% 25% Improved 66% 61% No change 7% 14%
Rollings et al[22]	Acute	Patient report of marked-to-complete relief at 8 days: Carisoprodol 69% Orphenadrine 69%

tial for side effects, and personal history of efficacy. In a meta-analysis of the risks of NSAIDs, it was concluded that the overall risk of serious gastrointestinal bleeding in patients who take NSAIDs is about one per 1,000 patients, with the risk being significantly greater in patients older than 65 years of age.[9]

The other medications commonly used for the treatment of patients with low back pain are the ''muscle relaxants.'' The mechanism by which these medications produce their therapeutic effect is unclear, but it almost certainly is not due to myographically demonstrated relaxation of the muscles. Recently, the English language randomized controlled trials, published through 1992, of patients with low back pain who were treated with muscle relaxants were reviewed and are summarized in Table 1. Participants in most of the studies were patients with acute low back pain. Most studies reported improvement in pain as an outcome measure. The treatment comparisons studied included muscle relaxant versus other muscle relaxants, placebo, barbiturates, or NSAID, and NSAID and muscle relaxant versus NSAID only.[4,10-22] These studies were analyzed according to these classifications and, when warranted, results from similar studies were statistically combined using a random effects model. The risks of the use of muscle relaxants, which are the side effects of the drug, were also assessed. A total of 14 study reports were analyzed; data on side effects were included in 11, statements about side effects were made in two, and side effects were not mentioned at all in one. Drowsiness and dizziness were the two most commonly occurring side effects in the patients who were treated with muscle relaxants. The percentage of patients who reported experiencing these symptoms in all trials that compared muscle relaxant use with placebo use, and for whom data on side effects were reported, are compared in Table 2. The frequency with which at least one side effect occurred was also reported for several studies. The cumulative data from these trials are shown in Table 2. Drowsiness, dizziness, and at least one side effect are much more likely to occur when a patient is treated with a muscle relaxant than with a placebo and are presumably caused by the drug.

The following conclusions were drawn about the use of muscle relaxants for low back pain patients. Muscle relaxants are probably, but not certainly, more effective than placebos in relieving pain; however, there is insufficient evidence to support whether muscle relaxants are more or less effective than NSAIDs at reducing pain. Data from a single study that examined this question showed no difference between treatments.

There is insufficient evidence to support whether the addition of a muscle relaxant adds anything to the efficacy of an NSAID. Data from two trials in which cyclobenzaprine was studied showed no clinically significant differences.

Based on these conclusions, the routine use of muscle relaxants as first-line agents for the relief of low back pain cannot be justified. Muscle relaxants should probably be reserved for situations in which a trial of a nonnarcotic analgesic has not produced acceptable pain relief or if the patient's prior experience with muscle relaxants is highly favorable.

Spinal Manipulation

Spinal manipulation is a form of manual therapy that involves the movement of a joint past its usual end range of motion but not past its anatomic range of motion. This area has been termed the ''paraphysiologic zone.'' Movement of the joint is frequently accompanied by an audible cracking or popping sound that is of unknown origin. There are two classifications of spinal manipulation. The type of spinal manipulation chosen depends on the lever arm used to help the practitioner apply the load necessary for the manipulation. ''Long lever low velocity'' manipulations, or ''nonspecific'' manipulations, use one of the long bones of the limbs (frequently the femur) to amplify the load applied by the clinician's hands to one or several spinal joints. ''Short lever high velocity'' manipulations, also sometimes called ''specific spinal adjustments,'' usually con-

Table 2 Side effects

| | % Reporting | | | |
Symptom	Muscle Relaxant Group	Placebo Group	Difference	95% Confidence Interval
Drowsiness	26%	11%	15%	9%, 22%
Dizziness	34%	7%	27%	20%, 35%
At least one side effect	55%	23%	32%	23%, 41%

sist of a short, forceful thrust by the practitioner on a specific vertebral transverse process, thus moving the specific joint. Long lever manipulations have been associated most often with the practice of osteopathy and popular methods of physical therapy. Short lever manipulations are usually associated with the practice of chiropractic. However, there is considerable overlap between practitioners, and the type of practitioner does not necessarily determine the type of manipulation practiced.

In 1992, Shekelle and associates[23] reviewed controlled trials of spinal manipulation as therapy for patients with low back pain. They reported that there are sufficient data regarding patients with acute uncomplicated low back pain to conclude that treatment with spinal manipulation is of benefit relative to the treatments to which it has been compared. There was insufficient evidence to draw a conclusion for patients with chronic back pain. Since completion of the review by Shekelle and associates,[23] data from eight clinical trials have been published that compare treatment including spinal manipulation with various alternative treatments for patients with low back pain (Table 3).[24-36] The results of these trials are mixed. Patients with acute low back pain were included in four studies. In one study of patients who were thought to have sacroiliac joint dysfunction, no benefits were found in using spinal manipulation to relieve pain.[29] In another study, it was demonstrated that the addition of spinal manipulation to exercise therapy improved functional outcomes (and pain) measured after 1 month.[32] In two other "pragmatic" studies, multiple therapies that included spinal manipulation were compared with conventional nonmanipulative therapy.[28,30] It was demonstrated in both studies that treatments that included manipulation benefit the patient. In one study that specifically included patients with subacute low back pain, a nonsignificant trend toward improvement in pain in the group receiving manipulation was shown.[33] In the one study that specifically compared spinal manipulation to an artfully conducted sham, a benefit in terms of pain relief immediately following the manipulation was shown for patients with chronic back pain.[35] The benefit, however, was not sustained once treatment was stopped. In two other long-term follow-up studies of patients treated with manipulation by either physiotherapists or chiropractors, better outcomes at 1 to 3 years were reported for the patients who received manipulation.[28,36] These new trials do not substantially alter the conclusions reached in the meta-analysis conducted previously by Shekelle and associates[23] that spinal manipulation is of value in relieving pain in patients with acute symptoms and its value in treating chronic back pain is yet to be determined. The principal remaining concerns about using lumbar spinal manipulation to treat

443

Table 3 Randomized controlled trials of spinal manipulative therapy for low back pain (LBP) since 1991

Reference	Patients Enrolled*	Manipulative Treatment*	Comparison Treatment*	Sample Size	Results*
Herzog et al[24]	Pain duration of > 1 month; SI joint problems	Chiropractic SMT	"Back school" therapy delivered by physiotherapist	29	SMT no better than, and possibly worse than, back school in functional recovery at 4 weeks
Koes et al[25-28]	Subacute and chronic LBP and neck pain	SMT delivered by physiotherapists	1) Physiotherapy-non SMT 2) GP treatment 3) Diathermy	256	SMT and physiotherapy better than GP treatment or diathermy at 12 weeks, SMT slightly better than physiotherapy at 1 year
Wreje et al[29]	Acute and subacute LBP, SI joint problem, no sciatica	"Muscle energy technique" delivered by physician	Transverse friction rub	37	No difference in pain, but less sick leave and less use of acetaminophen in the manipulative treatment group measured 3 weeks after a single treatment
Blomberg et al[30,31]	Acute and subacute LBP, no sciatica	SMT with exercises, cortisone injections, and auto-traction	Conventional treatment by physiotherapists	101	Significant benefit for many activities of daily living and physiologic measures at 4 months for the manipulated group
Erhard et al[32]	Acute and subacute LBP	SMT by physiotherapist, with exercises	Extension exercises	24	Significant improvement in oswestry score at 5 days and 1 month for the SMT group
Pope et al[33] Hsieh et al[34]	LBP of 3 weeks to 6 months' duration, no sciatica	Chiropractic SMT	1) Soft-tissue massage 2) Transcutaneous muscle stimulation 3) Corset	164	No difference between groups, nonsignificant improvement in pain for the SMT group, measured at 3 weeks
Triano al[35]	Chronic LBP	Chiropractic SMT	1) Sham manipulation 2) Back education program	184	No difference between groups measured 2 weeks after 2 weeks of treatment
Meade et al[36]	Variety of low back pain syndromes	Chiropractic care including SMT	Hospital-based physiotherapy care, some including SMT	741	Significant benefit for chiropractic patients measured up to 3 years after treatment

*SI = sacroiliac; SMT = spinal manipulation therapy; GP = general practitioner idiopathic low back pain are its efficacy relative to other therapies and how many manipulations are necessary to achieve a response.

Summary

Sufficient data exist to prompt the recommendation that nonnarcotic analgesics or spinal manipulation as pain-relieving therapy be used for patients with idiopathic low back pain. The relative effectiveness and cost effectiveness of these two options, and the value of adding muscle relaxants to either regimen, remain to be determined.

References

1. Amlie E, Weber H, Holme I: Treatment of acute low-back pain with piroxicam: Results of a double-blind placebo-controlled trial. *Spine* 1987;12:473–476.
2. Postacchini F, Facchini M, Palieri P: Efficacy of various forms of conservative treatment in low back pain: A comparative study. *Neuro-Orthop* 1988;6:28–35.
3. Berry H, Bloom B, Hamilton EB, et al: Naproxen sodium, diflunisal, and placebo in the treatment of chronic back pain. *Ann Rheum Dis* 1982;41:129–132.
4. Basmajian JV: Acute back pain and spasm: A controlled multicenter trial of combined analgesic and antispasm agents. *Spine* 1989;14:438–439.
5. Koes BW, Scholten RJPM, Mens JMA, et al: Efficacy of NSAIDs for low back pain: An updated systematic review of randomized clinical trials, in van Tulder MW, Koes BW, Bouter LM (eds): *Low Back Pain in Primary Care: Effectiveness of Diagnostic and Therapeutic Interventions.* Amsterdam, The Netherlands, EMGO Institute, 1996.
6. Brown FL Jr, Bodison S, Dixon J, et al: Comparison of diflunisal and acetaminophen with codeine in the treatment of initial or recurrent acute low back strain. *Clin Ther* 1986;9(suppl):52–58.
7. Muncie HL Jr, King DE, DeForge B: Treatment of mild to moderate pain of acute soft tissue injury: Diflunisal vs. acetaminophen with codeine. *J Fam Pract* 1986;23:125–127.
8. Wiesel SW, Cuckler JM, Deluca F, et al: Acute low-back pain: An objective analysis of conservative therapy. *Spine* 1980;5:324–330.
9. Gabriel SE, Jaakkimainen L, Bombardier C: Risk for serious gastrointestinal complications related to use of nonsteroidal anti-inflammatory drugs: A meta-analysis. *Ann Intern Med* 1991;115:787–796.
10. Arbus L, Fajadet B, Aubert D, et al: Activity of tetrazepam [Myolastan (R)] in low back pain: A double-blind trial vs. placebo. *Clin Trials J* 1990;27:258–267.
11. Baratta RR: A double-blind study of cyclobenzaprine and placebo in the treatment of acute musculoskeletal conditions of the low back. *Curr Ther Res* 1982;32:646–652.
12. Basmajian JV: Cyclobenzaprine hydrochloride effect on skeletal muscle spasm in the lumbar region and neck: Two double-blind controlled clinical and laboratory studies. *Arch Phys Med Rehabil* 1978;59:58–63.
13. Borenstein DG, Lacks S, Wiesel SW: Cyclobenzaprine and naproxen versus naproxen alone in the treatment of acute low back pain and muscle spasm. *Clin Ther* 1990;12:125–131.
14. Boyles WF, Glassman JM, Soyka JP: Management of acute musculoskelatal conditions: Thoracolumbar strain or sprain: A double-blind evaluation comparing the efficacy and safety of carisoprodol with diazepam. *Today's Ther Trends* 1983;1:1–16.
15. Casale R: Acute low back pain: Symptomatic treatment with a muscle relaxant drug. *Clin J Pain* 1988;4:81–88.
16. Dapas F, Hartman SF, Martinez L, et al: Baclofen for the treatment of acute low-back syndrome: A double-blind comparison with placebo. *Spine* 1985;10:345–349.

17. Gold RH: Orphenadrine citrate: Sedative or muscle relaxant? *Clin Ther* 1978;1:451–453.
18. Hindle TH III: Comparison of carisoprodol, butabarbital, and placebo in treatment of the low back syndrome. *Calif Med* 1972;117:7–11.
19. Hingorani K: Diazepam in backache: A double-blind controlled trial. *Ann Phys Med* 1966;8:303–306.
20. Klinger NM, Wilson RR, Kanniainen CM, et al: Intravenous orphenadrine for the treatment of lumbar paravertebral muscle strain. *Curr Ther Res* 1988;43:247–254.
21. Middleton RS: A comparison of two analgesic muscle relaxant combinations in acute back pain. *Br J Clin Pract* 1984;38:107–109.
22. Rollings HE, Glassman JM, Soyka JP: Management of acute musculoskeletal conditions: Thoracolumbar strain or sprain. A double-blind evaluation comparing the efficacy and safety of carisoprodol with cyclobenzaprine hydrochloride. *Curr Ther Res* 1983;34:917–928.
23. Shekelle PG, Adams AH, Chassin MR, et al: Spinal manipulation for low-back pain. *Ann Intern Med* 1992;117:590–598.
24. Herzog W, Conway PJ, Willcox BJ: Effects of different treatment modalities on gait symmetry and clinical measures for sacroiliac joint patients. *J Manipulative Physiol Ther* 1991;14:104–109.
25. Koes BW, Bouter LM, van Mameren H, et al: The effectiveness of manual therapy, physiotherapy, and treatment by the general practitioner for nonspecific back and neck complaints: A randomized clinical trial. *Spine* 1992;17:28–35.
26. Koes BW, Bouter LM, van Mameren H, et al: A randomized clinical trial of manual therapy and physiotherapy for persistent back and neck complaints: Subgroup analysis and relationship between outcome measures. *J Manipulative Physiol Ther* 1993;16:211–219.
27. Koes BW, Bouter LM, van Mameren H, et al: A blinded randomized clinical trial of manual therapy and physiotherapy for chronic back and neck complaints: Physical outcome measures. *J Manipulative Physiol Ther* 1992;15:16–23.
28. Koes BW, Bouter LM, van Mameren H, et al: Randomised clinical trial of manipulative therapy and physiotherapy for persistent back and neck complaints: Results of one year follow up. *Br Med J* 1992;304:601–605.
29. Wreje U, Nordgren B, Aberg H: Treatment of pelvic joint dysfunction in primary care: A controlled study. *Scand J Prim Health Care* 1992;10:310–315.
30. Blomberg S, Hallin G, Grann K, et al: Manual therapy with steroid injections: A new approach to treatment of low back pain. A controlled multicenter trial with an evaluation by orthopedic surgeons. *Spine* 1994;19:569–577.
31. Blomberg S, Svardsudd K, Tibblin G: Manual therapy with steroid injections in low-back pain: Improvement of quality of life in a controlled trial with four months' follow-up. *Scand J Prim Health Care* 1993;11:83–90.
32. Erhard RE, Delitto A, Cibulka MT: Relative effectiveness of an extension program and a combined program of manipulation and flexion and extension exercises in patients with acute low back syndrome. *Phys Ther* 1994;74:1093–1100.
33. Pope MH, Phillips RB, Haugh LD, et al: A prospective randomized three-week trial of spinal manipulation, transcutaneous muscle stimulation, massage and corset in the treatment of subacute low back pain. *Spine* 1994;19:2571–2577.
34. Hsieh CY, Phillips RB, Adams AH, et al: Functional outcomes of low back pain: Comparison of four treatment groups in a randomized controlled trial. *J Manipulative Physiol Ther* 1992;15:4–9.
35. Triano JJ, McGregor M, Hondras MA, et al: Manipulative therapy versus education programs in chronic low back pain. *Spine* 1995;20:948–955.
36. Meade TW, Dyer S, Browne W, et al: Randomised comparison of chiropractic and hospital outpatient management for low back pain: Results from extended follow up. *Br Med J* 1995;311:349–351.

Chapter 28

Surgical Indications for Chronic Idiopathic Low Back Pain

Harry N. Herkowitz, MD
Kanwaldeep S. Sidhu, MD

Introduction

The treatment of mechanical low back pain without associated radiculopathy remains a challenge for the orthopaedic surgeon. The lifetime incidence of low back pain in the general population is estimated to be 60% to 80%.[1,2] For most patients with idiopathic low back pain, spontaneous resolution of symptoms typically occurs within a few weeks. Although the etiology of the pain is better defined in patients with herniated disks, spondylolisthesis, spinal stenosis, or tumors, the "pain generator" associated with lumbar disk degeneration is quite controversial. The socioeconomic impact of this "disease," however, is not in doubt.[3]

The lumbar spine is the site of the most expensive industrial injuries, and pain is the most common cause of disability in adults younger than 45 years of age.[4] Low back pain accounted for 15 million office visits in 1990, ranking it the fifth most common cause for all physician visits.[5] The annual incidence of lumbar spine surgery in the United States is approximately 165 operations per 100,000 persons.[5,6] Lumbar fusion ranks as the second most common lumbar spine procedure (25 lumbar fusions per 100,000 persons).[5] A large percentage of these fusions are performed for mechanical lower back pain or "disk degeneration." The failure rate for lumbar fusions is estimated to be in the 20% to 40% range.[7]

The direct and indirect costs of low back pain were analyzed by Frymoyer and Cats-Baril in 1990.[2] The estimated direct costs related to hospitalization, surgery, physicians, physical therapy, and medication exceeded $24 billion. The indirect costs related to lost productivity were estimated to exceed $27 billion. The available data clearly prove that the socioeconomic effect of low back disorders is indeed tremendous.

The degenerative disorders of the lumbar spine that occasionally require surgical intervention include herniated disks, spinal stenosis, degenerative spondylolisthesis, degenerative scoliosis, and degenerative disk disease. The most controversial among them is the treatment of idiopathic low back pain associated with lumbar degenerative disk disease.

There is little debate as to whether patients with chronic mechanical low back pain are indeed experiencing pain. For the orthopaedic surgeon who has followed this subgroup of low back pain patients in the office, it is obvious that their ability to be productive at work or even perform their activities of daily living is severely limited by their affliction. The difficulty in treating patients with idiopathic low back pain lies in the accurate identification of the ''pain generator.'' Data from several cadaveric and magnetic resonance imaging (MRI) studies have demonstrated that lumbar disk degeneration is a physiologic process associated with aging.[8-10] Most patients with lumbar disk degeneration are asymptomatic.

Which degenerated disks are painful? What is the biochemical or neurogenic pain mediator? Which patients with chronic idiopathic low back pain are good surgical candidates? Can surgical treatment provide results better than the natural history of diskogenic pain? It is because of the lack of conclusive data to answer the above questions that the surgical treatment of idiopathic low back pain is controversial.

What is the Pain Generator?

Disk degeneration is physiologic and mostly asymptomatic. Holt[11] found disk degeneration on the radiographs of 80% of adults studied, although 53% had no history of low back pain. Miller and associates[9] reported on 600 autopsy specimens and found that 90% of all disks had evidence of degeneration by age 50 years.

With the advent of MRI, varying stages of lumbar disk degeneration have been identified.[10] Paajanen and associates[10] noted that 34% of healthy male volunteers without low back pain demonstrated significant disk degeneration on MRI. Boden and associates[8] demonstrated abnormal disks in 28% of subjects without back pain or sciatica.

Buirski[12] prospectively analyzed abnormal MR images in 892 patients with chronic low back pain. They identified six patterns of lumbar disk degeneration.

The signals associated with MRI images of any tissue are related to its water content or ''hydration.'' On T2-weighted images, a normal hydrated disk should appear white. Dehydration, or disk degeneration, appears ''dark'' on T2-weighted images, giving rise to the term ''black disk disease.'' The anatomic architecture of a degenerated disk typically is disrupted from normal; therefore, the term ''internal disk derangement'' has been used as a diagnosis for patients with idiopathic low back pain associated with disk degeneration. The various names that have been used interchangeably for patients with chronic idiopathic low back pain include degenerative disk disease, diskogenic low back pain, internal disk derangement, and black disk disease.

What causes a degenerated disk to become painful? Because diskogenic low back pain has a somatotopic rather than dermatomal pattern, it is difficult to localize the exact level of pathology by performing a physical examination. The outer anulus is the only innervated part of the intervertebral disk.[13,14] The recurrent sinuvertebral nerve is postulated to be involved in the mechanism of pain transmission along the spinal column.[1] The nerve is a derivative of the postganglionic rami communicantes and branches into segments that ascend or descend one or more adjacent levels of the vertebral column. The branches of the sinuvertebral nerve accompany the venus plexus into the vertebral body end plates.[1] The nerve endings found in both the posterior longitudinal ligament

(PLL) and the outer lamina of the anulus are the terminal branches of the sinu-vertebral nerve. Malinsky[13] has described five types of nerve endings, includ-ing the nociceptive, pain-producing free nerve endings, which may fire in re-sponse to painful stimuli. Thus, evidence in the literature does suggest that components of the disk (outer anulus, PLL) may have the ability to respond to stimuli by painful efferent discharge.[13,14]

A peripheral lesion in the anulus fibrosus, despite a normal nucleus pulposus, can cause pain. The ability of small annular tears to cause nuclear degeneration has been demonstrated in the animal model.[14,15] Also, the material contained in the nucleus may be a source of inflammation itself.[14,16,17]

The nuclear material in a healthy disk without annular tears or fissures is never exposed to the innervated outer third of the anulus. End plate failure under com-pressive loads may expose the avascular nucleus to the systemic circulation. In a histologic study, McCarron and associates[14] injected autologous nucleus pul-posus into the epidural space of dogs. A control group of dogs underwent an epidural injection with saline. An inflammatory reaction to the injected nuclear material was observed only in the experimental group. One inflammatory com-ponent of human nucleus pulposus is phospholipase A_2 (PLA_2). It is found in high concentration in human disks and its inflammatory potential may be re-lated to its ability to liberate arachidonic acid from cell membranes.[16,17] Results of in vivo studies in which purified disk PLA_2 was used have demonstrated its potential to act as an inflammagen both directly, and by its ability to generate other inflammatory mediators, such as prostaglandins, leukotrienes, and lyso-phospholipids.[16,17]

Thus, the available data in the literature suggest that the disk is innervated and capable of being a source of pain. The pain originating from a disk may be related to the potentially inflammatory contents of the nucleus pulposus, or it may be a representation of the noxious discharge from the free nerve endings in the outer anulus. There is no reasonable explanation as to why most degen-erated disks are asymptomatic. Therefore, there is a diagnostic dilemma. Is a single ''black disk'' on MRI the source of pain? Which disk in the setting of multilevel disk degeneration is painful?

The answers to the above questions are very important for appropriate selec-tion of patients who would benefit from surgical treatment of idiopathic low back pain. Surgery typically involves arthrodesis across the degenerated disk space. Arthrodesis across several motion segments for multilevel disk degeneration typically is associated with poor outcomes. If surgical treatment for black disk disease is to be successful, it should be limited to a single level lumbar disk that has been identified as the pain generator. Diskography may have a role in iden-tifying that disk.

Diskography

Diskography frequently is performed in patients who are being considered for lumbar spine fusion for chronic idiopathic low back pain. However controver-sial, it is the only diagnostic modality that may provide a cause and effect re-lationship between a degenerated disk and pain.

The technique involves injection of a radiopaque contrast material into the nucleus pulposus of an awake patient (Fig. 1). The results of diskography de-

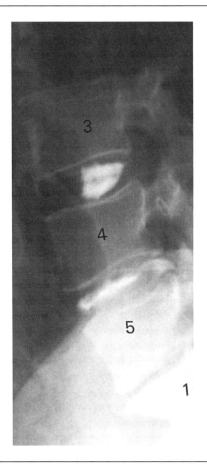

Fig. 1   *Diskography at L3-4, L4-5, and L5-S1 with injection of dye into each of the disk spaces.*

pend on the presence or absence of familiar back pain reproduction after the injection of contrast material into a radiographically abnormal disk. If injection of the dye material into the nucleus of an abnormal disk simulates the patient's back pain symptoms, then the diskogram is considered to be positive.

If nonsurgical treatment of a patient with chronic low back pain and a positive diskogram has failed, then that patient may be a candidate for surgery. It is important to perform diskography at more than one level. A negative diskogram at one or two control levels (normal on MRI) may add to the predictive value of a positive diskogram at a degenerated motion segment.

The ability of diskography to predict a successful outcome following surgery is controversial. It is an invasive test that should be performed on an awake patient with minimal sedation.[18] The results of diskography are quite dependent on the patient response regarding reproduction of "familiar" low back pain symptoms. However, the pain may be related to introduction of a needle into the disk space. It has also been hypothesized that the fluid volume injected increases pressures at the end plates.[19] Then, end plate deflection related to the injection may transfer the stresses to the vertebral body, thereby causing an increased intraosseous pressure,[19] which may cause pain. This mechanism may be responsible for positive diskograms at levels that appear normal on MRI.

The psychologic component of diskography should also be considered. Patients who had elevated hysteria or hypochondriasis scores on the Minnesota Multiphasic Personality Inventory (MMPI) were more likely to have positive diskograms at normal appearing levels than were controls.[20]

Holt,[21] in a study of asymptomatic prison volunteers, concluded that there was a 37% false positive rate with lumbar diskography. Several authors have since criticized Holt's data analysis, patient selection, and technique of diskography.[22,23] Walsh and associates[24] reported a 0% false positive rate and 100% specificity in ten asymptomatic volunteers after use of modern techniques of diskography. A prospective study of 195 patients with diskogenic pain and preoperative diskography was reported by Calhoun and associates.[22] Of the patients with positive preoperative diskograms at the fused level, 89% had significant pain relief, compared to 52% of patients with a negative diskogram. Horton and Daftari[25] prospectively studied 25 patients with nonradicular back pain. All underwent diskography and MRI. The authors concluded that MRI did not replace diskography as a diagnostic modality. For single level black disk, with a specific pattern of degeneration (black disk with annular tear) as visualized on MRI, diskography was unnecessary (Fig. 2). The MRI alone was felt to be adequate for the diagnosis of diskogenic pain at that level. The authors recommended diskography for multilevel black disk disease on MRI, in order to localize the segment or segments that are the pain generators. Simmons and associates[26] re-

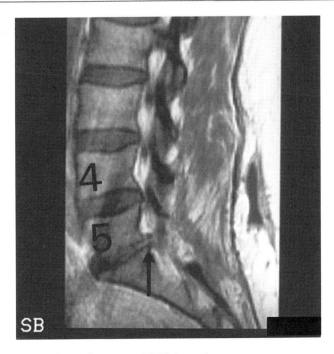

Fig. 2   *Dark disk with annular tear at L5-S1 (arrow).*

ported on 164 consecutive patients with chronic diskogenic low back pain. MRIs were performed before diskography in each case. MRI and diskography correlated in only 55% of the patients. At each disk level, MRI correlated with diskography in 80% of the disks. Of the disks that were abnormal on MRI, 37% had negative diskograms. A positive diskogram occurred in 7% of the disks that appeared normal on MRI.

In conclusion, the ability of diskography to select patients for surgical treatment of idiopathic low back pain is controversial. However, it is the only test available for dynamic evaluation of a disk. It is an invasive procedure and its accuracy and specificity depend on subjective pain response as determined by the patient. It is a preoperative test, and should be performed only after adequate attempts at conservative care have failed. It does not have a role in patients whose lumbar disks all appear normal on MRI.

Response to Preoperative Immobilization as a Criterion for Patient Selection

If a particular motion segment is believed to be the pain generator, then preoperative immobilization may relieve the symptoms. The surgical treatment for diskogenic pain, that is, arthrodesis, acts as an internal brace of a particular motion segment. If the patient's symptoms are relieved by external bracing, may the surgeon extrapolate that the symptoms would benefit from an internal surgical arthrodesis?

Rask and Dall[27] reported on 45 patients who were placed in a pantaloon cast preoperatively; 69% of the patients experienced significant pain relief. Of the patients (the 31 who experienced pain relief in the cast) who underwent arthrodesis, 74% had significant pain relief. However, the surgical and nonsurgical groups had no significant difference in functional improvement. Ordeberg and associates[28] reported on 77 patients who underwent presurgical immobilization by the use of a spinal external fixator. Sixty-three of the 77 patients experienced pain relief after external fixation. However, at 5-year follow-up, only 50% of the patients who underwent surgery had significant pain relief.

The available data in the literature do not support the use of preoperative immobilization as a diagnostic entity for selecting patients who would benefit from surgical treatment of idiopathic low back pain.

Psychologic and Secondary Gain Issues

The reasons for failure of lumbar fusion operations include improper diagnosis, poor patient selection, psychosocial factors, incorrect indications, inadequate surgical technique, and complications inherent with the surgical procedure.[29] In order to minimize the risk of failure of surgery for idiopathic low back pain, proper patient selection is extremely important.[29,30]

When the pathologic entity being treated is discrete and obvious, both clinically and radiographically, such as radiculopathy associated with an extruded disk herniation (on MRI), then it is assumed that most patients who are treated for it shall benefit from the treatment. This is not so when the primary reason for treatment is "pain." The perception of pain varies significantly from one person to the next and even among various ethnic groups. It is a combination of individual neurochemistry, psychosocial factors, personality, and social, familial, and economic factors.[31] The final outcome of a technically successful surgical procedure may be compromised if pain persists postoperatively as a result of psychosocial factors.[32] Unfortunately, when treating idiopathic low back pain, most surgical decisions are based on subjective perceptions of pain—pain experienced during diskography, pain associated with work activities, and pain during activities of daily living.

Symptoms of depression and anxiety are quite common in patients with chronic back pain.[32] It is unknown whether the depression is a result of chronic pain or the pain exists as a result of depression. Polatin and associates[33] assessed 200 chronic low back pain patients for current and lifetime psychiatric syndromes. They reported that 77% of the patients met lifetime DSM-III-R diagnostic criteria for psychiatric illness. Fifty-nine percent of the patients demonstrated current symptoms for at least one psychiatric diagnosis. The most common diagnoses were depression, substance abuse, and anxiety disorders. Over 50% of the patients had personality disorders. More than half had symptoms related to their psychiatric diagnoses before the onset of low back pain. The authors[33] concluded that certain psychiatric diagnoses, such as substance abuse and anxiety disorders, appear to precede chronic low back pain, whereas others, such as depression, may develop either before or after the onset of low back pain.

Various self-administered questionnaires have been used to assess the psychologic profiles of chronic low back pain patients. These include the MMPI, Cornell Medical Index, Middlesex Hospital Questionnaire, Eysenck Personality Inventory, Melzack Pain Questionnaire, and more. High scores on the hypochondriasis and hysteria scales on the MMPI have been associated with poor surgical results.[20] Despite the large number of psychologic questionnaires available, their ability to predict surgical outcome remains suspect because of the high number of false positives.

Workers' compensation and secondary gain issues may tend to influence a patient's perception of pain and may also diminish the incentive for pain relief.[34] These socioeconomic factors are unrelated to the anatomic pathology that may be responsible for pain. However, they do influence the outcome of surgical treatment. If a successful surgical outcome means that a worker may have to return to an unpopular occupation or lower economic standard of living, then there may be a minimal incentive for clinical improvement. Similarly, if resolution of symptoms associated with chronic low back pain may result in a plaintiff losing a potentially profitable litigation, then the outcome of treatment may be significantly biased. In conclusion, psychologic factors and secondary gain issues should be resolved prior to recommending surgical treatment for idiopathic low back pain.

Selection of Surgical Candidates

The indications of surgical treatment of diskogenic low back pain are very limited. Long lumbar fusions in patients with multilevel disk degeneration typically are failures and are not recommended.

The benefits of surgical treatment (arthrodesis) must outweigh the risk associated with surgery. Moreover, the long-term data from outcome studies following fusion for diskogenic pain must be an improvement over the natural history of idiopathic low back pain. This area is where the literature lacks conclusive data. There are no long-term prospectively randomized studies that compare surgical treatment of idiopathic low back pain with nonsurgical measures. In addition, the natural history of diskogenic low back pain is relatively unknown. Rhyne and Smith[35] reported on the outcome of diskogram-positive low back pain that was not treated surgically. Twenty-five single-level, diskogram-positive patients were evaluated at an average follow-up of 4.9 years; 68% had improved without surgery. Of the 32% that had not improved, 66.7% had an underlying psychiatric diagnosis. The authors concluded that diskogenic low back pain improves in patients without psychiatric diagnosis. In addition, outcome without surgery appears to be equal to or better than outcome after surgical treatment for diskogenic pain.

The following surgical indications should be considered for patients with chronic idiopathic low back pain:[29,36] (1) unremitting pain and disability for more than 1 year; (2) failure of trial of aggressive physical conditioning and conservative treatment lasting more than 4 months; (3) advanced single-level disk degeneration on MRI with a concordant pain response on diskograpy; and (4) absence of psychiatric or secondary gain issues.

An ideal surgical candidate would be a professionally satisfied, psychologically normal individual who has diskogram-concordant single-level disk degeneration on MRI. The ideal pattern of disk degeneration on MRI would be a dark disk with an annular tear (Fig. 2). The symptoms should have been present for more than 1 year, and the patient should have failed a trial of aggressive conservative treatment.

The reported success rates of arthrodesis for diskogenic pain range from 50% to 80%. Appropriate patient selection and a thorough preoperative discussion of expectations significantly influence the outcome of surgical treatment.[29] Randomized prospective studies are needed to evaluate the role of arthrodesis in the treatment of idiopathic low back pain.

Surgical Treatment of Idiopathic Low Back Pain

For appropriately selected patients with chronic diskogenic pain, the recommended surgical treatment is arthrodesis. Fusion across a diseased motion segment may be accomplished through several techniques. These techniques include posterolateral intertransverse process fusion, anterior lumbar interbody fusion (ALIF), posterior lumbar interbody fusion (PLIF), and anterior and posterior fusion (global fusion).

The role of segmental instrumentation using pedicle screws is also controversial. Data from retrospective and prospective randomized trials suggest that instrumentation, when used as an adjunct to arthrodesis, may improve the fusion rate (Fig. 3). The role of instrumentation in multilevel fusions, trauma, tumor, and scoliosis surgery is less controversial; however, its efficacy for single-level fusions is uncertain. The use of instrumentation is associated with a higher complication rate when compared to in situ fusion, and thus, the benefits associated with its use must outweigh the risks.

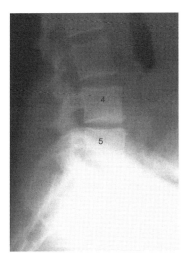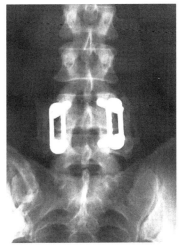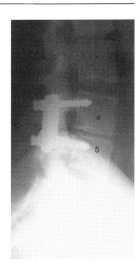

Fig. 3   **Left**, *Lateral radiograph depicting loss of disk height at L4-5 with sclerosis and end plate changes consistent with disk degeneration.* **Center**, *Postoperative anteroposterior radiograph depicting L4-5 fusion with pedicular instrumentation and solid arthrodesis.* **Right**, *Postoperative lateral radiograph.*

The rationale for surgical treatment of idiopathic low back pain is based on two theories. Posterolateral fusion limits motion across a degenerated motion segment, and this limit may be sufficient to minimize the symptoms associated with low back pain originating from that region. Instrumentation, when used as an adjunct to posterolateral fusion, may confer immediate stability to the spinal motion segment being fused.

However, motion can still occur along the anterior column despite a solid posterior fusion. Posterolateral fusion does not remove the postulated pain generator in internal disk derangement disorder, namely the intervertebral disk itself. Whether the disk itself needs to be removed in order to achieve a cure for diskogenic pain is controversial. Success rates around 70% to 85% have been reported for surgical treatment of diskogenic pain by posterolateral fusion with pedicular instrumentation.[37]

Some authors believe that minimizing motion at the disk space by posterolateral fusion may not be enough to accomplish a ''cure'' for diskogenic pain.[38-44] The reasons for this belief are twofold. First, the disk itself may be a source of pain and as such needs to be completely eliminated, and second, anterior motion and diskogram-concordant pain have been shown to occur despite a solid posterior fusion.[45] Reduction of motion across the disk by posterolateral fusion may not be sufficient to prevent displacement of biochemical substances from the central nucleus pulposus to the richly innervated peripheral anulus. Procedures that eliminate the disk as a potential pain generator include ALIF, PLIF, and global fusions. Satisfactory results have been reported in 80% to 95% of the patients with diskogenic pain treated with PLIF or global fusions.[41-43,46] Most series reported in the literature for these surgical techniques have used instrumentation as an adjunct for both PLIF and global fusions.[41-43,46] Anterior

455

interbody fusions alone have reported success rates of 70% to 75% for disko-genic pain.[39,47] The addition of instrumentation for anterior interbody fusions is not typically indicated.

Posterolateral Intertransverse Process Fusion

Bilateral posterolateral intertransverse process fusion of the spine is the most frequently used technique of lumbar arthrodesis.[29] Advantages of this technique include (1) high probability of obtaining a solid fusion; (2) the ability to perform fusion in the presence of a previous laminectomy; (3) the ability to avoid iatrogenic stenosis by placement of bone graft away from the midline; and (4) low risk of injury to the neural elements.

The pseudarthrosis rate after posterolateral fusions is estimated to be from 5% to 25%.[48] For a primary, single-level in situ arthrodesis (Fig. 4), a 10% to 15% pseudarthrosis rate is usual. The rate of pseudarthrosis increases with the number of levels being fused and with revision surgery. For a two- to three-level posterolateral fusion without instrumentation, a 20% to 35% pseudoar-throsis rate is to be expected.[29,48] Data from recent prospective trials suggests that the addition of instrumentation may lower the pseudarthrosis rate.[37,49,50] The pseudarthrosis rate for an instrumented single-level posterolateral fusion is reported to be in the 5% to 10% range (Fig. 5).[29,49] Whereas a solid arthrodesis does not guarantee a successful clinical outcome, a lumbar pseudarthrosis is as-sociated with a higher incidence of unsuccessful results.

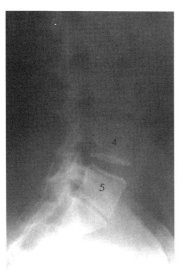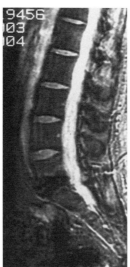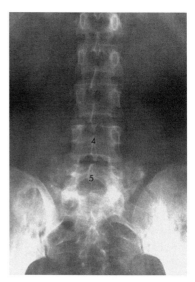

Fig. 4   **Left**, *Lateral radiograph (preoperative) depicting degenerative changes at L5-S1 in-terspace with complete loss of disk height.* **Center**, *Sagittal T2 magnetic resonance image showing a black disk at L5-S1. The other disk spaces appear normal.* **Right**, *Postoperative anteroposterior radiograph depicting a L5-S1 in situ arthrodesis without instrumentation.*

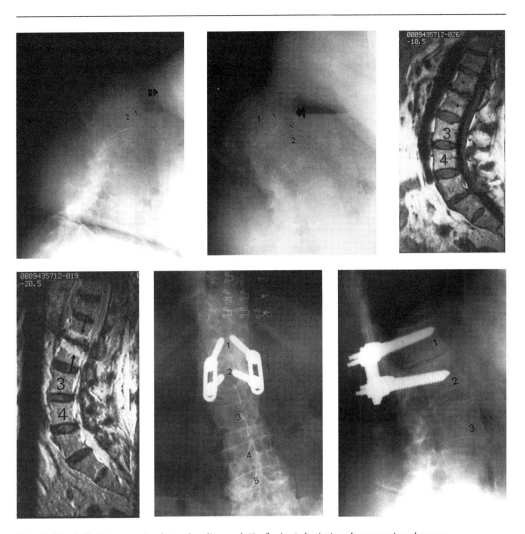

Fig. 5   **Top left**, *Preoperative lateral radiograph (in flexion) depicting degenerative changes at the L1-2 interspace.* **Top center**, *Preoperative lateral radiograph (in extension). There is no translational instability in flexion-extension.* **Top right**, *Sagittal T1 MRI depicting a degenerated disk at L1-2 with end plate sclerotic changes (asterisk).* **Bottom left**, *Sagittal T2 MRI depicting a black disk at L1-2 with typical end plate sclerotic changes (arrows).* **Bottom center**, *Postoperative AP radiograph after single level L1-2 fusion with instrumentation. The dotted lines reveal the bilateral intertransverse fusion mass.* **Bottom right**, *Postoperative lateral radiograph depicting fusion with instrumentation at L1-2.*

Dawson and associates[51] retrospectively reported on 58 patients who underwent in situ posterolateral fusions without instrumentation for diskogenic pain. The patients achieved a 92% fusion rate. The clinical success rate was reported as being between 70% and 80%. The authors acknowledged a 50% failure rate for patients undergoing revision surgery. In addition, the pseudarthrosis rate for floating fusions (not involving the sacrum) was 45%. Hellstadius[52] and Shaw and Taylor[53] reported retrospectively on their patients who underwent in situ posterolateral fusion without instrumentation. The pseudarthrosis rates in their series were 26% and 27%, respectively.

Wood and associates[37] reported on 28 patients who underwent lumbar fusion with instrumentation for degenerative disk disease. Their study was a multicenter trial involving the use of a pedicle screw/plate system. The minimum follow-up was 2 years. The authors used literature controls and concluded that "patients with degenerative disk disease who underwent fusion without pedicle screw instrumentation were over 24 times more likely to have a pseudarthrosis than comparable patients implanted with the screw/plate system." The pseudarthrosis rate in this series was 0%, and 75% of the patients had "improvement" in their back pain at 2-year follow-up. In a prospective, randomized trial, Zdeblick[49] reported on 49 patients who underwent fusion for diskogenic pain. The group that underwent posterolateral fusion with pedicular instrumentation had 95% good/excellent clinical outcome compared to 71% for the in situ fusion group. In addition, the fusion rate in the instrumented group was 93%, compared to 45% in the in situ fusion group. This difference was statistically significant.

Lorenz and associates[54] retrospectively reviewed 47 patients who underwent single-level posterolateral fusion with and without instrumentation for degenerative disk disease. Pseudarthrosis rates in the noninstrumented and instrumented groups were 58% and 0%, respectively. Pain improvement was 41% in the in situ fusion group, compared to 77% in the instrumented group. Of the instrumented group, 72% returned to work compared to 31% of the noninstrumented group. The authors concluded that "fusion rate for patients exhibiting single level disk disease improves with spinal fixation."[54]

Grubb and associates[55] prospectively reported on one- and two-level fusions for degenerative disk disease. Forty-nine patients underwent fusion without instrumentation, and 52 had fusion with compression U rod instrumentation. The pseudarthrosis rate without instrumentation was 35% compared to 6% with instrumentation. In both groups, a solid arthrodesis was associated with decreased pain at follow-up and higher return to work. The authors concluded that their data "warrants the use of instrumentation in one and two level lumbosacral fusions."

Temple and associates[56] retrospectively reported on 39 patients who underwent posterolateral fusion with Steffee instrumentation. Twelve of 39 patients had surgery for diskogenic pain. The authors reported 67% good/excellent results with an overall pseudarthrosis rate of 8%.

In summary, posterolateral fusion for appropriately selected patients with diskogenic pain is successful in 60% to 80% of the patients. The use of pedicular instrumentation may lower the pseudarthrosis rate and possibly improve the clinical outcome. Instrumentation is recommended for multilevel fusions and is indispensable for revision surgery patients. Available data suggest, but do not conclusively prove, that the addition of instrumentation may be beneficial for single-level fusions.[37,49,50] Further prospective, randomized trials need to be done to address this issue definitively.

Anterior Lumbar Interbody Fusion

This technique involves an anterior approach to the lumbar spine with complete excision of the disk and end plates. Corticocancellous bone graft is then inserted between the contiguous vertebral bodies (Fig. 6). Instrumentation is usually not recommended for single level ALIF.[29]

The advantages of ALIF include (1) complete excision of the disk space; (2) placement of the bone graft under compression along the anterior vertebral col-

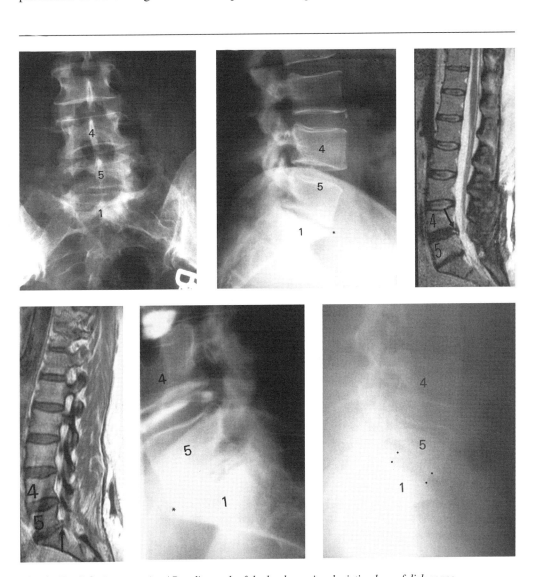

Fig. 6   **Top left,** *Preoperative AP radiograph of the lumbar spine depicting loss of disk space height at L5-S1.* **Top center,** *Lateral radiograph showing disk degeneration at L5-S1 (asterisk).* **Top right,** *Sagittal MRI revealing disk degeneration at L4-5 with a partial annular tear (arrow).* **Bottom left,** *Sagittal MRI showing black disk at L5-S1 with a complete annular cleft posteriorly (arrow).* **Bottom center,** *Diskogram at L3-4, L4-5 and L5-S1. The diskogram pattern is consistent with a normal disk at L3-4; abnormal disk at L4-5 (no pain) and abnormal disk at L5-S1 with familiar pain reproduction. Only L5-S1 was treated with ALIF (asterisk).* **Bottom right,** *Lateral radiograph depicting an ALIF at L5-S1 (the dots show the anterior and posterior limits of the autogenous corticocancellous bone graft).*

umn; (3) large surface area available for graft incorporation; (4) absence of complications related to the use of instrumentation; and (5) provision of a virgin site for arthrodesis in patients with previous posterior operations. The majority of the studies report pseudarthrosis rates ranging from 20% to 30%. The accepted fusion rates for one- and two-level anterior interbody fusion are 85% and 70%, respectively.[48]

Greenough and associates[39] reported on 150 patients who underwent ALIF for "intractable back pain." A solid bony fusion was attained in 76% of the patients. The clinical success rate was 68%. The noncompensation patients had higher return to work and higher clinical success rates than the compensation patients. Newman and Grinstead[47] reported on 36 patients who underwent ALIF for internal disk disruption. Twenty-eight of 36 patients had anterior surgery at a single level. Eight patients had two-level fusions. At follow-up, 89% of the patients had a solid arthrodesis and 86% had good/excellent outcomes. Fujimaki and associates[57] reported on 150 ALIFs performed primarily for diskogenic pain. The fusion rate in this series was 96%, with greater than 90% of the patients returning to work. Raugstad and associates[58] reported on 47 cases of ALIF for spondylolisthesis or degenerative disk disease. Their clinical success rate was 82%.

Blumenthal and associates[38] reported on 34 patients who underwent single level ALIF for diskogenic low back pain. The fusion rate in their series was 73%. Of the patients, 74% had good/excellent results at follow-up. Gill and Blumenthal[59] retrospectively assessed 53 patients who underwent ALIF at the lumbosacral junction. All patients had positive diskograms. However, the MRI was consistent with disk degeneration in only 39 of 53. Fourteen patients had normal MRI images. The authors reported a 75% success rate in the group of patients with positive MRI and diskography. The clinical success in the normal MRI and positive diskography patients was only 50%. Goldner and associates[60] reported on 100 patients who were similarly treated with ALIF for internal disk derangement. The clinical success rate in this series was 78%, with a 91% fusion rate. Knox and Chapman[40] reported on 22 patients who underwent ALIF for diskogram concordant low back pain. All two-level fusions had poor results, and only 35% of the single-level fusions did well. The overall failure rate in this series was 65%.

In summary, for appropriately selected patients, single-level ALIF for diskogenic pain is successful in approximately 70% to 75% of the patients. The pseudarthrosis rate for single level ALIF is higher than that for posterolateral fusion with instrumentation, PLIF, or global fusion.[37,48]

Posterior Lumbar Interbody Fusion

PLIF was introduced by Cloward in 1945. The technique involves a wide posterior decompression and complete disk excision by retraction of the dural sleeve and nerve roots. Through the posterior exposure, bone graft is placed anteriorly between the contiguous vertebral bodies.[61] The pseudarthrosis rate is reported to range from 6% to 27%.[48] Several modifications of the original technique have been described. It is recommended that posterior pedicular instrumentation be used as an adjunct to PLIF.[46] This may lower the pseudarthrosis rate and prevent graft dislodgement.

The proponents of PLIF suggest that the technique has the following advantages: (1) total excision of the source of pain, namely the intervertebral disk; (2) possible restoration of disk height with an anterior bone graft; (3) a biomechanical advantage in having the site of arthrodesis under compression along the anterior column; and (4) achievement of nerve root decompression.[29]

Disadvantages of PLIF include the following: (1) necessity of a wide, destabilizing posterior decompression; (2) risk of canal compromise from posterior extrusion of the graft; (3) risk of injury to the nerve roots, and postoperative epidural fibrosis due to wide decompression and significant retraction of the neural elements; and (4) destabilization of the anterior column by performing a radical diskectomy. Also, the posterior column is destabilized by a radical decompression.[29]

Wetzel and Larocca[44] reported on 12 patients with failed PLIF. They concluded that the extensive manipulation of the neural elements required during the surgery may result in chronic radiculopathy due to endoneural fibrosis. This radiculopathy may be a major symptomatic problem for which there is no solution. In addition, it is recommended that the three-column instability resulting from a PLIF be stabilized by the addition of instrumentation. Schechter and associates[62] reported on 25 patients who underwent single level PLIF for diskogram concordant diskogenic low back pain. They achieved good/excellent results in 89% of the patients, with an overall fusion rate of 95%. Lin and associates[63] reported on 46 patients with diskogenic back pain treated by PLIF. There were 89% good or excellent results. Collis[64] reported on 25 patients with internal disk derangement treated by PLIF. A 96% fusion rate and 100% satisfactory clinical outcome were reported by the authors. Another series of 62 patients with diskogenic low back pain treated with PLIFs was reported by Lee and associates.[42] All patients in this series had positive diskograms at the level involved. Satisfactory clinical outcome was observed in 89% of the patients. The fusion rate was 94%, with 82% of the patients returning to work at follow-up. Posterior instrumentation was not used in this series.

In summary, PLIF is a technically challenging surgical procedure that has a limited role, if any, in primary lumbar fusions for diskogenic pain. It may have a limited role in revision surgery in which standard intertransverse process fusion is associated with a higher pseudarthrosis rate. In this situation, PLIF may facilitate a combined anterior-posterior fusion through a single approach. PLIF also may be associated with lower morbidity compared to the two approaches needed for global fusions. Further prospective, randomized trials in which varying surgical techniques are compared may be needed to determine the definitive role of PLIF.

Combined Anterior-Posterior Fusions (Global Fusion)

This technique combines the two approaches of ALIF and posterolateral intertransverse process fusion. Pedicular instrumentation typically is recommended as an adjunct to the posterior fusion.[41,43] Proponents of global fusion report a low pseudarthrosis rate of 5% to 10% for one- and two-level fusions.[41,43,48] Retrospective studies indicate clinical success rates in the range of 75% to 85% in treating diskogenic pain.[41,43,65]

O'Brien and associates[43] reported on combined anterior-posterior fusions with instrumentation in 150 patients. The diagnoses included in this series were primarily failed back syndrome and diskogenic pain. Clinical improvement was reported in 86% of the patients. Kozak and O'Brien,[41] in another retrospective series, reported on 69 patients who underwent global fusions for internal disk derangement. This group included both primary and revision surgery patients. The authors reported a greater than 90% fusion rate for one- and two-level fusions. The fusion rate dropped to 77% for three-level fusions. Satisfactory clinical results were achieved in 80% of the patients. Clinical success was achieved in 77% of the revision surgery patients.

Linson and Williams[65] reported on 51 consecutive patients who underwent ALIF and global fusion for diskogenic pain. All patients had preoperative diskograms. The overall success rate for "achieving measurable diminution of preoperative pain" was 80%. The clinical success rate for patients with single-level disk degeneration, who were treated only with ALIF, was 78%. All patients who underwent global fusions had at least one previous failed lumbar surgery. The clinical success rate in this group was 69%. The authors also used ten control patients who met the criteria for surgery but did not undergo the operation. The clinical success rate in this nonsurgical group was only 10%.

Most proponents of global fusions recommend the addition of posterior instrumentation in compression. This instrumentation not only prevents anterior graft ejection, it may also lower the pseudarthrosis rate by applying compressive axial loads across the anterior graft and by stabilizing the involved motion segment.

In summary, global arthrodesis for diskogenic pain involves a radical diskectomy and may lower the pseudarthrosis rate to less than 5%. However, the added morbidity of the two surgical procedures must be justified by improved clinical results over standard posterolateral fusion techniques. For appropriately selected patients with diskogenic low back pain, clinical success rates for global fusions range from 80% to 90% in most retrospective series.

Complications of Spinal Instrumentation

The use of spinal instrumentation is associated with a steep learning curve and significant risks. It is associated with a higher rate of infection (3% to 6%), neurologic injury (1% to 5%), instrumentation failure (6% to 10%) and reoperation (20%) compared to in situ fusions.[66]

The cohort study sponsored by the North American Spine Society (NASS) for the use of pedicular instrumentation reported an overall complication rate of 5% related to the use of instrumentation.[66] The complication rate related to the use of instrumentation both in the cohort study and in the literature is given in Table 1.

Pedicular instrumentation should be used only by experienced surgeons who are well versed with the pitfalls associated with its use. Its occasional use in inexperienced hands may be associated with an unacceptably high complication rate.

Table 1 Complications related to the use of instrumentation

Complication	Cohort Study	Literature
Instrumentation failure	10%	6%
Pedicle fracture	1%	2%
Vascular injury	0.5%	—
Neurologic deficit	< 0.5%	5%
Infection	3%	6%
Reoperation rate	20%	—

Experimental Arthrodesis Techniques

In order to minimize the morbidity associated with anterior approaches for ALIF or global fusions, laparoscopic techniques are being explored for use by the spine surgeon. Laparoscopic ALIFs have been performed at the L5-S1 levels in small series.[67]

Metallic devices referred to as ''cages,'' filled with cancellous autograft, are being used for reconstruction of the anterior column following anterior diskectomy.[67] The theoretical advantages of ''cages'' include: (1) metallic structural support along the anterior column; (2) indirect decompression of the neuroforamina by insertion of a metallic distractor (cage) anteriorly; (3) eliminating the necessity of structural cortical autograft or allograft in order to maintain anterior column height; (4) potential for bony ingrowth across the porous, mesh-like ''cage'' walls; and (5) the ability to insert an autograft filled cage into the L5-S1 interspace via a laparoscope.

Regan and associates[67] reported on their initial experience with transperitoneal laparoscopic disketomy and fusion of the L5-S1 interspace. Twelve patients underwent anterior L5-S1 fusion for diskogram concordant idiopathic low back pain. Custom titanium cages filled with autograft were used anteriorly in eight of 12 patients. There were no major complications in this series.

Genetic engineering may play a significant role in future techniques of arthrodesis. Recombinant human bone morphogenetic protein (BMP) is capable of osteoinduction and has been used successfully in animal models. Boden and associates[68] reported on the use of BMP for posterolateral intertransverse process fusion in an animal model. The fusion rate was 100% in the animals arthrodesed with BMP compared to 42% in the autograft group. Biomechanical testing of segments arthrodesed with BMP revealed stiffer and stronger fusions than in the autograft animals. Current studies using BMP for ALIF in animal models are in progress. This may signal the beginning of the era of biologic spine fusion.

Summary

The treatment of chronic idiopathic low back pain is a tremendous challenge for the orthopaedic surgeon. The estimated direct and indirect costs of low back disorders exceed $50 billion per year.

Lumbar disk degeneration as visualized on MRI is physiologic and is a normal result of aging. Surgical treatment is rarely indicated for diskogenic pain.

Lumbar fusions across several motion segments for multilevel disk degeneration are associated with poor outcomes. The difficulty associated with the treatment of chronic diskogenic pain, lies in the identification of the true pain generator.

Anatomic studies have demonstrated that the outer third of the anulus fibrosus is richly innervated with free nerve endings. These are nociceptive and may respond to physiologic stimuli by painful efferent discharge. Diagnosis of disk degeneration on the basis of MRI alone is associated with a high false positive rate. In one study, greater than 30% of asymptomatic subjects were found to have significant disk abnormalities on MR images.

The only provocative in vivo test available for identification of the pain source is the diskogram. Its role, however, is quite controversial. The results of diskography are highly dependent on the technique employed and the subjective pain response of the patient. However, in the absence of other definitive tests for in vivo evaluation of diskogenic pain, the role of diskography is indispensable.

The natural history of diskogenic pain is relatively unknown. In some series, there has been 67% improvement in patients with untreated diskogenic pain at 5-year follow-up. A large percentage of patients who did not improve during the follow-up period had underlying psychiatric diagnoses. In reports of surgical treatment of chronic diskogenic pain there was clinical success in 60% to 90% of the patients. Therefore, further prospective, randomized trials comparing conservative and surgical treatment of diskogenic pain are needed in order to determine whether surgery can improve over the natural history of diskogenic pain.

The entity and symptom being treated in these patients is pain. The perception of pain differs from patient to patient and varies among different ethnic groups. Also, psychosocial factors and secondary gain issues, such as workers compensation and litigation, may alter a patient's pain perception and response to treatment. As such, these issues need to be resolved prior to surgical treatment of diskogenic pain. Patient selection is extremely important to prevent failures of surgical treatment.

The surgical treatment of diskogenic pain is arthrodesis across the involved motion segment. Arthrodesis may be accomplished by a wide variety of techniques including posterolateral fusion, ALIF, PLIF, and combined anterior-posterior fusion. The role of instrumentation as an adjunct to arthrodesis is controversial. Early trends from prospective, randomized trials suggest that it may lower the pseudarthrosis rate. It is very useful for multilevel fusions and in revision surgery. However, its use is associated with a higher complication rate than in situ fusions. Circumstances under which surgical treatment for chronic diskogenic pain may be recommended are given above.

At the time of this writing, bone screws placed posteriorly into vertebral elements have not been cleared for use in this specific manner by the Food and Drug Administration (FDA). These are Class III devices. This category includes screws placed transfacetally, within pedicles, or in articular, lateral masses. Some bone screws for use within the sacrum have been approved as Class II devices. Some companies have received Class II clearance for use of screws in lumbar pedicles specifically to supplement fusions in the treatment of grade III and IV spondylolisthesis with the proviso that these devices are removed after the arthrodesis has healed. Anterior vertebral body screws (cervical, thoracic, and lumbar) are Class II devices and can be used as labeled in vertebral bodies. Many of the posterior screw-based devices have been shown in laboratory and clinical testing to be useful and may be used in an off-label manner if the physician feels this is appropriate and important for the treatment of the patient. As with all surgeries, informed consent should explain the procedure and why a particular technique has been chosen, as well as its risks and benefits. The question of whether informed consent regarding pedicle screws must include a discussion of the device's FDA clearance status is currently being litigated in several jurisdictions. In cases that have been included in the multidistrict litigation in the Eastern District of Pennsylvania, this additional requirement has not been imposed.

References

1. Fischgrund JS, Montgomery DM: Diagnosis and treatment of discogenic low back pain. *Orthop Rev* 1993;22:311–318.
2. Frymoyer JW, Cats-Baril WL: An overview of the incidences and costs of low back pain. *Orthop Clin North Am* 1991;22:263–271.
3. Kelsey JL, White AA III: Epidemiology and impact of low-back pain. *Spine* 1980;5:133–142.
4. Hart LG, Deyo RA, Cherkin DC: Physician office visits for low back pain: Frequency, clinical evaluation, and treatment patterns from a U.S. national survey. *Spine* 1995;20:11–19.
5. Davis H: Increasing rates of cervical and lumbar spine surgery in the United States, 1979-1990. *Spine* 1994;19:1117–1124.
6. Cherkin DC, Deyo RA, Loeser JD, et al: An international comparison of back surgery rates. *Spine* 1994;19:1201–1206.
7. Turner JA, Ersek M, Herron L, et al: Patient outcomes after lumbar spinal fusions. *JAMA* 1992;268:907–911.
8. Boden SD, Davis DO, Dina TS, et al: Abnormal magnetic-resonance scans of the lumbar spine in asymptomatic subjects: A prospective investigation. *J Bone Joint Surg* 1990;72A:403–408.
9. Miller JA, Schmatz C, Schultz AB: Lumbar disc degeneration: Correlation with age, sex, and spine level in 600 autopsy specimens. *Spine* 1988;13:173–178.
10. Paajanen H, Erkintalo M, Kuusela T, et al: Magnetic resonance study of disc degeneration in young low-back pain patients. *Spine* 1989;14:982–985.
11. Hult L: Cervical, dorsal and lumbar spinal syndromes. *Acta Orthop Scand* 1954;17(suppl):1–102.
12. Buirski G: Magnetic resonance signal patterns of lumbar discs in patients with low back pain: A prospective study with discographic correlation. *Spine* 1992;17:1199–1204.
13. Malinsky J: The ontogenetic development of nerve terminations in the intervertebral discs of man. *Acta Anat* 1959;38:96–113.
14. McCarron RF, Wimpee MW, Hudkins PG, et al: The inflammatory effect of nucleus pulposus: A possible element in the pathogenesis of low back pain. *Spine* 1987;12:760–764.
15. Howe JF: A neurophysiological basis for the radicular pain of nerve root compression, in Bonica JJ, Liebeskind JC, Albe-Fessard D, et al (eds): *Advances in Pain Research and Therapy: Proceedings of the Second World Congress on Pain.* New York, NY, Raven Press, 1979, vol 3, pp 647–657.
16. Franson RC, Saal JS, Saal JA: Human disc phospholipase A2 is inflammatory. *Spine* 1992;17(suppl 6):S129–S132.
17. Saal JS, Franson RC, Dobrow R, et al: High levels of inflammatory phospholipase A2 activity in lumbar disc herniations. *Spine* 1990;15:674–678.
18. Simmons EH, Segil CM: An evaluation of discography in the localization of symptomatic levels in discogenic disease of the spine. *Clin Orthop* 1975;108:57–69.
19. Heggeness MH, Doherty BJ: Discography causes end plate deflection. *Spine* 1993;18:1050–1053.

20. Southwick SM, White AA: The use of psychological tests in the evaluation of low-back pain. *J Bone Joint Surg* 1983;65A:560–565.
21. Holt EP Jr: The question of lumbar discography. *J Bone Joint Surg* 1968;50A:720–726.
22. Colhoun E, McCall IW, Williams L, et al: Provocation discography as a guide to planning operations on the spine. *J Bone Joint Surg* 1988;70B:267–271.
23. Simmons JW, Aprill CN, Dwyer AP, et al: A reassessment of Holt's data on: "The question of lumbar discography." *Clin Orthop* 1988;237:120–124.
24. Walsh TR, Weinstein JN, Spratt KF, et al: Lumbar discography in normal subjects: A controlled, prospective study. *J Bone Joint Surg* 1990;72A:1081–1088.
25. Horton WC, Daftari TK: Which disc as visualized by magnetic resonance imaging is actually a source of pain? A correlation between magnetic resonance imaging and discography. *Spine* 1992;17(suppl 6):S164–S171.
26. Simmons JW, Emery SF, McMillin JN, et al: Awake discography: A comparison study with magnetic resonance imaging. *Spine* 1991;16(suppl 6):S216–S221.
27. Rask B, Dall BE: Use of the pantaloon cast for the selection of fusion candidates in the treatment of chronic low back pain. *Clin Orthop* 1993;288:148–157.
28. Ordeberg G, Enskog J, Sjostrom L: Diagnostic external fixation of the lumbar spine. *Acta Orthop Scand* 1993;251(suppl):94–96.
29. Herkowitz HN, Sidhu KS: Lumbar spine fusion in the treatment of degenerative conditions: Current indications and recommendations. *J Am Acad Orthop Surg* 1995;3:123–135.
30. Hanley EN Jr, Spengler DM, Wiesel S, et al: Controversies in low back pain: The surgical approach, in Schafer M (ed): *Instructional Course Lectures 43*. Rosemont, IL, American Academy of Orthopaedic Surgeons, 1994, pp 415–423.
31. Esses SI, Huler RJ: Indications for lumbar spine fusion in the adult. *Clin Orthop* 1992;279:87–100.
32. Leavitt F, Garron DC: The detection of psychological disturbance in patients with low back pain. *J Psychosom Res* 1979;23:149–154.
33. Polatin PB, Kinney RK, Gatchel RJ, et al: Psychiatric illness and chronic low-back pain: The mind and the spine. Which goes first? *Spine* 1993;18:66–71.
34. Bigos SJ, Battie MC, Spengler DM, et al: A prospective study of work perceptions and psychosocial factors affecting the report of back injury. *Spine* 1991;16:1–6.
35. Rhyne AL III, Smith S: Outcome of unoperated discogram positive low back pain. Proceedings of the American Academy of Orthopaedic Surgeons 62nd Annual Meeting, Orlando, Florida. Rosemont, IL, American Academy of Orthopaedic Surgeons, 1995, p 258.
36. Srdjan M: The role of surgery for nonradicular low-back pain. *Curr Opin Orthop* 1994;5:37–42.
37. Wood GW II, Boyd RJ, Carothers TA, et al: The effect of pedicle screw/plate fixation on lumbar/lumbosacral autogenous bone graft fusions in patients with degenerative disc disease. *Spine* 1995;20:819–830.
38. Blumenthal SL, Baker J, Dossett A, et al: The role of anterior lumbar fusion for internal disc disruption. *Spine* 1988;13:566–569.
39. Greenough CG, Taylor LJ, Fraser RD: Anterior lumbar fusion: A comparison of noncompensation patients with compensation patients. *Clin Orthop* 1994;300:30–37.
40. Knox BD, Chapman TM: Anterior lumbar interbody fusion for discogram concordant pain. *J Spinal Disord* 1993;6:242–244.
41. Kozak JA, O'Brien JP: Simultaneous combined anterior and posterior fusion: An independent analysis of a treatment for the disabled low-back pain patient. *Spine* 1990;15:322–328.
42. Lee CK, Vessa P, Lee JK: Chronic disabling low back pain syndrome caused by internal disc derangements: The results of disc excision and posterior lumbar interbody fusion. *Spine* 1995;20:356–361.
43. O'Brien JP, Dawson MH, Heard CW, et al: Simultaneous combined anterior and posterior fusion: A surgical solution for failed spinal surgery with a brief review of the first 150 patients. *Clin Orthop* 1986;203:191–195.

44. Wetzel FT, LaRocca H: The failed posterior lumbar interbody fusion. *Spine* 1991;167:839–845.

45. Weatherley CR, Prickett CF, O'Brien JP: Discogenic pain persisting despite solid posterior fusion. *J Bone Joint Surg* 1986;68B:142–143.

46. Steffee AD, Sitkowski DJ: Posterior lumbar interbody fusion and plates. *Clin Orthop* 1988;227:99–102.

47. Newman MH, Grinstead GL: Anterior lumbar interbody fusion for internal disc disruption. *Spine* 1992;17:831–833.

48. Steinmann JC, Herkowitz HN: Pseudarthrosis of the spine. *Clin Orthop* 1992;284:80–90.

49. Zdeblick TA: A prospective, randomized study of lumbar fusion: Preliminary results. *Spine* 1993;18:983–991.

50. Zucherman J, Hsu K, Picetti G III, et al: Clinical efficacy of spinal instrumentation in lumbar degenerative disc disease. *Spine* 1992;17:834–837.

51. Dawson EG, Lotysch M III, Urist MR: Intertransverse process lumbar arthrodesis with autogenous bone graft. *Clin Orthop* 1981;154:90–96.

52. Hellstadius A: Experiences gained from spondylosyndesis operations with H-shaped bone transplantations in the case of degeneration of discs in the lumbar back. *Acta Orthop Scand* 1955;24:207–215.

53. Shaw EG, Taylor JG: The results of lumbosacral fusion for low back pain. *J Bone Joint Surg* 1956;38B:485–497.

54. Lorenz M, Zindrick M, Schwaegler P, et al: A comparison of single-level fusions with and without hardware. *Spine* 1991;16(suppl 8):S455–S458.

55. Grubb SA, Lipscomb HJ: Results of lumbosacral fusion for degenerative disc disease with and without instrumentation: Two-to-five year follow-up. *Spine* 1992;17:349–355.

56. Temple HT, Kruse RW, van Dam BE: Lumbar and lumbosacral fusion using Steffee instrumentation. *Spine* 1994;19:537–541.

57. Fujimaki A, Crock HV, Bedbrook GM: The results of 150 anterior lumbar interbody fusion operations performed by two surgeons in Australia. *Clin Orthop* 1982;165:164–167.

58. Raugstad TS, Harbo K, Oogberg A, et al: Anterior interbody fusion of the lumbar spine. *Acta Orthop Scand* 1982;53:561–565.

59. Gill K, Blumenthal SL: Functional results after anterior lumbar fusion at L5-S1 in patients with normal and abnormal MRI scans. *Spine* 1992;17:940–942.

60. Goldner JL, Urbaniak JR, McCollum DE: Anterior disc excision and interbody spinal fusion for chronic low back pain. *Orthop Clin North Am* 1971;2:543–568.

61. Rish BL: A critique of posterior lumbar interbody fusion: 12 years' experience with 250 patients. *Surg Neurol* 1989;31:281–289.

62. Schechter AN, France MP, Lee CK: Painful internal disc derangements of the lumbosacral spine: Discographic diagnosis and treatment by posterior lumbar interbody fusion. *Orthopedics* 1991;14:447–451.

63. Lin PM, Cautilli RA, Joyce MF: Posterior lumbar interbody fusion. *Clin Orthop* 1983;180:154–168.

64. Collis JS: Total disc replacement: A modified posterior lumbar interbody fusion. Report of 750 cases. *Clin Orthop* 1985;193:64–67.

65. Linson MA, Williams H: Anterior and combined anteroposterior fusion for lumbar disc pain: A preliminary study. *Spine* 1991;16:143–145.

66. Yuan HA, Garfin SR, Dickman CA, et al: A historical cohort study of pedicle screw fixation in thoracic, lumbar, and sacral spinal fusions. *Spine* 1994;19(suppl 20):2279S–2296S.

67. Regan JJ, Guyer RD, McAfee P, et al: Early clinical results of laparoscopic fusion of the L5-S1 disc space. *Orthop Trans* 1995;19:776–777.

68. Boden SD, Schimandle JH, Hutton WC: Spine fusion with recombinant human bone morphogenic protein: Beginning the era of biologic spine fusion. Proceedings of the American Academy of Orthopaedic Surgeons 62nd Annual Meeting, Orlando, FL. Rosemont, IL, American Academy of Orthopaedic Surgeons, 1995, p 259.

Directions for Future Research

Identify factors that influence risk of idiopathic low back pain and, in particular, recurrent episodes and extended disability.

Epidemiologic studies of idiopathic low back pain have been hindered by the ill-defined nature of the condition, inaccurate measures of suspected risk factors, and inadequate control of potentially confounding factors. More large-scale, cross-sectional studies using similar methodology are unlikely to lead to significant advances in knowledge.

Instead, epidemiologic studies are needed that (1) provide clearer definitions of the outcome (for example, filing of a back injury claim, seeking medical care for recurrent back symptoms, persistent symptoms lasting longer than 3 months with associated functional impairment or work loss; (2) use reliable, validated measures of exposure; and (3) adequately control for potentially confounding factors.

Also, studies are needed to test the effects of interventions on recurrences and the development of long-term disability. Costs need to be included in the data collection and considered in the assessment of interventions.

Perform randomized controlled studies of the efficacy of different types of surgical treatment for "diskogenic" low back pain.

A variety of surgical procedures are currently used to treat "diskogenic" low back pain. None of these methods has a documented superior outcome. Further, the choice between procedures (if any) cannot be made based on solid scientific information.

Following an acceptable definition of diskogenic low back pain, a prospective, randomized study should compare the outcomes between posterolateral, anterior, and combined arthrodeses and an active standardized nonsurgical treatment program. Special effort should be made to precisely define the inclusion criteria. Patients with single level degenerative disk "disease" documented by magnetic resonance imaging (MRI) and with concordant pain on diskography should be classified by demographic, clinical, and psychological criteria and randomly assigned to the four treatment areas. Appropriate outcome measures should include physician and patient measure of pain and function, patient satisfaction assessment and overall health status, and a cost analysis. Patients should be followed for at least 3 to 5 years to determine the effect of treatment on rate of recurrence.

Establish the therapeutic utility of diagnostic tests commonly used in the investigation of idiopathic low back pain.

Many diagnostic procedures are used in an effort to determine an anatomic diagnosis of back pain of unknown origin, but the reliability and therapeutic utility of these procedures is unknown. What needs to be established for each of these procedures is whether the information obtained is reliable and whether performing the test makes any difference to eventual outcome of therapy.

Efficacy studies should be conducted on the commonly used diagnostic tests. If these studies vindicate the test, they should be followed by effectiveness studies that assess whether the reliability and utility are sustained when the tests are performed in conventional practice. High priority tests are computed tomography, MRI, bone scans, diskography, and diagnostic blocks.

Identify the important factors associated with clinical instability in low back pain.

Abnormalities of the lumbar spine are important in the etiology of low back pain. The clinical entity of instability is poorly understood and defined. Because the entities of acute and chronic instability differ, their definitions and measurement techniques also should differ.

Therefore, in order to study these phenomena, a checklist should be established and validated (a modification of the checklist of White and Panjabi, which includes chronic anatomic changes noted on radiographs and defined by computed tomography and MRI) for the assessment and quantitation of chronic instability. Factors, including the anatomic components of the spinal stabilizing system, should be identified that, when altered, lead to pain. These factors should be quantitated using: (1) the aforementioned checklist, (2) electrodiagnostic and other muscle function studies, (3) imaging techniques, and (4) intervertebral kinematic studies. Patients should be studied in longitudinal and interventional (prospective, randomized, controlled) manners, using these techniques.

Study the efficacy and cost implications of nonsurgical treatments for idiopathic low back pain.

There is a plethora of nonsurgical treatments currently used for patients with idiopathic low back pain. There exist few data to support the selection of any particular therapy for individual patients. There also are few data to support the dose, duration, or frequency and repetition of therapy to be given. Considerable variations in the use of nonsurgical therapies have been documented. Besides potential differences in patient outcomes, these differences in use of therapies are associated with significant differences in the cost of patient care.

Studies about the efficacy and cost implications of nonsurgical treatments for idiopathic low back pain are needed. Examples of therapies for which more study is needed include medications, prescribed exercises, passive modalities, physical agents, manual therapy, and patient education. Because of the variability in the course of idiopathic low back pain, such efficacy studies should be randomized clinical trials. In the design of such trials, the following issues deserve attention: the enrollment of a well-defined patient population; the comparison of well-described therapies, including where feasible a placebo control; the use of clinically relevant outcome measures such as pain, functional status, and patient satisfaction; the measurement of such outcomes in an appropriate fashion (either by a blinded observer or the use of patient self-reports); and the costs, both direct and indirect, of therapy. Frequently, practitioners choose to provide multiple therapies or combinations of therapies to idiopathic low back pain patients. Investigators interested in studying multiple therapies should consider a factorial design to allow for the evaluation of each therapy independently. Investigators should be aware of the obstacles to the successful completion of such studies. These include the loss to follow-up of enrolled subjects, the use of cointerventions by subjects, and lack of subject compliance with assigned therapy.

Section Four

Basic and Applied Science Issues of Idiopathic Low Back Pain

Section Editor:
Joseph A. Buckwalter, MS, MD

Shirley Ayad, BSc, PhD
Michael T. Bayliss, PhD
John M. Cavanaugh, MS, MD
Christopher H. Evans, PhD
Robert J. Foster, ScD
James C. Iatridis, PhD
Brian Johnstone, PhD
James D. Kang, MD

Martin Krag, MD
James Martin, PhD
Van C. Mow, PhD
Theodore R. Oegema, Jr, PhD
Linda J. Sandell, PhD
Lori A. Setton, PhD
Mark Weidenbaum, MD

Overview

One of the critical unanswered questions concerning idiopathic low back pain is: Does age-related intervertebral disk degeneration cause pain? All disks undergo significant age-related changes and some disks in some individuals degenerate; that is, they undergo progressive alterations in structure and composition that lead to almost complete loss of disk function. Although disk aging and disk degeneration overlap, there also appear to be distinctions between these processes. Understanding these distinctions and the potential role of disk degeneration in idiopathic low back pain requires in-depth understanding of disk structure, composition, nutrition, cell and matrix biology, and mechanical function. In addition, it is necessary to understand the innervation of the spine, mechanical and biochemical changes in the intervertebral disk that may cause pain, and the relationships between animal models of disk degeneration and the degenerative process seen in human disks.

Human intervertebral disks consist of an outer anulus fibrosus and a central nucleus pulposus. The anulus consists of peripheral concentric rings of collagen lamellae and a larger inner area of fibrocartilage. The nucleus pulposus occupies the most central area of the disk and is separated from the inner fibrocartilaginous region of the anulus fibrosus by a narrow transition zone. In intervertebral disks of newborns and infants, the nucleus contains notochordal cells. During growth and development, these cells disappear and are replaced by a population of connective tissue cells. Anulus fibrosus cell populations include cells that appear to have primarily a fibroblastic phenotype as well as cells that have a more chondrocytic phenotype.

Collagens account for approximately 50% to 60% of the dry weight of the anulus fibrosus, 15% to 20% of the dry weight of the nucleus pulposus, and 50% to 70% of the cartilage end plate. In the anulus, the concentration of type I collagen decreases from approximately 80% of the total collagen in the outermost region to less than 1% in the nucleus. Over the same interval, the concentration of type II collagen increases from less than 1% to approximately 80% of the total collagen. The anulus also contains small amounts of collagen types III, V, IV, and VII. Type VI collagen makes up approximately 10% of the anulus fibrosus collagen. Type II collagen makes up approximately 80% of the total collagen of the nucleus. This tissue also contains small amounts of types III, IV, and VII collagen, and 15% to 20% of the total collagen of the nucleus is type VI collagen.

The contribution of proteoglycans to adult disk dry weight increases from about 10% to 20% in the outer regions of the anulus to approximately 50% in the central regions of the nucleus. Large aggregating proteoglycans contribute to disk stiffness in compression. The disk also contains a population of large nonaggregating proteoglycans and several small proteoglycans that appear to be involved in matrix organization and cell-matrix interactions. These small proteoglycans may also bind growth factors. Multiple noncollagenous proteins within the matrix of the intervertebral disk appear to help organize and stabilize the matrix and influence cell function. Throughout life the anulus is roughly

60% to 70% water, whereas the water concentration in the nucleus declines from approximately 80% to 90% at birth to approximately 70% in adults.

The innervation of the intervertebral disk is limited to the periphery. The annular surface has both simple free and encapsulated nerve endings, whereas small nerve fibers and free nerve endings penetrate the most superficial layers of the anulus. Nerves have not been seen in the more central disk regions. Facet joint capsules are richly innervated and nerve endings are also found within spinal ligaments. At this time the relationship between deformation of the intervertebral disk and stimulation of these nerves is uncertain. It is clear that a variety of chemicals, including hydrogen ions, adenosine triphosphate, excitatory amino acids, bradykinin, serotonin, histamine, prostaglandins, leukotrienes, and nitric oxide, can excite or sensitize nerve endings. There may be other mediators as well. Some of these mediators may be released from degenerating disks.

The mechanical behavior of the intervertebral disk is complex. The normal nucleus pulposus appears to function predominantly as a fluid under static loading conditions. The swelling pressure resulting from the high concentration of proteoglycans in the nucleus and inner anulus helps maintain disk height and contributes to the pressurization mechanism of load support and load transfer. The relatively high hydraulic permeability of the cartilage end plates serves to transfer loads in a uniform manner across the anulus fibrosus and nucleus pulposus. The high values for tensile modular stiffness and failure stress of the normal anulus fibrosus in the circumferential direction indicate that the anulus is well suited to resist large tensile stresses. In particular, the outer lamellar region of the anulus fibrosus, the region with the highest tensile modulus, is ideally suited to minimizing intervertebral disk bulging and anulus fibrosus strains generated during compression, bending, or torsional loading. Experimental measurements of the surface strain of the outer anulus indicate that the extension of the fibers and circumferential strain are relatively small (less than 5%), suggesting that the high tensile modulus of the outer anulus helps limit deformation of the tissue. In contrast, the lower modulus of the inner anulus may permit larger deformations in response to applied loadings. The elevated deformations in the inner anulus will give rise to viscoelastic dissipation through a fluid-dependent mechanism. This viscoelastic dissipation in the inner anulus fibrosus along with significant flow-independent dissipation resulting from deformations of the nucleus appear to be the dominant mechanisms for energy dissipation and shock absorption in the intervertebral disk.

The disk cells receive nutrition from two sources: blood vessels that lie on the surface of the anulus and occasionally penetrate a short distance into the outer layers of the anulus, and blood vessels within the vertebral bodies that lie against the cartilage end plates. The diffusion of nutrients and metabolites across the cartilage end plates appears to be the most important source of nutrition for the central disk. The large size of the disk and lack of a vascular supply leads to relatively high lactate concentrations and low pH in the central regions of the disk. With increasing age, there is a decline in the number of arterioles supplying the periphery of the disk and calcification or mineralization of the end plates. These changes may further compromise nutrition of the central disk, leading to a rising lactate concentration and a falling pH, factors that can compromise cell synthetic function and promote the production of free radicals and other mediators.

With aging of the human intervertebral disk, along with the decline in central disk nutrition, there is a progressive loss of notochordal cells and an apparent decrease in the concentration of viable connective tissue cells in the inner anulus and nucleus pulposus. In addition, water and proteoglycan concentrations decrease, the synthesis of collagens and proteoglycans may decrease, and there may be increased proteinase and free radical activity. Morphologic studies show accumulation of dense matrix material that may represent degraded matrix molecules. At the same time there is increased posttranslational modification of matrix proteins. A combination of these events, including declining disk nutrition, loss of proteoglycan organization and concentration, decline in cell numerical density and synthetic activity, and increased degradative enzyme activity relative to matrix synthesis, may lead to the loss of disk structure and function recognized as disk degeneration.

There are two basic types of animal models of disk degeneration: spontaneous disk degeneration and induced degeneration of normal disks. The animal models of spontaneous disk degeneration include the sand rat, the pin tail mouse, Chinese hamsters, and certain dogs and baboons. The sand rat develops spontaneous cysts and tears in the anulus, degeneration of the facet joint, and herniation of the nucleus pulposus. This animal model of spontaneous disk degeneration has been the most extensively studied. Models of induced degeneration have included disruption of the anulus fibrosus, facetectomy, forelimb amputations, repetitive electrical stimulation of muscles, and whole body vibration. Models that involve disruption of the outer anulus fibrosus have been the most extensively studied and appear to produce a process that resembles human disk degeneration in rabbits, dogs, monkeys, sheep, pigs, and goats.

Based on the available information, it appears that disk degeneration may contribute to low back pain through two mechanisms. First, significant loss of disk structure and function may alter loading of vertebral bodies, facet joints, muscles, and spinal ligaments, and thus cause pain due to alteration of the loads on these tissues and induction of degenerative changes in the facet joints. Second, disk degeneration may be associated with the release of cytokines, free radicals, prostaglandins, matrix degradation products, and other mediators that may sensitize nociceptive nerve endings. Important areas for future investigation include defining the cellular, biochemical, and mechanical events that lead to disk degeneration, developing and refining animal models that will allow investigation of specific aspects and mechanisms of disk degeneration, further characterization of the roles of the various populations of disk cells in maintaining and possibly repairing the disk, determining if disk cells and degenerating disk matrix may produce mediators with nociceptive effects, determining the role of alterations in disk nutrition on disk function, and clarifying the relationships between disk degeneration and low back pain.

Chapter 29
Animal Models for Human Disk Degeneration

Martin Krag, MD

Disk degeneration in humans is a widespread phenomenon that is at least closely related to, if not the proximate cause of, a variety of clinical problems that result in substantial pain and suffering and increased health care costs. The way in which this process develops and its exact interrelationship to these clinical problems (its pathophysiology) is not clearly understood.

Relevant to this understanding are a number of animal studies in which a naturally occurring process appears similar to that of disk degeneration or in which such a process is artificially produced. These studies are summarized below.

Naturally Occurring Disk Changes

Sand Rat

Using the sand rat (*Psammomys obesus*) as a model, Silberberg and associates[1] and Adler and associates[2] first described the spontaneous appearance of a high incidence of disk changes that appear very similar to those that occur in humans. The histologic changes in 39 animals from 2 to 30 months of age were described. The thoracic disks and vertebrae, knee joints, femoral heads, and sections of the tail were studied. At 2 months, the disks and vertebral bodies were fully developed. At 3 months, a few areas of vertebral growth plate cartilage degeneration had developed. At 6 months, these areas were more extensive. The nucleus pulposus (NP) in some animals had granular debris; the anulus fibrosus (AF) in others had less regularly oriented fiber bundles than in younger animals, and in one animal a small tear was seen. At 18 months, no further changes relative to 6 months were seen in the disk, although vertebral changes had progressed and facet joint degeneration was first noted. AF cysts, tears, and occasional bony bars were seen more frequently in the 18- to 30-month-old animals. There were NP herniations, which were sometimes quite large, into and through the AF or end plates, end plate spurring, and more extensive facet joint changes.

The sand rat is indigenous to eastern Mediterranean deserts and its natural diet is largely a high salt content shrub. According to Silberberg and associates,[1,2] this low water, high salt diet may somehow be related to altered metabolism, which is somehow related to abnormal function of the disk, especially of the NP. They point out that the sequence of disk changes seems to occur from

479

"inside out," that is, the NP changes develop first, facet changes come later, and end plate spurring occurs only after herniations develop. Silberberg[3] described the more rapid onset of these changes in sand rats fed a low fiber diet, previously noted to induce diabetes.

Moskowitz and associates[4] further studied the sand rat, fed a normal diet, by including radiographs along with histologic assessment, study of the lumbar as well as the thoracic spine, and measurements of serum glucose and insulin. Degeneration was seen radiographically in 10% of the 3-month-old and 50% of the 18-month-old animals. In addition, calcifications in the anterior longitudinal ligament were seen in some of the older animals. No hip or knee joint changes were seen. There was no correlation between glucose or insulin levels and degree of degeneration (although all the animals were maintained on a diet equivalent to the natural one, so a large spectrum of values was not seen). A preliminary study of breeding pairs that had early onset of degeneration resulted in offspring with even earlier onset, suggesting a strong hereditary component.

Ziv and associates[5] studied young healthy, old healthy, and young diabetic sand rats. Their measures included hydration, fixed charge density (FCD), and swelling pressure (assessed by hydration after equilibration in vitro with either 15 or 25 g% polyethylene glycol). Relative to the values in young healthy animals, all three of these measures were reduced in the disks of young diabetic rats and to a lesser extent in old healthy rats. No changes in hydration or FCD were seen in paraspinal muscle or vertebral cancellous bone. Even in the young healthy animals, the hydration and FCD values were 30% to 50% lower than in the common laboratory rat.

Ziran and associates[6] added biomechanical measures to study of the (nondiabetic) sand rat. The specimens used were functional spinal units with posterior elements removed. The measures used were peak force and force decay (1 versus 500 s) in response to a flexion-producing step displacement of the test machine crosshead. No statistically significant correlation was seen between these measures and radiographic or histologic measures in specimens from 3-, 9-, 15-, or 18-month-old animals. Nonetheless, a trend was noted toward a parabolic relation between peak force and radiographic grade.

Other Animals

Spontaneous onset of disk degeneration has been described in other animals as well. The pintail mouse (pBr strain mutated by exposure to methylcholanthrene) was studied by Berry.[7] Beginning at the age of 3 weeks, the NP in the subcervical disks underwent changes similar in appearance to those in humans (loss of mucopolysaccharides, assessed by increased ability for methylene blue staining to be cleared by methylsalicylate). This tendency was moderate in heterozygotes and very strong in mutant homozygotes. Based on this, it is believed that disk degeneration in humans also may be genetic. In contrast to the NP, there were no abnormalities noted in differentiation of the AF, although ossification adjacent to the end plate "sometimes occurred." Mason and Palfrey[8] described in detail a mutant mouse strain (BDL ky/ky) that has a high incidence of spontaneous development of disk degeneration and posterior herniation (20%). However, also occurring were kyphoscoliosis (the reason this strain was initially of interest), vertebral body wedging, end plate destruction, and spinal cord cystic lesions.

Praomys natalensis, a wild African rodent intermediate in size between the mouse and rat (and initially studied because of its high incidence of stomach cancer), was noted by Sokoloff and Stewart[9] also to have a high incidence of disk degeneration. The histologic appearance of 154 spines from animals 8 to 35 months of age was described. Degeneration was present in the majority of animals 9 months of age and older. For all age groups together, disk protrusions were present in 12% of the females and 52% of the males. Other abnormalities were also more common in males than in females. End plate osteophytes were uncommon. Aseptic necrosis of the vertebral secondary ossification centers and severe osteoarthritic changes in many diathrodial joints (especially elbow and knee) were seen in addition to disk changes. The osteoarthritic changes were not gender specific, and age-specific data were not given.

The Chinese hamster (*Cricetulus griseus*), noted to frequently develop diabetes, was studied by Silberberg and Gerritsen[10] to see if these animals developed the same ''hyperostotic spondylosis,'' which occurs more commonly in humans with diabetes than in those without. Histologic evaluations were performed on 43 animals with and 36 animals without diabetes. The former showed a higher incidence of spondylosis (60% versus 39% in the animals without diabetes) but, surprisingly, a lower incidence of disk herniation (9% versus 30%). Both spondylosis and disk degeneration increased with age.

The spontaneous development of disk degeneration in the dog was extensively described and the previous literature reviewed by Hansen.[11-13] He reviewed the canine disk structure and its susceptibility to herniation, both in certain chondrodystrophoid breeds (for example, bassett hound, beagle, and dachshund) and in others. Typically by 1 year of age, the NP becomes occupied by chondrocytes with a matrix containing an increased collagen content and decreased proteoglycan (PG) and water content. This matrix may become calcified after disk herniation, unlike the human disk. Ghosh and associates[14] have reviewed the variation in both collagenous and noncollagenous proteins with age, spinal level, and breed, both for chondrodystrophoid and nonchondrodystrophoid breeds. King and Smith[15] provided a useful comparison between dog and human disks, including the topic of degeneration.

A series of 645 dogs with disk herniations was reviewed by Goggin and associates.[16] Breed, gender, age at onset of herniation, and vertebral level involved were compared with a control population. The relative risk of disk herniation compared to the control group was 12.6 for dachshunds, 10.3 for Pekingese, 6.4 for beagles, and 2.6 for cocker spaniels.

Beagle disks from 30 animals of various ages were studied by Gillett and associates[17] radiographically, histologically, and in response to compressive loads. The histologic and mechanical age-related changes preceded the radiographic ones. In all three areas, the changes were similar to those reported by others to occur in humans.

The baboon (*Papio cynocephalus anubis*) recently was studied by Lauerman and associates.[18] A radiographic survey of the thoracic and lumbar spines of 126 normal adult baboons (age 6 to 30 years) in a large captive colony was performed. A highly statistically significant correlation was seen between age and both disk degeneration grade (Spearman correlation coefficient of 0.726, $p <$

0.0001) as well as kyphosis angle (coefficient of 0.633, $p < 0.0001$). A comparative analysis of humans was not presented.

Artificially Produced Disk Changes

Anterior Annulotomy

Rabbits The earliest work in this area was in the 1930s. Lob[19] apparently was the first to report experimental anterior disruption of an animal disk (study of posterior annulotomies in dogs and monkeys was reported 1 year earlier by Keyes and Compere,[20] as will be described). He noted after an anterior incision in the disk that disk degeneration gradually developed, similarly to that which occurs in humans, based on radiographic and unaided visual inspection. Filippi[21] added microscopic examination at various times after transversely sectioning the anterior portion of the AF. He described repair of the lesion, present partially at 40 days and fully at 100 days. However, such full healing has not been shown by any of the subsequent studies, beginning with the work of Key and Ford[22] on posterior annulotomies in dogs.

Smith and Walmsley[23] performed a similar study, prompted by the superficiality of healing seen after posterior annulotomy in the dog disk.[22] Fifty-five immature adult rabbits were grossly and microscopically examined at times ranging from 1 to 25 months after ventral annulotomy (transverse, mid-disk, 4-mm long, through the AF and into the NP) of a single lumbar disk. Ventral NP herniation occurred in all animals. The main findings were that (1) healing occurred only in the outermost portion of the lesion, and (2) progressive degeneration occurred throughout the disk, even though the lesion was only in the anterior part of the AF.

In 1970, Haimovici[24] used this experimental method to investigate the effect of repeated intramuscular injection of adrenocorticotropic hormone (ACTH), which was a treatment earlier reported to be useful for human disk herniations. An annulotomy similar to that of Smith and Walmsley was used, although the incision was longer (15 to 20 mm). ACTH was injected every second day for 1 month and every third day for another month. Gross, microscopic, and radiographic examinations were performed at 13, 26, 39, and 55 days. The changes seen by Smith and Walmsley were confirmed, and ACTH had no effect (although Higuchi and Abe[25] did note ultrastructural changes in the NP of otherwise intact mouse disks after repeated intramuscular hydrocortisone injections).

Ten years later, Lipson and Muir[26,27] first applied biochemical analyses to this line of investigation. In addition to a full-thickness stab through the anterior part of the AF (2 mm in length, similar to but shorter than that of Smith and Walmsley), they also studied a superficial scratch on its anterior surface. White New Zealand rabbits weighing 2.5 kg were examined at various times up to 6 months. From each animal, the NP and the anterior AF of intact disks and the central region of the lesioned disks were removed and analyzed. Biochemical measures included analysis of PG, water, and hyaluronic acid (HA) concentration as well as PG monomer size and percent aggregated PG relative to total PG content. Rabbit disks were similar to human disks in some measures (for example, similar water concentration and PG size) and different in others (for example, smaller HA concentration and percent aggregated PG). Gradual decreases developed over 12 months in all measures except PG size, after larger transient changes in the first few days or weeks. These changes were similar in many respects to the changes seen in disk degeneration in humans. No effect was seen from the scratch on the anterior anulus.

Urayama[28] focused on the topographic distribution of postannulotomy changes within the AF after an annulotomy of rabbit disks like that of Lipson and Muir.[26] Each AF was separated into nine specimens: outer, intermediate, and inner layers of each of the anterior, lateral, and posterior regions. At various times up to 32 weeks after surgery, specimens were examined by light microscopy, electron microscopy, and autoradiography. Relative to control disks, the greatest changes in the AF were in its inner layer, even more for light than for electron microscopic measures.

Sheep Because of their hypothesis that a peripheral "rim lesion" is an initiator of disk degeneration from "outside in" (Vernon-Roberts and Pirie[29] and Hilton and Ball[30]), Osti and associates[31] studied an only partial thickness anterior annulotomy. The annulotomy was 5 mm in depth, while the average full depth of AF was 7.5 mm. The annulotomy length was 5 mm at the surface. In contrast to the annulotomy used in previous work on rabbits, this one did not produce an immediate NP herniation. Surgery was performed on 2-year-old Merino sheep, which were then studied histologically at various times up to 18 months. By 1 to 2 months, fibrous healing developed in the peripheral but not (then or subsequently) in the inner portions of the annulotomy. By 4 to 6 months, disruption of the inner portion of the AF was seen along with degeneration and tracking of the NP along the annulotomy. Also, increased end plate ossification was seen in some disks. By 6 to 8 months, there was decreased disk height (often accompanied by increased end plate ossification) and some osteophyte formation. By 18 months, many of these changes were seen in all specimens. The magnitude of end plate changes was proportionate to the amount of disk height decrease and osteophyte development. Overall, the results were interpreted to support the "outside in" view of disk degeneration (in contrast to the "inside out" view that NP changes occur first, followed by secondary AF changes).

Further work[32] from the same laboratory dealt with end plate vascularity changes, using the same experimental method. The stab annulotomy was made a few millimeters off the midline, just below the cranial end plate and to the left in each of three randomly selected lumbar disks in each of 31 sheep that were 2 years of age. Disks from each animal were examined at 1 to 2, 4 to 12, or 18 to 24 months after surgery. Parasagittal slices of functional spine units were prepared (three slices across the left half and three across the right half of each specimen). The slice containing the lesion (cut slice), the corresponding slice on the opposite side (opposite slice), the corresponding slice at an adjacent control level (adjacent level control slice), and slices from control animals that had not undergone surgery (nonop control slice) were examined histologically.

The major findings were as follows: (1) In all slices, the vascularity was greater adjacent to the NP than to the anterior or posterior AF. (2) The cranial end plates were similar to the caudal end plates in all groups, even though the cuts were closer to the former. (3) The cut slices showed greater vascularity than did the control disks that had not undergone surgery, more so at 1 to 2 months than at later times. (4) The cut slices showed greater vascularity than did the opposite slices at all times. The first finding is consistent with the situation in humans, in spite of the fact that sheep are quadrupedal while humans are bipedal. The second finding shows that the effects of the cut are not strictly localized. The third and fourth findings show the reaction to the cut includes an increased vascularity. An unexpected additional result was that the cut slice was not different than the adjacent level control slice. Whether the changes in adjacent disks were produced by the presence of the cut itself (as the authors speculate) or by some other factor involved in the performance of the surgical procedure is not clear (no sham operation group was included in the study).

In a third study, Melrose and associates[33] investigated the biochemical changes resulting from this experimental method at 2, 4, 6, 8, 12, and 18 months after annulotomy of the L4-5 disk. The AF and NP from the cut and the uncut sides were analyzed separately. Analyses included water, collagen, and noncollagen protein content as well as PG content, extractability, aggregation, and size.

The major findings were as follows: (1) In the NP of the cut disks, there was an initial loss of PG aggregation, which recovered to normal by 8 months, by which time there was loss of PG and collagen content. (2) Also in the NP of the cut disks, there was an increase in noncollagen protein, a sizable portion of which derived from the serum. (3) In the adjacent, uncut disks, the NP showed loss of collagen and PG, although the AF was unchanged. As in the previous study, changes induced by the localized annulotomy occurred not only in the injured AF but also in the NP, and not only in the disk operated on but also in adjacent disks. As in the previous study, a sham surgery group was not included.

In a fourth study from this laboratory, Latham and associates[34] studied the biomechanical changes produced by this experimental method. The sheep were grouped into those with an annulotomy and those with sham surgery. Within each group, disks were tested either immediately or at 6 months. The annulotomies were along the lateral aspect of L2-3 and L4-5 and were each 4 mm deep and 10 mm long. Each L4-5 annulotomy was also spanned by a longitudinal metal plate, attached by two screws to each of the L4 and L5 vertebrae. Subject disks were tested with the plate (if present), with the plate removed, then again with the posterior elements removed. Test loads were anteriorly and posteriorly offset compressive forces and a pure moment about the longitudinal axis. Histologic examination of disks and facet joints was also performed.

The major results were that the annulotomy caused an initial drop in disk torsional stiffness, followed by a return toward normal at 6 months. The presence of the metal plate significantly increased the flexion and extension stiffness initially but not at 6 months. The (intact) L2-3 disks were not altered by the annulotomy initially, but were less stiff at 6 months. All incised disks showed changes at 6 months that were indicative of degeneration. The presence of a plate did not markedly reduce this histologic change, but did seem to reduce facet degeneration and did improve the mechanical recovery. Latham and associates[34] interpreted this as supporting the concept that healing of a naturally occurring annular tear may be improved by limiting disk motion.

Pigs Somewhat in parallel with these studies on sheep and prompted by the same view that disk degeneration may well be from outside in, Kääpä and associates[35,36] studied domestic pigs (*Sus scrofa*, aged 1 to 1.5 years and weighing 100 to 150 kg). Their lesion was a stab to a depth of 13 mm with a #11 scalpel blade, located not anterolaterally but at the midline anteriorly. In both studies, analyses were performed at 3 months after surgery. The first of these studies deals with collagen and the second with PG analyses.

In the first study,[35] the disk was divided into seven slices from front to back, each of which was analyzed for total collagen (hydroxyproline, Hyp), two key enzymes for collagen synthesis (prolyl 4-hydroxylase, PH, and galactosylhy-droxylysyl glucosyltransferase, GGT), and collagen cross-links (HP, hydroxy-pyridinium). In all the lesioned disks, degeneration of both the NP and AF had occurred. In the NP, Hyp concentration was increased, PH and GGT activity was increased, and water content was decreased. In the anterior portions of the AF, HP was decreased, while in the posterior portions there was no change. In the control disks, PH and GGT activity was significantly higher in the anterior relative to the posterior portions of the AF, and the HP value in humans is substantially higher than in the pig.

In the second study,[36] which focused on PG analyses, the disk was divided into 11 slices, each of which was analyzed for PG content and size distribution of its monomers, DNA, organic and inorganic ^{35}S, hexosamines, ratio of chondroitin 4-sulfate to chondroitin 6-sulfate, and ratio of chondroitin sulfate to keratan sulfate. A general decrease in inorganic ^{35}S was believed to indicate decreased solute transport, possibly from end plate ossification or disk stiffening from osteophytes. Organic ^{35}S was also decreased. DNA was increased in the anterior AF and in the NP, and this increase was thought to be from an increased number of cells, probably fibroblasts. A decrease in PG, seen also in humans with disk degeneration, was believed to be caused by either increased synthesis or decreased breakdown. The disk above the injured one (the L3-4) showed no changes except for a slight increase in ^{35}S, the cause of which is not clear.

A comparison of different procedures performed on the lumbar disks of Göttingen minipigs (age 2 to 3 years, weight 20 to 30 kg) was carried out by Pfeiffer and associates.[37] The procedures were as follows: (1) a somewhat more extensive annulotomy than that performed by Osti and associates;[31] (2) cutting of a window in the AF anterolaterally and removal of the NP using surgical rongeurs; (3) same as number 2 plus injection of HA and placement of a fibrin glue plug in the opening created; and (4) injection of chymopapain. Intradiskal pressure (IDP), assessed by peak and relaxation values, was measured before each procedure. Radiographs and histology were performed at 0, 3, 6, 12, and 24 weeks after surgery. After all four procedures, IDP approximately equaled one third of the preoperative value at 3 weeks and two thirds of it at later times. Also for all groups, degeneration was well developed by 3 weeks and progressed slightly later on. The results from group 3 were interpreted as showing some healing (fewer necrotic areas, more chondrocytes per cell cluster, slightly less loss of NP size and IDP).

Other Animals Apparently the earliest report of experimental annulotomy to produce disk degeneration is that of Keyes and Compere.[20] They viewed disk degeneration in humans as an ''inside out'' process, evidenced by their statement of intent to reproduce ''. . . the pathological conditions which clinically have been thought to be due to injuries or disease of the nucleus pulposus. . .''.[20] Although the bulk of their report dealt with human clinical and cadaveric disk specimens, they successfully studied 16 dogs and 2 monkeys, which had had one each of three different disk lesions performed. After annulotomy and NP curettage, the end plates developed osteophytes and marked sclerosis. After placement of a small drill hole obliquely through the vertebral body and central end plate into the NP, "cartilage nodules" were found similar to those "described by Schmorl." Finally, after a chisel cut extending from the vertebral body through the end plate, changes similar to those seen in humans with disk degeneration were regularly produced.

Also studying dogs, Hampton and associates[38] compared the gross and microscopic appearance of disks at 3, 6, 9, and 12 weeks after performing four different interventions (one on each of four adjacent lumbar disks): (1) removal of a 3 × 5 mm full thickness block of anulus, down to the NP; (2) same as number 1 plus removal of the NP; (3) same as number 2 plus curettage of the end plates; and (4) a stab wound through the AF, 5 mm long at the surface. Subsequent examinations showed that the cavity formed by interventions numbers 1, 2, and 3 was "filled with a large mass of fibrous tissue," whereas for number 4, the stab wound tracts showed no evidence of healing except for a small cap at the surface. These findings were interpreted to support concern that a spontaneously occurring fissure in the AF, similar to the stab wound, may not heal sufficiently to prevent "leakage of nuclear irritants." Hampton and associates[38] conjecture that this may be a model for "internal disk disruption."

A similar study was performed on goats.[39] The three interventions were also through the AF into the NP: (1) a 2.5 × 2.5 mm block; (2) a 2.5 mm × 2.5 mm cruciate stab with a #69 Beaver scalpel blade; and (3) a stab wound with a sharp-tipped 2.5 mm diameter trocar. Histologic appearance and strength of healing were examined. The latter was measured by the force needed to pull a 1.8 mm diameter sphere through the AF at the intervention site and also by the torsional stiffness of the disk (after posterior element removal). By pull-through testing, the trocar site was seen to be the strongest at 4 weeks but only equal to the others at 8 and 12 weeks. By torsion testing (both for peak angle and stiffness), there were no differences between the groups at any time, except that the stiffness at 4 weeks in group 1 was lower than that in the other two groups. Ethier and associates[39] concluded that these results argue for careful performance of surgery to minimize AF injury.

Posterior Annulotomy

Key and Ford[22] produced four different types of lesions in the posterior aspect of four lumbar disks in 14 adult dogs: (1) a small annular window and vigorous curettage of the NP and cartilage end plate; (2) same as number 1 but without disruption of the cartilage end plate; (3) a transverse annulotomy into the NP, approximately half the canal diameter in length; and (4) insertion and removal of a 20-gauge needle through the AF into the NP. Each animal was studied at a time between 2 days and 28 weeks after surgery.

The first two types of lesions resulted in disk changes similar to those seen in humans. The annulotomy occasionally resulted in a "well-developed rupture" of the NP. The absence of complete healing of the deep part of the annulotomy was also noted. This was in contrast to the results of Filippi[21] who had described healing of both the superficial and the deep parts of the annulotomy. Earlier authors[19,20] had not mentioned the topic of annulotomy healing. Finally, the 20-gauge needle puncture resulted in a NP herniation in 1 of 14 disks, which led to careful needle placement during lumbar punctures.

Some 40 years after Key and Ford's study, experimentally puncturing through the posterolateral AF was revisited.[40,41] Nguyen and associates[40] describe the method: creation percutaneously in dogs of either a "diskotomy" or a "diskectomy" through the AF just lateral to a lumbar pedicle. The former was done by cutting a cylindrical hole through the AF with a trephine (diameter and insertion depth not specified), the latter by also using a "nucleotome" (Surgical Dynamics Inc, Sunnyvale CA) to remove some of the central NP (amount not specified).

On magnetic resonance images (MRI) scans of ten disks (apparently, since the actual number is not clear), an unspecified number showed decreased T1-weighted signal intensity in adjacent bone marrow, one developed a NP herniation, and five showed a decreased disk height and increased T2-weighted signal intensity. No histologic assessment was reported. Although this work was undertaken in an effort to develop an experimental method for producing disk degeneration, this did not occur in four of the ten disks. This work was also performed in order to develop a method that was more consistent and produced less mortality and morbidity than did anterolateral annulotomy; however, no comparison was provided between that method and the author's method.

Sether and associates[41] described the MRI and the gross morphologic appearance of 15 disks that had undergone the "diskectomy" procedure (as well as disks from three dogs that had had acute NP herniations). Five types of MRI images (plus a sixth type for chondrodystrophoid calcification) are described; however, no validation of these types is provided.

Alteration of Annulotomy Healing

In addition to extensive studies of the effects of disk annulotomy, work from two different laboratories also includes studies of the effects of intervention to alter the subsequent healing process. The first of these, by Waters and Lipson,[42] involves the use of spinous process pins and polymethylmethacrylate to immobilize rabbit disks after anterior annulotomy. This treatment produced a substantial reduction in subsequent disk changes at 6 and 12 weeks. The authors[42] showed that this reduction did occur if the immobilization was begun at 1 or 2 days after the annulotomy, but did not occur if begun at 3, 5, 7, or 14 days after.

Parallel studies were done by Latham and associates[34] and Moore and associates[43] using anterior plating in sheep across one of two nonadjacent lumbar disks that had undergone partial thickness annulotomy. The former study deals with the biomechanical results and was previously described. The latter study deals with the histologic results. Although the hypothesis was that annulotomy healing would be improved and degeneration-like changes reduced in the plated disks, this in fact was not seen. According to these authors, the amount of immobilization was not sufficient or movement may not be the crucial factor in determining the reaction after annulotomy. The related earlier work of Waters and Lipson[42] showed opposite results.

Facetectomy

Sullivan and associates,[44] studying the lumbar spine of immature white rabbits, resected the inferior articular process on one side at one vertebral level and on the opposite side at the adjacent level. In 14 of their 39 animals, they also intraoperatively "... rotated the spine forcefully at the operated level...". Radiography (including diskography) and analysis of gross and microscopic morphology were performed at 2 weeks and 1, 2, 4, 6, 9, and 12 months.

Disk height was decreased at the surgical level in 50% of the disks at 6 months and 74% at 12 months. However, this decrease also was seen in 46% of the adjacent disks, which had not undergone surgery at 9 to 12 months (unfortunately, no nonsurgical or sham surgery controls were included). There was no difference between the 14 forcefully rotated and the 25 other animals. The disks in the transverse plane at 9 to 12 months showed thinning of the posterior AF, circumferential slits in the peripheral AF (possibly artefacts), and an increased area and decreased organization of the NP. The facet joints opposite to those operated on began to show degeneration at 6 months. These results support the authors' belief that "the main role of the posterior facet joint is to protect the disk against rotational stresses...".[44]

Cauchoix and associates[45] used a variation of this experimental method: they resected both "articular joints" at the same lumbar level. Disk narrowing and osteophytes gradually developed, and histology at 12 weeks after surgery showed substantial degeneration-like changes.

Stokes and associates,[46] interested in the mechanical and chemical changes from this experimental technique, performed resection of the entire facet joint (not just the inferior articular process). This was done on opposite sides, in some animals at adjacent levels and in others at the same level. A sham surgery group was included. Also, some animals were allowed high activity after surgery but others only low activity. Animals were studied at 2 weeks and 1, 6, and 12 months after surgery. An initial increase in flexibility was followed by a return toward normal, which was more rapid in the high than in the low activity group. No significant chemical (hexosamine, hydroxyproline) or morphologic changes were seen, in contrast to the two previous studies. The basis for this difference is not clear.

Forelimb Amputations (Bipedal Quadripeds)

Goff and Landmesser,[47] interested in developing a method for studying disorders of posture and building upon the previous work of Colton[48] and others, described the changes in bone dimensions, gait, and certain behavioral features in the Wistar rat and DBA strains of mice after neonatal midhumeral surgical amputations.

This work sparked interest in the following few years in using this method for the experimental production of disk degeneration.[49-52] For example, Yamada[52] describes work on 62 rats and 53 mice. Postural changes included reduction of the usual lumbar kyphosis, sometimes even reversal to lordosis. Changes in both the AF and NP gradually developed during 3 to 12 months and became even more conspicuous later on. Disk herniations developed in some of the bipedal but in none of the control animals.

Gloobe and Nathan[53] measured the distribution in normal and bipedal rats of vertebral osteophytes at various times up to 18 months. The incidence increased with age and was highest in the upper cervical and thoracic as well as thoracolumbar regions, but was higher in the bipedal than in the normal rats.

The electron (as well as light) microscopic changes in the NP of bipedal mice were described by Higuchi and associates.[54] Animals were examined at 3, 6, and 12 months. The disks in bipedal animals changed over time in a way similar to but more rapid than in normal animals (for example, 3 month bipedal resembled 6 month normal disks, 6 month bipedal resembled 12 month normal). By 12 months, "frequent" NP herniations were present.

Cassidy and associates[55] were primarily interested in vertebral and muscle changes in the lumbosacral region of bipedal rats. However, they also observed large disk herniations, all at the lumbosacral level, in five of 21 animals for a 24% incidence. They noted three other studies[49,50,52] to show a combined incidence of 32%, similar to their own results.

Other Interventions

Bercovici and Paraschivesco[56] injected hyaluronidase into the disks of dogs. The changes produced in some respects mimicked those that occur during disk degeneration.

Lindblom[57,58] bent the tails of rats into a "U" shape and maintained this either constantly or 12 hours per day for times from 2 weeks to 14 months then released the bend for times from 0 to 7 months. Degeneration of the AF did occur on the compression but not the tension side of the AF. Within the NP, increased cell vacuolization occurred.

A somewhat related although more indirect technique was used by Neufeld.[59] He attempted to produce increased lumbar lordosis, similar to that believed to be present in bipedal rats, by causing rats to ambulate along the inside surface of a fairly small diameter cylinder. At onset of the study (duration up to 5 months) the Sprague-Dawley rats were 5 months old. The results were conflicting: at about 1 month, disk height was decreased by radiography but increased by histology. At 3 and 5 months, this radiographic change was less than at 1 month.

Repetitive electrical stimulation of muscle contraction was used by Wada and associates[60] to try to produce spondylosis in the cervical spine of rabbits. They used five stimuli/minute over 10 hours for 0, 15, 30, and 60 days (the latter equivalent to about 200,000 cycles). This resulted in mild osteophytosis and extensive AF delamination by 60 days (although not by 15 or 30 days) but no changes in the NP. This result can be interpreted as supporting the idea that disk degeneration in humans develops primarily from "outside in" and not primarily from NP changes.

Exposure of rabbits to whole body vibration (4 Hz, 0.2 g, 3 hr/d, 5 d/wk) was investigated by Pedrini-Mille and associates.[61] Anterior annulotomy was performed on some lumbar disks and not others. A sham surgery group was included. Measured at 6 and 12 weeks were hexuronate (related to PG content), hydroxyproline (to estimate collagen content), and collagen hydroxylysinopyridinoline cross-links. Between vibrated and nonvibrated animals, there were no differences in any of these measures for the intact disks and no significant differences in hydroxyproline or cross-link concentration for the annulotomized disks. However, there was a greater hexuronate content for the annulotomized disks in the vibrated animals at both 6 and 12 weeks. The significance of this observation is not clear, although the authors conjecture that it may indicate an acceleration of degeneration after annulotomy.

Conclusion

Many methods have been applied to the development of experimental models of disk degeneration in humans. One can try to compare them based on how well they mimic human disk degeneration, but there are no agreed-upon parameters for doing so. Naturally occurring models have the drawback that the basis for the high rate of disk degeneration is not known. Although the interventions in artificial models are known, the relations of these to the true events leading to disk degeneration in humans are not. In any case, the usefulness of a particular model derives not from the extent to which it mimics reality (because that cannot be known in advance), but rather from the extent to which it facilitates the formulation and subsequent testing of hypotheses that lead to an improved understanding of that reality. Finally, it is not the model that should be viewed as having been "proven" or "validated," but rather the hypotheses that may arise from it.

Acknowledgment

This work was supported by the National Institutes of Health (grant # 8 RO1 AR44119-02) and the National Institute on Diseases Rehabilitation and Research (grant # USDE H133E30014). The authors gratefully acknowledge the assistance of Ms. Karen W. Gendron in manuscript preparation.

References

1. Silberberg R, Aufdermaur M, Adler JH: Degeneration of the intervertebral disks and spondylosis in aging sand rats. *Arch Pathol Lab Med* 1979;103:231–235.
2. Adler JH, Schoenbaum M, Silberberg R: Early onset of disk degeneration and spondylosis in sand rats (Psammomys obesus). *Vet Pathol* 1983;20:13–22.
3. Silberberg R: The vertebral column of diabetic sand rats (Psammomys obesus). *Exp Cell Biol* 1988;56:217–220.
4. Moskowitz RW, Ziv I, Denko CW, et al: Spondylosis in sand rats: A model of intervertebral disc degeneration and hyperostosis. *J Orthop Res* 1990;8:401–411.
5. Ziv I, Moskowitz RW, Kraise I, et al: Physicochemical properties of the aging and diabetic sand rat intervertebral disc. *J Orthop Res* 1992;10:205–210.
6. Ziran BH, Pineda S, Pokharna H, et al: Biomechanical, radiologic, and histopathologic correlations in the pathogenesis of experimental intervertebral disc disease. *Spine* 1994;19:2159–2163.
7. Berry RJ: Genetically controlled degeneration of the nucleus pulposus in the mouse. *J Bone Joint Surg* 1961;43B:387–393.
8. Mason RM, Palfrey AJ: Intervertebral disc degeneration in adult mice with hereditary kyphoscoliosis. *J Orthop Res* 1984;2:333–338.
9. Sokoloff L, Snell KC, Stewart HL: Degenerative joint disease in Praomys (Mastomys) natalensis. *Ann Rheum Dis* 1967;26:146–154.
10. Silberberg R, Gerritsen G: Aging changes in intervertebral discs and spondylosis in Chinese hamsters. *Diabetes* 1976;25:477–483.
11. Hansen H-J: A pathologic-anatomical interpretation of disc degeneration in dogs. *Acta Orthop Scand* 1951;20:280–293.
12. Hansen H-J: A pathologic-anatomical study on disc degeneration in dog: With special reference to the so-called enchondrosis intervertebralis. *Acta Orthop Scand Suppl* 1952;11:1–117.
13. Hansen H-J: Comparative views on the pathology of disc degeneration in animals. *Lab Invest* 1959;8:1242–1265.

14. Ghosh P, Taylor TK, Braund KG, et al: The collagenous and non-collagenous protein of the canine intervertebral disc and their variation with age, spinal level and breed. *Gerontology* 1976;22:124–134.
15. King AS, Smith RN: Comparison of the intervertebral disc in dog and man. *Vet Rec* 1955;67:135–149.
16. Goggin JE, Li AS, Franti CE: Canine intervertebral disk disease: Characterization by age, sex, breed, and anatomic site of involvement. *Am J Vet Res* 1970;31:1687–1692.
17. Gillett NA, Gerlach R, Cassidy JJ, et al: Age-related changes in the beagle spine. *Acta Orthop Scand* 1988;59:503–507.
18. Lauerman WC, Platenberg RC, Cain JE, et al: Age-related disk degeneration: Preliminary report of a naturally occurring baboon model. *J Spinal Disord* 1992;5:170–174.
19. Lob A: Die Zusammenhänge zwischen den Verletzungen der Bandscheiben und der Spondylosis deformans im Tierversuch. *Deut Ztschr Chir* 1933;240:421–440.
20. Keyes DC, Compere EL: The normal and pathological physiology of the nucleus pulposus of the intervertebral disc: An anatomical, clinical, and experimental study. *J Bone Joint Surg* 1932;14:897–938.
21. Filippi A: La guarigióne del disco intervertebrale dopo asportazione del nucleus pulposus negli animali da esperimento. *Chir Organi Mov* 1935;20:1–9.
22. Key JA, Ford LT: Experimental intervertebral-disc lesions. *J Bone Joint Surg* 1948;30A:621–630.
23. Smith JW, Walmsley R: Experimental incision of the intervertebral disc. *J Bone Joint Surg* 1951;33B:612–625.
24. Haimovici EH: Experimental disc lesion in rabbits: The effect of repeated ACTH administration. *Acta Orthop Scand* 1970;41:505–521.
25. Higuchi M, Abe K: Ultrastructure of the nucleus pulposus in the intervertebral disc after systemic administration of hydrocortisone in mice. *Spine* 1985;10:638–643.
26. Lipson SJ, Muir H: Vertebral osteophyte formation in experimental disc degeneration: Morphologic and proteoglycan changes over time. *Arthritis Rheum* 1980;23:319–324.
27. Lipson SJ, Muir H: Proteoglycans in experimental intervertebral disc degeneration. *Spine* 1981;6:194–210.
28. Urayama S: Histological and ultrastructural study of degeneration of the lumbar intervertebral disc in the rabbit following nucleotomy, with special reference to the topographical distribution pattern of the degeneration. *Nippon Seikeigeka Gakkai Zasshi* 1986;60:649–662.
29. Vernon-Roberts B, Pirie CJ: Degenerative changes in the intervertebral discs of the lumbar spine and their sequelae. *Rheumatol Rehab* 1977;16:13–21.
30. Hilton RC, Ball J: Vertebral rim lesions in the dorsolumbar spine. *Ann Rheum Dis* 1984;43:302–307.
31. Osti OL, Vernon-Roberts B, Fraser RD: Anulus tears and intervertebral disc degeneration: An experimental study using an animal model. *Spine* 1990;15:762–767.
32. Moore RJ, Osti OL, Vernon-Roberts B, et al: Changes in end plate vascularity after an outer anulus tear in the sheep. *Spine* 1992;17:874–878.
33. Melrose J, Ghosh P, Taylor TKF, et al: A longitudinal study of the matrix changes induced in the intervertebral disc by surgical damage to the anulus fibrosus. *J Orthop Res* 1992;10:665–676.
34. Latham JM, Pearcy MJ, Costi JJ, et al: Mechanical consequences of anular tears and subsequent intervertebral disc degeneration. *Clin Biomech* 1994;9:211–219.
35. Kääpä E, Holm S, Han X, et al: Collagens in the injured porcine intervertebral disc. *J Orthop Res* 1994;12:93–102.
36. Kääpä E, Holm S, Inkinen R, et al: Proteoglycan chemistry in experimentally injured porcine intervertebral disk. *J Spinal Disord* 1994;7:296–306.
37. Pfeiffer M, Griss P, Franke P, et al: Degeneration model of the porcine lumbar motion segment: Effects of various intradiscal procedures. *Eur Spine J* 1994;3:8–16.

491

38. Hampton D, Laros G, McCarron R, et al: Healing potential of the anulus fibrosus. *Spine* 1989;14:398–401.

39. Ethier DB, Cain JE, Yaszemski MJ, et al: The influence of anulotomy selection on disc competence: A radiographic, biomechanical, and histologic analysis. *Spine* 1994;19:2071–2076.

40. Nguyen CM, Haughton VM, Ho KC, et al: A model for studying intervertebral disc degeneration with magnetic resonance and a nucleotome. *Invest Radiol* 1989;24:407–409.

41. Sether LA, Nguyen C, Yu SN, et al: Canine intervertebral disks: Correlation of anatomy and MR imaging. *Radiology* 1990;175:207–211.

42. Waters PM, Lipson SJ: Modification of the degenerative response in experimental intervertebral disk herniation in rabbits. *J Spinal Disord* 1988;1:81–85.

43. Moore RJ, Latham JM, Vernon-Roberts B, et al: Does plate fixation prevent disc degeneration after a lateral anulus tear? *Spine* 1994;19:2787–2790.

44. Sullivan JD, Farfan HF, Kahn DS: Pathologic changes with intervertebral joint rotational instability in the rabbit. *Can J Surg* 1971;14:71–79.

45. Cauchoix J, El Yaacoubi M, Garcia-Romero C, et al: An experimental model of lumbar degenerated disc in rabbits. *Orthop Trans* 1984;8:431.

46. Stokes IA, Counts DF, Frymoyer JW: Experimental instability in the rabbit lumbar spine. *Spine* 1989;14:68–72.

47. Goff CW, Landmesser W: Bipedal rats and mice: Laboratory animals for orthopaedic research. *J Bone Joint Surg* 1957;39A:616–622.

48. Colton HS: How bipedal habit affects the bones of the hind legs of the albino rat. *J Exp Zool* 1929;53:1–11.

49. Sato Y: Studies on deformation of the spinal column in bipedal mice. *Shikoku Acta Med* 1959;15:1888–1890.

50. Ushikubo S: Study of intervertebral disc herniation in "Bipedal rat." *Shikoku Acta Med* 1959;15:1759–1780.

51. Yamada K, Sakamoto K, Ushikubo S, et al: Study of intervertebral disc herniation in bipedal rats. *Tokushima J Exp Med* 1960;7:93–103.

52. Yamada K: The dynamics of experimental posture: Experimental study of intervertebral disk herniation in bipedal animals. *Clin Orthop* 1962;25:20–31.

53. Gloobe H, Nathan H: Osteophyte formation in experimental bipedal rats. *J Comp Pathol* 1973;83:133–141.

54. Higuchi M, Abe K, Kaneda K: Changes in the nucleus pulposus of the intervertebral disc in bipedal mice: A light and electron microscopic study. *Clin Orthop* 1983;175:251–257.

55. Cassidy JD, Yong-Hing K, Kirkaldy-Willis WH, et al: A study of the effects of bipedism and upright posture on the lumbosacral spine and paravertebral muscles of the Wistar rat. *Spine* 1988;13:301–308.

56. Bercovici S, Paraschivesco E: Recherche experimentale sur la discopathie vertebrale degenerative. *Rev Rheum* 1958;25:487–499.

57. Lindblom K: Experimental ruptures of intervertebral discs in rats' tails: A preliminary report. *J Bone Joint Surg* 1952;34A:123–128.

58. Lindblom K: Intervertebral-disc degeneration considered as a pressure atrophy. *J Bone Joint Surg* 1957;39A:933–945.

59. Neufeld JH: Induced narrowing and back adaptation of lumbar intervertebral discs in biomechanically stressed rats. *Spine* 1992;17:811–816.

60. Wada E, Ebara S, Saito S, et al: Experimental spondylosis in the rabbit spine: Overuse could accelerate the spondylosis. *Spine* 1992;17(suppl 3):S1–S6.

61. Pedrini-Mille A, Weinstein JN, Found EM, et al: Stimulation of dorsal root ganglia and degradation of rabbit anulus fibrosus. *Spine* 1990;15:1252–1256.

Chapter 30

Proteoglycans of the Intervertebral Disk

Brian Johnstone, PhD
Michael T. Bayliss, PhD

Introduction

The functional properties of the tissues that make up the intervertebral disk depend largely on the structure of their extracellular matrices. Therefore, knowledge of the content, organization, and interactions of the molecules within these matrices is vital in order to characterize disk pathology and determine etiology. Apart from water, the major extracellular components of disk tissues are proteoglycans, collagens, and noncollagenous proteins. Recent general reviews of disk biochemistry covering all these components are available.[1,2] This chapter will concentrate on what is known about the biochemistry of disk proteoglycans, and the changes found with age, topography, and pathology.

Proteoglycans are a family of glycoproteins with a specialized type of glycosylation: they consist of a protein core to which is attached at least one glycosaminoglycan chain. They are found intracellularly, associated with the cell surface and in the extracellular matrix of all tissues studied. In the cartilaginous tissues of the spine, such as the intervertebral disk and the facet joints, only the extracellular proteoglycans have been studied. Extracellular proteoglycans play a role in many matrix functions. Large extracellular proteoglycans are one of the major structural components of the intervertebral disk, and their concentration and organization have considerable influence on its mechanical properties. The hydrophilic nature of these molecules allows the disk to hold water and withstand compressive loads. The cells of the disk are dependent on the water compartment that these proteoglycans maintain: it facilitates the supply of nutrients, chemical messengers, and hormones, and the clearance of waste products.

Proteoglycans are also involved in the organization of the collagens of the disk. Several proteoglycans, members of the "small" proteoglycan subfamily, have been shown to bind collagens and influence their fibril formation. The interactions of proteoglycans and collagens are very important for maintaining the organization of the extracellular matrix. It has also been shown that certain proteoglycans can bind growth factors, providing a mechanism for their extracellular storage. Growth factor binding to cell-associated proteoglycans appears to be an important step in the presentation of the factors to their cellular receptors. Proteoglycans are also important in both cell-cell and cell-matrix interactions, providing important links between the cell and its surrounding environment. The following sections specifically detail what is known about proteoglycans in the intervertebral disk.

Disk Proteoglycan Metabolism

Proteoglycans are constantly being turned over in the extracellular matrix of connective tissues. Turnover in the disk is slow, but without replacement the proteoglycan content would decrease and the disk's mechanical function would be impaired. The integrity of the disk, therefore, depends largely on the viability of its cells. However, the proteoglycan content of the human disk decreases markedly with age and also in degenerative conditions such as spondylolisthesis.[3] It is not known if this change in composition is the result of an increase in the rate of proteoglycan degradation or a decrease in the rate of synthesis. A better understanding of the mechanisms by which the cells synthesize and degrade the extracellular matrix may make it possible to differentiate between the normal aging process and pathologic degeneration of the disk.

The Effect of Hydration on Proteoglycan Synthesis

In earlier studies of various animal species, disk proteoglycan synthesis rates were calculated from the results of in vivo tracer tests.[4-7] However, values for human disks were always extrapolated from the in vitro values obtained for articular cartilage,[8] because of the problems associated with in vitro culture of disk tissues. When placed in aqueous medium, disk explants swell rapidly and lose proteoglycans;[9] thus, the concentration of proteoglycans around the cells decreases both through dilution and loss. Because proteoglycan synthesis rates measured in cell cultures[10,11] are influenced by the proteoglycan concentration, the rates measured in such an in vitro system will not reflect the synthesis rates that occur in vivo. Thus, in vitro methods for measuring proteoglycan synthesis in articular cartilage cannot be applied directly to slices of intervertebral disk.

Bayliss and associates[12] developed a culture system that limited the swelling and matrix loss from disk explants by balancing the potential swelling pressure of the proteoglycans in disk slices with the osmotic properties of polyethylene glycol included in the culture medium. This culture method provided the opportunity to examine the effects of hydration, and hence of changes in the pericellular environment, on the production of matrix macromolecules. Because the hydration of the disk varies during daily activity, such studies have physiologic significance. For rabbit, dog, and human explants, the rate of proteoglycan synthesis was greatest when the tissue was maintained at its in vivo hydration.[12,13]

Alterations in the ionic environment of articular cartilage have been shown to modulate the rate of proteoglycan synthesis and may also, in part, account for the effect of hydration on the metabolic activity of the disk.[14] The polyelectrolyte properties of proteoglycans control ionic concentrations through the Gibbs-Donnan equilibrium. An increase in proteoglycan concentration will cause an increase in cation concentration and a corresponding decrease in anion concentration. Furthermore, proteoglycans contribute to the steric exclusion of solutes from matrices; this effect is particularly marked for large solutes such as serum albumin, but even glucose is partly excluded from the normal disk.[15,16] Thus, changes in proteoglycan concentration will influence the concentration of nutrients and will certainly influence the manner in which newly synthesized proteoglycans can move through the matrix. Changes in hydration will also affect the thickness and shape of the tissue and, therefore, may alter the concentration of rapidly used metabolites such as oxygen.[17] The changes may also influence the shape of cells, which is known to modulate the biosynthesis of matrix macromolecules. Whether the changes in rate are in response to any or all of these alterations in the matrix is not known; they may result from a direct response to proteoglycan or hyaluronan concentration through cell surface receptors.

Proteoglycan Synthesis in the Human Disk: Variation With Age, Region, and Pathology

The average rate of synthesis in the adult human normal anulus is very low[13] and is only one third of that for adult articular cartilage (3 to 4×10^{-6} mmol/h/g and 9 to 11×10^{-6} mmol/h/g dry weight, respectively). Fetal and newborn nucleus pulposus have rates that are two to three times higher than the anulus from the same disk, whereas synthesis rates for adult anulus are five times less than those for immature anulus. Although these rates are directly comparable, they may not be a true reflection of the in vivo rates because the disks used were collected 18 to 24 hours postmortem. The period of time between death and in vitro incubation and the conditions of storage were shown to influence the measured rates of synthesis.[13]

There is considerable variation in the biosynthetic activity of cells in different regions of the disk. Rate measurement (Fig. 1) and autoradiographic studies indicated that the cells most actively synthesizing proteoglycan in the adult human disk are those in the midanulus region. Recently, Puustjärvi and associates[18] used a modified version of the polyethylene glycol culture method coupled with autoradiography to label slices of adult beagle disks and also found the incorporation highest in the midanulus. However, autoradiography of the human disk slices revealed that the most active cells in fetal disks are those in the inner regions of the anulus and nucleus.[13] This distribution of synthetic activity in immature disks was previously found in microautoradiographic studies of labeled immature rabbit disks,[19] and is in agreement with data from more recent studies that determined synthetic rates in young porcine and bovine disks, using either osmotic pressure or mechanical loading to counteract the disk's swelling pressure.[20,21] Why the distribution of proteoglycan synthesis should be different in adult disks is not known. It is clear, however, that the maximum biosynthetic activity in the midregion of the anulus is not directly related to cell number, hydration, or proteoglycan content. It is possible that the zone of active cells redistributes as the disk grows, or it could be that there is a change in the activity of chondrocytes in different regions in response to the age-related altered biomechanical loading of the adult disk.

The measurement of proteoglycan synthesis rates could be considered a useful tool for examining the contribution of proteoglycans to disk pathology. However, because of the heterogeneity of the disease processes and also the problems encountered in defining the biologic stage of disk degeneration, results of this kind of study have to be interpreted with caution. The rationale for measuring proteoglycan synthesis rates in pathologic disks is based on the assumption that cells in the diseased tissue will attempt to repair a defective matrix. Table 1 shows the results of our study on proteoglycan synthesis rates in anulus sections from disks of various pathologies. One appreciable difference is the much lower synthesis rate measured in the anterior anulus of L5-S1 spondylolisthetic disks, compared with rates from other disk disorders. This is not nec-

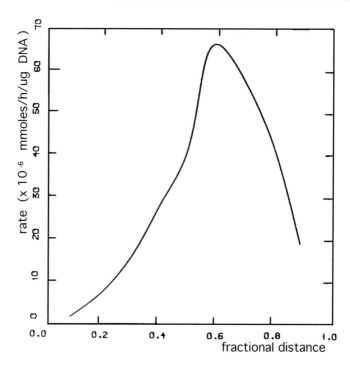

Fig. 1 *Variation in the rate of proteoglycan synthesis across the anterior anulus of a normal 32-year-old human disk at in vivo hydration. (Reproduced with permission from Bayliss MT, Johnstone B, O'Brien JP: Proteoglycan synthesis in the human intervertebral disc: Variation with age, region and pathology.* Spine *1988;13:972–981.)*

Table 1 Comparison of proteoglycan synthesis rates between adult disks of different pathologies for the L4-5 and L5-S1 spinal levels*

Pathology	L4-5	L5-S1
Spondylolisthesis	3.4 ± 1.8 (22)	0.8 ± 0.4 (11)
Posterior annular tear	4.8 ± 2.1 (11)	3.0 ± 1.6 (9)
Idiopathic low back pain	5.2 ± 2.9 (14)	4.8 ± 1.5 (11)

*The rates given are means ± standard deviations, with the number of measured disks in parentheses

essarily the expected result if one considers that evidence from work on cartilage indicates that the onset of degenerative conditions stimulates the synthetic activity of chondrocytes, presumably in an attempt at repair.[22,23] Because spondylolisthesis affects the anterior anulus from its onset, a stimulation of synthesis might be expected. However, it has also been shown that proteoglycan synthesis is decreased in the later stages of both cartilage[24] and disk degeneration.[23] Because disk degeneration is often rapid and severe in cases of spondylolisthesis,[25] it is possible that degeneration of the L5-S1 disks had already occurred. However, the anulus from L4-5 disks with the same clinically defined grade of degeneration had incorporation rates in the same range as the other groups studied. Perhaps the different mechanical forces acting on level L5-S1 have a greater effect on the biologic activity of these disks, causing them to degenerate faster. This is an important distinction; it cannot be assumed that there is a direct correlation between clinical assessment and biologic activity.

Disk Proteoglycan Structure

Large Interstitial Proteoglycans

Several studies have shown that the major large proteoglycan of the disk resembles aggrecan, the large proteoglycan of articular cartilage.[1,2] Aggrecan contains a large core protein of over 200,000 molecular weight, with three globular domains (termed G1, G2, G3). The N-terminal G1 is the hyaluronan binding domain. The chondroitin sulfate and keratan sulfate chains are attached mainly to a long linear region of the core protein between the G2 and G3 domains. No specific function has yet been ascribed to the G2 and G3 globular domains. The large proteoglycans of the disk have similar chondroitin sulfate-rich and keratan sulfate-rich domains to aggrecan and also possess the specific N-terminal globular region of the protein core (G1), which enables them to form large aggregates with hyaluronan and link protein.

Differences have been observed in the composition, molecular dimensions, and functional properties (aggregation) of large disk proteoglycans, depending on the topographic location and age of the specimen from which they were extracted. For example, keratan sulfate concentration is always greater in the nucleus than the anulus; in fact, its concentration in the adult nucleus pulposus is the highest found in any connective tissue.[26-28] The proportion of keratan sulfate relative to chondroitin sulfate increases with age in both cartilage and the intervertebral disk, but at all ages studied it is higher in the disk.[2] In addition, the molecular weight of the disk keratan sulfate chain is two to three times greater than that of articular cartilage. The functional significance of these differences is not known.

Aging and Biosynthesis The proportion of large proteoglycans that do not have the capability to aggregate with hyaluronan increases as a function of time in both articular cartilage and the intervertebral disk, but the proportion is always greater in the disk at any age, and increases to much higher levels than are ever seen in cartilage (Fig. 2). It is generally accepted that many of the changes in aggrecan structure are a consequence of enzymatic cleavage in the extracellular matrix and thus, the high content of nonaggregating, large proteoglycan in the disk represents turnover products that accumulate because of the relatively long pathway for diffusion that exists in the tissue. It is not known, however, what effect changes in the pattern of synthesis have on proteoglycan composition and structure.

Such changes are hard to discern within a population that includes the pool of accumulated large proteoglycan degradation products, the proportion of which increases with age. The answer is to study the structure of newly synthesized proteoglycans. In vivo data on the structure of newly synthesized proteoglycans in the disk has been obtained for some animal species.[4-7] In vitro studies are

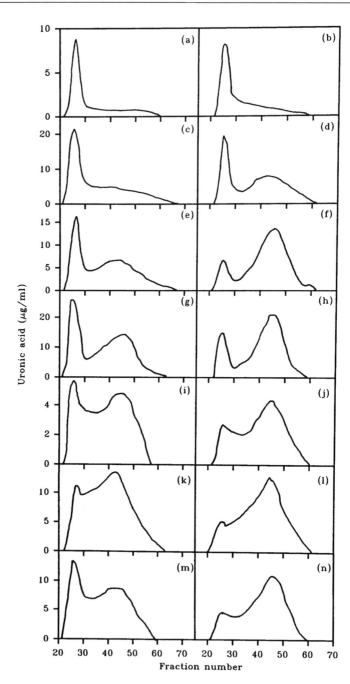

Fig. 2 *Sepharose CL-2B elution profiles of A1 fraction proteoglycans from the extracts of anulus fibrosus (left panels) and nucleus pulposus (right panels) of ages (a,b) fetal, (c,d) 15-month, (e,f) 9 years, (g,h) 20 years, (i,j) 38 years, (k,l) 48 years, and (m,n) 60 years. (Reproduced with permission from Johnstone B, Bayliss MT: The large proteoglycans of the human intervertebral disc: Changes in their biosynthesis and structure with age, topography, and pathology.* Spine *1995;20:674–684.)*

necessary for the study of human disks, and Oegema and associates[29] did analyze newly synthesized proteoglycans made by a single sample of human nucleus, but in that study no attempt was made to control tissue structure during culture. To overcome this problem, we used the in vitro method described earlier, which controls swelling and proteoglycan loss[12,13] during disk explant incubation. We carried out a large study of the changes in structure of the newly synthesized, large proteoglycans that occur with age, topography, and pathology, comparing them with those of the proteoglycans preexisting in the tissue. The results indicated that there were significant age-related changes in the newly synthesized large proteoglycans.[30]

The majority of newly synthesized large proteoglycans from newborn disks were extracted in a form capable of aggregation (Fig. 3). In young, postnatal disks, however, there was a significant decrease in aggregation in and, even though there was considerable variation between specimens, aggregation was reduced to a far greater extent in the extracts of all adult disks. The extracellular mechanism(s) by which aggrecan is consolidated into stable aggregates in situ is poorly understood. In adult articular cartilage it has been shown that extracellular maturation of the hyaluronan binding region (G1) of newly synthesized aggrecan occurs over a relatively long period of time in culture.[31,32] This process, which appears to involve the formation of intramolecular disulfide bonds in G1,[33,34] is essential for the conversion of aggrecan from a molecule with a low affinity to one with a high affinity for hyaluronan. It has been postulated that this may be one way of enabling aggrecan to escape the hyaluronan-rich pericellular zone before attaining its full aggregating potential in the intercellular space. Using pulse-chase radiolabeling we showed that this mechanism is also active in adult disk (Fig. 3). However, in newborn and immature disks, newly synthesized, large proteoglycans attained full aggregating potential during the initial 4-hour pulse-culture suggesting that either the process of maturation is absent or occurs at a much faster rate. The latter explanation seems the most likely and is consistent with the higher rate of proteoglycan synthesis in disks of this age,[12] and also with the need for a more rapid deposition of extracellular matrix during growth and development.

Aggregate Stability Proteoglycan aggregation is accomplished through a noncovalent interaction of the N-terminal G1 domain of core protein with a region of hyaluronan of 10 monosaccharides in length.[35,36] This aggregation is stabilized by link protein, a 40,000 to 50,000 molecular weight glycoprotein.[37] In previous studies of adult disk proteoglycans, aggregates were found to be less stable than those of articular cartilage.[38,39] In our studies, we found that both endogenous and newly synthesized proteoglycan aggregates purified from fetal anulus were unaffected by the addition of a large excess of hyaluronan-derived oligosaccharides, which dissociate nonlink stabilized aggregates by competing with endogenous hyaluronan chains for the binding of aggrecan (Fig. 4). Similarly, only a small proportion of aggregate from the 15-month-old disk was dissociated, whereas adult disk proteoglycan aggregates were almost completely dissociated. This age-related decrease in aggregate stability could be caused by changes in the quantity and/or quality of disk link protein. Earlier work suggested that there was less abundance of link protein in adult disks, but it has been shown that there is no such deficiency[40] and that the link protein of adult

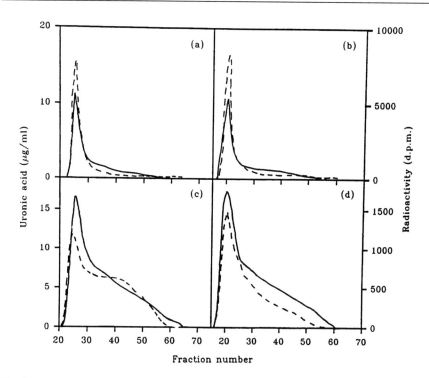

Fig. 3 *Sepharose CL-2B elution profiles of newly synthesized (dashed lines) and total A1 proteoglycans (solid lines) from (a,c) 4-hour pulse and (b,d) 4-hour pulse, 18-hour chase radiolabeled slices of normal anulus fibrosus of ages (a,b) fetal and (c,d) 73 years. (Reproduced with permission from Johnstone B, Bayliss MT: The large proteoglycans of the human intervertebral disc: Changes in their biosynthesis and structure with age, topography, and pathology. Spine 1995;20:674–684.)*

disks is much more degraded than that of both young disks and articular cartilage.[40,41]

Structural Heterogeneity In the adult human intervertebral disk, there are at least two aggregating and three nonaggregating large proteoglycan populations, as defined by differences in electrophoretic mobility and hydrodynamic size.[42,43] Our findings indicate that a single, high molecular weight, proteoglycan monomer is the major product synthesized at all ages by the cells of the intervertebral disk. Therefore, this molecule must then be converted into the lower molecular weight, faster migrating forms, by proteolytic degradation of the C-terminal chondroitin sulfate-rich region of the protein core, in the extracellular space. Cleavage of the N-terminal regions during the relatively long time the proteoglycan is resident in the tissue would generate the heterogeneous mixture of molecules that have lost their capacity to interact with hyaluronan. Attempts to confirm this hypothesis by performing short-term, pulse-chase experiments were unsuccessful because of the long half-life of the monomer, but this is still the most likely explanation for the decrease in size and increase in concentration of partially degraded, nonaggregating proteoglycans during aging.

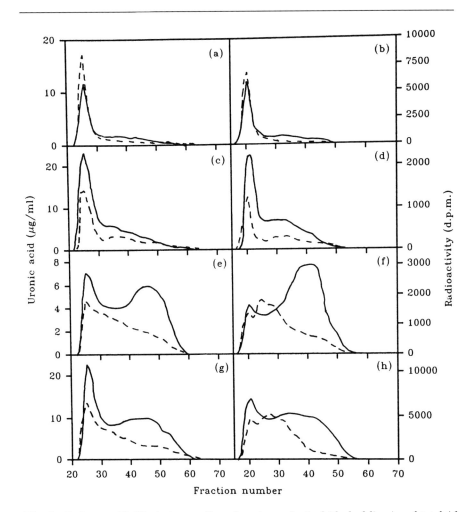

Fig. 4 *Sepharose CL-2B elution profiles of newly synthesized (dashed lines) and total A1 proteoglycans (solid lines). Without (a,c,e,g) and with (b,d,f,h) exogenous hyaluronan oligosaccharide addition. Extracts from radiolabeled normal anulus fibrosus of ages (a,b) fetal, (c,d) 15-month, (e,f) 38 years, and (g,h) 55 years. (Reproduced with permission from Johnstone B, Bayliss MT: The large proteoglycans of the human intervertebral disc: Changes in their biosynthesis and structure with age, topography, and pathology.* Spine *1995;20:674–684.)*

However, it should be emphasized that our results indicate that synthetic processes also contribute to the age-related changes in the large proteoglycan population. The aggregating proteoglycan synthesized by newborn disk has a hydrodynamic size greater than that synthesized by adult disk. Moreover, when adult disk was subdivided into different regions from the outer anulus to the nucleus pulposus, it was observed that in some regions more than one ^{35}S-labeled product was synthesized during the initial 4-hour pulse (Fig. 5). A subsequent chase-culture of these slices indicated that there was no redistribution of the ^{35}S-labeled bands, confirming that they did not arise from proteolytic deg-

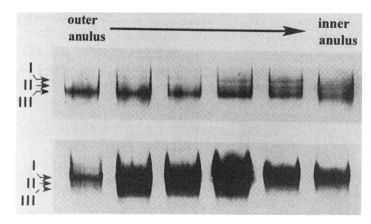

Fig. 5 *Composite gel electrophoresis of A1 proteoglycans from sagittal slices of a 4-hour pulse radiolabeled 45-year-old normal human anulus fibrosus. Upper panel, toluidine blue stain; lower panel, fluorograph of the same gel. The migration distances of I, II, and III, the three major electrophoretic subpopulations detected by toluidine blue, are indicated on both panels. (Reproduced with permission from Johnstone B, Bayliss MT: The large proteoglycans of the human intervertebral disc: Changes in their biosynthesis and structure with age, topography, and pathology.* Spine *1995;20:674–684.)*

radation during the 4-hour pulse culture. Thus, there is evidence of a direct contribution of biosynthesis to the age-related structural changes in the large proteoglycans of the intervertebral disks.

Multiple synthetic products can result from variable splicing of the mRNA for the proteoglycan core protein. This has been observed for aggrecan synthesized by articular cartilage chondrocytes,[44] but it was limited to the C-terminal, G3 region of the protein and therefore is unlikely to play a significant role in producing the extensive changes observed in the molecular size of the extracellular pool. Variation in glycosylation of the core protein would also change the hydrodynamic size and electrophoretic mobility. As discussed earlier there is considerable evidence for age-related changes in the glycosaminoglycan content of the endogenous proteoglycan pool. In our studies we found chondroitin sulfate chain size was constant during aging but variation in substitution of the newly synthesized molecules is possible.

For all of the parameters examined, we could find no differences between the large proteoglycans of normal and pathologic disks. It cannot be concluded, however, that there are no differences, or that large proteoglycans have no role in disk pathology. The studies described here are only the beginning of the complex task of defining the proteoglycans of the extracellular matrix of the disk, and as the following section illustrates, about which we still know very little.

Other Large Proteoglycans It is now known that aggrecan is a member of a subfamily of large proteoglycans capable of aggregation with hyaluronan.[45] We know that aggrecan is made in the disk, but we do not know whether other aggregating proteoglycans are also present. For example, versican, which was originally purified and characterized from fibroblast cultures,[46] also contains an

N-terminal hyaluronan binding domain and a C-terminal globular domain homologous to those of aggrecan. However, it lacks the G2 globular domain closest to the keratan sulfate-rich region, and does not contain any keratan sulfate chains. It is substituted with chondroitin sulfate, but to a much lesser extent than aggrecan. It was initially thought that this proteoglycan represented the fibrous tissue equivalent of aggrecan, but it is now appreciated that there are a family of related aggregating proteoglycans; no one molecule is necessarily tissue-specific, and more than one variant can be present in any particular tissue.[47] Because the outer anulus fibrosus is more like fibrocartilage than hyaline cartilage and its cells are much more fibroblast-like, it is possible that other large aggregating proteoglycans of the fibrous tissue-type are present there. In a preliminary report, Johnstone and associates[48] found immunohistochemical evidence of a versican-like proteoglycan in the matrix of the outer anulus of human disks. A more recent report has shown that mRNA for versican is present in the human disk.[49] The functional significance of the presence of this large proteoglycan in disk tissues is unknown.

Small Interstitial Proteoglycans

All of the small interstitial proteoglycans identified are members of a larger family of leucine-rich molecules.[50] Between seven and 24 amino acid sequence motifs, containing leucine in conserved positions, make up the majority of the protein core of these molecules. Biglycan, decorin, proteoglycan-Lb, and proteoglycan-100 all contain either dermatan sulfate or chondroitin sulfate glycosaminoglycan chains, whereas lumican and fibromodulin contain keratan sulfate chains.

Biglycan and decorin are present in cartilage, tendon, skin, and other connective tissues.[51,52] They can bind to other extracellular molecules and regulate their functions. For example, in tendon, skin, sclera, and cornea, decorin has been shown to be specifically associated with the "d" and "e" bands of collagen fibrils.[53] The decorin from tendon can inhibit the rate of type I and type II collagen fibrillogenesis in vitro.[54,55] It is unclear whether the biglycan core protein will bind collagens. One feature common to both biglycan decorin and the structurally related fibromodulin is the ability to bind TGF-β, suggesting a significant role for these molecules in tissue repair.[56] These low molecular weight proteoglycans account for only a small proportion of the total mass of proteoglycans present in cartilaginous tissues; however, they may be present in similar molar proportions to the large aggregating proteoglycans.[57]

Biglycan and Decorin in Disk Tissues Bianco and associates[58] have detected decorin mRNA in the anulus and nucleus of a 14- to 17-week-old human fetus using in situ hybridization. The expressed protein was also immunolocalized in the tissue. In an immunostaining study of the developing mouse spine, Bianco and associates[59] showed a difference in the staining patterns for the mature biglycan protein versus the initially synthesized form that contains a propeptide that is cleaved prior to secretion. The intracellular form was localized in the center of the developing vertebrae, whereas the secreted product was found in the intervertebral disks (excluding the notochordal remnant) and outer rims of the adjacent vertebrae. This implies that biglycan is synthesized in certain cells and deposited in the matrix surrounding others during development. This was not necessarily seen in other areas of the developing skeleton. Clearly, there is still much to understand about biglycan's functions during growth and development. In postnatal disks, Johnstone and associates[60] identified both biglycan and decorin in the tissues of human intervertebral disks of several ages (Fig. 6), and both were also recently isolated from ovine anulus and nucleus.[61]

In the anulus and nucleus of both species, these proteoglycans were found to be substituted with dermatan sulfate, a glycosaminoglycan not previously detected in the disk.[62] In contrast, Johnstone and associates[60] found that the biglycan and decorin of the cartilage end plate contained chondroitin sulfate. This finding raises an important structural difference between the cartilage end plate of the disk and articular cartilage, because dermatan sulfate-containing small proteoglycans are the prevalent form of decorin and biglycan found in articular cartilage.[63] The composition of the extracellular matrix of end plate has long been assumed to be like that of articular cartilage.[64,65] However, results of morphologic studies have indicated structural differences between the two tissues. The arrangement of cells in the mature end plate is very different from that of articular cartilage, in that no change in cell size, shape, or columnar arrangement is evident toward the bone.[66] Clearly the collagen arrangement differs, because the collagen fibers of the end plate enter the anulus fibrosus, rather than running parallel on the surface as found in articular cartilage. Moreover, biochemical studies indicate that as well as the differences in small proteoglycans, both the large proteoglycans[67,68] and the collagen types[69] are different from those of articular cartilage. Collectively, these data emphasize that the cartilage end plate

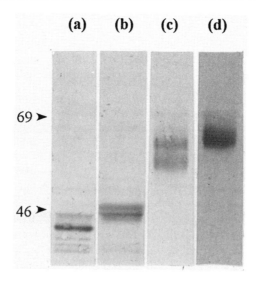

Fig. 6 *Immunolocation of the core proteins of the small proteoglycans biglycan (a), decorin (b), lumican (c), and fibromodulin (d) on Western blots of SDS-polyacrylamide separated anulus fibrosus extracts. For biglycan and decorin blots, the extracts were electrophoresed after chondroitinase ABC digestion, such that both deglycanated and nonglycanated forms are seen. Differential glycosylation of the core protein gives two forms of lumican, seen here as a doublet. Molecular weight markers are indicated.*

should be considered a connective tissue that is biochemically and morphologically distinct from articular cartilage.

Johnstone and associates[60] also found two nonproteoglycan forms (ie, core proteins lacking glycosaminoglycan chains) of both biglycan and decorin in all three regions of the intervertebral disk. These molecules are of similar size to the native core protein, and it is possible that at least some of them represent different synthesis products. However, N-terminal sequence data for one of the nonglycanated forms of decorin indicates it is a degradation product of glycanated protein. Furthermore, the concentration of these nonglycanated components increased with age, consistent with the hypothesis that they are created by degradation of glycanated precursors. Nonglycanated forms of decorin have been detected in other tissues, including human and porcine articular cartilage[70,71] and adult human skin.[72] Koob and Horoschak[73] found both the glycanated and nonglycanated forms of decorin were extractable from bovine connective tissues under the same conditions, indicating that they were both associated with collagen fibrils, a plausible finding because the glycosaminoglycan chain is not required for collagen binding.[55,74-76] There may be functional significance related to the distinct glycosylation patterns of these molecules. For example, the removal of the glycosaminoglycan chain-bearing portion may alter the role of decorin in collagen organization, and thereby alter the physiologic function of the tissue. Recent results suggest that biglycan may bind to type I collagen through its glycosaminoglycan chains.[77] This interaction may be broken by removal of the chain-bearing portion of biglycan.

Other Small Proteoglycans Two other small proteoglycans, lumican and fibromodulin, contain keratan sulfate glycosaminoglycan chains, which are attached to the core protein via an N-glycosidic linkage from N-acetylglucosamine to asparagine residues.[78,79] Like decorin, both proteoglycans have been found to influence collagen fibrillogenesis.[50] Lumican, in its proteoglycan form, was thought to be exclusive to the cornea. Other forms of lumican have been found in other tissues, but they lack keratan sulfate substitution of their N-linked oligosaccharides.[80] However, recent data indicate that there are age-related changes in the keratan sulfate substitution, both in embryonic development and postnatal life. In early embryonic cornea, lumican exists as a glycoprotein, but at later stages it is substituted with keratan sulfate.[81] In a recent study, the first to report the presence of lumican in cartilage, it was found that glycoprotein forms predominate in mature human articular cartilage.[82] It has also been found that nonproteoglycan forms of fibromodulin are present in mature tissues, including cartilage.[83] The functional significance of the age-related changes in glycosaminoglycan substitution is presently unknown. Both lumican and fibromodulin have been immunolocated in extracts of disk tissues (Fig. 6), and immunohistochemical staining of fibromodulin and lumican in porcine intervertebral disk tissues has been reported.[84]

Conclusion

The anatomic features of the intervertebral disk are a product of the interaction of diverse tissue structures that combine to provide each segment with its unique biomechanical properties. The morphologic characteristics of each region of the disk are a reflection of the highly organized, macromolecular components of the extracellular matrix. It is becoming increasingly apparent that in order to appreciate the pathologic processes leading to disk disorders, we must increase our knowledge of these components and their interactions as well as improving our understanding of the cells that synthesize and degrade them. There is no doubt that major changes do take place in the composition, concentration, and turnover of proteoglycans in a variety of lumbar disk disorders.[30] In this chapter we have considered the details of proteoglycan biochemistry as it relates to the human intervertebral disk; however, it is as yet unknown what role, if any, these molecules might have in initiating and/or exacerbating low back pain.

References

1. Bayliss MT, Johnstone B: Biochemistry of the intervertebral disc, in Jayson MIV (ed): *The Lumbar Spine and Back Pain*, ed 4. Edinburgh, Scotland, Churchill Livingstone, 1992, pp 111–131.
2. McDevitt CA: Proteoglycans of the intervertebral disc, in Ghosh P (ed): *The Biology of the Intervertebral Disc*. Boca Raton, FL, CRC Press, 1988, pp 151–170.
3. Roberts S, Beard HK, O'Brien JP: Biochemical changes of intervertebral discs in patients with spondylolisthesis or with tears of the posterior annulus fibrosus. *Ann Rheum Dis* 1982;41:78–85.
4. Davidson EA, Small W: Metabolism in vivo of connective-tissue mucopolysaccharides: I. Chondroitin sulfate C and keratosulfate of nucleus pulposus. *Biochim Biophys Acta* 1963;69:445–452.
5. Lohmander S, Antonopoulos CA, Friberg U: Chemical and metabolic heterogeneity of chondroitin sulfate and keratin sulfate in guinea pig cartilage and nucleus pulposus. *Biochim Biophys Acta* 1973;304:430–448.
6. Urban JP, Holm S, Maroudas A: Diffusion of small solutes into the intervertebral disc: An in vivo study. *Biorheology* 1978;15:203–221.
7. Venn G, Mason RM: Biosynthesis and metabolism in vivo of intervertebral-disc proteoglycans in the mouse. *Biochem J* 1983;215:217–225.
8. Maroudas A: Metabolism of cartilaginous tissue: A quantitative approach, in Maroudas A, Holborow EJ (eds): *Studies in Joint Disease,* ed 2. London, England, Pitman Medical, 1983, pp 59–85.
9. Urban JP, Maroudas A: Swelling of the intervertebral disc in vitro. *Connect Tissue Res* 1981;9:1–10.
10. Handley CJ, Brooks PR, Lowther DA: Extracellular matrix metabolism by chondrocytes: VI. Concomitant depression by exogenous levels of proteoglycan of collagen and proteoglycan synthesis by chondrocytes. *Biochim Biophys Acta* 1978;544:441–444.
11. Wiebkin OW, Muir H: Influence of the cells on the pericellular environment: The effect of hyaluronic acid on proteoglycan synthesis and secretion by chondrocytes of adult cartilage. *Philos Trans R Soc Lond B Biol Sci* 1975;271:283–291.
12. Bayliss MT, Urban JP, Johnstone B, et al: In vitro method for measuring synthesis rates in the intervertebral disc. *J Orthop Res* 1986;4:10–17.
13. Bayliss MT, Johnstone B, O'Brien JP: Proteoglycan synthesis in the human intervertebral disc: Variation with age, region and pathology. *Spine* 1988;13:972–981.
14. Urban JP, Bayliss MT: Regulation of proteoglycan synthesis rate in cartilage in vitro: Influence of extracellular ionic composition. *Biochim Biophys Acta* 1989;992:59–65.
15. Maroudas A: Nutrition and metabolism of the intervertebral disc, in White AA III, Gordon SL (eds): American Academy of Orthopaedic Surgeons *Symposium On Idiopathic Low Back Pain*. St Louis, MO, CV Mosby, 1982, pp 370–390.
16. Urban JP, Holm S, Maroudas A, et al: Nutrition of the intervertebral disc: An in vivo study of solute transport. *Clin Orthop* 1977;129:101–114.

17. Holm S, Maroudas A, Urban JP, et al: Nutrition of the intervertebral disc: Solute transport and metabolism. *Connect Tissue Res* 1981;8:101–119.
18. Puustjärvi K, Lammi MJ, Kiviranta I, et al: Flat bed scanner in the quantitative assay of 35SO4-incorporation by X-ray film autoradiography of intervertebral disc sections. *Histochemistry* 1993;99:67–73.
19. Souter WA, Taylor TK: Sulphated acid mucopolysaccharide metabolism in the rabbit intervertebral disc. *J Bone Joint Surg* 1970;52B:371–384.
20. Ishihara H, Tsuji H, Hirano N, et al: Effects of continuous quantitative vibration on rheologic and biological behaviors of the intervertebral disc. *Spine* 1992;17(3 suppl):S7–S12.
21. Oshima H, Ishihara H, Urban JP, et al: The use of coccygeal discs to study intervertebral disc metabolism. *J Orthop Res* 1993;11:332–338.
22. Carney SL, Billingham ME, Muir H, et al: Demonstration of increased proteoglycan turnover in cartilage explants from dogs with experimental osteoarthritis. *J Orthop Res* 1984;2:201–206.
23. Lipson SJ, Muir H: Proteoglycans in experimental intervertebral disc degeneration. *Spine* 1981;6:194–210.
24. Brocklehurst R, Bayliss MT, Maroudas A, et al: The composition of normal and osteoarthritic articular cartilage from human knee joints: With special reference to unicompartmental replacement and osteotomy of the knee. *J Bone Joint Surg* 1984;66A:95–106.
25. De Palma AF, Rothman RH (eds): *The Intervertebral Disc*. Philadelphia, PA, WB Saunders, 1970.
26. Antonopoulos CA, Fransson LA, Gardell S, et al: Fractionation of keratan sulfate from human nucleus pulposus. *Acta Chem Scand* 1969;23:2616–2620.
27. Pearce RH, Grimmer B: The chemical constitution of the proteoglycan of human intervertebral disc. *Biochem J* 1976;157:753–763.
28. Lyons G, Eisenstein SM, Sweet MB: Biochemical changes in intervertebral disc degeneration. *Biochim Biophys Acta* 1981;673:443–453.
29. Oegema TR Jr, Bradford DS, Cooper KM: Aggregated proteoglycan synthesis in organ cultures of human nucleus pulposus. *J Biol Chem* 1979;254:10579–10581.
30. Johnstone B, Bayliss MT: The large proteoglycans of the human intervertebral disc: Changes in their biosynthesis and structure with age, topography, and pathology. *Spine* 1995;20:674–684.
31. Bayliss MT, Ridgway GD, Ali SY: Differences in the rates of aggregation of proteoglycans from human articular cartilage and chondrosarcoma. *Biochem J* 1983;215:705–708.
32. Oegema TR Jr: Delayed formation of proteoglycan aggregate structures in human articular cartilage disease states. *Nature* 1980;288:583–585.
33. Plaas AH, Sandy JD: The affinity of newly synthesized proteoglycan for hyaluronic acid can be enhanced by exposure to mild alkali. *Biochem J* 1986;234:221–223.
34. Sandy JD, Plaas AH: Studies on the hyaluronate binding properties of newly synthesized proteoglycans purified from articular chondrocyte cultures. *Arch Biochem Biophys* 1989;271:300–314.
35. Hardingham TE, Muir H: Binding of oligosaccharides of hyaluronic acid to proteoglycans. *Biochem J* 1973;135:905–908.
36. Hascall VC, Heinegard D: Aggregation of cartilage proteoglycans: II. Oligosaccharide competitors of the proteoglycan-hyaluronic acid interaction. *J Biol Chem* 1974;249:4242–4249.
37. Neame PJ, Barry FP: The link proteins. *Experientia* 1993;49:393–402.
38. Tengblad A, Pearce RH, Grimmer BJ: Demonstration of link protein in proteoglycan aggregates from human intervertebral disc. *Biochem J* 1984;222:85–92.
39. Donohue PJ, Jahnke MR, Blaha JD, et al: Characterization of link protein(s) from human intervertebral-disc tissues. *Biochem J* 1988;251:739–747.
40. Liu J, Pearce RH, Mathieson JM, et al: Link protein quantitation and function in the human intervertebral disc. *Trans Orthop Res Soc* 1993;18:212.

507

41. Pearce RH, Mathieson JM, Mort JS, et al: Effect of age on the abundance and fragmentation of link protein of the human intervertebral disc. *J Orthop Res* 1989;7:861–867.

42. DiFabio JL, Pearce RH, Caterson B, et al: The heterogeneity of the non-aggregating proteoglycans of the human intervertebral disc. *Biochem J* 1987;244:27–33.

43. Jahnke MR, McDevitt CA: Proteoglycans of the human intervertebral disc: Electrophoretic heterogeneity of the aggregating proteoglycans of the nucleus pulposus. *Biochem J* 1988;251:347–356.

44. Baldwin CT, Reginato AM, Prockop DJ: A new epidermal growth factor-like domain in the human core protein for the large cartilage-specific proteoglycan: Evidence for alternative splicing of the domain. *J Biol Chem* 1989;264:15747–15750.

45. Kjellén L, Lindahl U: Proteoglycans: Structures and interactions. *Annu Rev Biochem* 1991;60:443–475.

46. Zimmermann DR, Ruoslahti E: Multiple domains of the large fibroblast proteoglycan, versican. *EMBO J* 1989;8:2975–2981.

47. Yanagishita M: Function of proteoglycans in the extracellular matrix. *Acta Pathol Japon* 1993;43:283–293.

48. Johnstone B, Roberts S, Menage J: The occurrence of versican in the human intervertebral disc. *Trans Orthop Res Soc* 1994;19:132.

49. Dours-Zimmermann MT, Zimmermann DR: A novel glycosaminoglycan attachment domain identified in two alternative splice variants of human versican. *J Biol Chem* 1994;269:32992–32998.

50. Kresse H, Hausser H, Schonherr E: Small proteoglycans. *Experientia* 1993;49:403–416.

51. Stanescu V: The small proteoglycans of cartilage matrix. *Semin Arthritis Rheum* 1990;20(suppl 1):51–64.

52. Rosenberg L, Tang LH, Choi HU, et al: Biological functions of dermatan sulphate proteoglycans, in Scott JE (ed): *Dermatan Sulphate Proteoglycans: Chemistry, Biology, Chemical Pathology.* London, England, Portland Press, 1993, pp 225–239.

53. Scott JE: Proteoglycan-fibrillar collagen interactions. *Biochem J* 1988;252:313–323.

54. Vogel KG, Paulsson M, Heinegard D: Specific inhibition of type I and type II collagen fibrillogenesis by the small proteoglycan of tendon. *Biochem J* 1984;223:587–597.

55. Hedbom E, Heinegard D: Interaction of a 59-kDa connective tissue matrix protein with collagen I and collagen II. *J Biol Chem* 1989;264:6898–6905.

56. Hildebrand A, Romaris M, Rasmussen LM, et al: Interaction of the small interstitial proteoglycans biglycan, decorin and fibromodulin with transforming growth factor beta. *Biochem J* 1994;302:527–534.

57. Roughley PJ, White RJ: Dermatan sulphate proteoglycans of human articular cartilage: The properties of dermatan sulphate proteoglycans I and II. *Biochem J* 1989;262:823–827.

58. Bianco P, Fisher LW, Young MF, et al: Expression and localization of the two small proteoglycans biglycan and decorin in developing human skeletal and non-skeletal tissues. *J Histochem Cytochem* 1990;38:1549–1563.

59. Bianco P, Riminucci M, Fisher LW: Biglycan and decorin in intact developing tissues: the in situ approach to their role in development, morphogenesis and tissue organization, in Scott JE (ed): *Dermatan Sulphate Proteoglycans: Chemistry, Biology, Chemical Pathology.* London, England, Portland Press, 1993, pp 193–205.

60. Johnstone B, Markopoulos M, Neame P, et al: Identification and characterization of glycanated and non-glycanated forms of biglycan and decorin in the human intervertebral disc. *Biochem J* 1993;292:661–666.

61. Melrose J, Ghosh P, Taylor TK: Proteoglycan heterogeneity in the normal adult ovine intervertebral disc. *Matrix Biol* 1994;14:61–75.

62. Inerot S, Axelsson I: Structure and composition of proteoglycans from human annulus fibrosus. *Connect Tissue Res* 1991;26:47–63.

63. Rosenberg LC, Choi HU, Tang L-H, et al: Isolation of dermatan sulfate proteoglycans from mature bovine articular cartilages. *J Biol Chem* 1985;260:6304–6313.
64. Eyre DR: Biochemistry of the intervertebral disc. *Int Rev Connect Tissue Res* 1979;8:227–291.
65. Ayad S, Weiss JB: Biochemistry of the intervertebral disc, in Jayson MIV (ed): *The Lumbar Spine and Back Pain*, ed 3. Edinburgh, Scotland, Churchill Livingstone, 1987, pp 100–137.
66. Roberts S, Menage J, Urban JP: Biochemical and structural properties of the cartilage end-plate and its relation to the intervertebral disc. *Spine* 1989;14:166–174.
67. Bishop PB, Pearce RH: The proteoglycans of the cartilaginous end-plate of the human intervertebral disc change after maturity. *J Orthop Res* 1993;11:324–331.
68. Jahnke MR, Caterson B: Immunochemical analysis of human neonatal and young adult intervertebral disc proteoglycans. *Trans Orthop Res Soc* 1986;11:419.
69. Roberts S, Menage J, Duance V, et al: Collagen types around the cells of the intervertebral disc and cartilage end-plate: An immunolocalization study. *Spine* 1991;16:1030–1038.
70. Sampaio L de O, Bayliss MT, Hardingham TE, et al: Dermatan sulphate proteoglycan from human articular cartilage: Variation in its content with age and its structural comparison with a small chondroitin sulphate proteoglycan from pig laryngeal cartilage. *Biochem J* 1988;254:757–764.
71. Roughley PJ, White RJ, Magny MC, et al: Non-proteoglycan forms of biglycan increase with age in human articular cartilage. *Biochem J* 1993;295:421–426.
72. Fleischmajer R, Fisher LW, MacDonald ED, et al: Decorin interacts with fibrillar collagen of embryonic and adult human skin. *J Struct Biol* 1991;106:82–90.
73. Koob TJ, Horoschak SA: Identification and partial characterization of small proteoglycan (PGII) lacking glycosaminoglycan in tendon. *Trans Orthop Res Soc* 1990;15:38.
74. Vogel KG, Koob TJ, Fisher LW: Characterization and interactions of a fragment of the core protein of the small proteoglycan (PGII) from bovine tendon. *Biochem Biophys Res Comm* 1987;148:658–663.
75. Uldbjerg N, Danielsen CC: A study of the interaction in vitro between type I collagen and a small dermatan sulphate proteoglycan. *Biochem J* 1988;251:643–648.
76. Brown DC, Vogel KG: Characteristics of the in vitro interaction of a small proteoglycan (PGII) of bovine tendon with type I collagen. *Matrix* 1989;9:468–478.
77. Pogány G, Hernandez DJ, Vogel KG: The in vitro interaction of proteoglycans with type I collagen is modulated by phosphate. *Arch Biochem Biophys* 1994;313:102–111.
78. Hassell JR, Blochberger TC, Rada JA, et al: Proteoglycan gene families. *Adv Mol Cell Biol* 1993;6:69–113.
79. Antonsson P, Heinegard D, Oldberg A: Posttranslational modifications of fibromodulin. *J Biol Chem* 1991;266:16859–16861.
80. Funderburgh JL, Funderburgh ML, Mann MM, et al: Arterial lumican: Properties of a corneal-type keratan sulfate proteoglycan from bovine aorta. *J Biol Chem* 1991;266:24773–24777.
81. Cornuet PK, Blochberger TC, Hassell JR: Molecular polymorphism of lumican during corneal development. *Invest Ophthalmol Vis Sci* 1994;35:870–877.
82. Grover J, Chen X-N, Korenberg JR, et al: The human lumican gene: Organization, chromosomal location, and expression in articular cartilage. *J Biol Chem* 1995;270:21942–21949.
83. Heinegård D, Larsson T, Sommarin Y, et al: Two novel matrix proteins isolated from articular cartilage show wide distributions among connective tissues. *J Biol Chem* 1986;261:13866–13872.
84. Markopoulos M, Johnstone B, Neame P, et al: Identification and immunolocalization of the small proteoglycans in porcine intervertebral disc tissues. *Trans Orthop Res Soc* 1994;19:133.

509

Chapter 31

The Role of Proteinases and Other Degradation Mechanisms in Idiopathic Low Back Pain

Theodore R. Oegema, Jr, PhD

Introduction

In the mature intervertebral disk, the anatomic constraints imposed by the calcified end plate and lack of vascularity on the inner two thirds of the anulus fibrosus and nucleus pulposus greatly limit not only the nutrition of these regions, but also the passage of degradation products.[1] The accumulation of a variety of matrix breakdown products from both abnormal and perhaps normal metabolic processes has been speculated to play a role in back pain. There are a few studies, such as one in which the influences of the nucleus pulposus on nerve conduction were tested directly and found to slow the rate of propagation,[2] and several experiments in which it was determined that the nucleus pulposus was chemotactic for peripheral macrophages.[3] However, it is still an important question whether the inner anulus fibrosus or nucleus pulposus extracellular matrix causes pain in a nonherniated disk that has a dramatically decreased nuclear magnetic resonance signal. In order to study this question, this topic will be addressed using a hierarchical approach. There will be a brief introduction to put the topic into perspective with reference to general reviews, followed by a discussion of information pertinent to the degeneration of the intervertebral disk, and, finally, a comparison with related tissues, such as articular cartilage. Knowledge in all areas of pathology, cell biology, and biochemistry of the disk lags behind that in other connective tissues. Therefore, many inferences on the roles these processes play in producing disk pain will have to be made indirectly from related tissues.

There are several means by which degradation products can cause pain. These include direct stimulation by the normal breakdown products of the nerves in the outer third of the anulus fibrosus; recruitment by the normal breakdown products of other cell types, such as macrophages or even annular cells, which then release pain-inducing products; or, less directly, the first alteration of the local environment inducing a change in disk cell phenotype, which then secondarily produces proinflammatory or nociceptive molecules. In the latter case, the degenerative process would be a prerequisite, but not sufficient for producing a painful disk. Although possible, it is unlikely that normal matrix fragments directly produce a pain response; it is more likely that pain production is mediated indirectly.

This chapter will review selected current literature to see if there is support for the hypothesis that the normal degenerative process leads to accumulation of matrix degradation products. These products, in turn, alter the cell-matrix interaction toward a more proinflammatory reactive state, and the cycle is accelerated. The hyperreactive cells would then be capable of persistently producing nociceptive substances after an unknown stimulation. The factors that determine susceptibility to the process could include both mechanical and genetic factors.

Free Radical Degradation of the Extracellular Matrix

In biology, two major free radical families that are capable of altering matrix molecules have been studied extensively. These two are the oxygen-derived free radicals (ODFR) and the free radicals from nitric oxide.

ODFRs have been implicated in the breakdown of the extracellular matrix in many tissues, in addition to their known participation in membrane phospholipid peroxidation, intracellular protein oxidation, and DNA damage.[4,5] In connective tissues, the effects of ODFRs have been extensively studied in rheumatoid arthritis,[4,6] where neutrophils present in the synovial fluid have been suggested to be the major source of ODFRs. The major steps in ODFR formation are shown in Figure 1.

The superoxide radical is produced in a number of normal enzymatic dehydrogenase reactions, such as aldehyde dehydrogenase, flavin dehydrogenase, and some peroxidases[7] (Outline 1). It is also generated in large amounts by several cell types such as neutrophils, in which superoxide production is an integral part of the host defense mechanism and is synthesized by a membrane-associated reduced nicotinamide adenine dinucleotide phosphate oxidase as part of an "oxidation burst."[5] Superoxide may also be generated during the oxidation of hypoxanthine to xanthine by the action of xanthine oxidase.

Xanthine oxidase is produced from xanthine dehydrogenase by a calcium-dependent proteinase, and hypoxanthine is derived from the salvage pathway for adenosine triphosphate. The production of both hypoxanthine and xanthine oxidase is greatly enhanced at low oxygen tension. This pathway is proposed to be a significant source of superoxide production in ischemia-reperfusion injuries and may be important in rheumatoid arthritis damage.[4] This type of injury could potentially contribute to disk degeneration, especially after early loss

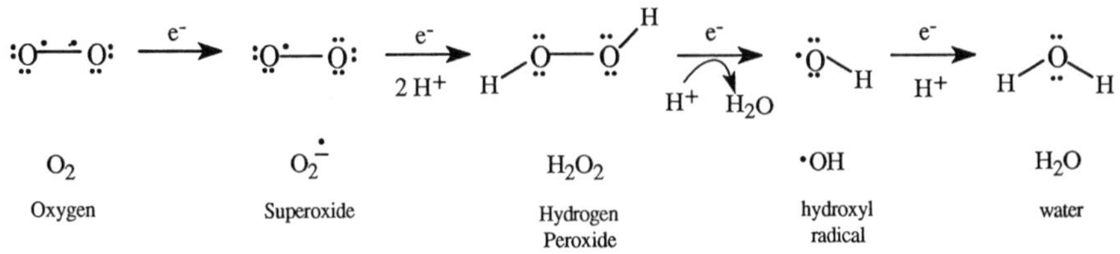

O_2	$O_2^{\cdot-}$	H_2O_2	$\cdot OH$	H_2O
Oxygen	Superoxide	Hydrogen Peroxide	hydroxyl radical	water

Fig. 1 *Steps in oxygen reduction and free radical formation.*

Outline 1 Mixed-function oxidation systems that catalyze the modification of enzymes

Enzyme systems
  NAD(P)H oxidases/NAD(P)H/Fe(III)/O_2
  Xanthine oxidase/hypoxanthine/Fe(III)/O_2
  Nicotinate hydroxylase/NADPH/Fe(III)O_2
  Cytochrome P_{450} reductase/cytochrome P_{450}/NADPH/Fe(III)O_2
  Redoxin reductase/redoxin/cytochrome P_{450}/NADH/Fe(III)O_2
Nonenzymatic systems
  Ascorbate/Fe(III)/O_2
  Thiol/Fe(III)O_2
  Fe(II)/O_2
  Fe(II)H_2O_2

(Reproduced with permission from Bomalaski JS, Lawton P, Browning JL: Human extracellular recombinant phospholipase A2 induces an inflammatory response in rabbit joints. *J Immunol* 1991;146:3904–3910.)

of proteoglycan, which could amplify the normal changes in blood flow and oxygen with daily loading.

Superoxide, hydrogen peroxide, singlet oxygen, and the hydroxyl radical can all cause various degrees of damage to biologic molecules, depending on their stability.[8] With most macromolecules, the superoxide radical is largely unreactive, while the hydroxyl radical reacts with most biologic compounds. However, at low pH, the superoxide radical can become protonated with a pK_a of 4.8.[9] This protonated form, like hydrogen peroxide, is membrane-permeable and is more reactive than the hydroxyl radical.[8]

Figure 2 shows the major steps in free radical scavenging. Normally, the superoxide radical will react with itself rapidly to form oxygen and hydrogen peroxide. This reaction is accelerated even more by superoxide dismutase so that superoxide radicals are usually present at less than 10^{-11} moles/l in cells and have very short half-lives of approximately 5 milliseconds.[4,10] Because of its rapid rate of diffusion, this radical or its products can cause damage well away from where it is generated, even with the short half-life.[4]

a) $\overset{\bullet}{O_2^-}$ + $\overset{\bullet}{O_2^-}$ $\longrightarrow$ H_2O_2 Superoxide Dismutase

b) $2\,H_2O_2$ $\longrightarrow$ $2H_2O$ + O_2 Catalase

c) $ROOH + H_2O_2$ $\longrightarrow$ $ROH + H_2O$ Glutathione Peroxidase
            2GSH   GS-SG

Fig. 2 *Major steps in free radical scavenging.*

The hydrogen peroxide then decomposes into $H_2O + O_2$, a reaction accelerated by catalase, or it can be broken down by various peroxidases, effectively removing the potential for damage. Glutathione peroxidase is perhaps the most important of the peroxidases. However, hydrogen peroxide can also give rise to the highly reactive hydroxyl radical via the enzymatic action of neutrophil myeloperoxidase or eosinophil peroxidase, which convert H_2O_2 into the reactive hypochlorous acid, which further reacts with superoxide to form a hydroxyl radical (Fig. 3). This pathway is limited to these cell types and is a significant component of the killing potential generated during the oxidation burst.[5]

The hydroxyl radical can also be produced by several nonenzymatic means, as shown in Figure 4. The first is the Haber-Weiss reaction, which without the metal ion catalysis could not make a quantitatively significant contribution in biologic systems.[4] However, by adding an intermediate metal-catalyzed Fenton-type reaction, the same net stoichiometry is obtained and the reaction is very efficient. The metal ion can be either iron or copper and the reducing equivalents can come from superoxide or a variety of easily oxidized metal-binding biologic molecules, including ascorbate and glutathione (see Outline 1). This reaction may make a significant contribution in the extracellular matrix generation of ODFR because H_2O_2 readily crosses the plasma membrane. It should also be noted that the oxygen produced from this reaction is in the singlet state and can also potentially participate in the oxidation of various biologic molecules.

Superoxide is also generated during the spontaneous metal ion-catalyzed remodeling of proteins glycated nonenzymatically with reducing sugars such as glucose in the Maillard reaction.[11] There is a metal ion independent pathway that can give rise to ODFR. It has been shown that nitric oxide can give rise to hydroxyl radicals via a nonmetal ion-dependent pathway[5] (Fig. 5). Quantitatively less than 1% to 4% of nitric oxide decays to a hydroxyl radical in this manner,[12] thus, the biologic significance is unknown but even peroxynitrite generated in this pathway is capable of protein modification.

pH Effects

If lipid peroxidation is used as a measure of ODFR production, then decreasing the pH from 7.4 to 6.5 increases peroxidation. The optimal range for ODFR seems to be 6.0 to 6.5. This may be because, although the Fenton reaction is not sensitive to pH in this range, the superoxide to hydrogen peroxide conversion is faster at lower pH[13] and more membrane-permeable protonated super-

a) $H_2O_2 + Cl^- \longrightarrow HOCl + H_2O$

b) $HOCl + O_2^{\cdot -} \longrightarrow \cdot OH + Cl^- + O_2$

Fig. 3 *Mechanisms of enzymatic hydroxyl formation.*

a) $\quad O_2^{\cdot-} + H_2O_2 \longrightarrow {}^1O_2 + {}^{\cdot}OH + OH^-$

$\qquad\qquad\qquad\qquad\qquad\quad$ singlet oxygen

b) $\quad O_2^{\cdot-} + Fe^{3+} \longrightarrow {}^1O_2 + Fe^{2+}$

$\qquad H_2O_2 + Fe^{2+} \longrightarrow {}^{\cdot}OH + OH^- + Fe^{3+}$

Fig. 4   *Mechanisms of nonenzymatic enhancing hydroxyl radical formation.*

a) $\qquad {}^{\cdot}NO + O_2^{\cdot-} \longrightarrow ONOO^-$

b) $\qquad ONOO^- + H^+ \longrightarrow ONOOH$

c) $\qquad ONOOH \longrightarrow {}^{\cdot}NO_2 + {}^{\cdot}OH$

Fig. 5   *Nitric oxide radical chemistry.*

oxide is formed.[14] The lower pH seen in a degenerative disk (as low as 6.1) will increase the potential for free radical damage.[1]

Quantitatively, in most biologic systems, the hydroxyl radical is the most damaging. Its presence along with superoxide and H_2O_2 has been identified in articular cartilage.[4,6] In fact, primed chondrocytes are capable of undergoing sustained release of ODFR species that exceeds that of the neutrophils.[15,16] Cells derived from the disk can also produce both nitric oxide (Fig. 6) and ODFR in culture (unpublished observation), but production in vivo needs to be quantitated.

Effects of Oxygen-Derived Free Radical Production

Radical damage to the phospholipid in membranes includes lipid cross-linking and cleavage of unsaturated lipid into small fragments such as malon-dialdehyde and pentane.[17] Lipid-protein adducts accumulate as fluorescent products called lipofuscin in lysosomes, and high concentrations may affect cell behavior.[17] Lipofuscin is found in high concentrations in degenerative disk.[18,19] A recent report found that ODFRs can nonenzymatically generate isoleukotrienes, oxidized arachidonic acid products that have leukotriene B_4 activity,[20] and once released by phospholipase A_2 may have relevance to the painful disk because phospholipase A_2 can cause inflammation in normal joints.[20,21]

515

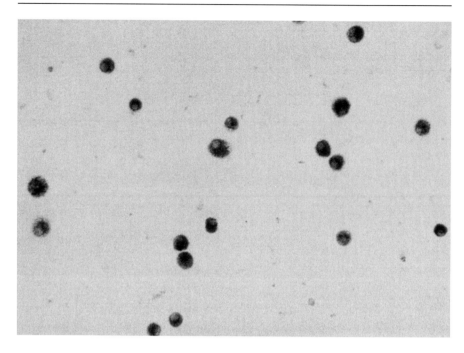

Fig. 6 *Photograph of cultured human anulus fibrosus cells stained for nitric oxide production. Cells were dissociated from a grade 3 degenerative disk and placed in alginate bead culture[87] and after 3 days were reacted with nitroblue tetrazolium in the presence of either NADPH (shown) or NADH (not shown). The cells stained positively in both cases indicating their ability to form both nitric oxide and oxygen-derived free radical.*

In addition to its oxidative effects on intracellular proteins,[22] ODFR also reacts with extracellular matrix proteins.[23] Because the metal ions involved in the Fenton reaction can be bound to specific sites on protein and the nascent hydroxyl radical is highly reactive, the damage will occur near the metal binding site. Thus, many of the modifications occur in specific sites in these proteins.[22] Table 1 shows typical reactions with amino acids.[7,22]

The reactivity of ODFRs with a number of extracellular matrix proteins in solution has been determined. Collagen is unusually reactive to ODFRs, and can even be degraded by superoxide to small fragments.[4,23] Fibronectin, in addition to being cleaved, can form high molecular weight complexes from the dimerization of tyrosines.[24]

Because of synovial fluid changes in rheumatoid arthritis, the reaction of ODFR with hyaluronate has been carefully investigated. The hydroxyl radical effectively degrades hyaluronate to small fragments.[4,25] ODFR damage to hyaluronate has been postulated to be one of the reasons for the small amount of rheumatoid arthritic synovial fluid hyaluronate and the basis for the observed decrease in viscosity. In cartilage, there is age-related accumulation of hyaluronate and a shift toward small size.[26,27] Because there has never been a demonstration of a hyaluronidase in cartilage, free radical damage also has been sug-

Table 1 Metal ion catalyzed protein modification

Type of Residue	Yield
Arginyl	Glutamylsemialdchyde residues
Prolyl	Glutamylsemialdehyde and cis/*trans*-4-hydroxy prolyl residues
Lysyl	α-Aminoadipylsemialdehyde residues
Histidyl	Asparaginyl/aspartyl residues
Cysteinyl	S-protein-protein cross links; or mixed disulfide protein S-S-R
Methionyl	Methionylsulfoxide residues
Tyrosyl	Tyrosyl-tyrosyl cross links

(Reproduced with permission from Bomalaski JS, Lawton P, Browning JL: Human extracellular recombinant phospholipase A2 induces an inflammatory response in rabbit joints. *J Immunol* 1991;146:3904–3910.)

gested as a reason for this shift, although in vivo mechanical forces could also contribute.[27]

In contrast to unsulfated hyaluronate, sulfated glycosaminoglycans such as chondroitin sulfate are good ODFR scavengers[4] and their loss with degeneration would decrease these protective effects. The effect of ODFR on the protein component of proteoglycans is detrimental. Reaction of aggrecan with H_2O_2 results in loss of the ability to bind hyaluronate and also causes changes in link protein.[28,29] Although chondrocytes are capable of producing a burstlike production of ODFR in a number of inflammatory situations, how much these radicals contribute to matrix degradation is still under investigation. Likewise, disk cells in culture can release nitric oxide (Fig. 6) and ODFR, and the enhanced accumulation of lipofuscin[18,19] speaks to the presence of ODFR in degenerative disk; however, the role of ODFR in disk generation and its contribution to pain production need to be evaluated quantitatively.

Role of Proteinases in Extracellular Matrix Catabolism

Four major proteolytic mechanisms have been proposed for the normal turnover of noncalcified extracellular matrix.[30] They are: (1) matrix metalloproteinases (MMP); (2) the plasminogen-plasmin cascade; (3) phagocytosis and degradation by lysosomal enzymes; and (4) the polymorphonuclear proteinases systems including neutrophil elastase and collagenase.

Except possibly during the rapid expansion of the nucleus pulposus in the developing disk,[31] there is no compelling evidence (such as cells containing fibrillar collagen fragments in vacuoles as seen in remodeling scars) for mechanism 3 (phagocytosis) in the degenerative disk. Likewise, the disk does not normally contain polymorphonucleocytes/macrophages, except in pathologic states such as in nonsequestered herniations, so mechanism 4 is not relevant.[32] As in most connective tissues, there is convincing but incomplete evidence for participation of mechanisms 1 and 2 in matrix turnover in the disk.

517

Metalloproteinases and Matrix Degradation

There is an expanding family of MMPs that are believed to play a major role in normal and pathologic extracellular matrix protein turnover.[30,33-36] MMPs have been cloned and sequenced, and for some, substrate specificity is known. The zinc-dependent metalloproteinases follow a common structural motif. They are synthesized as an inactivated proform whose activity is controlled via a cysteine switch, are activated in vivo by the proteolytic removal of a 10 kd propeptide, and can be activated in vitro via mercuric salts such as 4-aminophenyl mercuric acetate. All members of the family, which are numbered in order of discovery, contain a conserved presumptive Zn^{+2} binding active site of HEXGHXXGAXH, a conserved free cysteine site, and except for the simplest member MMP-7 (punctuated metalloproteinase [PUMP], matrilysin) contain additional sequences that contribute to specificity.[30] The whole family is effectively inhibited by α_2 macroglobulin, but more importantly, by the family of three tissue inhibitors of metalloproteinase (TIMP-1, -2, and -3). TIMP-1 and/or TIMP-2 are present in most connective tissues at molar concentrations greater than that of the MMPs.[36,37]

The original member of the family is fibroblast or interstitial collagenase (MMP-1). This enzyme degrades the fibrillar collagens of types I, II, and III at a highly conserved site in the triple helix to give fragments of three fourths to one fourth length. This led to the optimistic view that there might be other MMPs with extreme substrate specificity. In general, except for the inability to degrade fibrillar collagens, this has not been the case. Although there are a limited number of bonds, typically on the carboxy side of hydrophobic residues, that can be cleaved by any MMP, the specificity for the matrix protein depends more on the sequence of the substrate, its accessibility to the enzyme, time, and concentration than on the specific protein. The most specific MMPs are the collagenases. Along with MMP-1, MMP-8 (neutrophil collagenase) and MMP-13 (collagenase 3) are capable of attacking fibrillar types I, II, and III collagen. Other less specific enzymes are characterized as gelatinases (MMP-2 and MMP-9) or enzymes with broad specificity such as stromelysin 1, 2, and 3 (MMP-3, MMP-10, MMP-11), MMP-7 (PUMP or matrilysin), and neutrophil elastase or MMP-12.

The three major areas of interest in MMP research that impact intervertebral disk research are: the factor that controls their synthesis, their activation and inactivation; and quantitatively, the importance of each enzyme in normal and abnormal matrix turnover.[30,36,38]

In cartilage, there is direct evidence of the presence of interstitial collagenase (MMP-1), stromelysin (MMP-3), 72 kd gelatinase (MMP-2) and 92 kd gelatinase,[38] and more recently, MMP-8[39] and MMP-13.[40] Their properties are briefly described here.

MMP-1 is synthesized by a wide variety of cell types, including chondrocytes,[41] as a protein of 57 to 52 kd. While capable of containing up to three N-linked chondrocytes, it is frequently nonglycosylated.[42] MMP-1 is easily activated by plasmin, trypsin, and stromelysin. MMP-8, or neutrophil collagenase, is about the same size protein as MMP-1, but is heavily glycosylated and has a 72 kd in the neutrophil. It is activated by stromelysin or ODFR, but is only poorly activated by plasmin and trypsin. Both collagenases have the ability to cleave fibrillar types I, II, and III collagen although with some differences in rate[43] as well as VII, VIII, and X, but not types V, VI, IX, or XI, and a number of noncollagenous proteins including proteinase inhibitors, such as α1-proteinase inhibitor and α1 antitrypsin. MMP-13 was originally thought to be orthologous to MMP-1 in the rat, but was recently shown to be different than human MMP-1.[44] This enzyme has been shown to be present in cartilage and elevated in osteoarthrosis.[40] It may be a major player in collagen turnover, because it has significant activity on both types I and II collagens.

MMP-2 is unusual in that it is poorly activated by plasmin or stromelysin.[45] Pro 72 kd collagenase binds a mole of TIMP-2 at a site other than the active site, and this bound TIMP-2 is important for its activation. Recent evidence demonstrates that 72 kd collagenase is converted to its active 64 kd and 62 kd forms by a membrane-bound metalloproteinase (MT-MP) and the process requires the presence of TIMP- 2.[46,47] This integral membrane metalloproteinase (MT-MP) has been cloned, sequenced, and overexpressed in COS cells.[48] The MT-MP, which is activated by urokinase plasminogen activator (uPA), will rapidly activate MMP-2 with the presence of TIMP-2.[49] Both MT-MP and MMP-2 are inhibited by additional TIMP-1 or TIMP-2. The MMP-2 has a broad substrate specificity and, in addition to degrading denatured collagen, it will degrade native types IV and V collagen, fibronectin, laminin, and aggrecan. In contrast to MMP-1, MMP-3, MMP-7, and MMP-9, MMP-2 lacks the 12-(O-tetra-decanoyl)-phorbol-13-acetate (PMA) response element that binds activator protein-1 (AP-1) so it is not upregulated by epidermal growth factor (EGF), tumor necrosis factor-alpha (TNF-α), interleukin-1 beta (IL-1β), and PMA.[34] In fibroblasts, it is constitutively expressed and is unexpectedly upregulated by transforming growth factor-beta (TGF-β),[50] a growth factor that suppresses the synthesis of most MMPs.

MMP-3 (stromelysin, transin, or proteoglycanase) and the related MMP-10 or transin-2 stromelysin-2 and the related stromelysin-3 (MMP-11) destroy a wide variety of matrix proteins including fibronectin, decorin, aggrecan, link protein, and collagen types IV, V, VII, IX, and XI. Type II collagen is cut inside the cross-links present in nonhelical teliopeptides, so the action of stromelysin can loosen the type II fibrillar structure.[51] On activation, MMP-3 goes from a 51 kd to a 41 kd protein and then is processed to active 21 kd and 25 kd proteins.[30,35] It has been postulated to be a key proteinase in cartilage matrix turnover and MMP activation. However, there may be significant overlap with other activation pathways, such as with the MT-MP system.

MMP-9 or 92 kd gelatinase will degrade gelatin, type V collagen, and aggrecan and can be activated by plasmin or stromelysin and inhibited by TIMP-1 and TIMP-2. All of the metalloproteinases can degrade aggrecan at a limited number of sites.[52] The major site is between N341 and F342 (human sequence)[52] and MMP-8 will also cleave between E373 and A374 (the aggrecanase site).[53] In cartilage, these represent the major earliest released fragments of aggrecan.[54,55]

Plasminogen-Plasmin Pathway

The plasminogen-plasmin pathway has been extensively investigated in a variety of tissues, and plasmin in some tissues plays a major role in turnover of the extracellular matrix.[30,56] The basic cascade involves the activation of tissue plasminogen activator (tPA) or uPA, serine endopeptidases that are present on cell membranes as inactive proforms. After conversion to their active forms, they then activate plasminogen to plasmin. Both tPA and uPA are effectively inhibited by plasminogen activator inhibitors 1 and 2, and plasmin is inhibited by α_2 macroglobulin and a variety of serine proteinase inhibitors, α_1 antitrypsin and anti-α_1 proteinase. Plasmin can degrade in a limited fashion a wide variety of proteins, including fibronectin and aggrecan. Plasmin activates stromelysin and thus crosses over into the regulation of the MMP pathway. In articular cartilage, the plasminogen-plasma pathway is present and uPA and tPA expression and activation are carefully regulated.[57-59]

Other proteinases that may participate include calpain. This normally intracellular calcium-dependent proteinase has a minor membrane form, may be able to degrade molecules near the cell surface, has been found in chondrocytes,[60,61] and may be involved in mineralization. Its presence or role in disk degeneration is unknown.

Proteinases in the Intervertebral Disk

In older studies of the intervertebral disk, a collagenogelic and two gelatinolytic mercuric ion-activatable ethylenediaminetetraacetic acid (EDTA)-sensitive proteolytic activates have been identified[62,63] that are present as zymogens.[64] The most recent in-depth study has been the identification of stromelysin in the human disk.[65] Stromelysin was present and upregulated by IL-1β in culture, and collagenase was present in lower amounts than in cartilage. Further evidence of the activity of stromelysin in disk is that link protein 3, which is known to accumulate in older intervertebral disk sampled,[66] was shown to be cleaved between the same amino terminal His 16/Leu 17 site[65] in which stromelysin cleaves native link proteins 1 and 2 in vitro.[67] The total number of MMP that contribute to the disk metabolism and their quantitative importance needs to be determined.

Melrose and Ghosh[68] have reviewed the pre-1970 literature on endogenous proteinases and found that there is good evidence for the presence of autolysis proteinases active at low pH. Because Dziewiatkowski and associates[69] used hemoglobin, an excellent substrate for cathepsin D at pH 3.8,[70] which is well in the pH range of cathepsin D, Melrose and Ghosh concluded that this enzyme is present in the disk. This belief is supported by the data of Naylor and associates.[71] This latter group also identified the presence of cathepsin B in the disk based on the use of synthetic substrate.[72] Both of these enzymes would only be expected to be active at a pH below 6.0. However, these low pHs are present in the pathologic disk because lactate is present as a result of the anaerobic metabolism of the disk, even in the presence of oxygen[1] and where a pH as low as 6.1 could be present in the central nucleus. Sedowofia and associates[62,63] also found an elastase-like activity that others have shown to be elevated in degenerative disk and proposed to react with leukocyte elastase antisera.[73] In immature porcine disk, the neutral proteinases were not inhibited by EDTA, but actually had increased activity.[74] This also has not been explained. A latent plasmin-like proteinase[64] also was found for which the novel name "diskinogen" has been proposed.

Disk Proteinase Inhibitors

The disk normally contains a variety of proteinase inhibitors whose highest concentration is in the nucleus.[75,76] These include inhibitors of plasmin, trypsin and chymotrypsin, neutrophil-elastase, and cathepsin G. An unusual secretory leukocyte proteinase inhibitor[77] has also been identified and shown to be synthesized by the disk cells, but with a lower concentration in degenerative disk.[68] Because disk extracts are analogous to cartilage in that they inhibit metalloproteinases, TIMP(s) are also expected to be present.

Accumulated Matrix Protein Fragments and Disk Biology

The disk, especially the nucleus pulposus, contains a significant amount of degraded molecules including those from aggrecan (see chapter by Johnstone), link protein,[66] and collagen. Hollander and associates[78] have developed a sensitive enzyme-linked immunosorbent assay (ELISA) for denatured versus native collagen. They used a monoclonal antibody to an epitope in the sequence of the CNBr'11B fragment of type II collagen in combination with differential digestion with proteinase K to release total collagen, and trypsin to release nonhelical collagen.[78] Using this assay, they were able to demonstrate that there is considerable nonhelical collagen in both older anulus fibrosus and nucleus fibrosus and even more than that of the corresponding articular cartilage.[79] This result would be consistent with extensive clipping by collagenase, but retention of the fragments within the fibrils, possibly because of the high level of normal crosslinks.

Not all of the collagen fragments are associated with the fibrils. For example, as shown in Figure 7, *left*, extract from a grade 3 degenerative disk contains multiple fragments that react with an antisera to cyanogen bromide (CNBr)-digested type II collagen. There may be a general accumulation of matrix protein fragments because fibronectin fragments are also readily detected in the same extract (Fig. 7, *right*).

The presence of degraded matrix proteins is not the only sign of a degradation pathway. The disk also contains amyloid that is formed by proteolysis of precursor proteins.[68] Amyloid increases with degeneration.[19] Many of the matrix molecules may also be modified in advanced glycation,[11] where sugars condensed with amino acid side chains have gone on to form complex products such as pentosidine, pyrrole, and pyrazidine derivatives, or may be products of lipid oxidation. For example, Hormel and Eyre[80] documented specific modifications typical of such reactions for type II collagen. This type of modification could change mechanical as well as blocking sites for cell-matrix interactions.[80] In addition, advanced glycan products, as defined earlier, are capable of directly altering cell-matrix interactions by binding to specific receptors[81] and have been shown to influence chondrocyte metabolism.[82]

It is very clear that extracellular matrix fragments may have significantly different biologic properties. For example, aggrecan synthesis by articular chondrocytes is more efficiently depressed by hyaluronate fragments than by the native molecule.[25] Fibronectin fragments will significantly upregulate a number of catabolic responses of the chondrocyte, including stromelysin production.[83]

521

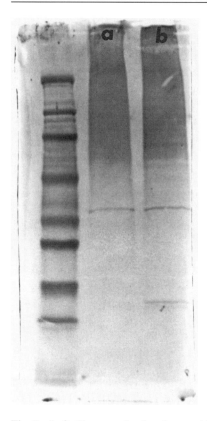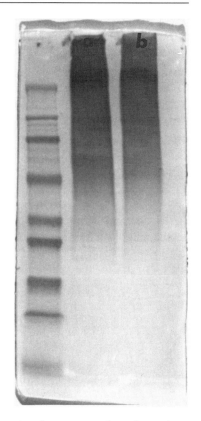

Fig. 7 *Left,* Photograph of an immunoblot demonstrating the presence of a collagen fragment in degenerative human intervertebral disk. Human anulus fibrosus (A) and nucleus pulposus (B) from a disk with grade 3 degeneration were extracted with 4 M guanidine hydrochloride in the presence of proteinase inhibitors and the proteoglycans removed in cesium chloride density centrifugation. After reduction, the D4 fractions were electrophoresed in 4% to 15% linear polyacrylamide gel with SDS in the presence of sodium dodecyl sulfate. The transblots were incubated with rabbit antisera to CNBr-treated type II collagen peptides, then a peroxidase-conjugated goat secondary antibody, and finally developed with $H_2O_2Ni^{+2}$, diaminobenzidine. The molecular weights standards from top to bottom are: 204, 121, 82, 50.2, 34.2 28.11, 19.4, and 7.3 kDa. **Right,** Photograph similar to left, except with a change in the primary antisera to rabbit anti-human fibronectin.

The term "dynamic reciprocity" was coined by Bissell in 1982 to capture the paradigm of the interplay between the cell and its extracellular matrix and how changes in one lead to changes in the other.[84] This is important because, in cartilage, chondrocytes show a strong dependence on cell shape to maintain the differentiated phenotype,[85,86] and loss of spherical shape leads to dedifferentiation and a switch from type II to types I and III collagens. Details of the molecular aspects of dynamic reciprocity are just starting to be understood. It is known that a significant component of the signaling involves cooperative interactions between integrins and other membrane proteins, such as proteoglycans and extracellular matrix macromolecules.[87] In the stable mature tissue, this interplay leads to normal matrix turnover with no net change. It is possible that, during disk degeneration, increased levels of extracellular matrix protein fragments exceed the normal range and force changes in phenotype of the multiple cell types present in the disk[88] with concomitant expression of new genes and suppression of others. This leads to an inability to restore the original matrix and further decline in the quality of the disk.

In summary, there is sound evidence that a variety of matrix protein breakdown products accumulate in the degenerated disk as a result of diverse pathways. Extrapolation studies of other tissues suggest that these products could have detrimental effects on disk cells and alter their metabolism, changing the "nature of the dynamic reciprocity" of the tissue and enhancing further degeneration. This concept needs to be tested directly and its possible relevance to the painful disk ascertained.

Acknowledgments

The author wishes to acknowledge the helpful discussions about the clinically painful disk with Dr. James W. Ogilvie, and the efforts of Jeffrey A.C. Borgia in developing Figures 1 through 5 and compositional assistance; Sandra Johnson for the unpublished results in Figures 6 through 8; and Andrea Chatfield for preparation of the manuscript. This work was supported by NIH grant AR32145.

References

1. Holm S, Maroudas A, Urban JP, et al: Nutrition of the intervertebral disc: Solute transport and metabolism. *Connect Tissue Res* 1981;8:101–119.
2. Olmarker K, Rydevik B, Nordborg C: Autologous nucleus pulposus induces neurophysiologic and histologic changes in porcine cauda equina nerve roots. *Spine* 1993;18:1425–1432.
3. Stromberg J, Zachrisson P, Olmarker K, et al: Inflammatory reactions induced by locally applied nucleus pulposus. *Trans Orthop Res Soc* 1995;20:72.
4. Greenwald RA: Oxygen radicals, inflammation, and arthritis: Pathophysiological considerations and implications for treatment. *Semin Arthritis Rheum* 1991;20:219–240.
5. Rosen GM, Pou S, Ramos CL, et al: Free radicals and phagocytic cells. *FASEB J* 1995;9:200–209.
6. Henrotin Y, Deby-Dupont G, Deby C, et al: Active oxygen species, articular inflammation and cartilage damage, in Emerit I, Chance B (eds): *Free Radicals and Aging.* Basel, Switzerland, Birkhauser Verlag, 1992, pp 308–322.
7. Stadtman ER: Metal ion-catalyzed oxidation of proteins: Biochemical mechanism and biological consequences. *Free Radic Biol Med* 1990;9:315–325.
8. Bedwell S, Dean RT, Jessup W: The action of defined oxygen-centred free radicals on human low-density lipoprotein. *Biochem J* 1989;262:707–712.
9. Behar D, Czapski G, Rabani J, et al: The acid dissociation constant and decay kinetics of the perhydroxyl radical. *J Phys Chem* 1970;74:3209–3213.
10. Yu BP: Oxidative damage by free radicals and lipid peroxidation in aging, in Yu BP (ed): *Free Radicals in Aging.* Boca Raton, FL, CRC Press, 1993, pp 57–88.
11. Wolff SP: Free radicals in glycation, in Yu BP (ed): *Free Radicals in Aging.* Boca Raton, FL, CRC Press, 1993, pp 123–142.
12. Lemercier J-N, Squadrito GL, Pryor WA: Spin trap studies on the decomposition of peroxynitrite. *Arch Biochem Biophys* 1995;321:31–39.
13. Halliwell B, Gutteridge JMC (eds): Protection against oxygen radicals in biological systems: The superoxide theory of oxygen toxicity, in *Free Radicals in Biology and Medicine.* Oxford, England, Clarendon Press, 1985, pp 67–138.

14. Halliwell B, Gutteridge JM: Oxygen free radicals and iron in relation to biology and medicine: Some problems and concepts. *Arch Biochem Biophys* 1986;246:501–514.

15. Tiku ML, Liesch JB, Robertson FM: Abstract: Chondrocytes produce oxygen radicals after treatment with concanavalin A, gamma interferon or tumor necrosis factor. *Arthritis Rheum* 1988;31:S69.

16. Tiku ML, Liesch JB, Robertson FM: Production of hydrogen peroxide by rabbit articular chondrocytes: Enhancement by cytokines. *J Immunol* 1990;145:690–696.

17. Marzabadi MR, Yin D, Brunk UT: Lipofuscinogenesis in a model system of cultured cardiac myocytes, in Emerit I, Chance B (eds): *Free Radicals and Aging*. Basel, Switzerland, Birkhauser Verlag, 1992, pp 78–88.

18. Ishii T, Tsuji H, Sano A, et al: Histochemical and ultrastructural observations on brown degeneration of human intervertebral disc. *J Orthop Res* 1991;9:78–90.

19. Yasuma T, Arai K, Suzuki F: Age-related phenomena in the lumbar intervertebral discs: Lipofuscin and amyloid deposition. *Spine* 1992;17:1194–1198.

20. Harrison KA, Murphy RC: Isoleukotrienes are biologically active free radical products of lipid peroxidation. *J Biol Chem* 1995;270:17273–17278.

21. Bomalaski JS, Lawton P, Browning JL: Human extracellular recombinant phospholipase A2 induces an inflammatory response in rabbit joints. *J Immunol* 1991;146:3904–3910.

22. Stadtman ER, Starke-Reed PE, Oliver CN, et al: Protein modification in aging, in Emerit I, Chance B (eds): *Free Radicals and Aging*. Basel, Switzerland, Birkhauser Verlag, 1992, pp 64–72.

23. Monboisse JC, Borel JP: Oxidative damage to collagen, in Emerit I, Chance B (eds): *Free Radicals and Aging*. Basel, Switzerland, Birkhauser Verlag, 1992, pp 323–327.

24. Vissers MC, Winterbourn CC: Oxidative damage to fibronectin-I: The effects of the neutrophil myeloperoxidase system and HOCl. *Arch Biochem Biophys* 1991;285:53–59.

25. McNeil JD, Wiebkin OW, Betts WH, et al: Depolymerisation products of hyaluronic acid after exposure to oxygen-derived free radicals. *Ann Rheum Dis* 1985;44:780–789.

26. Ng CK, Handley CJ, Preston BN, et al: The extracellular processing and catabolism of hyaluronan in cultured adult articular cartilage explants. *Arch Biochem Biophys* 1992;298:70–79.

27. Ng CK, Handley CJ, Preston BN, et al: Effect of exogenous hyaluronan and hyaluronan oligosaccharides on hyaluronan and aggrecan synthesis and catabolism in adult articular cartilage explants. *Arch Biochem Biophys* 1995;316:596–606.

28. Roberts CR, Mort JS, Roughley PJ: Treatment of cartilage proteoglycan aggregate with hydrogen peroxide: Relationship between observed degradation products and those that occur naturally during aging. *Biochem J* 1987;247:349–357.

29. Roberts CR, Roughley PJ, Mort JS: Degradation of human proteoglycan aggregate induced by hydrogen peroxide: Protein fragmentation, amino acid modification and hyaluronic acid cleavage. *Biochem J* 1989;259:805–811.

30. Birkedal-Hansen H, Moore WG, Bodden MK, et al: Matrix metalloproteinases: A review. *Crit Rev Oral Biol Med* 1993;4:197–250.

31. Taylor JR, Twomey LT: The development of the human intervertebral disc, in Ghosh P (ed): *The Biology of the Intervertebral Disc: Volume 1*. Boca Raton, FL, CRC Press, 1988, pp 39–82.

32. Gronblad M, Virri J, Tolonen J, et al: A controlled immunohistochemical study of inflammatory cells in disc herniation tissue. *Spine* 1994;19:2744–2751.

33. Matrisian LM: The matrix-degrading metalloproteinases. *Bioessays* 1992;14:455–463.

34. Woessner JF Jr: Matrix metalloproteinases and their inhibitors in connective tissue remodeling. *FASEB J* 1991;5:2145–2154.

35. Woessner JF Jr: The family of matrix metalloproteinases. *Ann N Y Acad Sci* 1994;732:11–21.

36. Murphy G, Docherty AJ: The matrix metalloproteinases and their inhibitors. *Am J Respir Cell Mol Biol* 1992;7:120–125.

37. Vincenti MP, Clark IM, Brinckerhoff CE: Using inhibitors of metalloproteinases to treat arthritis: Easier said than done? *Arthritis Rheum* 1994;37:1115–1126.

38. Tyler JA, Bolis S, Dingle JT, et al: Mediators of matrix catabolism, in Kuettner KE, Schleyerbach R, Peyron JG, et al (eds): *Articular Cartilage and Osteoarthritis*. New York, NY, Raven Press, 1992, pp 251–264.

39. Cole A, Chubinskaya S, Huch K, et al: Abstract: Neutrophil collagenase (MMP-8) is expressed by human osteoarthritic chondrocytes. *Transactions of the 2nd Combined Meeting of the Orthopaedic Research Societies of USA, Japan, Canada, and Europe 1995*, San Diego, CA, 1995. Rosemont, IL, Orthopaedic Research Society, in press.

40. Reboul P, Pelletier J-P, Hambor J, et al: Collagenase 3/MMP-13 is selectively expressed by chondrocytes and its synthesis is increased in human OA cartilage: Role in OA pathophysiology. *Orthop Res Soc*, in press.

41. Lefebvre V, Peeters-Joris C, Vaes G: Production of gelatin-degrading matrix metalloproteinases ('type IV collagenases') and inhibitors by articular chondrocytes during their dedifferentiation by serial subcultures and under stimulation by interleukin-1 and tumor necrosis factor alpha. *Biochim Biophys Acta* 1991;1094:8–18.

42. Nagase H, Brinckerhoff CE, Vater CA, et al: Biosynthesis and secretion of procollagenase by rabbit synovial fibroblasts: Inhibition of procollagenase secretion by monensin and evidence for glycosylation of procollagenase. *Biochem J* 1983;214:281–288.

43. Hasty KA, Jeffrey JJ, Hibbs MS, et al: The collagen substrate specificity of human neutrophil collagenase. *J Biol Chem* 1987;262:10048–10052.

44. Freije JMP, Diez-Itza I, Balbin M, et al: Molecular cloning and expression of collagenase-3, a novel human matrix metalloproteinase produced by breast carcinoma. *J Biol Chem* 1994;269:16766–16773.

45. Kleiner DE Jr, Stetler-Stevenson WG: Structural biochemistry and activation of matrix metalloproteinases. *Curr Opin Cell Biol* 1993;5:891–897.

46. Brown PD, Kleiner DE, Unsworth EJ, et al: Cellular activation of the 72 kDa type IV procollagenase/TIMP-2 complex. *Kidney Int* 1993;43:163–170.

47. Strongin AY, Marmer BL, Grant GA, et al: Plasma membrane-dependent activation of the 72-kDa type IV collagenase is prevented by complex formation with TIMP-2. *J Biol Chem* 1993;268:14033–14039.

48. Sato H, Takino T, Okada Y, et al: A matrix metalloproteinase expressed on the surface of invasive tumour cells. *Nature* 1994;370:61–65.

49. Strongin AY, Collier I, Bannikov G, et al: Mechanism of cell surface activation of 72-kDa type IV collagenase: Isolation of the activated form of the membrane metalloprotease. *J Biol Chem* 1995;270:5331–5338.

50. Tryggvason K, Huhtala P, Tuuttila A, et al: Structure and expression of type IV collagenase genes. *Cell Differ Dev* 1990;32:307–312.

51. Wu JJ, Lark MW, Chun LE, et al: Sites of stromelysin cleavage in collagen types II, IX, X, and XI of cartilage. *J Biol Chem* 1991;266:5625–5628.

52. Hardingham TE, Fosang AJ: The structure of aggrecan and its turnover in cartilage. *J Rheumatol* 1995;43(suppl):86–90.

53. Fosang AJ, Last K, Neame PJ, et al: Neutrophil collagenase (MMP-8) cleaves at the aggrecanase site E373-A374 in the interglobular domain of cartilage aggrecan. *Biochem J* 1994;304:347–351.

54. Hughes CE, Caterson B, Fosang AJ, et al: Monoclonal antibodies that specifically recognize neoepitope sequences generated by ''aggrecanase'' and matrix metalloproteinase cleavage of aggrecan: Application to catabolism in situ and in vitro. *Biochem J* 1995;305:799–804.

55. Loulakis P, Shrikhande A, Davis G, et al: N-Terminal sequence of proteoglycan fragments isolated from medium of interleukin-1-treated articular-cartilage cultures: Putative site(s) of enzymic cleavage. *Biochem J* 1992;284:589–593.

56. Baricos WH, Cortez SL, el-Dahr SS, et al: ECM degradation by cultured human mesangial cells is mediated by a PA/plasmin/MMP-2 cascade. *Kidney Int* 1995;47:1039–1047.

57. Serni U, Fibbi G, Anichini E, et al: Plasminogen activator and receptor in osteoarthritis. *J Rheumatol* 1995;43(suppl):120–122.

58. Fibbi G, Serni U, Matucci A, et al: Control of the chondrocyte fibrinolytic balance by the drug piroxicam: Relevance to the osteoarthritic process. *J Rheumatol* 1994;21:2322–2328.

59. Campbell IK, Wojta J, Novak U, et al: Cytokine modulation of plasminogen activator inhibitor-1 (PAI-1) production by human articular cartilage and chondrocytes: Down-regulation by tumor necrosis factor alpha and up-regulation by transforming growth factor-B basic fibroblast growth factor. *Biochim Biophys Acta* 1994;1226:277–285.

60. Yasuda T, Shimizu K, Nakagawa Y, et al: m-calpain in rat growth plate chondrocyte cultures: Its involvement in the matrix mineralization process. *Dev Biol* 1995;170:159–168.

61. Fujimori Y, Shimizu K, Suzuki K, et al: Immunohistochemical demonstration of calcium-dependent cysteine proteinase (calpain) in collagen-induced arthritis in mice. *Z Rheumatol* 1994;53:72–75.

62. Sedowofia KA, Tomlinson IW, Weiss JB, et al: Collagenolytic enzyme systems in human intervertebral disc: Their control, mechanism, and their possible role in the initiation of biomechanical failure. *Spine* 1982;7:213–222.

63. Sedowofia SKA, Tomlinson I, Jayson MIV, et al: Abstract: Identification of collagenase and other neutral proteinases in human intervertebral discs. *Ann Rheum Dis* 1979;38:573.

64. Melrose J, Ghosh P, Taylor TK: Neutral proteinases of the human intervertebral disc. *Biochim Biophys Acta* 1987;923:483–495.

65. Liu J, Roughley PJ, Mort JS: Identification of human intervertebral disc stromelysin and its involvement in matrix degradation. *J Orthop Res* 1991;9:568–575.

66. Pearce RH, Mathieson JM, Mort JS, et al: Effect of age on the abundance and fragmentation of link protein of the human intervertebral disc. *J Orthop Res* 1989;7:861–867.

67. Nguyen Q, Liu J, Roughley PJ, et al: Link protein as a monitor *in situ* of endogenous proteolysis in adult human articular cartilage. *Biochem J* 1991;278:143–147.

68. Melrose J, Ghosh P: The noncollagenous proteins of the intervertebral disc, in Ghosh P (ed): *The Biology of the Intervertebral Disc, Volume 1*. CRC Press, Boca Raton, FL, 1988, pp 189–237.

69. Dziewiatkowski DD, Tourtellotte CD, Campo RD: Degradation of protein-polysaccharide (Chondromucoprotein) by an enzyme extracted from cartilage, in Quintarelli G (ed): *The Chemical Physiology of Mucopolysaccharides*. London, England, J & A Churchill, 1968, pp 63–79.

70. Barrett AJ, McDonald JK: Cathepsin D, in Barrett AJ, McDonald JK (eds): *Mammalian Proteinases: A Glossary and Bibliography. Volume I: Endopeptidases*. New York, NY, Academic Press, 1980, pp 338–350.

71. Naylor A, Shentall RD, West DC: Current investigations on the biochemical aspects of intervertebral disc degeneration and herniation, in Hartmann F, Hartung C, Zeidler H (eds): *Biopolymere und Biomechanik von Bindegewebssystemen*. Berlin, Germany, Springer-Verlag, 1974, p 77.

72. Barrett AJ: An improved color reagent for use in Barrett's assay of Cathepsin B. *Anal Biochem* 1976;76:374–376.

73. Fujita K, Nakagawa T, Hirabayashi K, et al: Neutral proteinases in human intervertebral disc: Role in degeneration and probable origin. *Spine* 1993;18:1766–1773.

74. Tomlinson I, Jayson MIV, Weiss JB: Abstract: Unusual collagenase and gelatinase enzymes in immature pig intervertebral discs. *Ann Rheum Dis* 1979;38:573.

75. Andrews JL, Melrose J, Ghosh P: A comparative study of the low-molecular mass serine proteinase inhibitors of human connective tissues. *Biol Chem Hoppe Seyler* 1992;373:111–118.

76. Knight JA, Stephens RW, Bushell GR, et al: Neutral proteinase inhibitors from human intervertebral disc and femoral head articular cartilage. *Biochim Biophys Acta* 1979;584:304–310.

77. Jacoby AS, Melrose J, Robinson BG, et al: Secretory leucocyte proteinase inhibitor is produced by human articular cartilage chondrocytes and intervertebral disc fibrochondrocytes. *Eur J Biochem* 1993;218:951–957.

78. Hollander AP, Heathfield TF, Webber C, et al: Increased damage to type II collagen in osteoarthritic articular cartilage detected by a new immunoassay. *J Clin Invest* 1994;93:1722–1732.

79. Hollander AP, Heathfield TF, Liu J, et al: Enhanced damage to type II collagen in normal adult human intervertebral discs compared to femoral articular cartilage. *J Orthop Res* 1996;14:61–66.

80. Hormel SE, Eyre DR: Collagen in the ageing human intervertebral disc: An increase in covalently bound fluorophores and chromophores. *Biochim Biophys Acta* 1991;1078:243–250.

81. Shaw SM, Crabbe MJ: Non-specific binding of advanced-glycosylation end-products to macrophages outweighs specific receptor-mediated interactions. *Biochem J* 1994;304:121–129.

82. Pokharna HK, Monnier V, Boja B, et al: Lysyl oxidase and Maillard reaction-mediated crosslinks in aging and osteoarthritic rabbit cartilage. *J Orthop Res* 1995;13:13–21.

83. Xie DL, Hui F, Meyers R, et al: Cartilage chondrolysis by fibronectin fragments is associated with release of several proteinases: Stromelysin plays a major role in chondrolysis. *Arch Biochem Biophys* 1994;311:205–212.

84. Bissell MJ, Hall HG, Parry G: How does the extracellular matrix direct gene expression? *J Theor Biol* 1982;99:31–68.

85. von der Mark K, Gauss V, von der Mark H, et al: Relationship between cell shape and type of collagen synthesised as chondrocytes lose their cartilage phenotype in culture. *Nature* 1977;267:531–532.

86. Benya PD, Shaffer JD: Dedifferentiated chondrocytes reexpress the differentiated collagen phenotype when cultured in agarose gels. *Cell* 1982;30:215–224.

87. Huhtala P, Humphries MJ, McCarthy JB, et al: Cooperative signaling by $\alpha5\beta1$ and $\alpha4\beta1$ integrins regulates metalloproteinase gene expression in fibroblasts adhering to fibronectin. *J Cell Biol* 1995;129:867–879.

88. Chelberg MK, Banks GM, Geiger DF, et al: Identification of heterogeneous cell populations in normal human intervertebral disc. *J Anat* 1995;186:43–53.

Chapter 32

Cytokines, Nitric Oxide, Prostaglandin E$_2$, and Idiopathic Low Back Pain

James D. Kang, MD
Christopher H. Evans, PhD

Introduction

Idiopathic low back pain continues to be a significant clinical and economic problem that causes major disability.[1-6] Although the exact pathophysiology of low back pain is unknown, intervertebral disk degeneration is believed to be an important factor.[4,7-9] Previous studies have described the changes in extracellular matrix of the intervertebral disk with respect to aging and degeneration,[7-11] but very little has been written on the possible roles of various cytokines and other inflammatory mediators in disk degeneration and low back pain. Because it is well known that there is a net loss of proteoglycans with disk degeneration, understanding the exact biochemical regulatory mechanisms related to this phenomenon would be beneficial in understanding the etiology of and possibly treating low back pain.

This chapter will review the current knowledge of cytokines and other mediators of inflammation with respect to the intervertebral disk and discuss their possible roles in the pathophysiology of low back pain.

Cytokines

Cytokines are low molecular weight proteins that mediate communication between cells during normal as well as abnormal biologic processes. They perform their functions, usually within a short distance from the cells that secrete them, either in an autocrine fashion (influencing the same cell that produced the cytokine) or in a paracrine fashion (influencing adjacent cells). Cytokines bind to specific membrane receptors on target cells, subsequently leading to alterations in gene expression.

The generic term *cytokine* includes, for example, colony stimulating factors, growth factors, chemotactic factors (chemokines), interleukins (ILs), and interferons. However, classifying cytokines in this manner is often confusing because of their multiple physiologic functions. For example, some ILs primarily regulate cell growth and differentiation, whereas some growth factors have proinflammatory properties. Some of the more important cytokines grouped by their primary physiologic function are shown in Table 1.

Table 1 Functional classification of cytokines

Colony-stimulating factors (CSFs)
GM-CSF (granulocyte–macrophage CSF)
G-CSF (granulocyte CSF)
M-CSF (macrophage CSF or CSF-1)
IL-3 (interleukin-3)
Erythropoietin

Growth and differentiation factors
PDGF (platelet-derived growth factor)
EGF (epidermal growth factor)
FGF (fibroblast growth factor)
TGF-β (transforming growth factor-beta)

Immunoregulatory cytokines
IL-2 (interleukin-2)
IL-4 (interleukin-4)
IL-5 (interleukin-5)
IL-7 (interleukin-7)
IL-9 (interleukin-9)
IL-10 (interleukin-10)
IL-11 (interleukin-11)
IFN-γ (interferon-gamma)

Proinflammatory cytokines
TNF–α (tumor necrosis factor-alpha)
IL-1 (interleukin-1)
IL-6 (interleukin-6)
IL-8 (interleukin-8)

(Reproduced with permission from Schumacher HR (ed): *Primer on the Rheumatic Diseases*, ed 10. Atlanta, GA, Arthritis Foundation, 1993, pp 46–50.)

Extensive research into the regulation of these cytokines has shown that these agents operate as a complex network that is difficult to investigate or regulate therapeutically because of extensive redundancy and overlap of function. In addition, cytokines influence each others' functions in additive synergistic or inhibitory fashions. However, the cytokine network is normally self-regulating, with pathophysiologic consequences arising from either a dysregulated action or an inappropriate production of certain cytokines.

The clinical relevance of cytokines in the field of orthopaedics has predominantly been in the field of articular cartilage biochemistry. In particular, the proinflammatory cytokines (tumor necrosis factor-alpha [TNF-α], IL-1, IL-6) and growth factors such as transforming growth factor-beta (TGF-β) have received much attention in the literature with specific reference to articular cartilage turnover.[12-23] The exact function of these agents in normal physiology is still unclear, but their role in pathophysiologic inflammation and tissue necrosis has been extensively investigated.

TNF-α is produced by monocytes, macrophages, lymphocytes, synovial cells, and articular chondrocytes as well as a variety of transformed cell lines. Its production is stimulated by endotoxin, viral infections, and other cytokines, such as IL-lα. It induces collagenase and prostaglandin E$_2$ (PGF$_2$) production in synovial fibroblasts and accelerates the release of matrix components from cartilage. It is present in rheumatoid synovium and may be an important inducer of IL-l in this disease. In addition to the catabolic process, TNF-α also has been shown to inhibit the biosynthesis of new proteoglycans by chondrocytes. For these reasons, TNF-α can be potentially very damaging to cartilage.[23]

The IL-1 family consists of IL-1α, IL-1β, and IL-1 receptor antagonist protein (IL-lra). IL-lα and IL-lβ bind to the same receptors and produce the same biologic responses. In humans, IL-1α is primarily membrane bound while IL-lβ is the major secreted product. They are produced by synovial fibroblasts, chondrocytes, macrophages, and other cells involved in inflammation. Similar to TNF-α, IL-l accelerates the breakdown of cartilage matrix by stimulating the production of matrix metalloproteinases (MMP) and inhibiting the biosynthesis of proteoglycans. Therefore, IL-1 can also be extremely damaging to articular cartilage. In contrast, IL-1ra has been shown to be protective of cartilage breakdown by binding to the specific IL-1 receptors and inhibiting the effects of IL-1.[19]

IL-6 also appears to play an important role in acute inflammatory diseases. It is produced by synovial cells in response to IL-1 and TNF-α, but its exact regulatory function has not been clearly defined. It is also produced by chondrocytes in vast amounts, and evidence indicates that IL-6 induces the synthesis of tissue inhibitor of metalloproteinases.[21] IL-6 may also be necessary, but not sufficient, for the suppression of matrix biosynthesis by IL-1.[22]

TGF-β is among the most studied of growth factors and has particular relevance in orthopaedics.[14,17,19] It has the paradoxical capability of enhancing or inhibiting the differentiation of fibroblasts, and depending on the circumstances, may enhance or inhibit inflammatory responses. However, it is generally agreed that TGF-β is an immunosuppressive molecule with the ability to promote repair.[19] In articular cartilage, TGF-β has an impressive ability to promote cartilage repair in vivo by stimulating proteoglycan synthesis and inhibiting the production of MMP.[17]

Nitric Oxide

Nitric oxide (NO) is a novel mediator that has been shown to play a role in immune regulation, inflammation, and of particular interest, in the pathophysiology of arthritis.[24-31] As a possible mediator of inflammation, NO has been shown to have paradoxical effects. As a proinflammatory agent, it has been shown to be a strong vasodilator and to cause increased vascular leaking. On the contrary, in certain circumstances, NO has demonstrated anti-inflammatory effects by its ability to inhibit the synthesis of PGE$_2$, thromboxane, and IL-6. In articular cartilage, proteoglycan synthesis is inhibited by IL-1 through a mechanism that at least partly involves the induction of NO synthesis.

Prostaglandin E$_2$

PGE$_2$ is an arachidonic acid metabolite that plays an important role in mediating inflammation. The anti-inflammatory nature of nonsteroidal anti-inflammatory drugs is believed to be largely related to their ability to inhibit PGE$_2$ synthesis. PGE$_2$ is a potent vasodilator and acts with other vasoactive mediators such as histamines and kinins to increase vascular permeability. In articular cartilage, PGE$_2$ may be a possible intermediary in the suppression of proteoglycan synthesis by IL-1.[22] It also stimulates osteoclastic bone resorption, suggesting that bone erosion in chronic inflammation may be mediated in part by PGE$_2$.[23] Finally, PGE$_2$ has also been shown to induce hyperalgesia.

Intervertebral Disk Metabolism

Because of the importance of cytokines, NO, and PGE$_2$ in the biochemistry of inflammation as well as in articular cartilage matrix metabolism, the question arises as to whether these agents are involved in intervertebral disk metabolism.

The intervertebral disk is an avascular tissue populated by poorly characterized cells in an extensive extracellular matrix. The matrix of the central nucleus pulposus is rich in proteoglycans, whereas the annulus fibrosus is predominantly collagenous.[7,11] With aging, the content of proteoglycans significantly decreases, and this is thought to be an important factor in intervertebral disk degeneration. Because articular cartilage and intervertebral disk share similar characteristics with respect to their matrix composition, it seems reasonable to suggest that the biochemical regulatory mechanisms of matrix turnover and synthesis are also similar.

Kang and associates[32] obtained 18 herniated lumbar disk specimens from 15 patients undergoing surgical diskectomy for persistent radiculopathy and cultured the disks in vitro to determine whether various biochemical agents were being produced. The specimens were cultured and incubated for 72 hours, and the media were subsequently collected for biochemical analysis. Biochemical assays for MMP, NO, PGE$_2$, and a variety of cytokines were performed. As a control group, eight lumbar disk specimens were obtained from four patients undergoing anterior surgery for scoliosis and traumatic burst fractures, and similar biochemical analyses were performed. The culture media from the herniated lumbar disks showed increased levels of MMP activity compared to that of the control disks. Similarly, the levels of NO, PGE$_2$, and IL-6 were significantly higher in the herniated disks compared to that of the control disks (Table 2). IL-1α, IL-1β, and IL-1ra, TNF-α, and substance P were not detected in the culture media of either the herniated or control disks. It was concluded that herniated lumbar disks were spontaneously producing increased amounts of MMPs, NO, PGE$_2$, and IL-6, and that these products may be intimately involved in the biochemistry of disk degeneration as well as the pathophysiology of radiculopathy.

Other studies have also demonstrated similar findings from herniated disk specimens. Saal and associates[33] and Franson and associates[34] studied high phospholipase A$_2$ (PLA$_2$) levels in herniated disks and speculated that the activity of this enzyme was important in vivo because of its inflammatory potential.

Table 2 Summary of biochemical agents produced by intervertebral disks

Study Group	Gelatinase (U/ml)	Collagenase (U/ml)	Caseinase (U/ml)	Nitrite (nmol/g wet weight)	IL-6 (pg/ml)	PGE$_2$ (ng/ml)
Control (n = 8)	1.05 ± 0.96	0 ± 0	0.110 ± 0.091	51.33 ± 6.91	174 ± 218	1.71 ± 1.88
Herniated (n = 18)	5.76 ± 3.62	0.316 ± 0.49	0.432 ± 0.153	132.21 ± 38.66	30401 ± 43480	20.85 ± 32.84
P values	< 0.0008	< 0.14 (NS)	< 0.0024	< 0.000036	< 0.035	< 0.0056

NS = not significant; IL-6 = interleukin-6; PGE$_2$ = prostaglandin E$_2$
(Reproduced with permission from Kang JD, Georgescu HI, Larkin L, et al: Herniated lumbar intervertebral discs spontaneously produce matrix metalloproteinases, nitric oxide, interleukin–6, and prostaglandin E2. *Spine* 1996;21:271–277.)

PLA$_2$ is the enzyme responsible for the liberation from membranes of arachidonic acid, which may ultimately lead to the production of prostaglandins and leukotrienes. Willburger and Wittenberg[35] also found that herniated disks release prostaglandins. Gronblad and associates[36] studied and immunohistochemically characterized the inflammatory cells in herniated disk tissue and were able to show cells that were producing IL-1β. They suggested that inflammation was important in disk tissue pathophysiology and in diskogenic pain mechanisms.[36]

In a later study, Kang and associates[37] measured the in vitro production of NO, IL-6, PGE$_2$ and MMPs by normal human intervertebral disks both under resting conditions and following the addition of human recombinant IL-1β (hr-IL-1β). They showed that, similar to articular cartilage, human intervertebral disk cells responded vigorously to IL-1β with an increase in production of these biochemical agents. In addition, the most significant conclusion was that disk cells not only synthesize NO and IL-6, but that the endogenously produced NO had a large inhibitory effect on IL-6 production. These observations again point to the complex nature of the regulatory interactions that exist between these mediators.

Other authors have also shown that intervertebral disk cells are responsive to stimulation with various cytokines. Yoo and associates (unpublished data, 1995) have shown that cells from the nucleus pulposus respond to TGF-β stimulation by increasing their production of proteoglycans. They hypothesized that TGF-β may modulate repair of the damaged intervertebral disks by its effect on matrix macromolecule synthesis. Thompson and associates[38] investigated the role of growth factors on canine intervertebral disks and similarly showed that these cells responded to various growth factors by increasing their proteoglycan synthesis rate by up to five times. These investigators speculated that exogenous application of certain growth factors to enhance disk tissue repair could be of great clinical significance in treating degenerative disk disease.

Based on these studies, it seems certain that intervertebral disk cells are capable of producing and responding to various cytokines, NO, and PGE$_2$. What remains uncertain is the exact functional roles these agents have on disk degeneration and low back pain.

Disk Degeneration

Based on our knowledge of cartilage biochemistry, speculations can be made as to the functional role of these various biochemical agents on intervertebral disk metabolism. It is well known that with aging, the degenerating interverte-bral disk loses its water content,[7,9-11] and this is believed to be because of the progressive loss of the highly negatively charged proteoglycans. The produc-tion of these cytokines in a degenerating disk would imply that these agents are intimately involved in the biochemistry of progressive proteoglycan loss.

For example, because proteoglycan synthesis in articular cartilage is inhib-ited by IL-1 through a mechanism that at least partly involves the induction of NO synthesis, it seems plausible that NO may also be involved in the inhibi-tion of proteoglycan synthesis by disk cells. Similarly, both IL-6 and PGE_2 are possible additional intermediaries in the suppression of proteoglycan synthesis by IL-1, and therefore may also be involved in the biochemical process of disk degeneration.

Disk degeneration may also occur because of matrix catabolism via the pro-duction of degradative enzymes such as MMPs.[39-44] In particular, the produc-tion of stromelysin, which degrades the core protein of the proteoglycan struc-ture, may have a direct effect on the integrity of the disk matrix. Because cytokines such as IL-1 have been shown to stimulate disk cells into producing increased amounts of MMPs, the functional role of cytokines may be of great importance in the pathophysiology of disk degeneration.

Facet Degeneration

Although evidence is currently lacking, it is conceivable that the facet joint is also a source for production of cytokines and inflammatory mediators. The facet joint is a diarthrodial joint and therefore is surfaced with articular carti-lage and encased by a synovial lining. As the facet joint undergoes degenera-tion, the various cytokines and mediators of inflammation that have been dis-cussed may also be produced and possibly add to the pathophysiology of clinical low back pain.[35,45]

Possible Role in Low Back Pain

What role do cytokines, NO, and PGE_2 have in clinical low back pain? If it is assumed that disk degeneration plays an important role in low back pain, these biochemical agents may have an indirect role in low back pain by being in-volved in the net loss of proteoglycans. However, it is possible to hypothesize that these proinflammatory agents are also directly involved in the production of low back pain.[46] If degenerating disks are producing increased levels of these inflammatory mediators, the mediators may directly affect the nerve endings that have been shown to exist in the outer anulus fibrosus and the longitudinal ligaments.[47-51] In addition, the production of cytokines and other inflammatory mediators by degenerating facet joints may also contribute to low back pain by directly sensitizing nerve endings in the facet capsules and the paraspinal muscles.[35,52] Finally, these cytokines may also directly affect the nearby dorsal root ganglion and spinal nerve root. In addition to possibly being involved in the pathophysiology of radiculopathy,[53-58] the effects on the dorsal root gan-glion may be part of the pathophysiology of low back pain. A hypothetical model

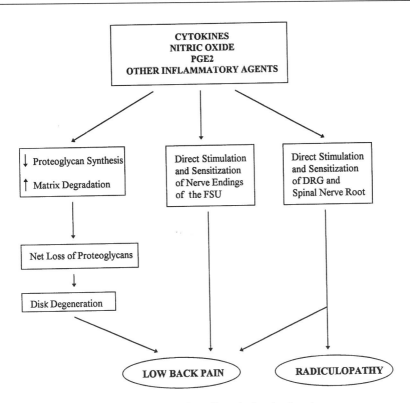

Fig. 1 *Hypothetical model of the role of cytokines in low back pain.*

for the role of cytokines in the pathophysiology of low back pain is illustrated in Figure 1.

Conclusion

Studies have shown that human intervertebral disks are capable of producing certain cytokines, NO, and PGE$_2$. These agents have been shown to be involved in the breakdown of articular cartilage, and therefore, it is plausible that they are also involved in the degeneration of intervertebral disk. In addition, these inflammatory agents may have some direct effect on sensitizing various nerve endings that exist within and around the functional spinal unit. Their exact role in idiopathic low back pain is uncertain, but their presence in degenerating disks should stimulate more investigations in order to clarify the mechanisms of low back pain.

References

1. Cunningham LS, Kelsey JL: Epidemiology of musculoskeletal impairments and associated disability. *Am J Public Health* 1984;74:574–579.
2. Deyo RA, Tsui-Wu YJ: Descriptive epidemiology of low-back pain and its related medical care in the United States. *Spine* 1987;12:264–268.

3. Frymoyer JW, Donaghy RM: The ruptured intervertebral disc: Follow-up report on the first case fifty years after recognition of the syndrome and its surgical significance. *J Bone Joint Surg* 1985;67A:1113–1116.

4. Frymoyer JW, Gordon SL (eds): *New Perspectives on Low Back Pain.* Park Ridge, IL, American Academy of Orthopaedic Surgeons, 1989.

5. Mixter WJ, Barr JS: Rupture of the intervertebral disc with involvement of the spinal canal. *N Engl J Med* 1934;211:210–215.

6. White AA III, Gordon SL (eds): American Academy of Orthopaedic Surgeons *Symposium on Idiopathic Low Back Pain.* St. Louis, MO, CV Mosby, 1982.

7. Coventry MB, Ghormley RK, Kernohan JW: The intervertebral disc: Its microscopic anatomy and pathology. Part II: Changes in the intervertebral disc concomitant with age. *J Bone Joint Surg* 1945;27A:233–247.

8. Gower WE, Pedrini V: Age-related variations in protein-polysaccharides from human nucleus pulposus, annulus fibrosus, and costal cartilage. *J Bone Joint Surg* 1969;51A:1154–1162.

9. Lipson SJ, Muir H: Experimental intervertebral disc degeneration: Morphologic and proteoglycan changes over time. *Arthritis Rheum* 1981;24:12–21.

10. Adams P, Muir H: Qualitative changes with age of proteoglycans of human lumbar discs. *Ann Rheum Dis* 1976;35:289–296.

11. Coventry MB, Ghormley RK, Kernohan JW: The intervertebral disc: Its microscopic anatomy and pathology. Part I: Anatomy, development, and physiology. *J Bone Joint Surg* 1945;27A:105–112.

12. Allen JB, Manthey CL, Hand AR, et al: Rapid onset synovial inflammation and hyperplasia induced by transforming growth factor beta. *J Exp Med* 1990;171:231–247.

13. Bandara G, Lin CW, Georgescu HI, et al: The synovial activation of chondrocytes: Evidence for complex cytokine interactions involving a possible novel factor. *Biochim Biophys Acta* 1992;1134:309–318.

14. Centrella M, McCarthy TL, Canalis E: Transforming growth factor-beta and remodeling of bone. *J Bone Joint Surg* 1991;73A:1418–1428.

15. Dingle JT, Knight CG: The role of the chondrocyte microenvironment in the degradation of cartilage matrix, in Verbruggen G, Veys EM (eds): *Degenerative Joints.* Amsterdam, The Netherlands, Elsevier Science, 1985, vol 2, pp 69–77.

16. Hickery MS, Palmer RMJ, Charles IG, et al: The role of nitric oxide in IL-1 and TNF-α-induced inhibition of proteoglycan synthesis in human articular cartilage. *Trans Orthop Res Soc* 1994;19:77.

17. Hunziker EB, Rosenberg L: Induction of repair in partial thickness articular cartilage lesions by timed release of TGF-b. *Trans Orthop Res Soc* 1994;19:236.

18. Kandel RA, Petelycky M, Dinarello CA, et al: Comparison of the effect of interleukin-6 and interleukin-1 on collagenase and proteoglycan production by chondrocytes. *J Rheumatol* 1990;17:953–957.

19. Kuettner KE, Goldberg VM (eds): *Osteoarthritic Disorders.* Rosemont, IL, American Academy of Orthopaedic Surgeons, 1995.

20. Lefebvre V, Peeters-Joris C, Vaes G: Modulation by interleukin-1 and tumor necrosis factor alpha of production of collagenase, tissue inhibitor of metalloproteinases and collagen types in differentiated and dedifferentiated articular chondrocytes. *Biochim Biophys Acta* 1990;1052:366–378.

21. Lotz M, Guerne PA: Interleukin-6 induces the synthesis of tissue inhibitor of metalloproteinases-1/erythroid potentiating activity (TIMP-1/EPA). *J Biol Chem* 1991;266:2017–2020.

22. Nietfeld JJ, Wilbrink B, Helle M, et al: Interleukin-1 induced interleukin-6 is required for the inhibition of proteoglycan synthesis by interleukin-1 in human articular cartilage. *Arthritis Rheum* 1990;33:1695–1701.

23. Schumacher HR Jr, Klippel JH, Koopman WJ (eds): *Primer on The Rheumatic Diseases,* ed 10. Atlanta, GA, The Arthritis Foundation, 1993.

24. Evans CH: Nitric oxide: What role does it play in inflammation and tissue destruction? *Agents Actions* 1995;47(suppl):107–116.

25. Evans CH, Stefanovic-Racic M, Lancaster J: Nitric oxide and its role in orthopaedic disease. *Clin Orthop* 1995;312:275–294.

26. Green LC, Wagner DA, Glogowski J, et al: Analysis of nitrate, nitrite, and [15N] nitrate in biological fluids. *Anal Biochem* 1982;126:131–138.

27. Meller ST, Cummings CP, Traub RJ, et al: The role of nitric oxide in the development and maintenance of the hyperalgesia produced by intraplantar injection of carrageenan in the rat. *Neuroscience* 1994;60:367–374.

28. Stadler J, Harbrecht BG, Di Silvio M, et al: Endogenous nitric oxide inhibits the synthesis of cyclooxygenase products and interleukin-6 by rat Kupffer cells. *J Leukoc Biol* 1993;53:165–172.

29. Stadler J, Stefanovic-Racic M, Billiar TR, et al: Articular chondrocytes synthesize nitric oxide in response to cytokines and lipopolysaccharide. *J Immunol* 1991;147:3915–3920.

30. Stefanovic-Racic M, Stadler J, Evans CH: Nitric oxide and arthritis. *Arthritis Rheum* 1993;36:1036–1044.

31. Taskiran D, Stefanovic-Racic M, Georgescu H, et al: Nitric oxide mediates suppression of cartilage proteoglycan synthesis by interleukin-1. *Biochem Biophys Res Commun* 1994;200:142–148.

32. Kang JD, Georgescu HI, Larkin L, et al: Herniated lumbar intervertebral discs spontaneously produce matrix metalloproteinases, nitric oxide, interleukin-6, and prostaglandin E2. *Spine* 1996;21:271–277.

33. Saal JS, Franson RC, Dobrow R, et al: High levels of inflammatory phospholipase A2 activity in lumbar disc herniations. *Spine* 1990;15:674–678.

34. Franson RC, Saal JS, Saal JA: Human disc phospholipase A2 is inflammatory. *Spine* 1992;17(suppl 6):S129–132.

35. Willburger RE, Wittenberg RH: Prostaglandin release from lumbar disc and facet joint tissue. *Spine* 1994;19:2068–2070.

36. Gronblad M, Virri J, Tolonen J, et al: A controlled immunohistochemical study of inflammatory cells in disc herniation tissue. *Spine* 1994;19:2744–2751.

37. Kang JD, Stefanovic-Racic M, Larkin L, et al: Nitric oxide production by human intervertebral disc in response to interleukin-1 and its effects on interleukin-6 production. *Trans Orthop Res Soc* 1995;20:351.

38. Thompson JP, Oegema TR Jr, Bradford DS: Stimulation of mature canine intervertebral disc by growth factors. *Spine* 1991;16:253–260.

39. Fujita K, Nakagawa T, Hirabayashi K, et al: Neutral proteinases in human intervertebral disc: Role in degeneration and probable origin. *Spine* 1993;18:1766–1773.

40. Hecht AC, Riviere L, Wright M, et al: The role of a novel serine protease in mammalian articular cartilage degradation. *Trans Orthop Res Soc* 1994;19:50.

41. Liu J, Roughley PJ, Mort JS: Identification of human intervertebral disc stromelysin and its involvement in matrix degradation. *J Orthop Res* 1991;9:568–575.

42. Melrose J, Ghosh P, Taylor TK: Neutral proteinases of the human intervertebral disc. *Biochim Biophys Acta* 1987;923:483–495.

43. Sedowofia KA, Tomlinson IW, Weiss JB, et al: Collagenolytic enzyme systems in human intervertebral disc: Their control, mechanism, and their possible role in the initiation of biomechanical failure. *Spine* 1982;7:213–222.

44. Woessner JF Jr, Gunja-Smith Z: Role of metalloproteinases in human osteoarthritis. *J Rheumatol* 1991;27(suppl):99–101.

45. Wehling P, Bandara G, Evans CH: Synovial cytokines impair the function of the sciatic nerve in rats: A possible element in the pathophysiology of radicular syndromes. *Neuro-Orthop* 1989;7:55–59.

46. McCarron RF, Wimpee MW, Hudkins PG, et al: The inflammatory effect of nucleus pulposus: A possible element in the pathogenesis of low-back pain. *Spine* 1987;12:760–764.

47. Bogduk N, Tynan W, Wilson AS: The nerve supply to the human lumbar intervertebral discs. *J Anat* 1981;132:39–56.

48. Jackson HC II, Winkelmann RK, Bickel WH: Nerve endings in the human lumbar spinal column and related structures. *J Bone Joint Surg* 1966;48A:1272–1281.

537

49. Nade S, Bell E, Wyke BD: Abstract: The innervation of the lumbar spinal joints and its significance. *J Bone Joint Surg* 1980;62B:255.

50. Roofe PG: Innervation of annulus fibrosus and posterior longitudinal ligament: Fourth and fifth lumbar level. *Arch Neurol Psychiat* 1940;44:100–103.

51. Shinohara H: Lumbar disc lesion, with special reference to the histological significance of nerve endings of the lumbar discs. *Nippon Seikeigeka Gakka Zasshi* 1970;44:553–570.

52. Giles LG, Taylor JR: Innervation of lumbar zygapophyseal joint synovial folds. *Acta Orthop Scand* 1987;58:43–46.

53. Bobechko WP, Hirsch C: Auto-immune response to nucleus pulposus in the rabbit. *J Bone Joint Surg* 1965;47B:574–580.

54. Gertzbein SD, Tile M, Gross A, et al: Autoimmunity in degenerative disc disease of the lumbar spine. *Orthop Clin North Am* 1975;6:67–73.

55. Marshall LL, Trethewie ER: Chemical irritation of nerve-root in disc prolapse. *Lancet* 1973;2:320.

56. Marshall LL, Trethewie ER, Curtain CC: Chemical radiculitis: A clinical, physiological and immunological study. *Clin Orthop* 1977;129:61–67.

57. Rydevik B, Brown MD, Ehira T, et al: Abstract: Effects of graded compression and nucleus pulposus on nerve tissue: An experimental study in rabbits. *Acta Orthop Scand* 1983;54:670–671.

58. Smyth MJ, Wright V: Sciatica and the intervertebral disc: An experimental study. *J Bone Joint Surg* 1958;40A:1401–1418.

Chapter 33

Collagens of the Intervertebral Disk: Structure, Function, and Changes During Aging and Disease

Shirley Ayad, BSc, PhD
Linda J. Sandell, PhD

Introduction

Our concept of "collagen" has changed dramatically over the past 20 years and it is becoming increasingly difficult to define what is a collagen and what is not.[1,2] The two criteria that classify a protein as a collagen are: (1) it must contain at least one domain with the characteristic triple helical structure, and (2) it must be an integral component of the extracellular matrix. The triple helix is comprised of three polypeptide (α-) chains, each exhibiting the repeating triplet $[Gly-X-Y]_n$ structure, where X and Y can be any amino acid but approximately 20% to 22% are the amino acids proline and hydroxyproline, respectively. Glycine is the only amino acid small enough to fit into the center of the helix, and hydroxyproline forms hydrogen bonds that stabilize the helix. Lysine and hydroxylysine in both helical and nonhelical regions are important for the formation of stable crosslinks between the different collagens in many of their supramolecular assemblies. Hydroxylysine is also a potential attachment site for galactose or glucosyl-galactose.

At least 19 collagen types are encoded by at least 33 genes, and many of these are present in the intervertebral disk[3] (Table 1). Further structural diversity of the collagens arises at both pre- and posttranslational levels. Variants of the same α-chain can arise via alternative splicing of exons or the use of an alternate promoter to give distinct mRNAs. Following translation, the α-chains are subjected to different levels of hydroxylation and glycosylation with both simple and complex sugars, and at least three collagen types can be posttranslationally modified with a glycosaminoglycan moiety and can be classified as proteoglycans. Further complexity arises according to the selection of identical or distinct α-chains to form homo- or heterotrimers, respectively, and some collagen types exist in several chain isoforms. Thus, collagens exist in a number of structural isoforms, each finely tuned to suit a particular function. This fine-tuning can vary within the same collagen in different tissues or in the same tissue at different developmental stages and different physiologic states. The majority of this chapter will concentrate on the collagens of the mature spinal column; however, a section on the potential role of collagens in development is presented.

Table 1 The genetically distinct collagens of the intervertebral disk

Class	Type	Molecules	α-chain Mr. x 10⁻³	Tissue Distribution
Fibrillar	I	[α1(I)]₂ α2(I)	95	Anulus fibrosus
	II	[α1(II)]₃	95	Anulus fibrosus Nucleus pulposus Cartilage end plate
	III	[α1(III)]₃	95	Traces in all 3 regions
	V/XI	[α1(V)]₂ α2(V) [α1(V) α2(V) α3(V)] [α1(XI) α2 (XI) α3(XI)] mixed molecules of V and XI	120-145	Heterotypic fibrils of V with I and XI with II, but mixed molecules of V/XI with I and/or II possible
Microfibrillar	VI	[α1(VI) α2(VI) α3(VI)]	α1/α2 = 140 α3 = 200-280	Largely pericellular in all 3 regions
Fibril-associated (FACITs)	IX	[α1(IX) α2(IX) α3(IX)]	α1 = 66 (short form) or 84 (long form), α2 = 66 (non-glycanated) or 66-115 (glycanated) α3 = 72	Long form in cartilage end plate, long and short forms in anulus fibrosus and nucleus pulposus
	XII	[α1(XII)]₃	220 (short form) 340 (long form) Long form can be glycanated	Unknown
	XIV	[α1(XIV)]₃	220 Can be glycanated	Unknown
Short-chain	X	[α1(X)]₃	59	Calcifying regions of end plate cartilage

Domain Organization and Supramolecular Assembly in the Extracellular Matrix

Newly synthesized collagens consist of both collagenous (COL) and noncollagenous (NC) domains and are modified in different ways outside the cell.[4] In the case of the major fibril-forming collagens I, II, and III, the molecules are synthesized as large precursor (pro) collagens comprising a relatively long continuous helical COL domain, at the ends of which are NC domains (propeptides) (Fig. 1, *top*). The propeptides are cleaved extracellularly by specific enzymes and the resulting (processed) molecules then spontaneously aggregate to form the fibrils. Collagens V and XI are also synthesized as procollagens but are only partially processed prior to assembly. For most other collagens, little or no processing can be demonstrated and the term "procollagen" is not used. These collagens differ significantly from the fibrillar collagens in the number, length, and complexity of the COL and NC domains.

Heterotypic Fibrils It is important to note that pure "type I" or "type II" collagen fibrils do not exist and that all fibrils are *heterotypic*, comprising at least three different collagens.[5,6] In general, collagens V and XI form a fibrillar core within the major fibers but their N-terminal propeptide domains that remain after partial processing project from the fibril surface. Other collagens, known as fibril associated collagens with interrupted triple helices (FACITs), which include collagens IX, XII and XIV, then associate with the outer fibril surface (Fig. 1, *bottom*).[7]

Microfibrils Microfibrils, composed entirely of collagen VI, form an interconnecting network between the major collagen fibers and other matrix macro-

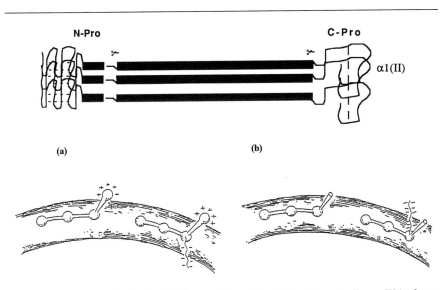

Fig. 1   Top, *Heterotypic fibrils of collagens II and XI and the different collagen IX isoforms.* **Bottom,** *Schematic diagram showing major fibrils of collagens II and XI with (a) long form of collagen IX (with positively charged noncollagenous (NC4) domain) or (b) short form of collagen IX, on the outer fibril surface. Both the long and short forms can exist as glycanated (with a negatively charged glycosaminoglycan chain) or nonglycanated species.*

molecules and, particularly in cartilaginous tissues, between the extracellular matrix and the cells.[8]

Collagens of the Intervertebral Disk

For detailed reviews on the earlier biochemical studies on the disk, the reader is referred to Eyre,[9] Ayad and Weiss,[10] Eyre,[11] and Bayliss and Johnstone.[12] The intervertebral disk is a unique and very specialized connective tissue, comprising three morphologically distinct regions: the fibrous anulus fibrosus, the gelatinous nucleus pulposus, and the cartilaginous end plates. Collagen accounts for approximately 50% to 60%, 15% to 20%, and 50% to 70% of the dry weight of the anulus fibrosus, nucleus pulposus, and cartilage end plate, respectively. However, the amount varies considerably in different anatomic sites within each of these three regions, in general being highest in the outer anulus and the end plate nearest the bone and lowest in the nucleus pulposus and cartilage end plate nearest the nucleus. The major fibrils of the anulus are organized in a parallel array in concentric lamellae around a central nucleus that contains randomly organized fibrils. It is not surprising that the collagens within the three distinct matrices are different. In general, the anulus fibrosus contains collagens I, II, III, V, VI, IX, and XI characteristic of both cartilage and fibrous tissues such as tendon, whereas the nucleus pulposus and the end plates contain collagens II, VI, IX, and XI found in cartilage (Table 1). The presence of the different collagens was first established after chemical modification of the tissues by either cyanogen bromide or pepsin digestion, or by immunolocalization using anticollagen antibodies. It should be stressed that, with few exceptions, the structures of the native intact forms of the disk collagens have not been determined unequivocally but have been inferred only from known structures in other tissues. Given the structural diversity that is possible, this is certainly not a valid assumption as recent studies have shown.

Fibrillar Collagens

Types I, II, and III Collagens The collagen content decreases across the disk from the outer anulus to the nucleus and is accompanied by a radial change in the distribution of collagens I and II: the collagens vary inversely in their proportions across the disk, with the outer section of the anulus fibrosus containing exclusively collagen I and the nucleus pulposus containing collagen II.[13,14] The degree of posttranslational modifications of both collagens I and II is higher in the disk than in other tissues. The disk collagens contain a higher hydroxylysine and hydroxylysine glycoside content as well as a higher disaccharide to monosaccharide ratio.[9,15-17] Although the significance of these changes is not known, it has been postulated that the increased glycoside content results in greater fibril stability, increased hydration (hence increased swelling pressure) and limits fibril diameters and fibril packing.[17] The presence of collagens I and II in the anulus fibrosus raises the possibility that the heterotypic fibrils may be even more complex and contain both these major collagens, in addition to V/XI and FACIT collagens. In this respect, recent crosslinking studies[18] have shown that although most of the collagens I and II form their own heterotypic fibrils, a proportion can copolymerize in the same fibril or at least crosslink with each other after lateral fusion of fibrils. Moreover, an antiparallel arrangement was observed for some of the collagen I molecules, possibly indicating the lateral fusion of adjacent antiparallel fibrils. This arrangement may allow fibril branching and an increased mechanical strength of the anulus.[18]

Type III collagen has also been detected around the cells in all three regions of the disk in immunofluorescence studies, but reports of its actual extraction are limited.[14,19,20]

Two forms of type II collagen can be synthesized from the single COL2A1 gene: a long form containing the NH_2-propeptide (encoded by exon 2) and a short form without the NH_2-propeptide.[21] In the vertebral column, as in other cartilaginous structures, these two splice forms are developmentally regulated with the long form (type IIA) predominant in chondroprogenitor cells and the short form (type IIB) predominant in cartilage.[22] In addition to the presence of type IIA in precartilage, it is also present in the notochord, a structure thought to induce chondrogenesis, and in the somites, structures that are precursors to vertebrae and intervertebral disk. A further discussion of development of the intervertebral disk will be presented later. In terms of fibril formation, both type IIA and type IIB collagens can form fibrils although there is some evidence that they may differ in final diameter. In mature disks, the type II collagen fibrils are primarily derived from the type IIB procollagen splice form.

Types V and XI Collagens   Collagens V and XI were originally thought to be present in noncartilaginous and cartilaginous tissues, respectively, but it is now known that the α-chains of the two collagens can form mixed molecules and that there is probably only one collagen V/XI family with many isoforms.[6,23,24] Because early reports have classified the two collagens separately, they will be designated here as collagens V and XI. Collagen XI is found in the nucleus pulposus whereas both collagens V and XI are found in the anulus.[10,11] Because collagen V forms copolymers with type I collagen[5] and collagen XI copolymerizes with collagen II,[6,25] it is possible that collagens V and XI will follow radial distribution patterns similar to those of collagens I and II, respectively.[11] However, mixed molecules cannot be ruled out, particularly in the anulus.

Collagens V and XI possess a carboxy propeptide that is similar in both size and the way it is processed to that of collagens I-III. However, the aminopropeptide of the different collagen V/XI α-chains varies considerably in size and in the degree and mode of processing and probably plays a role in controlling the ultimate diameter of the major collagen fibrils with which they copolymerize.[26,27] The aminopropeptide domains project from the surface of the fibrils and therefore (like FACITs) have the potential to interact with other matrix components. Recent evidence suggests that complex alternative splicing of the aminopropeptide domain occurs to give tissue-specific forms.[28,29] In particular, the α1 and α2 chains of collagen XI from cartilage lack an acidic region that is present in noncartilaginous tissues. Whether cartilage- and/or noncartilage-specific forms are present in the disk tissues is not known.

FACIT Collagens

Type IX Collagen   Collagen IX is the best characterized of the FACITs and occurs almost exclusively in cartilaginous tissues and vitreous humor.[6,30] In these tissues it not only interacts with the collagen II fibril surface but is covalently crosslinked to, and bridges, the fibrils, thereby stabilizing the collagenous net-work.[31] Recent studies have indicated that the collagen IX monomers are also covalently linked to each other, increasing the stability of this network still fur-ther.[32] Collagen IX is comprised of three short triple-helical domains (COL1-3) interspersed by four nonhelical domains (NC1-4), and the individual α-chains are genetically distinct (Fig. 2). It can exist in both glycanated and nonglycan-ated forms according to the presence or absence, respectively, of a glycosami-noglycan (GAG) chain on the NC3 domain of the α2 chain.[33,34] Two further isoforms of collagen IX are possible depending on the presence or absence of the large amino-terminal NC4 domain on the α1(IX) chain, giving rise to long and short forms respectively. The NC4 domain, which, together with the COL3 domain, projects away from the fibril surface, is positively charged. It therefore has the potential to interact with the negatively charged proteoglycans and/or hyaluronan in the cartilage matrix[35] (Fig. 3). The short form is caused by the use of an alternative promoter and alternative splicing in the gene encoding the α1(IX) chain.[36]

The proportion of collagen IX to collagen II in the nucleus pulposus is simi-lar to that in hyaline cartilage. Similarly, the lower levels of collagen IX present in the anulus fibrosus is proportional to the lower levels of collagen II.[11] Col-lagen IX is probably present on the outside of the "collagen II" fibrils as in other cartilages. Recent studies have shown that both the short and long forms of collagen IX are present in the anulus fibrosus and nucleus pulposus, the short form predominant particularly in the nucleus.[37] The short form's predominance in the nucleus is consistent with observations that this form is secreted by the notochord, believed to be the precursor of the nucleus, at least in the early stages of development.[38,39] It would appear that the short form is predominant in tis-sues in which there are few collagen fibrils that are randomly organized, as in

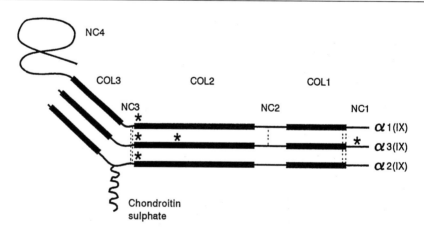

Fig. 2 *Domain structure of collagen IX. Schematic diagram of collagen IX showing the three collagenous triple helical domains (COL1-3) interspersed between four noncollagenous do-mains (NC1-4). Crosslinking sites are indicated by an asterisk and disulfide bonds by the dotted lines. A chondroitin sulfate glycosaminoglycan chain can be attached to the NC3 do-main of the α2(IX) chain.*

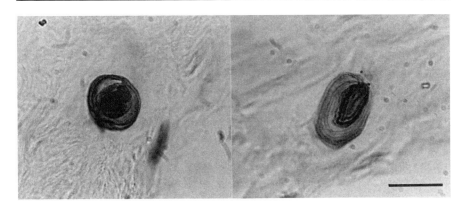

Fig. 3 *Immunoperoxidase localization of collagen VI in the nucleus pulposus of the human intervertebral disk. Collagen VI is localized in the pericellular microenvironment of the chondrocytes (often in the form of discrete concentric rings). Bar represents 30 μm. (Reproduced with permission from Roberts S, Ayad S, Menage PJ: Immunolocalisation of type VI collagen in the intervertebral disc.* Ann Rheum Dis *1991;50:787–791.)*

the nucleus pulposus and also the vitreous humor.[40,41] Only the long form is present in the cartilage end plate and both short and long forms exist as glycanated and nonglycanated species in the disk.[37]

Types XII and XIV Collagens Two further members of the FACITs, collagens XII and XIV, were originally believed to be the analogues of collagen IX and to be present only in noncartilaginous tissues in association with collagen I-containing fibrils.[7] However, recent studies have demonstrated their presence as both glycanated and nonglycanated forms in fetal cartilage.[42] Collagens XII and XIV are homotrimers and contain two collagenous domains (COL1-2) interspersed by three noncollagenous (NC1-3) domains. The amino-terminal NC3 domain is extremely large and contains motifs characteristic of adhesive glycoproteins.[43,44] Alternative splicing of the pre-mRNA encoding the NC3 domain of the α1(XII) chain gives rise to two variants: a large variant carrying the GAG chain(s) in an extended NC3 domain and predominating in cartilage and a smaller nonglycanated variant. In contrast to collagen IX, current evidence suggests that collagens XII and XIV are not covalently crosslinked to the major fibrils and consequently are extracted easily from tissues. Collagens XII and XIV have also been found in the intervertebral disk but have not been fully characterized.[18]

Type VI Collagen Collagen VI is a component of most, if not all, connective tissues and occurs as thin microfibrils adjacent to the major collagen fibrils and to cells.[8] It is essentially a glycoprotein with a short triple helix (approximately one third the length of collagen I) and large nonhelical N- and C-terminal domains and exists largely in the form of a heterotrimer comprising three distinct α1(VI), α2(VI), α3(VI) chains. The N- and C-terminal domains of each of the three α-chains are extremely complex and comprise several structural motifs characteristic of adhesive glycoproteins. The α3(VI) chain is the most complex of all three chains because of extended N- and C-terminal domains, being

545

approximately twice the size of the other two chains. Several structural variants also arise because of alternative splicing at the N-terminal domain of the α3(VI) chain and at the C-terminal end of the α2(VI) chain. Differential expression of specific domains within collagen VI could modulate the interactions that occur during self-assembly of the monomers into microfibrils as well as interactions with other macromolecules and cells.

Collagen VI is preferentially localized to the pericellular microenvironment of the chondrocyte and the surrounding fibrillar capsule which together constitute the chondron, believed to be the functional metabolic unit in cartilage.[45,46] Electron-microscopic studies have shown that collagen VI provides a close functional interrelationship between the chondrocyte, its pericellular environment, and the load-bearing extracellular matrix of adult cartilage. Collagen VI is also localized preferentially to the chondrons in all three regions of the disk but is more pronounced in the nucleus pulposus[20,47] (Fig. 3). Its presence in the nucleus pulposus explains the preponderance of unusual banded structures (sometimes called "zebra" collagen, "Luse bodies," or "fibrous-long-spacing (FLS) collagen" that were observed previously via electron microscopy[48,49] and that are now known to result from the lateral aggregation of collagen VI microfibrils.[8] Collagen VI has been isolated from the disk in an intact form using a specific *Streptomyces* hyaluronidase.[50] This study provided the first evidence for the interaction of collagen VI with hyaluronan in a cartilaginous tissue. Collagen VI was found to be abundant in the disk, especially the nucleus pulposus, where it accounts for 20% of the total collagen (bovine) in agreement with localization studies.[20,47,49] In the anulus fibrosus it accounts for 5% of the total collagen, although amounts may vary with species because it was localized to a greater extent in the interterritorial matrix in the bovine tissue compared to human.[20,47]

Type X Collagen Collagen X is produced largely by the hypertrophic chondrocytes within the growth plates at the ends of developing long bones. It appears to be a marker for cartilage that calcifies and is subsequently replaced by bone by endochondral ossification.[51] However, there is no conclusive evidence for a direct relationship between this collagen and the mechanism of calcification. Collagen X comprises a short triple helix (approximately half the length of collagens I-III), a small amino terminal domain, and a large globular carboxy terminal domain. Collagen X has not been extracted from, or localized in, the intervertebral disk but is probably a component of the end plate cartilage that is replaced by vertebral bone.

Collagen Crosslinking in the Disk The heterotypic fibrils (but not the collagen VI microfibrils) are stabilized by covalent bonds derived by the chemical modification of lysine/hydroxylysine residues.[31] Crosslinks involving only two molecules are replaced by more stable trifunctional hydroxypyridinium crosslinks. Human disk collagens contain a higher concentration of these mature crosslinks than any other connective tissue, the highest concentration occurring in the nucleus pulposus where there may be a greater need for fiber reinforcement to the gel matrix.[11,50]

Biosynthesis of Extracellular Matrix Components by Cells of Intervertebral Disk

Until recently, few studies have been done using the cells of the disk. Johnstone and Bayliss[52] have now established a technique whereby slices of disk tissue can be maintained in organ cultures. Using this technique, proteoglycan synthesis was examined in human disks of various ages and pathologies. The results indicate that biosynthetic changes can contribute significantly to the increased heterogeneity observed in the matrix proteoglycans on aging. In particular, they found that a single, high molecular weight proteoglycan is the major [^{35}S]-labeled synthetic product of disk cells at all ages; however, the monomer made by fetal and newborn disk cells was larger than that of adults. Furthermore, adult disk cells made other minor large [^{35}S]-labeled products that varied depending on the origins of the disk.

Disk cells have been liberated from the extracellular matrix and cultured on agarose beads in studies by Maldonado and Oegema.[53] Although cultured as one population of disk cells, there was evidence for at least two phenotypically distinct phenotypic populations of cells in the intervertebral disk: a large notochordal cell and a smaller chondrocyte-like cell. They found that most all cells synthesized significant amounts of matrix as evidenced by Alcian Blue staining. By immunohistochemical analysis, the matrix contained chondroitin 6-sulfate, and keratan sulfate was also present in the majority of the matrices around cells. Later Chelberg and associates[54] cultured the cells from the nucleus pulposus and anulus fibrosus separately. The majority of cells cultured produced both keratan sulfate and chondroitin sulfate, a few cells produced only detectable levels of one or the other, while a significant population produced neither. Unlike the fairly even distribution of proteoglycan synthesis, the synthesis of collagen types I and II was more discreetly localized. The majority of cells from the anulus fibrosus produced both types I and II collagen, while the majority of cells from the nucleus pulposus produced type II collagen. These authors also noted that the percentage of cells in the nucleus that stained positively for collagens was higher than those staining for proteoglycan. Clearly, this is an area that deserves more attention if repair of disk tissue is desired.

Development of the Vertebral Column

Many vertebral anomalies originate as derangements of the mesenchymal, cartilaginous, and osseous models found during development. The most frequently encountered conditions are spina bifida, hemi- and wedged vertebrae, and fusions. Notochordal elements can persist in the disk or vertebral bodies where they can result in a neoplastic chordoma found particularly in the sacrococcygeal or spheno-occipital regions (Fig. 4). The vertebrae develop from specialized epithelialized mesenchymal segments (somites) composed of regions of dermatome (destined to differentiate into skin), myotome (muscle) and sclerotome (skeleton). Early in development, the cells of the sclerotome spread out and around the notochord to form a perichordal sheath. The sclerotome itself segregates into two parts, a loose cephalic and dense caudal zone of cells. The intersegmental artery and spinal nerve go through the cephalic loose zone. The dense caudal sclerotomal area develops into the neural arch. Dense and loose zones also appear in the cellular sheath of the notochord with the loose cephalic zone becoming the vertebral centrum and the dense caudal area the intervertebral disk. The centrum surrounds the notochord, developing into the vertebral body. The neural processes extend dorsally on each side of the neural tube and eventually unite to complete the neural arch. Chondrification of the vertebral

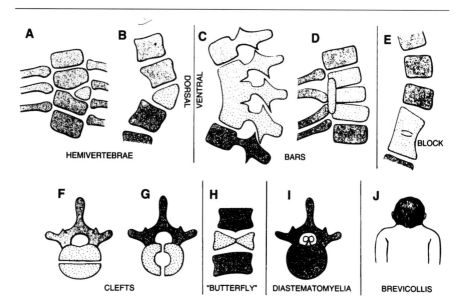

Fig. 4   **A** *through* **J**, *Examples of vertebral anomalies. (Reproduced with permission from O'Rahilly R, Muller F: The skeletal system and the limbs, in O'Rahilly R, Muller F (eds): Human Embryology and Teratology. New York, NY, Wiley-Liss, 1992, pp 233–252.)*

column is believed to be induced by the notochord and neural tube at 6 weeks in the human embryo, and ossification of the vertebrae begins around 9 weeks. The patterning of the vertebral column and subsequent cartilage and bone formation is under the complex control of a variety of cytokines, growth factors, and "patterning" genes. A description of these factors is beyond the scope of our present discussion but the reader is referred to the literature.[55,56]

The intervertebral disk develops from the dense cellular zones of the perichordal sheath. Cellular aggregations in the notochord appear at the level of the disk; while in the centra, the notochord degenerates into a mucoid streak. The nucleus pulposus arises out of these notochordal expansions (Fig. 5). Eventually, by about 10 years of age, the notochordal cells degenerate.

During development of the vertebral column, specialized collagens are synthesized and incorporated into the extracellular matrix. In general, type I collagen is produced specifically by mesenchymal cells, periosteum, and bone, while type II collagen is characteristic of cartilage. In development of endochondral bones of the skeleton, selected mesenchymal cells differentiate into prechondrocytes, then chondrocytes, the cells that synthesize cartilage. Eventually, the cartilage model is replaced by bone synthesized by cells originating in the periosteum or from the vasculature. Figure 6 shows cells synthesizing mRNA encoding these two collagens during development of the vertebral column in a 57-day-old embryo. Type I is synthesized by the cells of the intervertebral disk that will form the anulus fibrosus. At this time during development, both type II procollagen splice forms can be observed. Type IIA procollagen mRNA, containing a large NH_2-propeptide, is characteristic of prechondrocytes and perichondrial tissue, while the shorter form, type IIB procollagen mRNA, is syn-

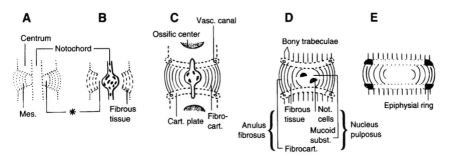

Fig. 5 *Summary of the development of an intervertebral disk.* **A,** *At 6 weeks the centra are separated peripherally by mesoderm and centrally (asterisk) by what some believe to be specialized cartilage.* **B,** *At the end of the embryonic period, the notochord is expanded in the area of the disk, and the periphery is an anulus fibrosus.* **C,** *In the fetal period, the nucleus is composed of notochordal cells and mucoid tissue.* **D,** *Newborn.* **E,** *At 33 years the distinction between nucleus and anulus is less well defined and the notochordal compartment has been replaced by fibrocartilage. Mes, mesenchyme. (Reproduced with permission from O'Rahilly R, Muller F: The skeletal system and the limbs, in O'Rahilly R, Muller F (eds): Human Embryology and Teratology. New York, NY, Wiley-Liss, 1992, pp 233–252.)*

thesized by chondrocytes resident in the cartilaginous vertebral body. Figure 7 shows the distribution of the type IIA procollagen in the notochordal remnants of the developing nucleus pulposus and the fibrous tissue of the developing anulus fibrosus of a 69-day-old embryo. The nucleus pulposus and inner anulus can be viewed as a continuation or specialization of the vertebral body cartilage anlage, while the outer anulus is derived from surrounding tissue. In the vertebral body, the notochord has degenerated into a mucoid streak as described previously, while distinct notochordal cells can be observed in the intervertebral area as shown diagrammatically in Figure 5.

Collagen Changes in Aging and Degeneration

Spinal pain may be associated with disk herniation because of degeneration of the nucleus pulposus, or to ruptures in the annular lamellus in the absence of disk herniation.[57,58] However, this view is controversial, as Hirsch and Schajowicz[59] found that no ruptures occur in the anulus fibrosus in the absence of advanced structural changes in the nucleus pulposus, while Vernon-Roberts and Pirie[60] observed peripheral annular tears and concluded that the tears were more likely to be the result of direct trauma to the disk. It is clear, however, that when the nucleus pulposus loses its weightbearing properties, and thereby its stability, through degeneration, the annular fibers can be damaged by loading and trauma.

Changes with age are more evident in the nucleus pulposus than in the anulus fibrosus. The nucleus becomes more fibrous, mainly because of the increase in the amount of noncollagenous proteins at the expense of the proteoglycans and the accompanying decrease in hydration. The demarcation between the inner anulus and nucleus becomes less distinct, and the two regions mesh. Both

549

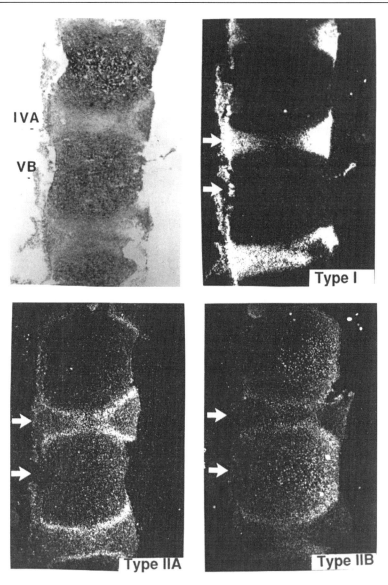

Fig. 6   *Serial sections of vertebral tissue hybridized with types I and II collagen probes, stained with cresyl violet and observed by bright-field optics* (**top left**) *and dark-field optics* (**top right, bottom left, bottom right**). **Top left,** *Tissue architecture can be seen. The centrum/vertebral body (VB) contains rounded cells producing abundant extracellular matrix that stains pink with cresyl violet. The intervertebral area (IVA) is made up of cells that are fibroblastic in appearance and stain blue with cresyl violet. Arrows indicate the position of VB and IVA. No extracellular matrix staining is observed in the IVA. Type I collagen mRNA is found in the intervertebral area* (**bottom left**) *and type IIB hybridized with cells in the vertebral body. Exposure times were: 3 days* (**top right**)*; 2 weeks* (**bottom left**)*; and 1 week* (**bottom right**). *Bar, 0.2 mm. (Reproduced with permission from Sandell LJ, Morris N, Robbins JR, et al: Alternatively spliced type II procollagen mRNAs define distinct populations of cells during vertebral development: Differential expression of the amino-propeptide. J Cell Biol 1991;114:1307–1319.)*

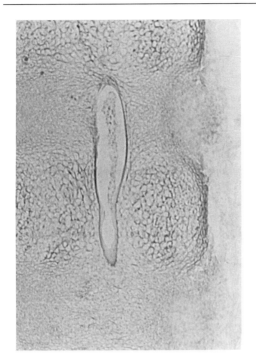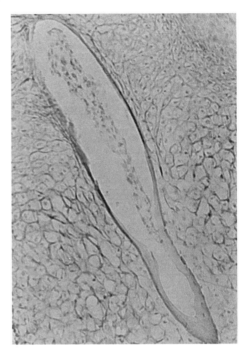

Fig. 7 *Immunolocalization of type IIA procollagen in a 57-day-old embryo. Antiserum was raised in rabbits against recombinantly expressed NH2-propeptide. Reactivity was detected with a biotin-labeled goat anti-rabbit second antibody.* **Left,** *Note positive staining particularly in the notochordal sheath and surrounding the perichondrium. Bar, 0.2 mm.* **Right,** *Higher magnification showing notochordal sheath staining and cells of the notochord.*

the nucleus and anulus become yellow because of an increase in sugars on the collagen molecules that are introduced nonenzymatically and take part in covalent crosslinking.[61] Nonenzymatic glycation is favored in the large avascular disks where oxygen tension is low. These modifications may contribute to disk degeneration and impaired function of the disk. Because degenerative changes can occur as early as the third decade, it is very difficult to differentiate between normal aging and degeneration. Moreover, because degenerative changes are distributed unevenly within the disk, interpretation of gross biochemical analyses is difficult.

Few studies have been carried out to assess changes in the different collagens with age and degeneration. However, although the total collagen content of the anulus fibrosus remains fairly constant with age, the relative proportions of collagens I and II vary with anatomic site: the ratio of collagen I to II increases in the outer anulus of the posterior segment but decreases in the outer lamellae of the anterior segment.[62] In an early study, it was also shown that collagen I synthesis increased in both the anulus and the nucleus of the normal disk above the degenerated disk.[63] It was suggested that the normal disk had compensated for the defective disk by synthesizing the (arguably) stronger collagen I fibrils at the expense of collagen II. Both immunochemical and biochemical techniques

551

indicate an increase in collagen III in the degenerative compared to the normal disk and the reversion to a more "immature" state.[19,20,64]

The structural diversity of both FACIT collagens and collagen VI and their ability to interact with other matrix components and cells make them ideally suited as "matrix organizers." Consequently, any modification in their structure (by synthesis of defective molecules or by enzymatic modification) could have a profound effect on matrix integrity. Disk degeneration resembles osteoarthrosis in several respects. Both show an early reparative phase with an accompanying cell proliferation, followed by a degradative phase in which there is a loss of proteoglycans. Osteophytes are also a feature of both diseases. In addition, disk degeneration is always accompanied by osteoarthrotic changes in the apophyseal joints. Changes in both collagen VI and IX have been observed in osteoarthrosis: collagen VI collagen increases and is deposited in the pericellular matrix of individual cells within the proliferating cell clones and collagen IX collagen decreases.[65] The decrease in collagen IX, which may be caused by degradation by stromelysin,[66] would result in a loosening of the fibrillar network and increased tissue swelling.[32]

Changes in the deposition of collagen VI have been observed in pathological specimens of the intervertebral disk removed at operation compared with normal autopsy specimens.[19,47] The increased deposition of collagen VI supports previous observations that there is an increase in unusual banded structures with a periodicity of 110 nm, which are characteristic of the lateral aggregates of collagen VI.[48,49]

Collagen X is also reexpressed in osteoarthrosis, in both the newly formed osteophytes and in regions that are not apparently calcifying.[67,68] It is therefore likely that collagen X will be reexpressed in the degenerating disk.

Models of Disk Degeneration

Changes in the metabolism of proteoglycans in animal models of disk degeneration resemble those of the human disease.[69] Less information is known about the collagen changes in these models. The metabolism of collagen was recently studied in an experimental model of disk injury.[70] To induce injury in the disks of domestic pigs, a retroperitoneal incision was made in the anterior part of the anulus fibrosus of disk L4-L5. The animals were killed 3 months postoperatively and the injured disks and intact disks from different animals were observed and removed for chemical analysis. Morphologically, healing was accomplished by granulation tissue with normal lamellar architecture being partially destroyed; small blood vessels had grown into the anterior anulus. Large osteophytes were observed at the ventral edges of the vertebral bodies. The nucleus pulposus was small and the normally white and translucent matrix was replaced by yellowish to brownish fibrous material. The morphology was normal only in the posterior and lateral parts of the anulus fibrosus. Various parameters of collagen metabolism were measured: total hydroxyproline concentration, the activities of two key enzymes in collagen biosynthesis, prolyl 4-hydroxylase and galactosylhydroxylysyl glucosyltransferase, and mature collagen crosslinks. The results show that while there is a slight increase in synthesis rate in the anterior anulus fibrosus, the predominant effect was seen in the nucleus fibrosus where collagen synthesis was accelerated significantly when compared to the normal rate. There is also an actual increase in collagen content in the nucleus pulposus that is greater than that accounted for by an increase in water content as previously thought.[15] This investigation, along with previous studies, suggests that during disk degeneration, the collagen concentration in the nucleus pulposus increases, thus partly explaining the fibrosus of the nucleus pulposus. Subsequent studies detected an increase in mRNA levels for collagens I and III in the anulus fibrosus but no changes were observed in the nucleus pulposus.[71] A decrease in the concentration of collagen crosslinks was observed; however, this may be related to the immature nature of the newly synthesized collagen which is not yet fully crosslinked. At any rate, the low crosslink concentration, together with a dispersed lamellar structure, suggests that the injured part of the anulus is less able to withstand mechanical forces than the normal disk and that loading and tension may damage the lamellar structures even more. Interestingly, Herbert and associates[63] observed that, during disk degeneration, new collagen was synthesized in the anulus fibrosus and nucleus pulposus in adjacent disks but not in the degenerated disk itself. Increased collagen synthesis has also been observed in human osteoarthritis that may parallel the severity of the disease.[72]

Acknowledgment

The authors thank Drs. Anush Oganisian and Yong Zhu for original data presented in Figure 7 and Margo Weiss for expert assistance in the preparation of the manuscript. The study was supported in part by National Institutes of Health Research Grant AR36994 LJS and the Department of Veterans Affairs.

References

1. van der Rest M, Garrone R: Collagen family of proteins. *FASEB J* 1991;5:2814–2823.
2. Kielty CM, Hopkinson I, Grant ME: Collagen: The collagen family. Structure, assembly, and organization in the extracellular matrix, in Royce PM, Steinmann BU (eds): *Connective Tissue and Its Heritable Disorders: Molecular, Genetic, and Medical Aspects*. New York, NY, Wiley-Liss, 1993, pp 103–147.
3. Ayad S, Boot-Handford RP, Humphries MJ, et al: *The Extracellular Matrix Facts Book*. London, England, Academic Press, 1994.
4. Bruckner P, van der Rest M: Structure and function of cartilage collagens. *Microsc Res Tech* 1994;3:78–84.
5. Birk DE, Silver FH, Trelstad RL: Matrix assembly, in Hay ED (ed): *Cell Biology of Extracellular Matrix*, ed 2. New York, NY, Plenum Press, 1991, 221–254.
6. Brewton RG, Mayne R: Heterotypic type II, IX, and XI fibrils: Comparison of vitreous and cartilage forms, in Yurchenco PD, Birk DE, Mecham RP (eds): *Extracellular Matrix Assembly and Structure*. San Diego, CA, Academic Press, 1994, pp 129–170.
7. Shaw LM, Olsen BR: FACIT collagens: Diverse molecular bridges in extracellular matrices. *Trends Biochem Sci* 1991;16:191–194.
8. Timpl R, Chu M-L: Microfibrillar collagen type VI, in Yurchenco PD, Birk DE, Mecham RP (eds): *Extracellular Matrix Assembly and Structure*. San Diego, CA, Academic Press, 1994, pp 207–242.
9. Eyre DR: Biochemistry of the intervertebral disc. *Int Rev Connect Tissue Res* 1979;8:227–291.
10. Ayad S, Weiss JB: Biochemistry of the intervertebral disc, in Jayson MIV (ed): *The Lumbar Spine and Back Pain*, ed 3. Edinburgh, Scotland, Churchill Livingstone, 1987, pp 100–137.

11. Eyre DR: Collagens of the disc, in Ghosh P (ed): *The Biology of the Intervertebral Disc*. Boca Raton, FL, CRC Press, 1988, vol 1, pp 171–188.

12. Bayliss MT, Johnstone B: Biochemisty of the intervertebral disc, in Jayson MIV (ed): *The Lumbar Spine and Back Pain*, ed 4. Edinburgh, Scotland, Churchill Livingstone, 1992, pp 111–131.

13. Eyre DR, Muir H: Types I and II collagens in intervertebral disc: Interchanging radial distributions in annulus fibrosus. *Biochem J* 1976;157:267–270.

14. Beard HK, Ryvar R, Brown R, et al: Immunochemical localization of collagen types and proteoglycan in pig intervertebral discs. *Immunology* 1980;41:491–501.

15. Eyre DR, Muir H: Quantitative analysis of types I and II collagens in human intervertebral discs at various ages. *Biochim Biophys Acta* 1977;492:29–42.

16. Grynpas MD, Eyre DR, Kirschner DA: Collagen type II differs from type I in native molecular packing. *Biochim Biophys Acta* 1980;626:346–355.

17. Yang CL, Rui H, Mosler S, et al: Collagen II from articular cartilage and annulus fibrosus: Structural and functional implication of tissue specific posttranslational modifications of collagen molecules. *Eur J Biochem* 1993;213:1297–1302.

18. Wu J-J, Knigge PE, Eyre DR: Evidence for copolymeric and anti-parallel cross-linking of collagens I and II in the intervertebral disc. *Trans Orthop Res Soc* 1994;19:131.

19. Roberts S, Menage J, Duance V, et al: Type III collagen in the intervertebral disc. *Histochem J* 1991;23:503–508.

20. Roberts S, Menage J, Duance V, et al: Collagen types around the cells of the intervertebral disc and cartilage end-plate: An immunolocalization study. *Spine* 1991;16:1030–1038.

21. Ryan MC, Sandell LJ: Differential expression of a cysteine-rich domain in the amino-terminal propeptide of type II (cartilage) procollagen by alternative splicing of mRNA. *J Biol Chem* 1990;265:10334–10339.

22. Sandell LJ, Morris N, Robbins JR, et al: Alternatively spliced type II procollagen mRNAs define distinct populations of cells during vertebral development: Differential expression of the amino-propeptide. *J Cell Biol* 1991;114:1307–1319.

23. Eyre D, Wu JJ: Type XI or 1α2α3α collagen, in Mayne R, Burgeson RE (eds): *Structure and Function of Collagen Types*. Orlando, FL, Academic Press, 1987, pp 261–281.

24. Fessler JH, Fessler LI: Type V collagen, in Mayne R, Burgeson RE (eds): *Structure and Function of Collagen Types*. Orlando, FL, Academic Press, 1987, pp 81–103.

25. Mendler M, Eich-Bender SG, Vaughan L, et al: Cartilage contains mixed fibrils of collagen types II, IX, and XI. *J Cell Biol* 1989;108:191–197.

26. Thom JR, Morris NP: Biosynthesis and proteolytic processing of type XI collagen in embryonic chick sterna. *J Biol Chem* 1991;266:7262–7269.

27. Moradi-Ameli M, Rousseau J-C, Kleman J-P, et al: Diversity in the processing events at the N-terminus of type-V collagen. *Eur J Biochem* 1994;221:987–995.

28. Oxford JT, Doege KJ, Morris NP: Alternative exon splicing within the amino-terminal nontriple-helical domain of the rat pro-α1(XI) collagen chain generates multiple forms of the mRNA transcript which exhibit tissue-dependent variation. *J Biol Chem* 1995;270:9478–9485.

29. Zhidkova NI, Justice SK, Mayne R: Alternative mRNA processing occurs in the variable region of the pro-alpha 1 (XI) and pro-alpha 2 (XI) collagen chains. *J Biol Chem* 1995;270:9486–9493.

30. van der Rest M, Mayne R: Type IX collagen, in Mayne R, Burgeson RE (eds): *Structure and Function of Collagen Types*. Orlando, FL, Academic Press, 1987, pp 195–221.

31. Eyre D: Collagen cross-linking amino acids. *Methods Enzymol* 1987;144:115–139.

32. Wu J-J, Woods PE, Eyre DR: Identification of cross-linking sites in bovine cartilage type IX collagen reveals an antiparallel type II-type IX molecular relationship and type IX to type IX bonding. *J Biol Chem* 1992;267:23007–23014.

33. Ayad S, Marriott A, Brierley VH, et al: Mammalian cartilage synthesizes both proteoglycan and non-proteoglycan forms of type IX collagen. *Biochem J* 1991;278:441–445.

34. Yada T, Arai M, Suzuki S, et al: Occurrence of collagen and proteoglycan forms of type IX collagen in chick embryo cartilage: Production and characterization of a collagen form-specific antibody. *J Biol Chem* 1992;267:9391–9397.

35. Vasios G, Nishimura I, Konomi H, et al: Cartilage type IX collagen-proteoglycan contains a large amino-terminal globular domain encoded by multiple exons. *J Biol Chem* 1988;263:2324–2329.

36. Nishimura I, Muragaki Y, Olsen BR: Tissue-specific forms of type IX collagen-proteogly can arise from the use of two widely separated promoters. *J Biol Chem* 1989;264:20033–20041.

37. Newall JF, Ayad S: Collagen IX isoforms in the intervertebral disc. *Biochem Soc Trans* 1995;23:517S.

38. Hayashi M, Hayashi K, Iyama K, et al: Notochord of chick embryos secretes short-form type IX collagen prior to the onset of vertebral chondrogenesis. *Dev Dyn* 1992;194:169–176.

39. Swiderski RE, Solursh M: Localization of type II collagen, long form $\alpha1(IX)$ collagen, and short form $\alpha1(IX)$ collagen transcripts in the developing chick notochord and axial skeleton. *Dev Dyn* 1992;194:118–127.

40. Bishop P, McLeod D, Ayad S: Extraction and characterization of the intact form of Bovine Vitreous Type IX Collagen. *Biochem Biophys Res Commun* 1992;185:392–397.

41. Yada T, Suzuki S, Kobayashi K, et al: Occurrence in chick embryo vitreous humor of a type IX collagen proteoglycan with an extraordinarily large chondroitin sulfate chain and short alpha 1 polypeptide. *J Biol Chem* 1990;265:6992–6999.

42. Watt SL, Lunstrum GP, McDonough AM, et al: Characterization of collagen types XII and XIV from fetal bovine cartilage. *J Biol Chem* 1992;267:20093–20099.

43. Yamagata M, Yamada KM, Yamada SS, et al: The complete primary structure of type XII collagen shows a chimeric molecule with reiterated fibronectin type III motifs, von Willebrand factor A motifs, a domain homologous to a noncollagenous region of type IX collagen, and short collagenous domains with an Arg-Gly-Asp site. *J Cell Biol* 1991;115:209–221.

44. Trueb J, Trueb B: The two splice variants of collagen XII share a common 5' end. *Biochim Biophys Acta* 1992;1171:97–98.

45. Ayad S, Evans H, Weiss JB, et al: Letter: Type VI collagen but not type V collagen is present in cartilage. *Collagen Relat Res* 1984;4:165–168.

46. Poole CA, Ayad S, Gilbert RT: Chondrons from articular cartilage: V. Immunohistochemical evaluation of type VI collagen organisation in isolated chondrons by light, confocal and electron microscopy. *J Cell Sci* 1992;103:1101–1110.

47. Roberts S, Ayad S, Menage PJ: Immunolocalisation of type VI collagen in the intervertebral disc. *Ann Rheum Dis* 1991;50:787–791.

48. Cornah MS, Meachim G, Parry EW: Banded structures in the matrix of human and rabbit nucleus pulposus. *J Anat* 1970;107:351–362.

49. Buckwalter JA, Maynard JA, Cooper RR: Banded structures in human nucleus pulposus. *Clin Orthop* 1979;139:259–266.

50. Wu J-J, Eyre DR, Slayter HS: Type VI collagen of the intervertebral disc: Biochemical and electron-microscopic characterization of the native protein. *Biochem J* 1987;248:373–381.

51. Schmid TM, Linsenmayer TF: Type X collagen, in Mayne R, Burgeson RE (eds): *Structure and Function of Collagen Types.* Orlando, FL, Academic Press, 1987, pp 223–259.

52. Johnstone B, Bayliss MT: The large proteoglycans of the human intervertebral disc: Changes in their biosynthesis and structure with age, topography, and pathology. *Spine* 1995;20:674–684.

53. Maldonado BA, Oegema TR Jr: Initial characterization of the metabolism of intervertebral disc cells encapsulated in microspheres. *J Orthop Res* 1992;10:677–690.

54. Chelberg MK, Banks GM, Geiger DF, et al: Identification of heterogeneous cell populations in normal human intervertebral disc. *J Anat* 1995;186:43–53.

555

55. Slack JM: Embryonic induction. *Mech Dev* 1993;41:91–107.
56. Erlebacher A, Filvaroff EH, Gitelman SE, et al: Toward a molecular understanding of skeletal development. *Cell* 1995;80:371–378.
57. Crock HV: Internal disc disruption: A challenge to disc prolapse fifty years on. *Spine* 1986;11:650–653.
58. Vanharanta H, Guyer RD, Ohnmeiss DD, et al: Disc deterioration in low–back syndromes: A prospective, multi–center CT/discography study. *Spine* 1988;13:1349–1351.
59. Hirsch C, Schajowicz F: Studies on structural changes in the lumbar annulus fibrosus. *Acta Orthop Scand* 1952;22:184–231.
60. Vernon-Roberts B, Pirie CJ: Degenerative changes in the intervertebral discs of the lumbar spine and their sequelae. *Rheumatol Rehabil* 1977;16:13–21.
61. Hormel SE, Eyre DR: Collagen in the ageing human intervertebral disc: An increase in covalently bound fluorophores and chromophores. *Biochim Biophys Acta* 1991;1078:243–250.
62. Brickley-Parsons D, Glimcher MJ: Is the chemistry of collagen in intervertebral discs an expression of Wolff's law? A study of the human lumbar spine. *Spine* 1984;9:148–163.
63. Herbert CM, Lindberg KA, Jayson MIV, et al: Changes in the collagen of human intervertebral discs during ageing and degenerative disc disease. *J Mol Med* 1975;1:79–91.
64. Adam M, Deyl Z: Degenerated annulus fibrosus of the intervertebral disc contains collagen type III. *Ann Rheum Dis* 1984;43:258–263.
65. Ayad S, Brierley VH, Marriott A, et al: Characterization of the collagens in normal and osteoarthrotic human articular cartilage. *Trans Orthop Res Soc* 1991;16:249.
66. Wu J-J, Lark MW, Chun LE, et al: Sites of stromelysin cleavage in collagen types II, IX, X, and XI of cartilage. *J Biol Chem* 1991;266:5625–5628.
67. Hoyland JA, Thomas JT, Donn R, et al: Distribution of type X collagen mRNA in normal and osteoarthritic human cartilage. *Bone Miner* 1991;15:151–163.
68. Walker GD, Fischer M, Gannon J, et al: Expression of type-X collagen in osteoarthritis. *J Orthop Res* 1995;13:4–12.
69. Lipson SJ, Muir H: Proteoglycans in experimental intervertebral disc degeneration. *Spine* 1981;6:194–210.
70. Kaapa E, Holm S, Han X, et al: Collagens in the injured porcine intervertebral disc. *J Orthop Res* 1994;12:93–102.
71. Kaapa E, Zhang LQ, Muona P, et al: Expression of type I, III, and VI collagen mRNAs in experimentally injured porcine intervertebral disc. *Connect Tissue Res* 1994;30:203–214.
72. Lippiello L, Hall D, Mankin HJ: Collagen synthesis in normal and osteoarthritic human cartilage. *J Clin Invest* 1977;59:593–600.

Chapter 34

Mechanical Behavior of the Intervertebral Disk and the Effects of Degeneration

Mark Weidenbaum, MD
James C. Iatridis, PhD
Lori A. Setton, PhD
Robert J. Foster, ScD
Van C. Mow, PhD

Introduction

The enormous socioeconomic consequences of low back pain have been well described. Approximately 50% to 70% of adults experience at least one episode of low back pain over their lifetime.[1-4] Disorders of the intervertebral disk have been some of the most widely supported and intensely investigated mechanisms for low back pain, although evidence for an indisputable link between clinical symptoms and disk degeneration remains elusive.[5-14] Many patients with low back pain have radiographic evidence of disk degeneration in the lumbar spine, such as loss of disk height, loss of lordosis, and anterior, posterior, or lateral subluxation.[8,11,15-17] Furthermore, degenerative changes in lumbar intervertebral disks, such as tears and fissures of the anulus fibrosus, are potential factors in many painful spinal conditions.[5-9,11,16,18,19] However, there is histopathologic evidence of lumbar disk degeneration in nearly all people at some point in life,[20] so that the incidence of low back pain may not be as high as that of disk degeneration. Importantly, there is an increased incidence of disk degeneration in asymptomatic patients as they grow older, suggesting that a natural relationship may exist between disk degeneration and physiologic aging.

It is widely accepted that intervertebral disk degeneration may contribute to symptomatic pathology in the lumbar spine; however, the mechanisms for this involvement are still being studied. Although the mechanical behavior of the motion segment has been the subject of frequent study, an overall understanding of the load-deformation characteristics of the intervertebral disk in situ does not bring with it knowledge of the internal stresses, strains, pressures, and flow fields responsible for the successful performance or failure of each component of the disk. We will present an overview of mechanics for the normal intervertebral disk, with an emphasis on the material behavior of its substructures (anulus fibrosus, nucleus pulposus, and cartilage end plate). Changes in the material behavior of these substructures during degeneration will lead to altered mechanics for the entire disk and the functional motion segment.

By studying the mechanical behaviors and contributions of these components to the entire intervertebral disk, we hope to construct a composite image of disk mechanics that will provide important information about pathways for progressive disk degeneration and pathology for the entire lumbar spine. A brief review of the structure and composition of the nondegenerate and degenerate intervertebral disk as it relates to the mechanical behavior of the disk also is presented. This review is followed by an introduction to the mechanics of the spinal motion segment and how they are altered with degeneration. We also give an overview of the material properties of the nondegenerate disk in swelling, tension, compression, and shear. Finally, what is known of alterations in material properties of the disk substructures with degeneration is presented, followed by a discussion of potential pathways to disk degeneration suggested by the available data.

Structure and Composition

Intervertebral Disk Structure

The spinal motion segment is comprised of a three-joint complex consisting of the intervertebral disk (IVD) and two zygoapophyseal or facet joints. The mechanics of all three joints are coupled so that degeneration-related changes in one joint will alter the mechanics for the others. The IVD is composed of three major substructures: anulus fibrosus (AF), nucleus pulposus (NP), and cartilage end plate (CEP) (Fig. 1). In the lumbar spine, the IVD assumes a kidney shape in the horizontal plane with the NP centered posteriorly. The composition and structure of each component is quite distinct, suggesting a unique mechanical role for each component. Nondegenerate disks are commonly described as having a gelatinous and shiny NP that is easily delineated from the surrounding AF. The AF has discrete fibrous lamellae that are devoid of macroscopic ruptures. Together, these lamellae appear as a layered composite with adjacent lamina varying at approximately ± 30° to the horizontal axis (Fig. 2). The CEP is a thin layer of hyaline cartilage that surrounds the cranial and caudal surfaces of the central regions of the disk. The orientation of the collagen

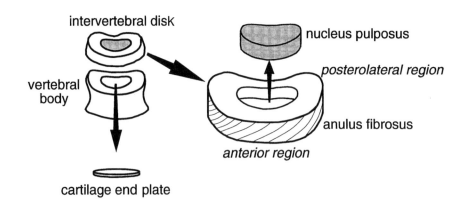

Fig. 1 *Schematic diagram of the spine, intervertebral disk, and the disk substructures, including anulus fibrosus, nucleus pulposus, and cartilage end plate.*

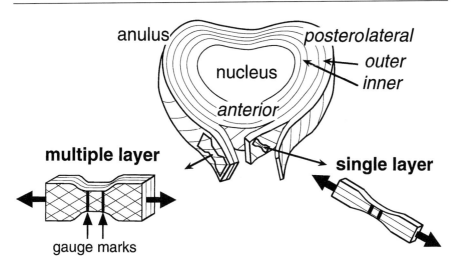

Fig. 2 *Schematic diagram of the intervertebral disk displaying the lamellar organization and the harvesting of single and multiple layer tensile test specimens. Diagram shows dumbbell-shaped test specimens, with multiple layer samples tested in the circumferential direction and single layer samples tested in a direction parallel to the predominant fiber orientation.*

fibers and chondrocytes in the CEP have been shown to vary considerably with depth in the cartilage layer, assuming a zonal organization not unlike that observed for articular cartilage.[21,22]

Intervertebral Disk Composition

A detailed overview of the composition for the IVD is presented elsewhere in this book. Briefly, the disk is composed mostly of water (65% to 90% wet weight) with significant quantities of collagen (15% to 65% dry weight), proteoglycan (10% to 60% dry weight), and other matrix proteins (15% to 45% dry weight).[23,24] Differences in disk composition and structure distinguish its different regions. Significant variation in composition from outer to inner regions has been reported, with water and proteoglycan content being greatest in the NP and inner AF, while collagen content is greatest in the outer AF. At least eight types of collagen have been identified in the IVD.[23-26] The outer AF is predominantly type I collagen, whereas the inner AF is mostly type II, with a decreasing ratio of type I to type II from outer to inner AF. The collagen composition of the CEP is almost exclusively type II and is similar in concentration and organization to that of articular cartilage.[22,27] In addition, a highly heterogeneous population of aggregating and nonaggregating proteoglycans exists in the disk. Several molecular types of glycosaminoglycan have been identified in the disk, including chondroitin-6 sulfate, chondroitin-4 sulfate, keratan sulfate, biglycan, decorin, versican, and hyaluronan.[23,24,28-33] The proteoglycan aggregate structure and relative composition of these constituents varies significantly with position in the IVD and with patient aging and disk degeneration.

Effects of Degeneration on Structure and Composition of the Intervertebral Disk

Degeneration and age-related changes in both the biochemical composition and structure of each IVD component have been widely reported.[18,20,21,23-26,28,29,31,34-45] Changes in the disk substructures with degeneration have also been noted as changes in geometry or signal intensity in radiographic and magnetic resonance imaging (MRI) studies of the intact spine.[15,23,46,47] In general, as the disks degenerate, the NP changes to a more consolidated fibrous structure and is less clearly demarcated from the AF. Mucinous material is deposited between the lamellae of the AF, and focal defects become apparent in the CEP. Changes in the vertebral bodies include early chondrophytes or osteophytes at the margins of the vertebral bodies. The severely degenerated IVD is characterized by a loss of disk material and prevalent fissures and disruptions throughout the NP and AF. In more advanced stages of degeneration, there is a greater incidence of associated bony changes radiographically, such as sclerosis of the vertebral and cartilage end plate, osteophyte formation, vertebral sclerosis, and apophyseal joint malalignment and hypertrophy. Thus, IVD degeneration may be suspected when there is radiographic evidence of bony changes.

With increasing degeneration, hydration decreases for both the NP and AF, accompanied by a decrease in proteoglycan content and significant alterations in proteoglycan structure. Proteoglycans from degenerate populations reportedly have been larger in hydrodynamic size and richer in keratan sulfate than proteoglycans from young tissue.[28,31] Although the collagen content in the disk appears to remain relatively constant with degeneration, alterations in the distribution of collagen types I and II have been reported.[23,24,31,34,45,48] Age-related changes in the morphology, histology, biochemistry, and radiographic or MRI appearance of the IVD often cannot be differentiated from degenerative changes.[18,20,34,37,39-43,45,46,49,50]

Although aging and degeneration must be considered as separate processes, high correlations between age and degenerative grade indicate that they occur simultaneously. To date, this correlation makes it impossible to differentiate alteration related to one mechanism versus the other. Determination of the differences between aging and degenerative changes in the IVD will provide further insight as to which causes low back pain, and thus open the possibility for new methods of prophylactic care.

Mechanics of the Intervertebral Disk

Structural Testing of the Spine and Motion Segment

Numerous mechanical studies of the "total" motion segment (vertebral body-disk-vertebral body units) have been performed to assess the in situ structural response to a variety of loading modes, such as compression, tension, flexion, extension, lateral bending, shear, and torsion.[51-72] These studies have resulted in documentation of some fundamental mechanical characteristics for the motion segment and IVD, such as viscoelasticity, nonlinear behaviors, and a sensitivity to environmental factors such as temperature and humidity. Although the results of the individual studies vary widely because of the different loading conditions used, the overall results of these studies gave evidence that torques and rotations applied to the nondegenerate disk are related to deformation of the AF, while compressive forces arc more related to deformation of the vertebral body and end plates and disk bulging. Reports of studies of motion segments with IVDs that were aged or degenerated indicated increased deformability, decreased nucleus pressure, reduced magnitudes of stiffness and fatigue strength, altered failure properties, and changes in the viscoelastic effects of the motion segment compared to nondegenerate IVDs.[52,57,59,60,62,64,66,73,74] These studies indicate that disk degeneration may be involved in altered mechanics for the various motion segments and spine.

Experimental models of IVD degeneration have been developed in combination with motion segment testing, to more precisely quantify the contribution of the IVD to motion segment mechanics. Surgical alterations of the disk, such as partial removal of AF or NP, or cutting to induce an AF tear, have been used as a means of determining the role of each disk component in load support.[55,58,67,70,73-79] In an early study, the uniaxial deformation response to a compressive load was studied in cadaveric motion segments before and after sequential injuries: the AF was punctured at a posterolateral site, and the NP and vertebral end plates removed.[78] In all cases, there was minimal change in the measured compressive stiffness at equilibrium. These findings, however, were not supported by later studies of the three-dimensional (3-D) motions of the IVD before and after surgical injury in response to various modes of applied loading.[55,67] Both major motions (mechanical response in the direction of applied load) and coupled motions (mechanical response about axes other than the axis of applied loading)[55,67] were altered after excision of a posterolateral portion of the AF, and even further by subsequent denucleation.[67] In studies of isolated nucleus injury, removal of the NP by excision or treatment with chymopapain was associated with increased motions at the level of injury, disk narrowing, altered deformation behavior of the AF, and decreased stiffness.[55,70,73,75,79] Injection of saline into the NP, however, caused a significant increase in intradiskal pressure and a decrease in segmental motion in various loading modes.[52,74] These results demonstrate that loss of fluid pressure will occur in response to denucleation or isolated AF injury and will affect the load response of the entire IVD. In general, it can be said that disturbance of one component of the IVD will affect the mechanical behavior of that component and the disk as a whole.

Finite Element Modeling

Another technique used to study the mechanical behavior of the IVD and motion segment is mathematical and numerical modeling.[27,56,80-96] Computational modeling is advantageous because it often is convenient and comparatively less costly to simulate pathology of the spine and IVD, based on known changes in anatomy or material properties with degeneration. Furthermore, computational modeling may be used to study loading conditions or material behavior that may not easily be achieved experimentally. Belytschko and associates[80] were the first to present details of a finite element analysis of a motion segment, assuming an axisymmetric geometry for the IVD. The NP was modeled as an incompressible and inviscid fluidlike material and the AF as a linearly elastic and orthotropic material. The model indicated that the mechanical stress-strain state of the NP is isotropic, while that of the AF was highly anisotropic. The "hoop" stress, or stress in the direction parallel to the anulus fibers, was greatest at the periphery of the IVD with a predicted value of 3.35 times the applied pressure.[80]

Other studies have used 3-D models with more realistic geometries of the IVD and vertebral bodies, either with or without the facet articulations.[83,86,89,90,96] In addition, a wide variety of material assumptions and material properties have been used. The most common manner of modeling the NP has been as an incompressible and inviscid material, although in some studies it has been modeled as a poroelastic solid.[85,91,93] Material models of the AF have been more varied, ranging from assumptions of linear and isotropic elastic material behaviors to assumptions of more complex fiber-reinforced composite models[56,80,83,86-90,92,95-97] and poroelastic models with a linearly or nonlinearly elastic solid component.[84,93,94,98] More recently, attempts were made to incorporate the effects for swelling of the IVD into finite element models.[85,94] In general, these studies have provided predictions for the internal stresses and deformations within the disk in response to many different loading conditions. Results of a number of numeric studies indicate that for nondegenerate disks loaded in compression, the AF will experience decreasing tensile strains from inner to outer layers. The addition of the putative swelling pressure in these models for the IVD led to predictions of increased stiffening of the disk, changes in the internal strains in the disk, and alterations in the magnitude and direction of fluid displacements.[85] The results of some models indicate that maximum fiber strain occurs in the posterior AF, and that the inner AF can deform inward or outward in the IVD, as a function of hydrostatic pressure in the disk.[85,90]

The effects of degeneration have also been modeled using finite element methods by parametrically varying the material properties of the IVD[80,89] or by simulating changes in fluid content.[92] The model predictions for simulated IVD pathology vary widely, but generally suggest a change in the loading pattern of the AF. In one study, finite element methods were used to examine propagation of tears by comparing predicted internal stresses and strains against a material failure criterion.[87] The results of this study indicate that the presence of discrete peripheral tears in the AF may have a role in the formation of concentric annular tears and in accelerating the degenerative process.

Clearly, the model predictions will necessarily depend on the assumed geometry, the nature of the stress-strain laws used to describe the constituent materials of the disks (ie, AF, NP, and CEP), and accuracy of the data for material coefficients associated with these laws. As an example, parametric studies performed to determine the sensitivity of finite element model predictions to geometric and material factors indicated that Young's modulus of cancellous bone and AF, and Poisson's ratio of the AF and CEP significantly affected the finite element predictions for disk height, lateral bulge, and NP pressure.[86,88,99] Therefore, the full usability of the finite element models will not be completely realized until realistic material models and geometries are used along with experimentally determined material properties.

Material Properties of the Nondegenerate Intervertebral Disk

Anulus Fibrosus

Swelling Behavior of the Anulus Fibrosus and Intradiskal Pressure Measurements The swelling pressure in the IVD and cartilaginous tissues arises from several sources. First, there exists an osmotic pressure difference between the interstitial fluid and external compartments because of an imbalance of ion concentrations caused by the presence of negatively-charged proteoglycans in the IVD. Second, there may exist a chemical expansion stress, or charge-to-charge repulsive force, which results from interactions between fixed charges on the proteoglycans.[94,100-103] The deformations caused by the swelling pressure are physically restrained by the fibrillar collagen network. Thus, the net swelling effect in a tissue will depend on the interaction between the swelling pressure, the integrity of the restraining collagen network, and the magnitude and directions of the applied mechanical loading.

The swelling behavior of the AF has been studied in several in vitro configurations. Osmotic pressure measurements made by Urban and Maroudas[102] equilibrated excised samples of AF and NP against polyethylene glycol (PEG) solutions of varying molecular weight and osmolarity. The fluid imbibition was found to be related to the concentration of negatively-charged proteoglycans per unit wet tissue weight of the tissue, as well as the osmotic pressure of the equilibrating PEG solution. From relationships between the proteoglycan concentration at equilibrium, and the PEG concentration, Urban and Maroudas[102] estimated osmotic pressures for the AF of 0.2 MPa. In another study, Glover and associates[104] developed an osmometer to directly measure the swelling pressure of the NP and AF in equilibration against solutions of known concentration. Using this method, the osmotic pressure of the AF was found to vary from 0.05 to 0.25 MPa.

In contrast to these osmometry techniques, other direct pressure measurements have been recorded using a pressure transducer in the IVD.[50, 52,64,74,77,79,105,106] In one of the earliest quantitative studies of intradiskal pressures, Naylor and Smare[105] placed a manometer needle into the center of motion segments that were immersed in water or normal saline. They found that the measured pressures of approximately 0.3 MPa depended on the concentration of "polysaccharide," the morphology of the NP, and the "elasticity" of the AF. Furthermore, they observed decreasing pressure values in older samples. Intradiskal pressures in this range have been confirmed by numerous studies that measured swelling pressures of 0.05 to 0.3 MPa under low loading conditions and as high as 1 to 3 MPa under high external loads on the motion segment.[50,52,64,74,77,79,105,106] Intradiskal pressure measured using pressure transducers in vivo ranged from 0.5 to 2 MPa and was dependent on loading conditions.[107,108] Intradiskal pressures were greater when sitting than when reclining, and when the trunk was loaded in rotation as compared to lateral flexion.

The swelling behavior of the AF has also been quantified in transient swelling experiments, because the rate of fluid imbibition is considered to reflect the integrity of the matrix and the diffusion characteristics and proteoglycan concentration of the tissue.[94,100,101] In our laboratory, we performed transient

563

swelling experiments on isolated cylindrical samples of human AF from the lumbar spine.[84,100] In these experiments, a perfectly confined AF sample was exposed to a change in the ion concentration of an external test bath, and the resulting transient change in force was recorded. At equilibrium, fluid no longer moved into the tissue, and the measured force was used to calculate an equilibrium swelling pressure, P_{SW}, for the AF. The magnitude of P_{SW} was found to be ~ 0.1 MPa and was similar to other values obtained using this testing configuration[84,94,98] and both pressure transducer and osmometry methods. The swelling pressure of the AF exhibited no significant effect of orientation for specimens aligned parallel and perpendicular to the axis of the spine,[84] thereby confirming the findings from studies using pressure transducer methods.[50,64] In contrast, the time constants governing the transient swelling behavior were found to be inhomogeneous (having regional variations from inner to outer AF)[100] and anisotropic (varying with orientation from radial to axial directions).[94] Further evidence of regional variations in the swelling behaviors was confirmed by free swelling measurements of the AF.[109] These regional variations may be related to the well-documented inhomogeneities in AF composition; however, the anisotropic nature of the transient swelling phenomena requires further quantitation.

Tensile Mechanical Behavior   An important component of IVD material testing has been the determination of properties of the AF in tension, because the anulus is likely to experience large tensile forces in vivo. Numerous studies have been investigations of the material properties of single and multiple layer samples (Fig. 2) of nondegenerate AF in uniaxial tension.[110-119] The investigators have documented that the tensile behavior of the AF is anisotropic, viscoelastic, nonlinear, inhomogeneous, and highly dependent on environmental factors, such as temperature and humidity of the test chamber. Most of these phenomena were first reported as observations in comprehensive studies by Galante[114] and Hirsch and Galante,[115] who studied the mechanical behavior of multiple layer AF samples subject to uniaxial tensile deformations and recorded the maximum elongation to failure, residual deformation, and energy dissipation properties for the tissue. All properties were found to depend on fiber orientation, sample thickness (ie, number of annular lamellae), position in the IVD, and extent of degeneration, with values of approximately 1 mm and 5 MJ/m^3 for maximum elongation and energy dissipation, respectively.[114] They also reported that these tensile properties for AF varied with humidity and temperature of the test chamber,[115] principally because of alterations in tissue water content.

In later studies, more knowledge was gained on the anisotropic, nonlinear, and viscoelastic behaviors of the AF in tension.[110-112,114,117-119] Significant nonlinear effects have also been observed for both single layer and multiple layer samples. In response to uniaxial deformations, a nonlinear "toe" region, or region of low force is observed for small tensile strains, followed by a near linear region at higher strains followed by an abrupt failure (Fig. 3). The failure stress (ϵ_f) and strain (σ_f) are denoted on the graph, along with the tensile modulus (E) (calculated as the slope of the stress-strain curve in the near linear region) and the strain energy density (SED) to failure (calculated as the area under the stress-strain curve). This behavior is characteristic of many collagenous tissues, including meniscus, tendon, ligaments, and articular cartilage.[120,121]

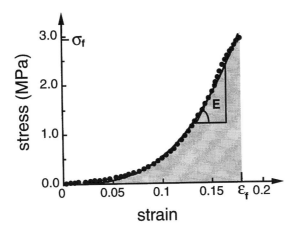

Fig. 3 *Stress-strain curve for a multiple layer anulus fibrosus in tension indicating a non-linear "toe" region at low strains and a near linear region at higher strains. The failure stress (σ_f) and failure strain (ϵ_f) are indicated on the plot. In addition, the tensile modulus (E) was calculated as the slope of the linear region of the curve while the strain energy density to failure (SED) was calculated as the area under the stress-strain curve (ie, the shaded region).*

The anisotropy and composite nature of the AF in tension also were investigated.[110-113,116-119] Specifically, values for tensile modulus have been reported that were as low as 0.2 MPa for specimens tested radially across the layers and as high as 645 MPa when tested along the principal fiber direction and assuming only the collagen component is load-sharing.[116] The tensile modulus and failure stresses are lowest for the AF when tested in the radial direction (the direction across the layers).[113,116] In general, the tensile modulus and failure stress are greatest when tested along the fiber direction[111,114,116,118] with reported values for the tensile modulus of single layer specimens tested in the range 60 to 140 MPa for human AF (Table 1).[118] Values for the tensile modulus of multiple layer AF specimens, when tested in the circumferential direction parallel to the layers, were lower with values in the range of 1 to 50 MPa, depending on test conditions and anatomic region (Table 2).[110,112,119]

Table 1 Tensile properties (mean ± standard deviation) of single layer anulus fibrosus

Nondegenerate*	Circumferential		Radial	
	Anterior	**Posterolateral**	**Outer**	**Inner**
E (MPa)*	123 ± 87	77 ± 57	124 ± 81	76 ± 64
σ_f (MPa)†§	7.9 ± 5.9	5.6 ± 2.4	8.3 ± 5.8	5.3 ± 2.3
ϵ_f (%)	9.1 ± 3.4	12.5 ± 7.2	10.0 ± 6.9	11.5 ± 4.6
SED (MJ/m³)	0.33 ± 0.31	0.36 ± 0.40	0.43 ± 0.47	0.26 ± 0.16

* E = tensile modulus; σ_f = tensile failure stress; ϵ_f = tensile failure strain; and SED = strain energy density to failure
† Significant effect of radial location ($p < 0.05$)
§ Significant effect of circumferential location ($p < 0.05$)

Table 2 Regional variations in tensile properties (mean ± standard deviation) of multiple layer anulus fibrosus

Condition*	Circumferential		Radial	
	Anterior	Posterolateral	Outer	Inner
Nondegenerate				
E (MPa)[†§]	16.8 ± 14.9	8.4 ± 9.0	20.1 ± 13.8	5.0 ± 5.6
σ_f (MPa) [†§¶]	1.4 ± 1.0	0.7 ± 0.8	1.6 ± 1.1	0.7 ± 0.6
ϵ_f (%)[†]	20.7 ± 6.5	19.2 ± 8.9	17.4 ± 7.1	21.5 ± 8.0
SED (MJ/m³) [†§¶]	0.10 ± 0.07	0.08 ± 0.10	0.12 ± 0.11	0.06 ± 0.05
ν[†¶]	1.3 ± 0.7	1.4 ± 0.6	1.2 ± 0.6	1.6 ± 0.6
Mildly degenerate				
E (MPa)	14.9 ± 15	5.4 ± 4.6	14.8 ± 14.6	5.2 ± 5.1
σ_f (MPa)	1.1 ± 0.7	0.5 ± 0.5	1.1 ± 0.8	0.6 ± 0.5
ϵ_f (%)	16.0 ± 7.0	20.1 ± 8.98	14.9 ± 9.4	20.1 ± 6.0
SED (MJ/m³)	0.07 ± 0.04	0.08 ± 0.10	0.08 ± 0.06	0.04 ± 0.03
ν	0.8 ± 0.9	1.1 ± 0.5	0.7 ± 0.8	1.2 ± 0.5
Severely degenerate				
E (MPa)	13.0 ± 12.2	5.9 ± 5.3	14.4 ± 11.3	4.1 ± 4.1
σ_f (MPa)	1.2 ± 0.8	0.4 ± 0.3	1.2 ± 0.8	0.6 ± 0.6
ϵ_f (%)	19.5 ± 11.9	20.2 ± 9.1	17.4 ± 11.5	21.8 ± 9.6
SED (MJ/m³)	0.07 ± 0.06	0.04 ± 0.04	0.06 ± 0.05	0.05 ± 0.05
ν	0.8 ± 0.7	0.5 ± 0.8	0.5 ± 0.9	0.9 ± 0.6

* E = tensile modulus; σ_f = tensile failure stress; ϵ_f = tensile failure strain; SED = strain energy density to failure; ν = Poisson's ratio

[†] Significant effect of radial location ($p < 0.001$)

[§] Significant effect of circumferential location ($p < 0.05$)

[¶] Significant effect of degeneration ($p < 0.05$)

The circumferential direction of loading is considered very important because this is the direction of tensile hoop stresses generated to resist swelling pressures from the NP.[50,122] The 1,000-fold difference in tensile modulus for samples tested along the fiber direction as compared to across the fibers gives dramatic evidence of the anisotropic behavior of the AF. In addition, the Poisson's ratio (ν, a measure of the transverse strain relative to the longitudinal strain in the test sample) was measured for the AF in tensile testing with values as high as 1.6, giving further evidence of the anisotropic nature of the AF in tension (Table 2).[110] Some of these variations may be attributed to experimental technique, however, because differences in the number of fibers that completely traverse the gauge region of test specimens will give rise to varying values for tensile stiffness.[111]

Inhomogeneities in AF composition have been clearly documented, with variations in water, collagen, and proteoglycan composition from inner to outer AF (radial direction), and from anterior to posterior AF (circumferential direction).[23-25] As previously discussed for swelling pressure effects in the AF, these inhomogeneities suggest that a variation in the material behavior of the AF may also exist in the radial and circumferential directions. Indeed, significant regional variations in the material properties of individual lamellae from nondegenerate AF have been reported, with larger tensile moduli for samples from anterior and outer regions (Table 1).[118] These regional variations have also been reported for multiple layer AF samples, with findings for higher tensile modulus and failure stress at the outer regions of the AF.[110,112,114] In addition, the anterior AF has been shown to have a larger tensile modulus and failure stress than the posterolateral regions.[110,112,114,118] Some of these regional variations in tensile properties are considered to be related to the regional variations in composition, such as higher content of collagen type I and lower content of water and proteoglycan at the outer AF.

It may be more difficult to understand the origin of the regional variation in tensile behavior from anterior to posterior regions on a compositional basis alone. Although a relationship between composition and tensile properties seems obvious, the complex structure of the AF obscures a simple relationship between compositional factors and the site-specific variations in tensile properties of AF. The circumferential variation in material properties, including a larger tensile modulus and failure stress in the anterior regions as compared to posterolateral regions, is intriguing given the higher proportion of disk herniations in the posterolateral region.[5,7,37,38,41] Furthermore, this finding is consistent with the conclusions of some investigators that posterior disk injury may be influenced by the regional variation in organization of laminate layers.[39,44,123] The combination of incomplete layers, increased fiber-interlacing angle, and ''loose'' interconnections of fibers of the posterior outer AF may be associated with the decreased tensile stiffness measured in that region. These findings support the concept that regional differences in material properties may be related to structural variations in the IVD, and that they may predispose the IVD to damage.

Compressive Mechanical Behavior   Compression is generally considered to be the dominant mode of loading for the AF as well as for the entire IVD in vivo.[122] In addition, radiographic studies on healthy human subjects indicate that the anterior portion of the IVD may compress by more than 25% during flexion as compared to standing erect[51,124] and may compress by more than 80% for degenerated disks.[124] Therefore, large compressive strains are present in the AF in the axial direction. These axial deformations coupled with the large swelling forces in the NP suggest that compressive deformations may be present in the radial direction as well.[50]

As a result, the mechanisms by which the AF responds to compressive loads and deformations are of great interest. The role of the interstitial fluid in the AF has been considered to be important for providing load support and energy dissipation in compression. Beginning in 1951 with observations by Virgin[72] of fluid flow through the IVD, the relationship between fluid motions and viscoelasticity of the entire IVD has been of interest. In our laboratory, we performed transient creep experiments on isolated cylindrical samples of human AF from the lumbar spine in order to quantify the role of fluid movement in the AF when it was loaded in compression.[98] In these experiments, an axial load was applied stepwise to a perfectly confined AF sample, and the resulting axial deformation of the sample was recorded. The transient deformation characteristics were found to be well described by the linear biphasic theory,[125] in which all viscoelastic effects are attributed to the frictional drag of interstitial fluid movement within the tissue solid matrix resulting from deformation. The compressive modulus (H_A) and hydraulic permeability (k) were quantified from a nonlinear least-squares regression fit of the theoretical model to the experimental behavior. Values for compressive moduli were 0.3 to 0.4 MPa and were greater in the outer than inner AF (Table 3). The hydraulic permeability was not found to vary with position in the disk, however, with a mean value of k = 0.25×10^{-15} m^4/N-s.

Under conditions of large strain, nonlinear effects were observed for the AF in compression.[84] In our laboratory, a biphasic mixture model was used to describe the mechanical behavior of the soft tissues in compressive stress-relaxation experiments,[126] and to determine parameters of the nonlinear compressive behavior of the AF.[84] The AF exhibited a nonlinear stress-strain relationship as well as a strain-dependent permeability effect in confined compression (Fig. 4).[84] The compressive modulus, determined from the slope of the stress-strain curve, increased with compressive strain, with a value at zero strain of $H_{Ao} \sim 0.56$ MPa and a value for the coefficient describing the nonlinear effects, $\beta \sim 2.3$. For comparison, articular cartilage had values for $H_{Ao} \sim 0.26$ MPa, roughly half that for AF, and a nonlinear stiffening coefficient with the same value ($\beta \sim 2.3$).[126] The permeability of the AF also exhibited nonlinear behavior (Fig. 4), and was described by a zero strain permeability $k_o \sim 0.2 \times 10^{-15}$ m^4/N-s, similar to the values determined under small strain conditions.[98] The exponential decrease in permeability with strain was related to strain as k $\sim$ $k_o$exp(Mϵ), where M is the nonlinear permeability coefficient, and ϵ is the Lagrangian finite strain. The value of ϵ is less than zero in compression indicating that the permeability decreases. Although the permeability of AF was relatively low compared to that of articular cartilage, the decrease in permeability with strain was relatively small as given by a value for the nonlinear permeability coefficient, M $\sim$ 1.4 (for comparison, $k_o \sim 1.9 \times 10^{-15}$ m^4/N-s and M $\sim$ 5.9, for articular cartilage).[126] Therefore, it appears that the material behavior of the AF may be well described by a linear biphasic mixture model for conditions of small strain, and that nonlinear effects may be more important for the compressive stiffness than for effects related to fluid movement through the tissue.

Although significant nonlinear and viscoelastic effects have been observed for the AF in compression, as well as with variations in position within the IVD, there is little evidence that the material properties of the AF in compression are anisotropic. In our study of the large deformation behavior of the AF in compression, there was no evidence of significant differences in any material parameters between specimens oriented in the axial and radial directions.[84] In a

Table 3 Regional variations in compressive modulus and hydraulic permeability of human anulus fibrosus (mean ± standard deviation)

Nondegenerate*	Circumferential		Radial	
	Anterior	Posterior	Outer	Inner
P_{sw} (MPa)	0.11 ± 0.05	0.14 ± 0.06	0.11 ± 0.07	0.12 ± 0.04
H_A† (MPa)	0.36 ± 0.15	0.40 ± 0.18	0.44 ± 0.21	0.27 ± 0.11
k(× 10^{-15} m^4/N-S)	0.26 ± 0.12	0.23 ± 0.09	0.25 ± 0.11	0.27 ± 0.13

*P_{sw} = equilibrium swelling pressure; H_A = compressive aggregate modulus; k = permeability
†Marginally significant effect of radial location (p = 0.055)

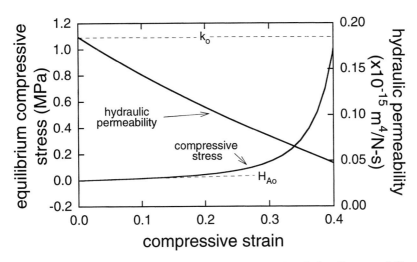

Fig. 4 *Nonlinear stress-strain relationship and strain-dependent hydraulic permeability of the anulus fibrosus in compression. The value of the zero-strain compressive modulus (H_{Ao}) was calculated as the slope of the stress-strain curve at zero compressive strain, while the value for the zero-strain permeability (k_o) was the hydraulic permeability in the absence of compressive strain.*

similar study, however, there was some evidence of differences in material behavior of the AF in radial and axial directions, although the exact nature of this difference could not be quantified.[94] In summary, the viscoelastic behavior of the AF in compression can be considered isotropic and nonlinear with evidence of radial and circumferential variations in material properties of the AF. The biphasic nature of viscoelasticity seems to be dominant under compressive loading.

Shear Mechanical Behavior Relatively few studies have investigated the shear behavior of the AF. In one study on the shear behavior of both the AF and NP, Bodine and associates[127] determined the dynamic shear modulus of cylindrical samples of AF to be 0.23 MPa at 100 Hz, increasing to 0.54 MPa as the sample dehydrated. More studies will be required to document the nonlinear, inhomogeneous, and viscoelastic behaviors of the AF in shear.

Nucleus Pulposus

Swelling Behavior In some of the earliest studies of the mechanical behavior of the IVD, the NP was observed to imbibe large amounts of water, swelling up to 200% of its initial volume.[128,129] In response to the considered importance of the enormous swelling propensity for the NP, several studies were conducted to measure its swelling pressure.[102-104,128,129] The osmotic pressure of isolated test samples of NP (from human, bovine, canine, and porcine IVDs) was determined to be in the same range as measurements of intradiskal pressure and osmotic pressures of AF (ie, 0.05 to 0.3 MPa).[102-104] Older studies using less advanced techniques tended to have much lower measured values for swelling pressure of the NP ($\sim$ an order of magnitude).[128,129] Intradiskal pressure measurements of the hydrostatic and swelling pressures in the NP have also been recorded using pressure transducer techniques (as previously discussed).

Tensile, Compressive, and Shear Behaviors Little is known of the material behaviors of the NP in loading modes other than isotropic pressurization. In one study, Panagiotacopulos and associates[130] examined the viscoelastic behavior of a nondegenerate NP sample in tension. The tensile relaxation modulus for the NP was determined to be 30 to 40 kPa; however, the number of measurements was limited because of problems encountered gripping the samples. To our knowledge, no other studies of the tensile behavior or compressive behaviors of the NP have been reported, presumably because of the difficulties handling and testing this tissue in tension.

There are also very few reported studies of the shear behavior of the NP. As previously described, Bodine and associates[127] studied the behavior of the NP in a dynamic simple-shear experiment. The dynamic shear modulus for the NP at 100 Hz was measured as 0.03 to 0.05 MPa at physiologic hydration (78%), and increased to 0.1 to 0.5 MPa with loss of hydration. In recent studies in our laboratory, the viscoelastic behavior of the human NP from the lumbar spine was studied in transient and dynamic pure-shear testing conditions.[131-133] A linearly viscoelastic model was used with a variable amplitude relaxation spectrum to describe the observed material behaviors, and to determine quantitative material parameters for this tissue. In response to a constant deformation in a stress-relaxation experiment, the shear stress of the NP decayed from large values at short times after loading (eg, 1 kPa) to values near zero at equilibrium (Fig. 5). This behavior is indicative of the fluidlike nature of the tissue. An instantaneous shear modulus, μ, was determined to be ~ 0.01 MPa. These values determined for the shear modulus of the NP are of the same order as the tensile relaxation modulus,[117] and dynamic shear modulus[127] reported in earlier studies.

In our experiments for the NP in dynamic shearing, the NP exhibited predominantly solidlike behaviors, with values for the loss angle (δ) less than 45°, and values of the magnitude of the dynamic shear modulus ($|G^*|$) of 0.01 to 0.02 MPa.[132,133] The average results of the dynamic frequency experiments for all nondegenerate NP specimens are shown in Table 4. Although the magnitude of dynamic shear modulus and tangent of the loss angle (tan δ) both increased with frequency, average values for both quantities were closer to values reported for biologic solids, such as meniscus and articular cartilage, than those for biologic fluids.[120,134] In general, the stress-relaxation behavior was well described by the linear viscoelastic model with variable amplitude relaxation spectrum (Fig. 5), so that it is tempting to conclude that the behaviors of the NP in

Table 4 Dynamic material properties of human lumbar nucleus pulposus in shear (mean ± standard deviation)

Nondegenerate*	Frequency (rad/s) 1	Frequency (rad/s) 10	Frequency (rad/s) 100
$|G^*|$ (kPa)	7.40 ± 11.6	11.3 ± 17.9	19.8 ± 31.4
δ (degrees)	23 ± 5	24 ± 5	30 ± 6

* $|G^*|$ = magnitude of dynamic shear modulus; δ = phase angle

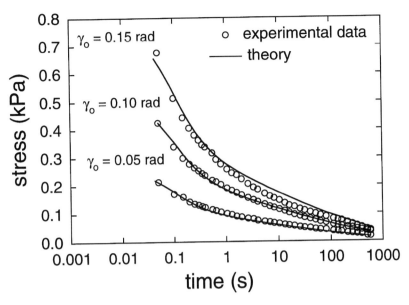

Fig. 5 *Shear stress-relaxation results for nucleus pulposus specimens when subjected to a strain amplitude of γ_o = 0.05, 0.10, and 0.15 rad. The experimental data relaxed to stress values near zero is indicative of the "fluidlike" behavior of the nucleus pulposus. The linear viscoelastic model with variable amplitude relaxation spectrum exhibited very good agreement with the experimental data for all stress-relaxation experiments.*

shear are largely linear and frequency-dependent. Many of the dynamic behaviors, however, were not well described by the viscoelastic model, so it is not yet clear if the assumptions of material linearity and frequency dependence are appropriate and adequate. More studies are required to fully document the mechanical behaviors of the NP before its mechanical role in the IVD can be fully understood.

Cartilage End Plate

Motion segment studies of the IVD have demonstrated that significant compressive deformations can be generated at the site of the CEP in situ.[53,56,68,69] Little is known, however, of the compressive behavior of the human CEP. Harvesting samples for mechanical testing is difficult because the cartilage end plate will undergo thinning and eventual calcification, beginning at a very early age.[21,35,37,49] We performed experiments on CEP from the baboon lumbar spine in order to quantify the compressive behaviors of this material.[27] As with the human AF studies,[98] one-dimensional compressive creep experiments were performed on cylindrical samples of CEP harvested from nondegenerate baboon IVDs. Similarities in structure and composition of articular cartilage and CEP suggested that the compressive behavior of the two tissues would also be similar. In contrast, we found that the compressive deformation response of the CEP was significantly prolonged and more rapid upon initial load as compared to articular cartilage. The prolonged deformation of the CEP in compressive creep experiments was attributed to fluid flow, as well as to intrinsic viscoelastic effects for the solid matrix of the CEP. Accordingly, a biphasic poroviscoelastic model was used to describe the compressive behavior of the CEP.[135] Values for compressive modulus for the CEP ($H_A \sim 0.4$ MPa) and hydraulic permeability ($k \sim 10^{-13}$ m^4/N-s) along with additional parameters (c, τ_1, τ_2) describing the intrinsic viscoelastic effects, were obtained. In general, the compressive behavior of the CEP, with a relatively high value for permeability as compared to AF,[98] was associated with rapid transport and pressurization of the interstitial fluid in response to loading and an increased emphasis on flow-independent viscoelastic effects. Fluid pressurization in the CEP may be important in the maintenance of a uniform stress distribution across the boundary between vertebral body and intervertebral disk.

Material Properties of the Degenerate Intervertebral Disk

The degenerative changes occurring in the intervertebral disk affect all components of the disk (AF, NP, and CEP) as well as other components of the motion segment (vertebral bodies and facet joints). To date, few data are available in the literature on the effects of IVD degeneration on the biomechanical behaviors of AF, CEP, and NP. An adequate understanding of the effects of altered joint loading, such as immobilization, fatigue, or impact, on the IVD is also lacking. The following section summarizes current knowledge on degeneration and the material properties of the IVD. There are, however, significant gaps in the existing knowledge on how the mechanics of individual disk components are affected by degenerative disk disease. Changes in composition and structure of the IVD with degeneration, however, suggest that there are likely to be associated changes in the mechanical behavior of the AF, NP, and CEP.

Anulus Fibrosus

Swelling Behavior Intradiskal pressure measurements generally decrease in magnitude with disk degeneration, with values as low as zero in severely degenerated disks.[50,74] Pressure transducer measurements taken in different directions (vertical and horizontal) indicated that nondegenerate disks behave isotropically with a uniform hydrostatic pressure in all directions, while severely degenerate disks had swelling pressures that were different in the vertical and lateral directions.[50,64] Decreases in the swelling pressure of AF with age have also been measured using confined swelling of isolated AF samples[100] and osmotic pressure techniques.[103] These findings for a reduction in swelling pressure and loss of isotropic pressurization with degeneration suggest an increase in nonisotropic stresses and deformations in the degenerate disk.

Tensile Mechanical Behavior Galante[114] demonstrated that the mechanical properties of the AF changed significantly with aging until maturity. While subsequent degenerative changes had a smaller effect, there was evidence of a significant increase in elongation and energy dissipation in the degenerate AF. Panagiotacopulos and associates[117,130] studied the effect of tissue hydration on tensile stiffness of AF, and observed increasing stiffness with loss of hydration in the AF. These findings led to the suggestion that, because of the observed decrease in hydration of the AF with age, the stiffness of the AF would also increase.

A study by Acaroglu and associates[110] was performed in order to determine the effects of degeneration and aging on the tensile mechanical behavior of the AF. The results of this study indicate that failure stress strain energy density, and Poisson's ratio were significantly lower in the degenerate AF, although evidence for changes in other measures of tensile behavior was not detected (Table 2). The degeneration- or age-related changes in the tensile properties of the AF were generally smaller in magnitude than the regional variations in tensile properties. This finding is interesting in light of the dramatic morphologic, histologic, and anatomic changes associated with both the aging and degeneration processes.[18,20,21,23,24,28,29,31,34,35,37-45] This study has shown, however, that degeneration is accompanied by specific variations in the tensile properties of the AF that may have a very specific effect on the mechanical behavior of the motion segment. For example, a decrease in both the failure stress and strain energy density to failure (SED) indicates that the degenerated AF will fail at lower stresses and require less energy to fail than the nondegenerate AF. A significant decrease in Poisson's ratio and decreasing trend in tensile modulus was also reported with degeneration[110] (Fig. 6). These alterations in material properties with degeneration will result in altered internal stresses within the AF, and the altered internal stresses may contribute to the etiology of IVD degeneration and failure. Furthermore, the causal relationship between these mechanical changes of the AF and AF failure is supported by the increased frequency of anulus tears and fissures in degenerated IVD.[9,37,41,45,56,87,136]

Degenerative grade correlated highly with age, as has been reported previously.[45,136] A previous study by Ebara and associates,[112] on tensile properties of nondegenerate AF indicated that significant but very low correlations were present between tensile properties and age. In the study by Acaroglu and associates,[110] on a population of IVDs of multiple degenerative grades, some ten-

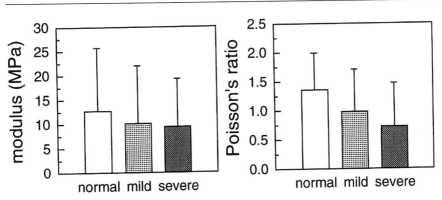

Fig. 6 *Effect of degeneration on tensile modulus (**left**) and Poisson's ratio (**right**) of multiple layer anulus fibrosus samples. The results indicated that degenerative level had a relatively small effect on tensile modulus (p = 0.06), but a highly significant effect on Poisson's ratio (p = 0.0004).*

sile properties that were apparently dependent on grade of degeneration also exhibited significant and low correlations with age. Conversely, the failure stress, which was significantly affected by degeneration, did not demonstrate a correlation with aging. Together, these results indicate that aging and degeneration may indeed be different processes, with degeneration having more deleterious effects than aging on the tensile behavior of the AF. However, the high correlation between age and degenerative grade along with the correlation between tensile properties and age indicates that these processes occur simultaneously.

Compressive and Shear Mechanical Behavior   The effect of degeneration on the compressive and shear behaviors of the AF remains largely uninvestigated. In a preliminary study, Best and associates[137] observed an effect of degeneration on the compressive modulus of the AF, with values of 0.34 MPa and 0.15 MPa for nondegenerate and degenerate specimens, respectively. In addition, the value for permeability increased more than an order of magnitude from 0.07×10^{-15} for the nondegenerate AF to 1.1×10^{-15} m^4/N-s for the degenerate specimens. These results suggest that the degenerate disk will exhibit a loss of hydrostatic pressurization on loading, resulting in a transfer of the load-carrying mechanism in the AF from pressurization to deformation-induced stresses on the solid matrix. Although no previous study on the effects of degeneration on the shear mechanical properties of the AF has been reported, Bodine and associates[127] indicated an increase in shear modulus with a loss of hydration. It may be speculated that losses in water content of the AF with degeneration may result in similar increases in the shear modulus of the degenerate AF.

Nucleus Pulposus

The marked morphologic and compositional changes reported in the NP with degeneration suggest significant and related changes in NP mechanics. Significant decreases in the intradiskal pressures and osmotic pressure of the degenerated IVD have been measured and were presented earlier in this chapter. In our laboratory, we investigated the effect of degeneration on the mechanical behavior of the NP in shear and found an increase in both instantaneous (0.01 to 0.02 MPa) and dynamic shear moduli (0.01 to 0.05 MPa) with grade of degeneration.[132] In addition, we observed a significant decrease in values of the phase angle δ (0.45° to 0.32°). These altered material parameters indicate dramatic changes in the mechanics of the degenerate NP, with suggestion of elevated stiffness, decreased dissipation, and a more solidlike behavior with degeneration. Importantly, the loss of a fluidlike nature with degeneration suggests a loss of the isotropic stress state in the NP. This mechanical change is likely to result in an increase in the anisotropic and nonuniform deformational behaviors of the entire IVD, and may be partly responsible for the induction of focal or site-specific damage in the disk.

Cartilage End Plate

To date, we have no knowledge of any studies that have investigated the effect of degeneration on the CEP mechanical properties. The most dramatic aging or degeneration-related changes in the CEP are a thinning and loss of the structure,[21,35,37,45] with some evidence of microfailure and invasion of a calcified cartilage. Damage to the CEP may significantly elevate its hydraulic permeability and allow rapid fluid exudation from the CEP on loading,[27] which would defeat any hydrostatic load-support mechanism provided by this structure. A loss of the CEP would lead to a nonuniform distribution of applied loads across the entire IVD, which may contribute to the development of site-specific damage in the disk.

Summary

In this review of IVD mechanics, we have presented a summary of the important information available on the material properties and behaviors of the substructures of the IVD and their changes with both degeneration and aging. A comprehensive picture of the mechanical function of the entire IVD emerges from this body of data. The nondegenerate NP appears to function predominantly as a biologic fluid under static loading conditions, generating large, hydrostatic pressures in the IVD. The relatively high hydraulic permeability of the CEP serves to transfer loads in a uniform manner across the AF and NP. In addition, the swelling pressure mechanisms arising from a high concentration of negatively-charged proteoglycans in this structure will serve to maintain disk height and additionally contribute to the pressurization mechanism of load support and transfer. The high values for the tensile modulus, stiffness, and failure stress of the nondegenerate AF in the circumferential direction indicate that the AF is well-suited to resisting large tensile stresses. In particular, the outer AF, the region with the highest tensile modulus, is ideally suited for minimizing IVD bulging and AF strains that will be generated during applied compression, bending, or torsional loading of the motion segment. Indeed, experimental measurements of the surface strain of the outer AF indicate that the extension of the fibers and circumferential strains are relatively small (< 5%), suggesting that the high tensile modulus of the outer AF serves to limit deformation in that tissue.[71] In contrast, the lower modulus of the inner AF may permit larger deformations in response to applied loadings, rather than restrict deformations as in the outer AF. These elevated deformations at the inner AF will give rise to viscoelastic dissipation through a flow-dependent mechanism.[98] This dissipation for the AF and significant flow-independent dissipation resulting from deformations of the NP[133] are likely to be the dominant mechanisms for energy dissipation and ''shock absorption'' in the entire IVD.

With this understanding of IVD mechanics, it is clear that changes in the material behaviors of the substructures of the IVD with aging or degeneration may predispose the IVD to failure in the absence of any change in the type, frequency, or magnitude of loading (Fig. 7, Pathway A). That intrinsic alterations in AF material properties could promote IVD degeneration was first suggested by Galante,[114] who reported that anulus failure was the result of early degenerative changes in the AF material. In 1983, Kirkaldy-Willis[138] suggested that the first of three ''stages of clinical evolution'' of disk degeneration included subtle alterations in the biochemistry and biomechanics of the motion segment, which predisposed the entire motion segment to further degeneration. Other investigators have supported this hypothesis that there are intrinsic material property differences with age or degeneration, and have specifically identified a localized ''weakening'' in the AF as the source of further degeneration.[42,139] In

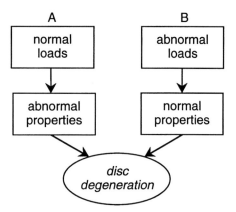

Fig. 7   *Flow diagram indicating two different proposed pathways to the etiology of disk degeneration or failure.*

this review of IVD material behaviors with aging and degeneration, we observed that the most significant degenerative changes appear to affect the NP and CEP, with comparatively minor changes to the AF. A scenario is suggested, therefore, that the loss of hydrostatic pressurization in both the NP and CEP with degeneration has a deleterious effect on the entire IVD. The loss of a uniform load transfer mechanism and an isotropic load support mechanism in the NP and CEP could be associated with increasing frequency of nonuniform stresses in the AF with degeneration, which may be associated with the development of focal stress concentrations and resulting material failure.

Although the available information does lend support to the hypothesis that intrinsic material property changes could predispose the IVD to degenerative disk disease with presentation of clinical symptoms, there are alternate scenarios for IVD degeneration. Many motion segment studies involving examination of the behavior of the IVD in response to altered joint loading have provided evidence that torsional forces applied to the joint may be associated with failure of the AF, while compressive forces may be related to end plate failure in vivo.[38,52,54,55,57-59,61,66,68-70,72,97] These findings are consistent with some epidemiologic surveys indicating that individuals exposed to repetitive lifting and twisting have a higher risk of developing disk prolapse.[140] In general, results of these studies point to the generally accepted notion that abnormal magnitudes or frequencies of externally applied loads may be related to clinical failure of the IVD in vivo. In this manner, these studies suggest another pathway in the etiology of disk degeneration or failure (Fig. 7, Pathway B). This advanced knowledge of the etiopathogenesis of IVD degeneration has been made possible by a large number of studies of motion segment mechanics and material behaviors of the IVD and its substructures, although more information is still required in order to understand how to inhibit or prevent IVD degeneration.

References

1. Andersson GBJ: Intervertebral disk: Clinical aspects, in Buckwalter JA, Goldberg VM, Woo SLY (eds): *Musculoskeletal Soft-Tissue Aging: Impact on Mobility.* Rosemont, IL, American Academy of Orthopaedic Surgeons, 1993, pp 331–347.
2. Deyo RA, Tsui-Wu YJ: Descriptive epidemiology of low-back pain and its related medical care in the United States. *Spine* 1987;12:264–268.
3. Kelsey JL, White AA III, Pastides H, et al: The impact of musculoskeletal disorders on the population of the United States. *J Bone Joint Surg* 1979;61A:959–964.
4. Praemer A, Furner S, Rice DP (eds): *Musculoskeletal Conditions in the United States.* Park Ridge, IL, American Academy of Orthopaedic Surgeons, 1992, pp 23–33.
5. Garfin SR, Herkowitz HN: The intervertebral disc: Disc disease–does it exist?, in Weinstein JN, Wiesel SW (eds): *The Lumbar Spine.* Philadelphia, PA, WB Saunders, 1990, pp 369–380.
6. Kirkaldy-Willis WH, Wedge JH, Yong-Hing K, et al: Pathology and pathogenesis of lumbar spondylosis and stenosis. *Spine* 1978;3:319–328.
7. Kurz L, Herkowitz HN: The pathogenesis and natural history of lumbar disc disease: Disc degeneration and herniation. *Semin Spine Surg* 1989;1:2–7.
8. Magora A, Schwartz A: Relation between low back pain and x-ray changes: 4. Lysis and olisthesis. *Scand J Rehabil Med* 1980;12:47–52.
9. Osti OL, Fraser RD: MRI and discography of annular tears and intervertebral disc degeneration: A prospective clinical comparison. *J Bone Joint Surg* 1992;74B:431–435.
10. Parkkola R, Rytökoski U, Kormano M: Magnetic resonance imaging of the discs and trunk muscles in patients with chronic low back pain and healthy control subjects. *Spine* 1993;18:830–836.
11. Vanharanta H, Sachs BL, Spivey MA, et al: The relationship of pain provocation to lumbar disc deterioration as seen by CT/discography. *Spine* 1987;12:295–298.
12. Vernon-Roberts B, Pirie CJ: Degenerative changes in the intervertebral discs of the lumbar spine and their sequelae. *Rheum Rehabil* 1977;16:13–21.
13. Wiesel SW, Tsourmas N, Feffer HL, et al: A study of computer-assisted tomography: 1. The incidence of positive CAT scans in an asymptomatic group of patients. *Spine* 1984;9:549–551.
14. Zucherman J, Derby R, Hsu K, et al: Normal magnetic resonance imaging with abnormal discography. *Spine* 1988;13:1355–1359.
15. Dupuis PR, Yong-Hing K, Cassidy JD, et al: Radiologic diagnosis of degenerative lumbar spinal instability. *Spine* 1985;10:262–276.
16. Frymoyer JW, Newberg A, Pope MH, et al: Spine radiographs in patients with low-back pain: An epidemiological study in men. *J Bone Joint Surg* 1984;66A:1048–1055.
17. Knutsson F: The instability associated with disc degeneration in the lumbar spine. *Acta Radiol* 1944;25:593–609.
18. Friberg S, Hirsch C: Anatomical and clinical studies on lumbar disc degeneration. *Acta Orthop Scand* 1949;19:222–242.
19. Schmorl G, Junghanns H (eds): *The Human Spine in Health and Disease.* New York, NY, Grune & Stratton, 1971.
20. Miller JA, Schmatz C, Schultz AB: Lumbar disc degeneration: Correlation with age, sex, and spine level in 600 autopsy specimens. *Spine* 1988;13:173–178.
21. Inoue H: Three-dimensional architecture of lumbar intervertebral discs. *Spine* 1981;6:139–146.
22. Roberts S, Menage J, Urban JP: Biochemical and structural properties of the cartilage end-plate and its relation to the intervertebral disc. *Spine* 1989;14:166–174.
23. Eyre D, Benya P, Buckwalter J, et al: The intervertebral disc: Basic science perspectives, in Frymoyer JW, Gordon SL (eds): *New Perspectives on Low Back Pain.* Park Ridge, IL, American Academy of Orthopaedic Surgeons, 1989, pp 147–207.

24. Pearce RH: Morphologic and chemical aspects of aging, in Buckwalter JA, Goldberg VM, Woo SLY (eds): *Musculoskeletal Soft-Tissue Aging: Impact on Mobility,* Rosemont, IL, American Academy of Orthopaedic Surgeons, 1993, pp 363–379.

25. Eyre DR: The intervertebral disc and spinal disease: Biochemical concepts, in Mayer TG, Mooney V, Gatchel RJ (eds): *Contemporary Conservative Care for Painful Spinal Disorders.* Philadelphia, PA, Lea & Febiger, 1991, pp 74–83.

26. Kaapa E, Han X, Holm S, et al: Collagen synthesis and types I, III, IV, and VI collagens in an animal model of disc degeneration. *Spine* 1995;20:59–67.

27. Setton LA, Zhu W, Weidenbaum M, et al: Compressive properties of the cartilaginous end plate of the baboon lumbar spine. *J Orthop Res* 1993;11:228–239.

28. Cole TC, Ghosh P, Taylor TK: Variations of the proteoglycans of the canine intervertebral disc with ageing. *Biochim Biophys Acta* 1986;880:209–219.

29. Jahnke MR, McDevitt CA: Proteoglycans of the human intervertebral disc: Electrophoretic heterogeneity of the aggregating proteoglycans of the nucleus pulposus. *Biochem J* 1988;251:347–356.

30. Johnstone B, Roberts S, Menage J: The occurrence of versican in the human intervertebral disc. *Trans Orthop Res Soc* 1994;19:132.

31. Lyons G, Eisenstein SM, Sweet MB: Biochemical changes in intervertebral disc degeneration. *Biochim Biophys Acta* 1981;673:443–453.

32. Markopoulos M, Yotovski P, Caterson B: Distribution of versican and aggrecan in porcine intervertebral disc tissues. *Trans Orthop Res Soc* 1995;20:69.

33. Roberts S, Caterson B, Evans H, et al: Proteoglycan components of the intervertebral disc and cartilage endplate: An immunolocalization study of animal and human tissues. *Histochem J* 1994;26:402–411.

34. Adams P, Eyre DR, Muir H: Biochemical aspects of development and ageing of human lumbar intervertebral discs. *Rheum Rehabil* 1977;16:22–29.

35. Bernick S, Cailliet R: Vertebral end-plate changes with aging of human vertebrae. *Spine* 1982;7:97–102.

36. Bernick S, Walker JM, Paule WJ: Age changes to the annulus fibrosus in human intervertebral discs. *Spine* 1991;16:520–524.

37. Coventry MB, Ghormley RK, Kernohan JW: The intervertebral disc: Its microscopic anatomy and pathology. Part II. Changes in the intervertebral disc concomitant with age. *J Bone Joint Surg* 1945;27:233–247.

38. Farfan HF, Huberdeau RM, Dubow HI: Lumbar intervertebral disc degeneration: The influence of geometrical features on the pattern of disc degeneration–A post mortem study. *J Bone Joint Surg* 1972;54A:492–510.

39. Harris RI, Macnab I: Structural changes in the lumbar intervertebral discs: Their relationship to low back pain and sciatica. *J Bone Joint Surg* 1954;36B:304–322.

40. Herbert CM, Lindberg KA, Jayson MIV, et al: Changes in the collagen of human intervertebral discs during ageing and degenerative disc disease. *J Mol Med* 1975;1:79–91.

41. Hirsch C, Schajowicz F: Studies on structural changes in the lumbar annulus fibrosus. *Acta Orthop Scand* 1952;22:184–231.

42. Jayson MI, Barks JS: Structural changes in the intervertebral disc. *Ann Rheum Dis* 1973;32:10–15.

43. Keyes DC, Compere EL: The normal and pathological physiology of the nucleus pulposus of the intervertebral disc: An anatomical, clinical, and experimental study. *J Bone Joint Surg* 1932;14A:897–938.

44. Marchand F, Ahmed AM: Investigation of the laminate structure of lumbar disc anulus fibrosus. *Spine* 1990;15:402–410.

45. Pearce RH, Grimmer BJ, Adams ME: Degeneration and the chemical composition of the human lumbar intervertebral disc. *J Orthop Res* 1987;5:198–205.

46. Pearce RH, Thompson JP, Bebault GM, et al: Magnetic resonance imaging reflects the chemical changes of aging degeneration in the human intervertebral disc. *J Rheumatol Suppl* 1991;27:42–43.

47. Schiebler ML, Camerino VJ, Fallon MD, et al: In vivo and ex vivo magnetic resonance imaging evaluation of early disc degeneration with histopathologic correlation. *Spine* 1991;16:635–640.
48. Brickley-Parsons D, Glimcher MJ: Is the chemistry of collagen in intervertebral discs an expression of Wolff's Law? A study of the human lumbar spine. *Spine* 1984;9:148–163.
49. Coventry MB, Ghormley RK, Kernohan JW: The intervertebral disc: Its microscopic anatomy and pathology. Part I: Anatomy, development, and physiology. *J Bone Joint Surg* 1945;27A:105–112.
50. Nachemson A: Lumbar intradiscal pressure: Experimental studies on post-mortem material. *Acta Orthop Scand Suppl* 1960;43:1–104.
51. Adams MA, Hutton WC: Prolapsed intervertebral disc: A hyperflexion injury. *Spine* 1982;7:184–191.
52. Andersson GB, Schultz AB: Effects of fluid injection on mechanical properties of intervertebral discs. *J Biomech* 1979;12:453–458.
53. Brinckmann P, Frobin W, Hierholzer E, et al: Deformation of the vertebral end-plate under axial loading of the spine. *Spine* 1983;8:851–856.
54. Brown T, Hansen RJ, Yorra AJ: Some mechanical tests on the lumbosacral spine with particular reference to the intervertebral discs: A preliminary report. *J Bone Joint Surg* 1957;39A:1135–1164.
55. Goel VK, Nishiyama K, Weinstein JN, et al: Mechanical properties of lumbar spinal motion segments as affected by partial disc removal. *Spine* 1986;11:1008–1012.
56. Hickey DS, Hukins DW: Relation between the structure of the annulus fibrosus and the function and failure of the intervertebral disc. *Spine* 1980;5:106–116.
57. Hirsch C, Nachemson A: New observations on the mechanical behavior of lumbar discs. *Acta Orthop Scand* 1954;23:254–283.
58. Kahmann RD, Buttermann GR, Lewis JL, et al: Facet loads in the canine lumbar spine before and after disc alteration. *Spine* 1990;15:971–978.
59. Kazarian LE: Creep characteristics of the human spinal column. *Orthop Clin North Am* 1975;6:3–18.
60. Keller TS, Spengler DM, Hansson TH: Mechanical behavior of the human lumbar spine: I. Creep analysis during static compressive loading. *J Orthop Res* 1987;5:467–478.
61. Keller TS, Holm SH, Hansson TH, et al: The dependence of intervertebral disc mechanical properties on physiologic conditions. *Spine* 1990;15:751–761.
62. Koeller W, Muehlhaus S, Meier W, et al: Biomechanical properties of human intervertebral discs subjected to axial dynamic compression-influence of age and degeneration. *J Biomech* 1986;19:807–816.
63. Krag MH, Seroussi RE, Wilder DG, et al: Internal displacement distribution from in vitro loading of human thoracic and lumbar spinal motion segments: Experimental results and theoretical predictions. *Spine* 1987;12:1001–1007.
64. McNally DS, Adams MA: Internal intervertebral disc mechanics as revealed by stress profilometry. *Spine* 1992;17:66–73.
65. Myers BS, McElhaney JH, Doherty BJ: The viscoelastic responses of the human cervical spine in torsion: Experimental limitations of quasi-linear theory, and a method for reducing these effects. *J Biomech* 1991;24:811–817.
66. Nachemson AL, Schultz AB, Berkson MH: Mechanical properties of human lumbar spine motion segments: Influence of age, sex, disc level, and degeneration. *Spine* 1979;4:1–8.
67. Panjabi MM, Krag MH, Chung TQ: Effects of disc injury on mechanical behavior of the human spine. *Spine* 1984;9:707–713.
68. Reuber M, Schultz A, Denis F, et al: Bulging of lumbar intervertebral discs. *J Biomech Eng* 1982;104:187–192.
69. Rolander SD, Blair WE: Deformation and fracture of the lumbar vertebral end-plate. *Orthop Clin North Am* 1975;6:75–81.
70. Seroussi RE, Krag MH, Muller DL, et al: Internal deformations of intact and denucleated human lumbar discs subjected to compression, flexion, and extension loads. *J Orthop Res* 1989;7:122–131.

71. Stokes IA: Surface strain on human intervertebral discs. *J Orthop Res* 1987;5:348–355.
72. Virgin WJ: Experimental investigations into the physical properties of the intervertebral disc. *J Bone Joint Surg* 1951;33B:607–611.
73. Krag MH, Pflaster DS, Johnson CC, et al: Effect of denucleation and degeneration grade on intervertebral disc stress relaxation. *Trans Orthop Res Soc* 1993;18:207.
74. Panjabi M, Brown M, Lindahl S, et al: Intrinsic disc pressure as a measure of integrity of the lumbar spine. *Spine* 1988;13:913–917.
75. Bradford DS, Oegema TR Jr, Cooper KM, et al: Chymopapain, chemonucleolysis, and nucleus pulposus regeneration: A biochemical and biomechanical study. *Spine* 1984;9:135–147.
76. Brinckmann P, Horst M: The influence of vertebral body fracture, intradiscal injection, and partial discectomy on the radial bulge and height of human lumbar discs. *Spine* 1985;10:138–145.
77. Brinckmann P, Grootenboer H: Change of disc height, radial disc bulge, and intradiscal pressure from discectomy: An in vitro investigation on human lumbar discs. *Spine* 1991;16:641–646.
78. Markolf KL, Morris JM: The structural components of the intervertebral disc: A study of their contributions to the ability of the disc to withstand compressive forces. *J Bone Joint Surg* 1974;56A:675–687.
79. Shea M, Takeuchi TY, Wittenberg RH, et al: A comparison of the effects of automated percutaneous discectomy and conventional discectomy on intradiscal pressure, disk geometry, and stiffness. *J Spinal Disord* 1994;7:317–325.
80. Belytschko T, Kulak RF, Schultz AB, et al: Finite element stress analysis of an intervertebral disc. *J Biomech* 1974;7:277–285.
81. Broberg KB, von Essen HO: Modeling of intervertebral discs. *Spine* 1980;5:155–167.
82. Furlong DR, Palazotto AN: A finite element analysis of the influence of surgical herniation on the viscoelastic properties of the intervertebral disc. *J Biomech* 1983;16:785–795.
83. Hakim NS, King AI: A three dimensional finite element dynamic response analysis of a vertebra with experimental verification. *J Biomech* 1979;12:277–292.
84. Iatridis JC, Setton LA, Mow VC, et al: Investigation of the anisotropic biphasic behavior of the annulus fibrosus in compression. *Trans Orthop Res Soc* 1995;20:70.
85. Laible JP, Pflaster DS, Krag MH, et al: A poroelastic-swelling finite element model with application to the intervertebral disc. *Spine* 1993;18:659–670.
86. Lin HS, Liu YK, Ray G, et al: Systems identification for material properties of the intervertebral joint. *J Biomech* 1978;11:1–14.
87. Natarajan RN, Ke JH, Andersson GB: A model to study the disc degeneration process. *Spine* 1994;19:259–265.
88. Rao AA, Dumas GA: Influence of material properties on the mechanical behaviour of the L5-S1 intervertebral disc in compression: A nonlinear finite element study. *J Biomed Eng* 1991;13:139–151.
89. Shirazi-Adl SA, Shrivastava SC, Ahmed AM: Stress analysis of the lumbar disc-body unit in compression: A three-dimensional nonlinear finite element study. *Spine* 1984;9:120–134.
90. Shirazi-Adl A, Ahmed AM, Shrivastava SC: A finite element study of a lumbar motion segment subjected to pure sagittal plane moments. *J Biomech* 1986;19:331–350.
91. Shirazi-Adl A: Effect of annulus composite representations on the response of a human disc: A poroelastic analysis. *Adv Bioeng* 1990;17:257–260.
92. Shirazi-Adl A: Finite-element simulation of changes in the fluid content of human lumbar discs: Mechanical and clinical implications. *Spine* 1992;17:206–212.
93. Simon BR, Wu JS, Carlton MW, et al: Structural models for human spinal motion segments based on a poroelastic view of the intervertebral disk. *J Biomech Eng* 1985;107:327–335.
94. Snijders H, Drost MR, Willems P, et al: Triphasic material parameters of canine annulus fibrosus, in Middleton J, Pande GN, Williams KR (eds): *Recent Advances*

in Computer Methods in Biomechanics and Biomedical Engineering. Clydach, Swansea, Wales, Books and Journals International, 1992, pp 220–229.

95. Spilker RL, Jakobs DM, Schultz AB: Material constants for a finite element model of the intervertebral disk with a fiber composite annulus. *J Biomech Eng* 1986;108:1–11.

96. Ueno K, Liu YK: A three-dimensional nonlinear finite element model of lumbar intervertebral joint in torsion. *J Biomech Eng* 1987;109:200–209.

97. Kulak RF, Schultz AB, Belytschko T, et al: Biomechanical characteristics of vertebral motion segments and intervertebral discs. *Orthop Clin North Am* 1975;6:121–133.

98. Best BA, Guilak F, Setton LA, et al: Compressive mechanical properties of the human annulus fibrosus and their relationship to biochemical composition. *Spine* 1994;19:212–221.

99. Suwito W, Keller TS, Basu PK, et al: Geometric and material property study of the human lumbar spine using the finite element method. *J Spinal Disord* 1992;5:50–59.

100. Best BA, Zhu WB, Jelsma R, et al: Equilibrium and transient swelling pressures of human annulus fibrosus. *Trans Orthop Res Soc* 1990;15:597.

101. Lai WM, Hou JS, Mow VC: A triphasic theory for the swelling and deformation behaviors of articular cartilage. *J Biomech Eng* 1991;113:245–258.

102. Urban JP, Maroudas A: Swelling of the intervertebral disc in vitro. *Connect Tissue Res* 1981;9:1–10.

103. Urban JPG, McMullin JF: Swelling pressure of the intervertebral discs: Influence of proteoglycan and collagen contents. *Biorheology* 1985;22:145–157.

104. Glover MG, Hargens AR, Mahmood MM, et al: A new technique for the in vitro measurement of nucleus pulposus swelling pressure. *J Orthop Res* 1991;9:61–67.

105. Naylor A, Smare DL: Fluid content of the nucleus pulposus as a factor in the disc syndrome: Preliminary report. *Br Med J* 1953;2:975–976.

106. Ranu HS: Measurement of pressures in the nucleus and within the annulus of the human spinal disc: Due to extreme loading. *Proc Inst Mech Eng (H)* 1990;204:141–146.

107. Andersson GB, Ortengren R, Nachemson A: Intradiscal pressure, intra-abdominal pressure and myoelectric back muscle activity related to posture and loading. *Clin Orthop* 1977;129:156–164.

108. Nachemson A, Morris JM: In vivo measurements of intradiscal pressure: Discometry, a method for the determination of pressure in the lower lumbar discs. *J Bone Joint Surg* 1964;46A:1077–1092.

109. Setton LA, Iatridis JC, Ehrlich RV, et al: A triphasic theory of swelling strains in human annulus fibrosus. *ASME Bioeng Conf* 1993;BED24:650–653.

110. Acaroglu ER, Iatridis JC, Setton LA, et al: Degeneration and aging affect the tensile behavior of human lumbar annulus fibrosus. *Spine* 1995;20:2690–2701.

111. Adams MA, Green TP: Tensile properties of the annulus fibrosus. *Euro Spine J* 1993;2:203–208.

112. Ebara S, Iatridis JC, Setton LA, et al: Tensile properties of non-degenerate human lumbar annulus fibrosus. *Spine* 1996;21:452–461.

113. Fujita Y, Lotz JC, Soejima O: Site specific radial tensile properties of the lumbar annulus fibrosus. *Trans Orthop Res Soc* 1995;20:673.

114. Galante JO: Tensile properties of the human lumbar annulus fibrosus. *Acta Orthop Scand Suppl* 1967;100:1–91.

115. Hirsch C, Galante J: Laboratory conditions for tensile tests in annulus fibrosus from human intervertebral discs. *Acta Orthop Scand* 1967;38:148–162.

116. Marchand F, Ahmed AM: Mechanical properties and failure mechanisms of the lumbar disc annulus. *Trans Orthop Res Soc* 1989;14:355.

117. Panagiotacopulos ND, Knauss WG, Bloch R: On the mechanical properties of human intervertebral disc material. *Biorheology* 1979;16:317–330.

118. Skaggs DL, Weidenbaum M, Iatridis JC, et al: Regional variation in tensile properties and biochemical composition of the human lumbar annulus fibrosus. *Spine* 1994;19:1310–1319.

581

119. Wu HC, Yao RF: Mechanical behavior of the human annulus fibrosus. *J Biomech* 1976;9:1–7.

120. Mow VC, Ratcliffe A, Chern KY, et al: Structure and function relationships of the menisci of the knee, in Mow VC, Arnoczky SP, Jackson DW (eds): *Knee Meniscus: Basic and Clinical Foundations*, New York, NY, Raven Press, 1992, pp 37–57.

121. Woo SL-Y, An KN, Arnoczky SP, et al: Anatomy, biology, and biomechanics of tendon, ligament, and meniscus, in Simon SR (ed): *Orthopaedic Basic Science.* Rosemont, IL, American Academy of Orthopaedic Surgeons, 1994, pp 45–87.

122. Schultz AB, Ashton-Miller JA: Biomechanics of the human spine, in Mow VC, Hayes WC (eds): *Basic Orthopaedic Biomechanics.* New York, NY, Raven Press, 1991, pp 337–374.

123. Tsuji H, Hirano N, Ohshima H, et al: Structural variation of the anterior and posterior anulus fibrosus in the development of human lumbar intervertebral disc: A risk factor for intervertebtral disc rupture. *Spine* 1993;18:204–210.

124. Ito M, Tadano S, Kaneda K: A biomechanical definition of spinal segmental instability taking personal and disc level differences into account. *Spine* 1993;18:2295–2304.

125. Mow VC, Kuei SC, Lai WM, et al: Biphasic creep and stress-relaxation of articular cartilage in compression: Theory and experiments. *J Biomech Eng* 1980;102:73–84.

126. Warden WH, Ateshian GA, Grelsamer RP, et al: Biphasic finite deformation material properties of bovine articular cartilage. *Trans Orthop Res Soc* 1994;19:413.

127. Bodine AJ, Ashany D, Hayes WC, et al: Viscoelastic shear modulus of the human intervertebral disc. *Trans Orthop Res Soc* 1982;7:237.

128. Charnley J: The imbibition of fluid as a cause of herniation of the nucleus pulposus. *Lancet* 1952;1:124–127.

129. Hendry NGC: The hydration of the nucleus pulposus and its relation to intervertebral disc derangement. *J Bone Joint Surg* 1958;40B:132–144.

130. Panagiotacopulos ND, Pope MH, Bloch R, et al: Water content in human intervertebral discs: Part II. Viscoelastic behavior. *Spine* 1987;12:918–924.

131. Iatridis JC, Setton LA, Blood DC, et al: Mechanical behavior of the human nucleus pulposus in shear. *Trans Orthop Res Soc* 1995;20:675.

132. Iatridis JC, Setton LA, Weidenbaum M, et al: Effects of degeneration and aging on the material behavior of the nucleus pulposus. *Ann Biomed Eng* 1995;23:S104.

133. Iatridis JC, Weidenbaum M, Setton LA, et al: Is the nucleus pulposus a solid or a fluid? Mechanical behaviors of the nucleus pulposus of the human intervertebral disc. *Spine* 1996;21:1174–1184.

134. Zhu W, Mow VC, Koob TJ, et al: Viscoelastic shear properties of articular cartilage and the effects of glycosidase treatments. *J Orthop Res* 1993;11:771–781.

135. Setton LA, Zhu W, Mow VC: The biphasic poroviscoelastic behavior of articular cartilage: Role of the surface zone in governing the compressive behavior. *J Biomech* 1993;26:581–592.

136. Thompson JP, Pearce RH, Schechter MT, et al: Preliminary evaluation of a scheme for grading the gross morphology of the human intervertebral disc. *Spine* 1990;15:411–415.

137. Best BA, Setton LA, Guilak F, et al: Permeability and compressive stiffness of annulus fibrosus: Variation with site and composition. *Trans Orthop Res Soc* 1989;14:354.

138. Kirkaldy-Willis WH (ed): *Managing Low Back Pain.* New York, NY, Churchill Livingstone, 1983.

139. Adams MA, Hutton WC: Gradual disc prolapse. *Spine* 1985;10:524–531.

140. Kelsey JL, Githens PB, White AA III, et al: An epidemiologic study of lifting and twisting on the job and risk for acute prolapsed lumbar intervertebral disc. *J Orthop Res* 1984;2:61–66.

Chapter 35

Neural Mechanisms of Idiopathic Low Back Pain

John M. Cavanaugh, MS, MD

Introduction

Idiopathic low back pain has confounded health care practitioners for decades. The cellular and neural mechanisms that lead to facet pain, diskogenic pain, and sciatica are not well understood. This chapter will focus on the neurophysiology and neuroanatomy of pain generation and persistence in spinal tissues, particularly the facet joints and intervertebral disks. Several issues will be addressed, including the following: (1) Mechanisms of nerve impulse generation in nociceptive nerve endings. (2) Mechanisms for persistent discharge of nociceptive impulses. These latter mechanisms include chemical sensitization of nerve endings (peripheral sensitization) as well as the sensitization of the dorsal horn neurons in the spinal cord (central sensitization). (3) Evidence for innervation, including nociceptive innervation, of the disk, facet, and paraspinal muscle tissues. (4) Evidence for disk, facet, and muscle pain based on pain provocation and/or relief in human subjects. (5) Facet, muscle, and disk neurophysiology data in animal models. (6) Proposed mechanisms of pain initiation and chronic pain generation in the lumbar spine. Generation of nociceptive impulses at nerve endings in spinal tissue will be discussed. Nociceptive impulses originating in nerve roots, dorsal root ganglia, neuromas, or other ectopic sites will not be addressed here.

Mechanisms of Pain Generation in Nerve Endings

The nerve endings of pain fibers (nociceptors), which are either small myelinated (A-delta [Aδ]) fibers (1 to 5 μm in diameter) or unmyelinated (C) fibers (0.5 to 2 μm in diameter), typically generate pain. The nerve endings of these fibers are free, or unencapsulated. Aδ and C fibers are also called group III and IV fibers, respectively. As can be seen in Table 1, not all C and Aδ fibers are pain fibers.[1] Some are fibers for temperature sensation, or pressure or crude touch sensations. In a normal state, pain fibers have high mechanical thresholds or are not responsive to mechanical stimuli. In the cat knee joint, unresponsive nociceptors have been termed silent nociceptors.[2] These are often small group IV fibers that do not respond even to forceful movements but

Table 1 Classification and function of sensory nerve fibers

Group	Function	Diameter (μm)	Conduction Velocity (m/s)
Group Ia	Muscle spindle Primary ending	13–20	80–120
Group Ib	Golgi tendon organs	12–18	70–110
Group II	Muscle spindle Secondary ending	5–12	20–70
Group III Aδ	Pricking pain Temperature Crude touch	1–5	2.5–20
Group IV C	Pain Itch Temperature Crude touch	0.5–2	0.5–2.5

(Adapted with permission from Guyton AC: Sensory receptors and their basic mechanisms of action, in Guyton AC (ed): *Textbook of Medical Physiology.* Philadelphia, PA, WB Saunders, 1981, pp 588–596.)

after inflammation respond vigorously to joint movement.[3] The functional role of a high threshold is to allow nociceptors to fire only when the stress to them is noxious. Thus, in healthy tissues, moderate stresses do not produce pain, but noxious stresses lead to pain, prompting measures to avoid impending tissue damage. Under pathologic conditions such as inflammation, nociceptors become sensitized and fire at lowered thresholds and silent nociceptors become responsive to mechanical stimulation.[2,3] In these cases, moderate stresses can be painful.

Pain fibers adapt slowly or not at all. That is, when they are subject to noxious stimulation, their firing rate decreases very slowly or remains constant. The behavioral correlative of this is demonstrated in experiments in thermal pain using human subjects, in which the temperature threshold to pain changes little over time.[4] On the other hand, it has been reported in human subjects that after prolonged noxious mechanical stimulation, the response of nociceptors adapts with time, but the experience of pain increases with time.[5] The receptive field of a mechanically responsive nociceptor can first be localized using noxious mechanical pressure. It can then be determined whether the nociceptor is responsive to other modalities, such as heat, cold, or chemical stimuli. Nociceptors responsive to more than one type of stimulus are called polymodal nociceptors. These include C-fiber mechano-heat nociceptors and A-fiber mechano-heat nociceptors.[6] Nociceptors responsive to heat and noxious mechanical stress have been extensively studied in skin. In deeper tissues such as muscles and joints, pain fibers that are responsive to noxious mechanical stress have also been characterized by their response to certain algesic chemicals, including bradykinin, serotonin, and histamine.[7-9]

Mechanotransduction in Nociceptors

In general, ion channels in cell membranes can be divided into those that are activated by changes in membrane potential (voltage-gated channels) and by chemicals (ligand-gated channels). Activation of inward currents or inactivation of outward currents will lead to increased excitability of the membrane (depolarization), and inhibition of inward currents or activation of outward currents will inhibit membrane excitability (hyperpolarization).[6]

The mechanism(s) by which pressure or stretch on nociceptive nerve endings may lead to activation of nociceptors has not been elucidated. Information on mechanical transduction in other cell types is available.[10-12] Sachs[12] reported that after stretch-activated channels are opened mechanically, sodium and other ions flow through the channels down electrical and concentration gradients, producing partial depolarization of the nerve ending. This partial depolarization, the generator potential, can lead to the opening of voltage-sensitive ion channels, which allow more sodium to enter the cell, leading to further depolarization. If the depolarization is of sufficient magnitude, a threshold is reached at which enough voltage-sensitive sodium channels open to initiate the action potential.

Mechanisms for the Persistence of Pain

Sensitization of Nerve Endings (Peripheral Sensitization)

Chemicals released in inflamed or damaged tissue can directly excite nociceptors or sensitize them to mechanical pressure. Sensitized nociceptors have lowered mechanical thresholds, so they fire in response to moderate rather than noxious mechanical pressure and have increased discharge rates at a given noxious pressure compared to the discharge rate in normal tissue. Chemicals that excite or sensitize nociceptors include hydrogen ions (low pH), capsaicin, adenosine triphosphate, excitatory amino acids, bradykinin, 5-hydroxytryptamine or serotonin, histamine, prostaglandins, leukotrienes, nitric oxide (NO), and hypertonic media. An excellent review of their actions on nociceptors is provided by Rang and associates.[6] Bradykinin is the most potent endogenous algesic chemical known. It activates nociceptors directly and sensitizes them to other stimuli. Both B1 and B2 bradykinin receptors have been identified.[13] The exposure of nociceptive nerve endings in disk, facet joint, and muscle to irritating chemicals such as these is likely to play a role in idiopathic low back pain.

Low pH may be particularly relevant to low back pain, as ischemia may produce muscle pain and it has been reported that the prolapsed disk can be low in pH.[14] Nachemson[14] reported that in 11 cases of prolapsed disk in which there was connective tissue reaction around the nerve root, mean pH was 6.8, while in 11 cases of no connective tissue reaction, mean pH was 7.2. In four disks with a more severe connective tissue reaction, mean pH was 6.1. Bulk fluid pH in inflamed joints has been reported to be as low as 6.6 to 6.8.[15] Low pH reportedly evokes prolonged activation of sensory nerves[16] and produces sharp, stinging pain in human subjects.[17] It appears that the action of hydrogen ions includes a prolonged nociceptor activation that involves a depolarizing electronic current with a slow rate of inactivation.[18]

Serotonin (5-HT), which is released from platelets and mast cells during tissue damage, sensitizes nociceptors to other stimulation[19] and enhances the pain produced by bradykinin.[20] Histamine, which is released from mast cells, is believed to cause itching in lower concentrations and pain in higher concentrations.[21] Prostaglandins are found in high concentrations in inflamed tissues. The main neural action of prostaglandins does not appear to be direct activation of nociceptors, but rather sensitization of nociceptors to noxious mechanical stimulation and algesic chemicals.[5]

Nitric oxide (NO) is formed from L-arginine following activation of nitric oxide synthase (NOS) by calcium and other cofactors.[22] Substance P (SP) and bradykinin stimulate vascular endothelial cells to release NO, which is a vasodilator. So far it is unclear how NO is involved in nociception.[5] Elevated levels of NO exist in herniated disk compared to controls,[23] and the disk is capable of producing NO.[24]

Raising the ionic concentration in the extracellular medium causes excitation of polymodal nociceptors but seldom of rapidly adapting mechanoreceptors.[25,26] This reaction is relevant to pain provocation trials in the lumbar spine: several studies report pain provocation in disk, facet, and interspinous ligaments by the injection of hypertonic saline or potassium.[27-29]

Phospholipase A_2 (PLA_2) is another chemical that may contribute to low back pain. It hydrolyses the sn-2 fatty acid (arachidonic acid) from a phospholipid.[30] This can lead to inflammatory tissue responses. In addition, PLA_2 may play a role in arthritis as it has been found in increased amounts in inflamed joint fluid effusions.[31] Saal and associates[32] reported that herniated human lumbar disk contains high levels of PLA_2, which is 20,000 to 100,000 times more active than any other PLA_2. Meyers and associates[33] reported that human disk and snake venom PLA_2 are neurotoxic when injected in rat sciatic nerves. Ozaktay and associates[34] demonstrated the effect of very low doses of snake venom PLA_2 on facet capsule receptive fields. The effect appeared to be dose related because 1,500 U injections resulted in greater reduction in nerve activity than 750 U injections, which initially caused nerve excitation. Taken together, these biochemical, histologic, and electrophysiologic data provide intriguing evidence for inflammatory and neurotoxic roles for PLA_2 in low back pain.

Inflammatory mediators include neuropeptides released from the nerves themselves. Substance P, one such 11-amino acid neuropeptide, has been studied extensively in relation to pain production. Substance P causes vasodilatation, plasma extravasation, and release of histamine from mast cells.[35] These actions are important in the inflammatory process, which can prolong pain. Substance P is also released centrally in the dorsal horn in response to noxious stimulation.[36,37] It produces a prolonged enhancement of the effects of glutamate in the dorsal horn,[38] and a combination of SP and N-methyl-D-aspartate (NMDA) enhances the responses of dorsal horn neurons to noxious and non-noxious mechanical stimulation.[39] Substance P has been demonstrated in nerves of lumbar spinal tissues, including the facet joint,[40-42] disk,[43-45] and posterior longitudinal ligament.[45,46] Yamashita and associates[47] demonstrated excitation and sensitization of nerves to spinal tissue (facet joint and paraspinal muscle) after exposure to SP. In this study SP may have had a direct effect on the nerve endings, or acted indirectly through its influence on vasodilatation, plasma extravasation, and histamine release from mast cells.

Some of the chemicals that may be irritating to the disk or nerve roots may originate in the herniated nucleus pulposus itself. These chemicals include hydrogen ions, NO, and PLA_2, as discussed earlier. McCarron and associates[48] demonstrated the inflammatory effect of autologous nucleus pulposus injected into the epidural space of the dog. Olmarker and associates[49] found that autologous nucleus pulposus produced inflammatory and degenerative changes in neural tissue of swine. Cavanaugh and associates[50] described excitation of dorsal roots in response to nucleus pulposus applied to the dorsal root ganglion.

Sensitization in Spinal Cord Pain Pathways (Central Sensitization)

It is likely that neurophysiologic and molecular changes that occur in the dorsal horn of the spinal cord play an important role in sensitization to and persistence of pain, including low back pain. A detailed review of synaptic transmission, neuroplastic changes, and membrane depolarization in the dorsal horn is beyond the scope of this chapter. Excellent reviews can be found elsewhere.[51-54] The dorsal horn can be sensitized by peripheral tissue injury or inflammation and nerve injury.[51] Under normal conditions, low intensity stimuli lead to activation of low threshold afferents which, after synapsing in the dorsal horn, lead to nonpainful sensations. When the dorsal horn is sensitized by injury or inflammation, this is no longer the case. Low threshold afferents can cause excitation of dorsal horn neurons, leading to pain. This phenomenon is called mechanical allodynia.[51] Activation of nociceptors causes a greater response from the sensitized dorsal horn neurons than would occur if the dorsal horn neurons were not sensitized, leading to increased pain (hyperalgesia). Dorsal horn sensitization appears to involve summation of slow synaptic potentials that are mediated by release of NMDA and neurokinin neurotransmitters such as SP, protein kinase activation and phosphorylation of membrane receptors, and increased synaptic membrane excitability.[51-54]

Neuroanatomic Evidence for Lumbar Pain

For a region of the lumbar spine to be a source of pain it must be innervated by nerve fibers that transmit the message of pain. Bogduk[55] reviewed the nerve distribution of lumbar spinal tissues and Stillwell[56] reported detailed findings on nerve distribution in the lumbar spine of monkeys. A diagram and description of the complex innervation of the lumbar spine is provided in Figure 1.

Facet Joint

The lumbar facet joints, also called the zygapophyseal joints, are paired synovial joints that are innervated by medial branches of the dorsal rami that exit the intervertebral foramen.[55,57,58] Typically, the joint is innervated from a branch at the same level and a branch originating from the foramen above.[55] Neuroanatomic studies reveal that the facet joint capsule is richly innervated,[27,59,60] containing both free and encapsulated endings, and can undergo extensive stretch under physiologic loading.[61] The facet can "bottom out" or "impinge" on the lamina below during spinal extension.[62]

Substance P, which is found in nociceptors, has been demonstrated in nerves in the capsular tissue of the lumbar facet joint[40,41] and also in erosion channels

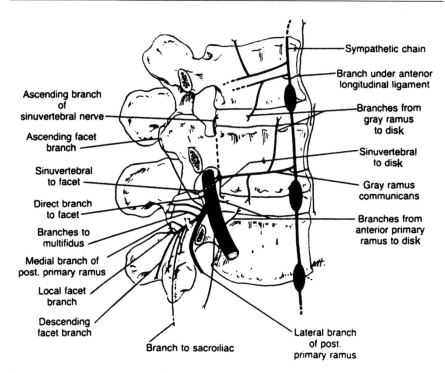

Fig. 1 *Segmental innervation of the lumbar spine. Disk innervation: Branches from the sympathetic chain innervate the lateral and anterior portions of the disk above and below. The recurrent sinuvertebral nerve, which is formed from the gray ramus communicans and mixed spinal nerves, innervates the posterior and posterolateral portions of the disk at two levels inside the spinal canal. The ventral ramus sends small branches to the disk at the level of nerve exit. Facet and erector spinae muscles: The posterior primary ramus sends medial branches to the facet at the level of nerve exit and to the facet below. Per some investigators there is also a branch to the facet above (as shown). There are also medial branches to multifidus muscle. Intermediate erector spinae muscle (longissimus) is innervated by the intermediate branches of posterior primary rami. Lateral erector spinae (iliocostalis) is innervated by lateral branches of erector spinae, which also innervate cutaneous tissue. (Reproduced with permission from Paris SV: Anatomy as related to function and pain.* Orthop Clin North Am *1983;14:475–489.)*

in subchondral bone and calcified cartilage of facet joints that have undergone degenerative changes.[43] Substance P has also been localized in the inferior recess and synovial folds of lumbar facet capsules[63] and in association with blood vessels in the joint tissue.[64]

Intervertebral Disk

A review of early literature indicates that little or no innervation of the disk anulus was reported,[65-67] while innervation of the superficial layers was reported in later studies. Two recent investigations describe sparse innervation of disk anulus in humans[68] and dogs,[69] but others have reported an apparently more densely innervated anulus,[44,59,70-72] even though the density was not quantified.

Some of the findings are as follows. Roofe[71] found many unmyelinated fibers in the L4-5 anulus that terminated in "naked nerve endings." Jackson and associates[59] reported innervation in the outer zones of the disk and in the loose connective tissue on its surface. In a study of 36 cadavers ranging in development from fctus to adult, Malinsky[70] found five types of unencapsulated nerve endings in the outer anulus. Ashton and associates,[44] using immunocytochemical techniques, found innervation to a depth of 3 mm in the anulus. Yoshizawa and associates[72] reported that the posterior longitudinal ligaments (PLL), anterior longitudinal ligaments (ALL), and outer half of the anulus were supplied with a profuse network of unmyelinated fibers. Endings included free terminals, bulbous endings, and occasional convoluted tangles or glomerular endings.[72]

A silver impregnation technique revealed an extensive distribution of fine nerve fibers in the superficial portions of the disk anulus and adjacent PLL attachments of the rabbit.[73] Typical nerve fiber diameters were 1 to 3 μm, indicating that they were unmyelinated and small myelinated fibers. In the disk, anulus nerve fibers were found in lateral, ventral, and dorsal regions. No nerve fibers were found in deeper regions of the disk or in the nucleus pulposus. A diagram of the nerve distribution is shown in Figure 2. The primary nerve structures seen within the anulus and on the annular surface were small single and branching fibers (Fig. 3). In addition, encapsulated endings were demonstrated on the annular surface and in the PLL but not within the anulus. These findings are in

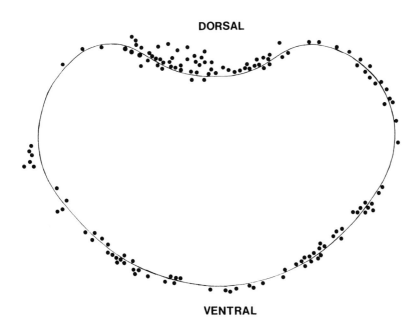

Fig. 2   *A diagram indicating location of nerves found in all rabbit disk sections studied. This is a composite of sections from nine lumbar disks (L5/L6 to L7/S1) in six rabbits. (Reproduced with permission from Cavanaugh JM, Kallakuri S, Ozaktay AC: Innervation of the rabbit lumbar intervertebral disk and posterior longitudinal ligament. Spine 1995;20:2080–2085.)*

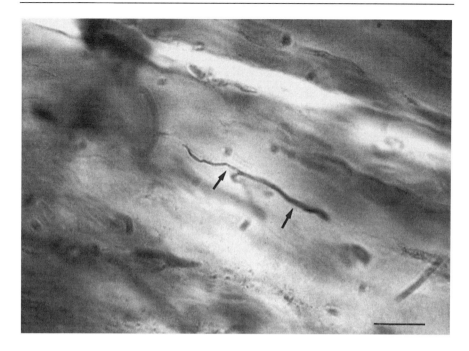

Fig. 3 *Small branching nerve fiber (arrows) on the surface of the rabbit disk. Average diameter of the terminal region is 0.5 μm. Scale bar = 10 μm. (Reproduced with permission from Cavanaugh JM, Kallakuri S, Ozaktay AC: Innervation of the rabbit lumbar intervertebral disk and posterior longitudinal ligament. Spine 1995;20:2080–2085.)*

agreement with other studies reporting a relatively dense innervation of the disk anulus[44,59,70-72] that does not extend deeper than superficial annular layers.[44,59,70,71]

Bogduk and associates,[68] investigating cadaveric disks, and Yoshizawa and associates,[72] in studying disks removed during surgery from back pain patients, reported a deeper annular innervation than previously reported.[59,70,71] It has been hypothesized that there is an expansion of nerve supply in vascular granulation tissue in degenerated disks.[27,72] Shinohara[74] reported granulation tissue and free nerve endings in the inner layers of anulus in degenerated disks. Kauppila[75] reported that the vascularity of the anulus increased significantly with disk degeneration.

Immunocytochemical studies lend credence to the belief that the disk is a source of pain. Substance P, calcitonin gene-related peptide, and vasoactive intestinal peptide immunoreactive nerve fibers have been found in the outer anulus of the rat[43,76] and human disks.[44,45]

Encapsulated and partially encapsulated nerve endings have been found on the external lateral surfaces of the anulus.[70] Many cholinesterase-positive end organs resembling the inner bulb of the Vater-Pacini corpuscle have been found in human fetal and neonate disk tissue.[59] Interestingly, these were concentrated primarily on the surface of the ventrolateral aspect of the disk anulus. Cavanaugh and associates[73] reported pacinian-type corpuscles on the ventral-lateral aspects of the disk surface adjacent to the ALL in the rabbit. The pacinian corpuscle is a rapidly adapting nerve ending to encode rate of movement.[1]

In summary, the human disk appears to be fairly densely innervated, but the innervation is limited to superficial layers in healthy disks. The annular surface contains both simple free and encapsulated nerve endings, while only small nerve fibers and free nerve endings have been visualized below the surface. A subpopulation of these is likely to signal pain.

Innervation of the Anterior and Posterior Longitudinal Ligaments

Innervation of the longitudinal ligaments has been described by several investigators.[59,66,68-73] The innervation of the PLL is extensive, and both free and glomerular-like terminations have been reported in this tissue.[71,72] However, the number of true encapsulated endings reported is sparse.[72,73] Korkala and associates[46] reported SP immunoreactivity in the human PLL. The extensive innervation of the PLL by fine nerve fibers and the presence of SP immunoreactivity implicate the PLL as a possible source of low back pain.

Clinical Evidence for Lumbar Pain Generators

Pain Provocation and Relief in Facet Joints

The existence of the facet syndrome is controversial, and it has been suggested that facet joint pathology plays an important role in low back pain.[29,77-79] Hirsch and associates[27] and Mooney and Robertson[29] produced low back pain with radiation to the posterior thigh by injecting hypertonic saline into facet joints. Kuslich and associates[80,81] reported that in a series of 193 patients undergoing lumbar spine surgery under progressive local anesthesia, 54% of patients had some sensation when the facet capsule was stimulated, and 20% had significant pain. On the other hand, Jackson and associates[82] performed facet injections on 454 patients without root tension signs and in whom conservative therapy had failed. A set of variables to select patients in whom injections were successful could not be determined. Thus, the facet syndrome is not a well-defined clinical entity and the significance of facet pain is controversial. Placebo effects and a lack of definitive diagnostic criteria for facet syndrome may contribute to the mixed success rate of these treatment modalities.

Schwarzer and associates[83] have put this problem in perspective in a recent study. In order to confirm true facet pain, they proposed that the pain be relieved with both a short-acting analgesic (lidocaine) and a longer acting analgesic (bupivacaine) injected into the medial nerve supplying the joint or into the joint itself. They then performed facet joint injections or medial branch blocks in 176 consecutive patients. Those who responded to the first series of blocks with lidocaine were given a confirmatory block with bupivacaine. Fifteen percent had a positive response to both and longer duration pain relief with bupivacaine, and were thus deemed to have facet pain. The clinical studies demonstrate that facet pain is difficult to diagnose, and pain relief with placebos makes it difficult to understand. The study of Schwarzer and associates[83] strongly suggests that facet pain does exist in approximately 15% of low back pain patients.

Pain Provocation and Relief in Intervertebral Disks

Hirsch and associates[27] injected 0.3 ml of 11% NaCl into the intervertebral disks of human subjects. A few seconds after injection, the subjects developed very severe pain with deep aching across the back and poor localization. Smyth and Wright[84] reported the case of a surgical patient who had backache produced by pulling on a nylon suture looped through the affected disk. Kuslich and associates[80,81] reported that 33% to 40% of back surgery patients studied under progressive regional anesthesia had significant pain when the affected central or lateral anulus was stimulated. On the other hand, almost two thirds of these patients being operated on for disk herniation or spinal stenosis had no disk pain.

Weinstein and associates[43] suggested that the pain associated with an abnormal diskogram may be related to the chemical environment of the disk and a sensitized state of nociceptors in the disk anulus. Derby and associates[85] performed an elegant study in 150 human subjects in which diskogram pressure was monitored simultaneously with radiopaque fluid localization in the disk, and pain severity was monitored in the patient. Pain was produced only when contrast reached the outer anulus through fissures in the anulus. In normal disks, pain occurred at an average of twice the pressure and in a smaller percentage than in degenerated disks. This study supports the existence of both mechanosensitive and chemosensitive nociceptors at the disk surface. The results suggest that the pain provocation during diskography is primarily caused by low pressure stimulation of an irritable outer anulus.

In a study of 32 patients, Nakamura and associates[86] recently reported that infiltration of L2 nerve roots with 1% lidocaine relieved back pain originating at the L4-5 and L5-S1 levels. These data supported their neuroanatomic study in the rat,[87] which provided evidence that the sensory innervation of the dorsal portion of the lower lumbar disks does not have its major pathway through the dorsal roots at that level, but rather through the sympathetic chain, entering the spine at the L2 level. The authors suggested that disk pain is a type of visceral pain.

Muscles and Tendons

The most common etiology of low back pain is often reported to be acute or chronic lumbosacral sprain or strain. However, the scientific evidence for low back pain originating from muscle is lacking.[88] Some patients with palpable abnormalities in their back muscles had increased myoelectric activity,[89-92] while Kraft and associates[93] found no increase in activity in areas of muscle spasm. There is neurophysiologic evidence for muscle nociceptors and reflex muscle activity when joints are stressed. This is presented in the following section.

Neurophysiologic Evidence of Lumbar Pain Sources

Facet Joint

Neuroanatomic and pain provocation studies provide evidence for the sources of lumbar pain. Additional evidence is provided by neurophysiologic studies in animal models, in which nerve discharge is recorded from the dorsal roots or spinal cord. Receptive fields in disk, facet, or muscle are characterized by their response to mechanical stimulation or chemical agents.

Facet Joint and Muscle Units in Control Animals Using the set-up shown in Figure 4, 30 mechanosensitive units have been identified at the facet joint and 27 others in the muscles and tendons near their insertion into the facet.[94,95] Of the 30 units at the facet joint, 13 were in the capsule, 15 in the border regions between capsule and muscle or tendon, and two in the ligamentum flavum (Fig. 5). Of the 30 units in the facet joint, two units (6.7%) had conduction velocities (CVs) < 2.5 m/s (group IV), 17 units 56.7%) had CVs of 2.5 to 20 m/s (group III), and 11 units (36.7%) had CVs > 20 m/s (group II). Nine units had thresholds > 6.0 g, 17 units had thresholds < 6.0 g, and four units were not examined. Eight units responded to joint movement caused by pulling on the isolated L5 lamina. Five of these were in the medial aspect of the facet joint. These units were most responsive to 1 to 2 mm of caudal-to-rostral stretch. The two units in the ligamentum flavum were most responsive to ventral-to-

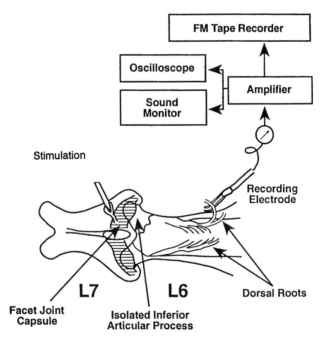

Fig. 4 *Diagram showing the set-up for rabbit lumbar facet joint neurophysiology studies reported in this chapter.[34,47,94,95,97–100] A laminectomy was performed at L4 and L5 or L5 and L6. The left L5 or L6 inferior articular process was left intact. Recordings were made from L5 or L6 dorsal roots whose proximal ends were cut from the spinal cord. In earlier studies[94,95,97] the response of nerves in facet joint and adjacent muscle to local pressure, loading and stretch was characterized. In later studies,[34,47,98–100] various chemicals involved in inflammation were applied to receptive fields in the facet joint capsule or adjacent muscle. (Reproduced with permission from Ozaktay AC, Cavanaugh JM, Blagoev DC, et al: Phospholipase A2-induced electrophysiologic and histologic changes in rabbit dorsal lumbar spine tissues.* Spine 1995;20:2659–2668.)

muscles and tendons   **facet joint capsule**

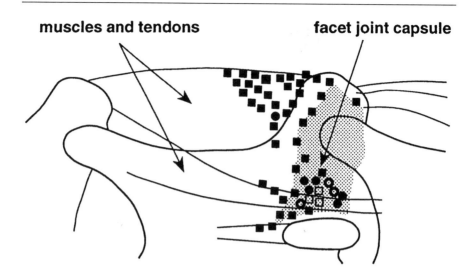

Fig. 5 *Diagram indicating the location of units that were characterized in the facet joint and adjacent tissue in control animals. Squares indicate units with thresholds less than 6 g and circles the units with thresholds greater than 6 g. Open circles indicate units that responded to stretch. (Reproduced with permission from Yamashita T, Minaki Y, Seiichi I, et al:* Somatosensory innervation of the lumbar spine and adjacent tissues. *Trends Compar Biochem Physiol 1993;1:219–227.)*

dorsal stretch. Of the 27 units in muscle and tendon, one unit (3.7%) had a CV < 2.5 m/s (group IV), 4 units (14.8%) had CVs of 2.5-20 m/s (group III), and 22 units (81.5%) had CVs > 20 m/s (group II). One unit had a threshold > 6.0 g and 26 units had thresholds < 6.09 g. Thus, the facet joint contained a much higher proportion of high-threshold, low CV units than muscle. It is these units that are likely to serve a pain function. In a study by Pickar and McLain,[96] the small fiber afferents in the cat facet showed directional sensitivity to stretch. Thresholds and receptive fields were similar to those reported in the rabbit.[94,95]

Response of Units to Spine Loading In a study reported by Avramov and associates,[97] the isolated rabbit spine in an in vitro loading chamber was loaded in tension. Compression, applied load, and nerve discharge were measured simultaneously. A constant finding during these experiments was a vigorous multiunit response to loading. During compressive loading, the spine underwent dorsal-lateral bending that caused the facet joints to articulate along the joint plane, stretching the facet joint capsule. Loading excited both units with spontaneous activity, as well as units that were silent before loading was initiated. Three patterns were observed: (1) phasic type mechanoreception; (2) slowly adapting low threshold mechanoreception; and (3) slowly adapting high-threshold mechanoreception.

In both the in vivo and in vitro experiments just described, nerves typically stopped firing when mechanical stimulus ceased, even if the stimulus was noxious. Thus, the results demonstrate the possible activation of pain generators in the facet joint but do not explain the persistence of pain. Therefore, studies were

undertaken to determine if neurogenic and non-neurogenic inflammatory mediators known to be released during tissue damage and inflammation result in
nerve sensitization or persistent discharge. Kaolin (a silica product) and carrageenan (a seaweed product) are commonly used to produce an acute tissue inflammation that releases histamine, bradykinin, and prostaglandins into tissue,
sensitizing nerve endings.

Cavanaugh and associates[98] injected 2% kaolin and 2% carrageenan into the
rabbit facet joint capsule or adjacent muscle and monitored neurophysiologic
response. Units were found in multifidus, rotatory, and intermamillary muscle,
or in the facet joint capsule and border regions at the junction of capsule and
muscle tendon insertions. For 30 units von Frey thresholds ranged from 0.05 to
17.3 g, with the lower threshold units primarily in muscle and the higher threshold units at the facet joint. Most of the units in this study were in group II (>
20 m/s) or group III (2.5 to 20 m/s). Spontaneous discharge rates (SDRs) were
monitored for 21 units in inflamed tissue and 21 units in controls. The average
SDR was 18.1 units/s (range 0 to 50) in the inflamed joints and 9.3 units/s (range
0 to 28) in the controls.

In a study reported by Ozaktay and associates,[99] 2% type II carrageenan was
injected into receptive fields in the rabbit facet joint and nerve discharge was
monitored for 3 hours. The multiunit spontaneous background discharge rate
showed increases over 150 minutes. The time course of single units, identified
as group II, III, IV, and silent units, was also investigated. Units that were previously silent appeared in the first 15 minutes and persisted beyond 75 minutes.
Thresholds of the characterized units decreased with time. Histologic examinations revealed inflammatory changes in carrageenan injected tissues, including
vasodilatation and edema in synovial capsule and leukocyte infiltration in the
perivascular space in surrounding muscle tissue. In controls injected with isotonic saline, no changes were observed.

Yamashita and associates[47] reported an increase in spontaneous discharge rate
after the injection of 10 μg SP into facet joint receptive fields in the rabbit. Most
of the units (83%) showed an increase in SDR after the injection; 54% of the
units showed immediate onset, and 29.2% of the units showed slow onset of the
excitation. One third of the units showed decreased von Frey thresholds after
the application of SP (Fig. 6). Substance P had an excitatory effect on both low
and high threshold units.

Because of high concentrations of PLA_2 reported in herniated disks and in
rheumatoid synovial joints, its possible effect on nerves in the joints of the lumbar spine is intriguing. Ozaktay and associates[34] reported dose-dependent effects of PLA_2 on sensory nerves in the rabbit facet joint. Four hundred, 750, or
1,500 U of PLA_2 (snake venom) in a buffered carrier solution was injected into
the receptive field of the lumbar facet joint or surrounding muscle in 18 anesthetized rabbits. The carrier solution was injected as control in four experiments. The threshold and unit activity was followed for 90 minutes (Fig. 7).
Only 1,500 U PLA_2 injections (n = 5) produced a significant decrease in spontaneous activity of multiunit nerve discharge over time. At 30 minutes, the characterized units were no longer mechanically responsive. In three of four experiments using 750 U PLA_2, the nerve discharge increased in response to mechanical
stimulation at 30 minutes and remained spontaneously active over time. After
400 U PLA_2 (n = 5) or control (n = 4) injections, spontaneous activity did not

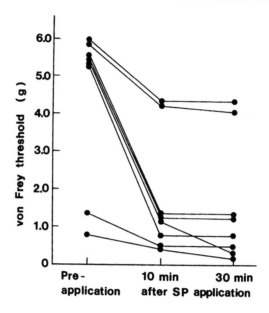

Fig. 6 *Changes in von Frey threshold of eight sensory neurons in the rabbit facet joint units and surrounding muscle units after injection of 10 μg SP into the receptive fields. (Reproduced with permission from Yamashita T, Cavanaugh JM, Ozaktay AC, et al: Effects of substance P on the mechanosensitive units in the lumbar facet joint and adjacent tissue. J Orthop Res 1993;11:205–214.)*

show any significant changes over time. Single unit data: Myelinated Aβ fibers (group II, n = 8) showed significant decrease in their activity after injection of 750 and 1,500 U PLA_2. Myelinated Aδ fibers (group III, n = 8), which may signal pain, became mechanically excited 30 minutes after 750 U PLA_2 injection. Two units that were neither spontaneously active nor mechanically responsive before PLA_2 injection were evoked mechanically 30 minutes after injection of 750 U PLA_2, and remained spontaneously active over time. These may be "silent nociceptors."[2,3]

Histologic examination revealed inflammatory changes as early as 2 hours after the PLA_2 injections, regardless of dose. In controls, no changes were observed either histologically or electrophysiologically.

Intervertebral Disk and Spinal Canal

Yamashita and associates[100] reported only three mechanically responsive group III units in the L5-6 rabbit anulus or at insertions of anulus fibrosus to vertebral bodies. These units had very high thresholds (164-279 g). In an independent study, Cavanaugh and associates[101] reported only occasional discharge after mechanically probing into the rabbit disk. In one experiment, vigorous discharges were obtained by applying the algesic (pain-producing) chemical serotonin over the spinal canal.[5] Thus, a portion of the fine unmyelinated and small myelinated fibers in the disk anulus may serve as silent no-

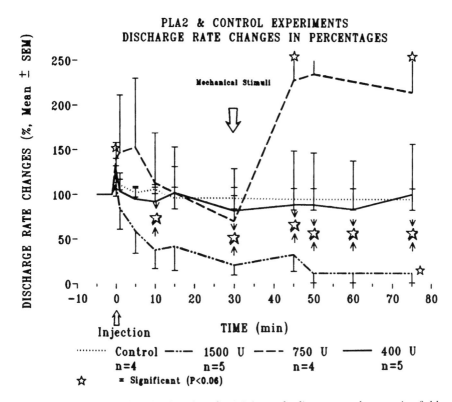

Fig. 7 *Response to PLA$_2$ injections into facet joint and adjacent muscle receptive fields. These plots show the average percentage change from the baseline multiunit SDR follow- ing the injections, over time. After injection of 1,500 U PLA$_2$, SDR showed a significant decrease within 10 min (p < 0.0001). After injection of 750 U PLA$_2$, the SDR shows an increase in the first 5 minutes (p < 0.012). Thirty minutes after the injection, the mechani- cal probing resulted in prolonged after-discharges (p < 0.047). After injection of 400 U of PLA$_2$, there was no significant change of SDR observed over time. The control injections did not produce any significant SDR changes over time. (Reproduced with permission from Ozaktay AC, Cavanaugh JM, Blagoev DC, et al: Phospholipase A2 induced electrophysi- ological and histological changes in rabbit lumbar dorsal lumbar spine tissues. Spine 1995;20:2659–2668.)*

ciceptors[2,3] that are not readily excited by mechanical stress, but that re- spond to algesic chemicals produced during tissue damage or inflammation. This dependence on an irritating chemical substance to activate a certain class of pain fibers may explain why Kuslich and associates[80,81] found the disks of some patients to be quite painful and other disks to be totally insensitive to stimulation.

As stated earlier, two recent studies[86,87] suggest that the primary sensory in- nervation of the posterior portion of the disk is a pathway through the sympa- thetic chain that enters the spinal cord at the L2 dorsal root level. If this is the major sensory pathway of the posterior disk, it provides an alternative reason for lack of mechanical response in segmental root recordings and suggests that sympathetic trunk or L2 root recordings need to be performed in an attempt to characterize receptive fields in the disk.

Neurophysiologic Studies in Muscle

Muscle is known to contain a large population of Aδ and C fibers. Mense and Meyer[102] characterized group III and IV units in the triceps surae muscle and calcaneal tendon of anesthetized cats. Group III included units that were low-threshold pressure-sensitive units (44%), nociceptive (33%), and contraction-sensitive (23%). Group IV units included nociceptive (43%), low-threshold pressure-sensitive (19%), contraction-sensitive (19%), and thermosensitive (19%) units. As a group, approximately 40% of these fibers appeared to serve a strict nociceptive function, while the rest appeared to be sensors of contraction and temperature. Yamashita and associates[94,95] reported activation of group III fibers in the multifidus muscle of the rabbit. These fibers generally had lower thresholds than the neurons of the facet joint, so they may have served functions similar to those of the contraction or pressure sensors reported by Mense and Meyer.[102]

Non-neurogenic pain mediators excite muscle units. Bradykinin, a nonapeptide, has been shown to be an excitant of muscle group III and IV afferent fibers.[103,104] Prostaglandin E$_2$ and 5-hydroxytryptamine enhance this action.[6] Carrageenan-induced myositis causes an increase in the background activity of group III and IV units in inflamed leg muscle and a lowering of threshold of group IV units.[105]

Reflex muscle spasm may play a role in low back pain. Cavanaugh and associates[106] reported that mechanical pressure to rat lumbar facet joints caused discharges in dorsal rami on the contralateral side, presumably from reflex motor afferents. Pedersen and associates[58] reported that mechanical stimulation of feline lumbar joints, fascia, ligaments, periosteum, and muscle was followed by reflex spasm of dorsal muscles, especially ipsilaterally. Thus, there is neurophysiologic evidence that stresses in the lumbar vertebrae cause reflex muscle activity in paraspinal muscles. This could increase mechanical stresses to the joints and muscles of the lumbar spine. If these tissues were already irritated by algesic chemicals, the added pressure could conceivably activate nociceptors.

Proposed Mechanisms for Chronic Low Back Pain

Based on the previously discussed neurobiologic, neuroanatomic, neurophysiologic, and clinical evidence, certain mechanisms of pain generation from lumbar tissues can be proposed.

Facet Pain

Facet capsular strain as a source of low back pain is supported by the following: (1) The facet capsule is richly innervated with C and Aδ fibers. (2) A large portion of these are high-threshold fibers, and thus likely to signal pain. (3) The fibers can be mechanically activated by local pressure and capsular stretch. (4) The fibers can be sensitized and/or excited by naturally occurring inflammatory agents, including SP and PLA$_2$. In addition, the potential for acute traumatic strain was demonstrated in biomechanical studies of facet joint capsule stretch in human cadaveric lumbar spines.[61]

Another possible pain mechanism in the facet joint is pressure to nerve endings in synovial folds or to nerve endings in osteoarthritic joints. The former is suggested by the existence of SP in synovial folds[63] and the latter by the report of SP in erosion channels and calcified cartilage of degenerated facet joints.[43] The lumbar facet joint can undergo the degenerative and inflammatory changes of rheumatoid arthritis or osteoarthritis. The facet joint can carry loads via lumbar extension, which bottoms out the superior articular process onto the lamina below.[62] This loading, if repetitive, may play a role in degenerative changes in the facet joint.

Based on the previously mentioned studies, it is recommended that injections for facet pain include the facet capsule as an injection site. Injection into the facet joint with overflow to the joint capsule may serve the same purpose. Injection of lidocaine to the capsule and surrounding tissue in the rabbit model caused cessation of all nerve activity from these tissues.[99] Injections confined to the joint space will not address irritation that may arise from the many nerve endings in facet capsule or adjacent muscle insertions.

In tissue damage or inflammation to posterior elements of the lumbar spine, the inflammatory cascade could cause prolonged nociceptor excitation, which can release SP from nerve endings, contributing to the cycle of pain. This peripheral hyperalgesia can lead to a sensitization of nerves in the spinal cord, leading to further persistence of pain. Nerve discharge from sensitized nerve endings in facet or paraspinal muscle may cause reflex muscle spasm, increasing the mechanical loads in the intervertebral joints, causing further stimulation of nociceptors. In addition, inflammatory or ischemic changes in contracted paraspinal muscles may activate nociceptors in the muscles themselves. The interplay of peripheral and central sensitization, increased loading caused by reflex muscle contraction, and the release of algesic chemicals from the nerves themselves suggests a vicious cycle propelled by mechanical stress and pain-producing chemicals. The net effect in the spinal cord may be central sensitization and expression of c-*fos* and c-*jun*, oncogenes that are expressed in the spinal cord in experimental studies of acute and chronic pain.[52] In polyarthritic rat and neuroma models, dense staining for c-*fos* in deeper lamina was found 3 to 4 weeks after initial insult. This suggests that deeper dorsal horn lamina contribute to hyperalgesia in chronic pain models.[52]

While the existence of the facet syndrome is controversial and no specific clinical signs and symptoms can successfully confirm a diagnosis of this syndrome, the latest work using double injections of local anesthetic strongly suggests that, in at least 15% of patients, low back pain originates in the facet joints.[83] It is only natural that a highly mobile, richly innervated synovial joint is a potential pain source. Pain originating from other synovial joints such as knee, ankle, and interphalangeal joints is well documented. In our studies, neurotoxicity was demonstrated in response to very low doses of snake venom PLA$_2$ injections on facet capsule receptive fields.[34] These data suggest inflammatory and neurotoxic roles for PLA$_2$ that may be relevant to diskogenic and facet pain. The longer term consequences of neurotoxicity may include neuroma formation and ectopic discharges from regenerating pain fibers.

Disk Pain

Based on early studies, it was once thought that the intervertebral disk had little or no innervation, so that the pain commencing after disk herniation must come from other nearby tissue.[107] However, the cumulative evidence of several studies using silver impregnation and immunocytochemistry techniques reveals that the surface of the disk is relatively well innervated, and the adjacent posterior longitudinal ligament probably more so. The existence in disk anulus of small nerve fibers and free nerve endings, and the demonstration that some of these fibers contain SP, supports the hypothesis of the disk as a potential source of pain. Pain provocation studies in the disks of awake patients suggests that the mechanisms of pain production are both mechanical and chemical.[80,81,85] Mechanical stimulation replicates the patients' disk pain in some cases. When disk pain is not replicated, it is possible that the nerves are not sensitized enough by chemical mediators for the mechanical stress to cause disk nociceptors to fire. However, because back pain is notoriously difficult to localize, an alternate explanation is that in some cases of reputed diskogenic pain, the pain did not originate in the disk in the first place. The neurophysiologic studies of the cat lumbar spine by Gillette and associates[108] demonstrate very large receptive fields with convergence from skin, muscle, and joint receptors to single sensory neurons in the spinal cord. This provides a plausible explanation for poor pain localization often seen in patients with low back pain.

Two intriguing findings that need further exploration for their potential role in disk pain are the growth of small blood vessels and nerves into deeper layers of the disk and the reports of a sensory pathway from the disk through the sympathetic chain. Could the ingrowth of new nerves and the degeneration of the disk itself allow disk compression to place higher stresses on nerve endings in the inner anulus than would typically be placed on the nerve endings in the tensile fibers of the outer anulus? In other words, are nerves in a degenerated disk compressed or pinched?

Low Back Pain: Mechanical or Chemical?

Persistent low back pain likely depends on both mechanical stress and chemical agents. The existence of inflammation in diskogenic pain has been controversial. Recent studies demonstrating the presence of inflammatory cells[109,110] and the control of sciatic pain using steroids[111] strongly suggest that inflammatory processes may be important factors in low back pain. If this is the case, the neural mechanisms previously described are likely to play an important role. After an initial inflammatory reaction or the release of algesic chemicals after tissue damage, peripheral and central sensitization of the pain pathway may occur. Because of its unique role in posture and weightbearing, and the potential forces imparted by body weight and the large mass of paraspinal muscles surrounding the intervertebral joints, the spine is under constant mechanical stress. If the pain pathway is chemically sensitized peripherally and/or centrally, the added mechanical stress is likely to play a role in activation of sensitized nociceptors.

Acknowledgments

I wish to thank Drs. A. Cuneyt Ozaktay, Toshihiko Yamashita, Albert I. King, and Thomas V. Getchell for their continued support of and significant contributions to the facet joint research reported in this paper. I also wish to thank Drs. Avram Avramov, Dimitar Blagoev, and Qing Hang Li for their valuable contributions to this work. I would also like to acknowledge Srinivasu Kallakuri and Suhas Naik for their technical assistance. This manuscript was partially supported by NIH Grant No. AR41739.

References

1. Guyton AC: Sensory receptors and their basic mechanisms of action, in Guyton AC (ed): *Textbook of Medical Physiology,* ed 6. Philadelphia, PA, WB Saunders, 1981, pp 588–596.
2. Schaible HG, Schmidt RF: Time course of mechanosensitivity changes in articular afferents during a developing experimental arthritis. *J Neurophysiol* 1988;60:2180–2195.
3. Grigg P, Schaible HG, Schmidt RF: Mechanical sensitivity of group III and IV afferents from posterior articular nerve in normal and inflamed cat knee. *J Neurophysiol* 1986;55:635–643.
4. Schmidt RF: Nociception and pain, in Schmidt RF (ed): *Fundamentals of Sensory Physiology,* ed 3. Berlin, Germany, Springer-Verlag, 1986, pp 117–143.
5. Adriaensen H, Gybels J, Handwerker HO, et al: Nociceptor discharges and sensations due to prolonged noxious mechanical stimulation: A paradox. *Hum Neurobiol* 1984;3:53–58.
6. Rang HP, Bevan S, Dray A: Nociceptive peripheral neurons: Cellular properties, in Wall PD, Melzack R, Bonica JJ (eds): *Textbook of Pain,* ed 3. Edinburgh, Scotland, Churchill Livingstone, 1994, pp 57–78.
7. Mense S: Sensitization of group IV muscle receptors to bradykinin by 5-hydroxytryptamine and prostaglandin E2. *Brain Res* 1981;225:95–105.
8. Schaible HG, Schmidt RF: Excitation and sensitization of fine articular afferents from cat's knee joint by prostaglandin E2. *J Physiol* 1988;403:91–104.
9. Neugebauer V, Schaible HG: Peripheral and spinal components of the sensitization of spinal neurons during an acute experimental arthritis. *Agents Actions* 1988;25:234–236.
10. French AS: Mechanotransduction. *Annu Rev Physiol* 1992;54:135–152.
11. Hille B (ed): *Ionic Channels of Excitable Membranes,* ed 2. Sunderland, MA, Sinauer Associates, 1992.
12. Sachs F: Biophysics of mechanoreception. *Membr Biochem* 1986;6:173–195.
13. Farmer SG, Burch RM: Biochemical and molecular pharmacology of kinin receptors. *Annu Rev Pharmacol Toxicol* 1992;32:511–536.
14. Nachemson A: Intradiscal measurements of pH in patients with lumbar rhizopathies. *Acta Orthop Scand* 1969;40:23–42.
15. Ward TT, Steigbigel RT: Acidosis of synovial fluid correlates with synovial fluid leukocytosis. *Am J Med* 1978;64:933–936.
16. Steen KH, Reeh PW, Anton F, et al: Protons selectively induce lasting excitation and sensitization to mechanical stimulation of nociceptors in rat skin, in vitro. *J Neurosci* 1992;12:86–95.
17. Lindahl O: Pain: A chemical explanation. *Acta Rheumatol Scand* 1962;8:161–169.
18. Bevan S, Yeats J: Protons activate a cation conductance in a sub-population of rat dorsal root ganglion neurones. *J Physiol* 1991;433:145–161.
19. Rueff A, Dray A: 5-hydroxytryptamine-induced sensitization and activation of peripheral fibres in the neonatal rat are mediated via different 5-hydroxytryptamine-receptors. *Neuroscience* 1992;50:899–905.
20. Richardson BP, Engel G, Donatsch P, et al: Identification of serotonin M-receptor subtypes and their specific blockade by a new class of drugs. *Nature* 1985;316:126–131.

21. Simone DA, Alreja M, LaMotte RH: Psychophysical studies of the itch sensation and itchy skin ('alloknesis') produced by intracutaneous injection of histamine. *Somatosens Mot Res* 1991;8:271–279.
22. Moncada S, Palmer RM, Higgs EA: Nitric oxide: Physiology, pathophysiology, and pharmacology. *Pharmacol Rev* 1991;43:109–142.
23. Kang JD, Georgescu HI, Larkin L, et al: Herniated lumbar and cervical intervertebral discs spontaneously produce matrix metalloproteinases, nitric oxide, interleukin-6, and prostaglandin E2. *Trans Orthop Res Soc* 1995;20:350.
24. Kang JD, Stefanovic-Racic M, Larkin LA, et al: Nitric oxide production by human intervertebral disc in response to interleukin-1 and its effects on interleukin-6 production. *Trans Orthop Res Soc* 1995;20:351.
25. Kumazawa T, Mizumura K: Chemical responses of polymodal receptors of the scrotal contents in dogs. *J Physiol* 1980;299:219–231.
26. Kumazawa T, Mizumura K, Sato J: Response properties of polymodal receptors studied using in vitro testis superior spermatic nerve preparations of dogs. *J Neurophysiol* 1987;57:702–711.
27. Hirsch C, Ingelmark BE, Miller M: The anatomical basis for low back pain: Studies on the presence of sensory nerve endings in ligamentous, capsular and intervertebral disc structures in the human lumbar spine. *Acta Orthop Scand* 1963;33:1–17.
28. Lewis T, Kellgren JH: Observations relating to referred pain, visceromotor reflexes and other associated phenomena. *Clin Sci* 1939;4:47–71.
29. Mooney V, Robertson J: The facet syndrome. *Clin Orthop* 1976;115:149–156.
30. Bomalaski JS, Clark MA: Phospholipase A2 and arthritis. *Arthritis Rheum* 1993;36:190–198.
31. Vishwanath BS, Fawzy AA, Franson RC: Edema-inducing activity of phospholipase A2 purified from human synovial fluid and inhibition by aristolochic acid. *Inflammation* 1988;12:549–561.
32. Saal JS, Franson RC, Dobrow R, et al: High levels of inflammatory phospholipasea A2 activity in lumbar disc herniations. *Spine* 1990;15:674–678.
33. Meyers R, Saal SJ, Franson R, et al: Human disc PLA2 induces neural injury: A histomorphometric study. *Orthop Trans* 1993;17:291.
34. Ozaktay AC, Cavanaugh JM, Blagoev DC, et al: Phospholipase A2 induced electrophysiologic and histologic changes in rabbit dorsal lumbar spine tissues. *Spine* 1995;20:2659–2668.
35. Rang HP, Bevan S, Dray A: Chemical activation of nociceptive peripheral neurones. *Br Med Bull* 1991;47:534–548.
36. Go VL, Yaksh TL: Release of substance P from the cat spinal cord. *J Physiol* 1987;391:141–167.
37. Oku R, Satoh M, Takagi H: Release of substance P from the spinal dorsal horn is enhanced in polyarthritic rats. *Neurosci Lett* 1987;74:315–319.
38. Willcockson WS, Chung JM, Hori Y, et al: Effects of iontophoretically released peptides on primate spinothalamic tract cells. *J Neurosci* 1984;4:741–750.
39. Dougherty PM, Willis WD: Enhancement of spinothalamic neuron responses to chemical and mechanical stimuli following combined micro-iontophoretic application of N-methyl-D-aspartic acid and substance P. *Pain* 1991;47:85–93.
40. el-Bohy A, Cavanaugh JM, Getchell ML, et al: Localization of substance P and neurofilament immunoreactive fibers in the lumbar facet joint capsule and supraspinous ligament of the rabbit. *Brain Res* 1988;460:379–382.
41. Ashton IK, Ashton BA, Gibson SJ, et al: Morphological basis for back pain: The demonstration of nerve fibers and neuropeptides in the lumbar facet joint capsule but not in ligamentum flavum. *J Orthop Res* 1992;10:72–78.
42. Beaman DN, Graziano GP, Glover RA, et al: Substance P innervation of lumbar spine facet joints. *Spine* 1993;18:1044–1049.
43. Weinstein J, Claverie W, Gibson S: The pain of discography. *Spine* 1988;13:1344–1348.
44. Ashton IK, Roberts S, Jaffray DC, et al: Neuropeptides in the human intervertebral disc. *J Orthop Res* 1994;12:186–192.

45. Konttinen YT, Gronblad M, Antti-Poika I, et al: Neuroimmuno-histochemical analysis of peridiscal nociceptive neural elements. *Spine* 1990;15:383–386.
46. Korkala O, Gronblad M, Liesi P, et al: Immunohistochemical demonstration of nociceptors in the ligamentous structures of the lumbar spine. *Spine* 1985;10:156–157.
47. Yamashita T, Cavanaugh JM, Ozaktay AC, et al: Effect of substance P on mechanosensitive units of tissues around and in the lumbar facet joint. *J Orthop Res* 1993;11:205–214.
48. McCarron RF, Wimpee MW, Hudkins PG, et al: The inflammatory effect of nucleus pulposus: A possible element in the pathogenesis of low-back pain. *Spine* 1987;12:760–764.
49. Olmarker K, Rydevik B, Nordborg C: Autologous nucleus pulposus induces neurophysiologic and histologic changes in porcine cauda equina nerve roots. *Spine* 1993;18:1425–1432.
50. Cavanaugh JM, Ozaktay AC, Vaidyanathan S: Mechano- and chemosensitivity of lumbar dorsal roots and dorsal root ganglia: An in vitro study. *Trans Orthop Res Soc* 1994;19:109.
51. Woolf CJ: The dorsal horn: State-dependent sensory processing and the generation of pain, in Wall PD, Melzack R, Bonica JJ (eds): *Textbook of Pain,* ed 3. Edinburgh, Scotland, Churchill Livingstone, 1994.
52. Yaksh TL, Malmberg AB: Central pharmacology of nociceptive transmission, in Wall PD, Melzack R, Bonica JJ (eds): *Textbook of Pain*, ed 3. Edinburgh, Scotland, Churchill Livingstone, 1994.
53. Dubner R, Basbaum AI: Spinal dorsal horn plasticity following tissue or nerve injury, in Wall PD, Melzack R, Bonica JJ (eds): *Textbook of Pain,* ed 3. Edinburgh, Scotland, Churchill Livingstone, 1994.
54. Coderre TJ, Katz J, Vaccarino AL, et al: Contribution of central neuroplasticity to pathological pain: Review of clinical and experimental evidence. *Pain* 1993;52:259–285.
55. Bogduk N: The innervation of the lumbar spine. *Spine* 1983;8:286–293.
56. Stillwell DL Jr: The nerve supply of the vertebral column and its associated structures in the monkey. *Anat Rec* 1956;125:139–169.
57. Paris SV: Anatomy as related to function and pain. *Orthop Clin North Am* 1983;14:475–489.
58. Pedersen HE, Blunck CFJ, Gardner E: The anatomy of lumbosacral posterior rami and meningeal branches of spinal nerves (sinu-vertebral nerves): With an experimental study of their functions. *J Bone Joint Surg* 1956;38A:377–391.
59. Jackson HC III, Winkelmann RK, Bickel WH: Nerve endings in the human lumbar spinal column and related structures. *J Bone Joint Surg* 1966;48A:1272–1281.
60. Ozaktay AC, Yamashita T, Cavanaugh JM, et al: Fine nerve fibers and endings in the fibrous capsule of the lumbar facet joint. *Trans Orthop Res Soc* 1991;16:353.
61. El-Bohy AA, Goldberg SJ, King AI: Measurement of facet capsular stretch. *1987 Biomechanics Symposium*. New York, NY, American Society of Mechanical Engineers, 1987, pp 161–164.
62. Yang KH, King AI: Mechanism of facet load transmission as a hypothesis for low-back pain. *Spine* 1984;9:557–565.
63. Giles LG, Harvey AR: Immunohistochemical demonstration of nociceptors in the capsule and synovial folds of human zygapophyseal joints. *Br J Rheumatol* 1987;26:362–364.
64. Gronblad M, Korkala O, Konttinen YT, et al: Silver impregnation and immunohistochemical study of nerves in lumbar facet joint plical tissue. *Spine* 1991;16:34–38.
65. Ikari C: Abstract: A study of the mechanism of low-back pain: The neurohistological examination of the disease. *J Bone Joint Surg* 1954;36A:195.
66. Jung A, Brunschwig A: Recherches histologiques sur l'innervation des articulations des corps vertébraux. *La Presse Medicale* 1932;40:316–317.
67. Wiberg G: Back pain in relation to the nerve supply of the intervertebral disc. *Acta Orthop Scand* 1949;19:211–221.

603

68. Bogduk N, Tynan W, Wilson AS: The nerve supply to the human lumbar intervertebral discs. *J Anat* 1981;132:39–56.

69. Forsythe WB, Ghoshal NG: Innervation of the canine thoracolumbar vertebral column. *Anat Rec* 1984;208:57–63.

70. Malinsky J: The ontogenetic development of nerve terminations in the intervertebral discs of man. *Acta Anat* 1959;38:96–113.

71. Roofe PG: Innervation of annulus fibrosus and posterior longitudinal ligament: Fourth and fifth lumbar level. *Arch Neurol Psychiat* 1940;44:100–103.

72. Yoshizawa H, O'Brien JP, Smith WT, et al: The neuropathology of intervertebral discs removed for low-back pain. *J Pathol* 1980;132:95–104.

73. Cavanaugh JM, Kallakuri S, Ozaktay AC: Innervation of the rabbit lumbar intervertebral disc and posterior longitudinal ligament. *Spine* 1995;20:2080–2085.

74. Shinohara H: Lumbar disc lesion, with special reference to the histological significance of nerve endings of the lumbar discs. *Nippon Seikeigeka Gakkai Zasshi* 1970;44:553–570.

75. Kauppila LI: Ingrowth of blood vessels in disc degeneration: Angiographic and histological studies of cadaveric spines. *J Bone Joint Surg* 1995;77A:26–31.

76. Ahmed M, Bjurholm A, Kreicbergs A, et al: SP- and CGRP-immunoreactive nervefibres in the rat lumbar spine. *Neuro Orthop* 1991;12:19–28.

77. Ghormley RK: Low back pain: With special reference to the articular facets, with presentation of an operative procedure. *JAMA* 1933;101:1773–1777.

78. Badgley CE: The articular facets in relation to low-back pain and sciatic radiation. *J Bone Joint Surg* 1941;23:481–496.

79. Shealy CN: Facet denervation in the management of back and sciatic pain. *Clin Orthop* 1976;115:157–164.

80. Kuslich SD, Ulstrom CL, Michael CJ: The tissue origin of low back pain and sciatica: A report of pain response to tissue stimulation during operations on the lumbar spine using local anesthesia. *Orthop Clin North Am* 1991;22:181–187.

81. Kuslich SD, Ahern JW: What tissues are responsible for low back pain and sciatica? Investigation of tissue sensitivity in humans. *Trans Orthop Res Soc* 1994;19:110.

82. Jackson RP, Jacobs RR, Montesano PX: Facet joint injection in low-back pain: A prospective statistical study. *Spine* 1988;13:966–971.

83. Schwarzer AC, Derby R, Aprill CN, et al: Pain from the lumbar zygapophysial joints: A test of two models. *J Spinal Disord* 1994;7:331–336.

84. Smyth MJ, Wright V: Sciatica and the intervertebral disc: An experimental study. *J Bone Joint Surg* 1958;40A:1401-1418.

85. Derby R, Kline G, Schwarzer A, et al: Relationship between intradiscal pressure and pain provocation during discography. *Orthop Trans* 1995;19:59–60.

86. Nakamura S, Takahasi K, Yamagata M, et al: Afferent pathway of low back pain: evaluation with L2-spinal-nerve infiltration. Proceedings of the International Society for the Study of the Lumbar Spine. Ontario, Canada, International Society for the Study of the Lumbar Spine, 1995, pp 18–22.

87. Nakamura S, Takahasi K, Yamagata M, et al: Innervation of the posterior portion of the annulus fibrosus. Proceedings of the International Society for the Study of the Lumbar Spine. Ontario, Canada, International Society for the Study of the Lumbar Spine, 1995, p 9.

88. Andersson G, Bogduk N, DeLuca C, et al: Muscle, Part A: Clinical perspectives, in Frymoyer JW, Gordon SL (eds): *New Perspectives on Low Back Pain.* Park Ridge, IL, American Academy of Orthopaedic Surgeons, 1989, pp 293–334.

89. Denslow JS, Clough GH: Reflex activity in the spinal extensors. *J Neurophysiol* 1941;4:430–437.

90. Elliott FA: Tender muscles in sciatica: Electromyographic studies. *Lancet* 1944;1:47–49.

91. Arroyo P Jr: Electromyography in the evaluation of reflex muscle spasm: Simplified method for direct evaluation of muscle-relaxant drugs. *J Fla Med Assoc* 1966;53:29–31.

92. Fischer AA, Chang CH: Electromyographic evidence of paraspinal muscle spasm during sleep in patients with low back pain. *Clin J Pain* 1985;1:147–154.

93. Kraft GH, Johnson EW, LaBan MM: The fibrositis syndrome. *Arch Phys Med Rehabil* 1968;49:155–162.

94. Yamashita T, Cavanaugh JM, el-Bohy AA, et al: Mechanosensitive afferent units in the lumbar facet joint. *J Bone Joint Surg* 1990;72A:865–870.

95. Yamashita T, Minaki Y, Seiichi I, et al: Somatosensory innervation of the lumbar spine and adjacent tissues. *Trends Compar Biochem Physiol* 1993;1:219–227.

96. Pickar JG, McLain RF: Responses of mechanosensitive afferents to manipulation of the lumbar facet in the cat. *Spine* 1995;20:2379–2385.

97. Avramov AI, Cavanaugh JM, Ozaktay CA, et al: The effects of controlled mechanical loading on group-II, III, and IV afferent units from the lumbar facet joint and surrounding tissue: An in vitro study. *J Bone Joint Surg* 1992;74A:1464–1471.

98. Cavanaugh JM, Yamashita T, Ozaktay AC, et al: An inflammation model of low back pain. Proceedings of the International Society for the Study of the Lumbar Spine. Ontario, Canada, International Society for the Study of the Lumbar Spine, 1990, p 46.

99. Ozaktay AC, Cavanaugh JM, Blagoev DC, et al: Effects of a carrageenan-induced inflammation in rabbit lumbar facet joint capsule and adjacent tissues. *Neurosci Res* 1994;20:355–364.

100. Yamashita T, Minaki Y, Oota I, et al: Mechanosensitive afferent units in the lumbar intervertebral disk and adjacent muscle. *Spine* 1993;18:2252–2256.

101. Cavanaugh JM, Avramov A, Ozaktay AC, et al: Initial electrophysiological studies of neurons of the lumbar spinal canal. *Orthop Trans* 1993;17:290.

102. Mense S, Meyer H: Different types of slowly conducting afferent units in cat skeletal muscle and tendon. *J Physiol* 1985;363:403–417.

103. Franz M, Mense S: Muscle receptors with group IV afferent fibres responding to application of bradykinin. *Brain Res* 1975;92:369–383.

104. Mense S: Nervous outflow from skeletal muscle following chemical noxious stimulation. *J Physiol* 1977;267:75–88.

105. Berberich P, Hoheisel U, Mense S: Effects of a carrageenan-induced myositis on the discharge properties of group III and IV muscle receptors in the cat. *J Neurophysiol* 1988;59:1395–1409.

106. Cavanaugh JM, El-Bohy A, Hardy WN, et al: Sensory innervation of soft tissues of the lumbar spine in the rat. *J Orthop Res* 1989;7:378–388.

107. Hirsch C: The reaction of intervertebral discs to compression forces. *J Bone Joint Surg* 1955;37A:1188–1196.

108. Gillette RG, Kramis RC, Roberts WJ: Characterization of spinal somatosensory neurons having receptive fields in lumbar tissues of cats. *Pain* 1993;54:85–98.

109. Gronblad M, Virri J, Tolonen J, et al: A controlled immunohistochemical study of inflammatory cells in disc herniation tissue. *Spine* 1994;19:2744–2751.

110. Saal JS: The role of inflammation in lumbar pain. *Spine* 1995;20:1821–1827.

111. Garfin SR, Rydevik BL, Brown RA: Compressive neuropathy of spinal nerve roots: A mechanical or biological problem? *Spine* 1991;16:162–166.

Chapter 36

Intervertebral Disk Degeneration and Back Pain

Joseph A. Buckwalter, MS, MD
James Martin, PhD

Intervertebral disks (Fig. 1) stabilize the spine by anchoring adjacent vertebral bodies to each other, and allow the movement between vertebrae that gives the spine its flexibility. They also absorb and distribute loads applied to the spine. All intervertebral disks undergo alterations in volume, shape, structure, and composition that can decrease spine motion and adversely alter the mechanical properties of the spine. These changes are part of the normal aging process. However, some intervertebral disks undergo an exceptionally severe age-related loss of structure and function that is best considered a form of degeneration that alters spine function and may contribute to the development of chronic or intermittent back pain.

Paralleling the changes in intervertebral disks, the frequency of spine stiffness and back pain increases with age. Children and adolescents rarely develop chronic or intermittent back and neck stiffness or spine-related pain that limits their mobility, but these problems are common in middle-aged and older people.[1] The relationship of these clinical problems to the age-related deterioration of intervertebral disks remains unclear, but no other component of the spine, and no other musculoskeletal soft-tissue structure, undergoes more dramatic alterations with age.[2-5] Perhaps for these reasons, many physicians attribute at least some back pain and stiffness to disk degeneration; yet, the causes of disk degeneration and the relationships between disk degeneration and pain remain poorly understood.

Recent work[2,3] has advanced understanding of the age-related changes in intervertebral disk structure, composition, function, metabolism, and nutrition, the mechanisms responsible for disk aging and degeneration, and factors that accelerate disk degeneration. This information makes it possible to develop potential answers to the following questions: What causes disk degeneration? Does disk degeneration contribute to chronic or intermittent back pain?

Intervertebral Disk Structure, Composition, and Function

Like other connective tissues, disks consist of a sparse population of cells and an abundant extracellular matrix formed by an elaborate framework of macromolecules filled with water. The cells synthesize the macromolecules

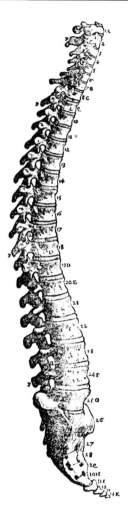

Fig. 1 *Drawing of the human spine from 1543 by Vesalius. The intervertebral disks unite adjacent vertebral bodies, but allow flexion, extension, and rotation. They also absorb and distribute loads.*

and then maintain and repair the framework created from these molecules. Structural integrity and mechanical properties of the disk are influenced by the macromolecules and their interactions with water. Because only the periphery of the disk has a blood supply, the nutrition of disk cells is dependent on the movement of nutrients and wastes through the matrix. This movement is dependent on the composition and organization of the macromolecular framework, and the matrix water content, which is largely determined by the proteoglycan concentration.[6,7]

Four concentrically arranged component tissues form the normal human intervertebral disk: (1) the outer anulus fibrosus, a ring of highly oriented, densely packed collagen fibril lamellae including collagen fibrils that insert into the vertebral bodies; (2) the larger fibrocartilaginous inner anulus fibrosus, which consists of a less dense collagenous matrix that lacks the lamellar organization of the outer anulus; (3) the transition zone, a thin zone of fibrous tissue between the inner anulus fibrosus and the nucleus pulposus; and (4) the central nucleus pulposus.[4] Vertebral end plates, initially consisting of hyaline cartilage and later during development of calcified cartilage and bone, form the superior and inferior boundaries of the disks. The cells of the cartilage end plates resemble chondrocytes found in other hyaline cartilages. The outer anulus contains fibroblast or fibrocyte-like cells, whereas the inner anulus and transition zone contain cells that more closely resemble chondrocytes.[4] Initially the nucleus pulposus contains a syncytium of notochordal cells (Fig. 2, *top left*). During growth and development, notochordal cells appear to separate from the syncytium and then disappear completely by early adult life, leaving scattered chondrocyte-like cells in their place (Fig. 2, *top right* and *bottom*).[4,8,9]

Normal disks have limited vascular and nerve supplies.[4] Blood vessels lie on the surface of the anulus and may penetrate a short distance into the outer layers. The blood vessels of the vertebral bodies lie directly against the end plates but do not enter the central regions of the disk. Simple and plexiform unmyelinated nerve endings and encapsulated nerve endings have been found on the surface of the anulus and small nerves with simple free nerve endings enter the outermost layers of the anulus, but nerves have not been identified within the central regions of the disk. Facet joint capsules and spinal ligaments have free and encapsulated nerve endings.

Collagens and proteoglycans are the primary structural components of the intervertebral disk's macromolecular framework.[10] Collagens provide form and tensile strength; proteoglycans, through their interactions with water, provide stiffness, resistance to compression, and viscoelasticity. The relative amounts of collagen and proteoglycan differ significantly in the matrices of disk component tissue.[4,10] Collagens account for as much as 70% of the dry weight of the outer anulus, but less than 20% of the dry weight of the central nucleus of younger individuals. In contrast, proteoglycans account for only a small percentage of the dry weight of the outer anulus, but as much as 50% of the dry weight of the nucleus in a child.

The matrices of the disk components also vary in the types of collagens that form part of their macromolecular framework.[10] The dense fibrous matrix of the outer anulus consists primarily of type I collagen (about 80%) along with small amounts of type V collagen (about 3%). Inside the outer anulus, the concentrations of type II collagen and proteoglycan progressively increase toward the center of the disk as the concentration of type I collagen decreases. In the nucleus the concentration of type II collagen reaches 80%, and type I collagen is absent. The nucleus also contains small amounts of type XI collagen, about 3%, and both anulus and nucleus contain small amounts, probably less than 2%, of type IX collagen. Disks contain remarkably high concentrations of type VI collagen, about 10% in the anulus and 15% or more in the nucleus. This collagen consists of fine filaments connected to dense transverse bands with central lucent areas.[11] The function of this collagen remains unknown, but its unusually high concentration in the disk suggests that it has a role in providing the unique mechanical properties of the disk matrix.

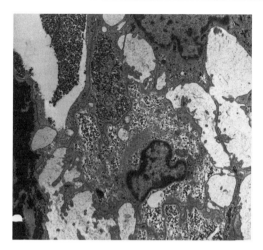
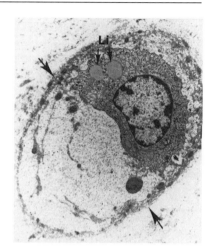
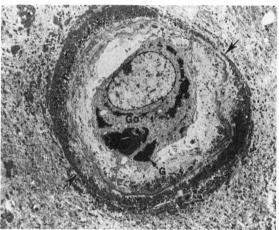

Fig. 2 *Transmission electron micrographs showing viable cells from human nucleus pulposus.* **Top left,** *Notochordal cells from a newborn. Note the elaborate interdigitation of the cell membranes, the regions of extracellular matrix surrounded by cell membranes, and the large amounts of intracellular glycogen.* **Top right,** *Chondrocyte-like cell from a 14-month-old infant. The arrows mark the edge of the accumulating pericellular granular material. Li, lipid deposits.* **Bottom,** *Chondrocyte-like cell from a 91-year-old patient. Go indicates Golgi membranes, G indicates glycogen, and the arrows mark the edge of the pericellular accumulation of electron dense material. Note the increased amount and density of the granular material in the matrix as compared with the micrograph from the 14-month-old patient. (Reproduced with permission from Buckwalter JA, Woo SL, Goldberg VM, et al: Soft-tissue aging and musculoskeletal function.* J Bone Joint Surg *1993;75A:1533–1548.)*

Proteoglycan aggregates consisting of central hyaluronan filaments and multiple attached aggrecan molecules exist in all the component tissues of disks from newborns and infants[5,12,13] (Fig. 3). Link proteins, small proteins that bind to aggrecan molecules and hyaluronan, stabilize the large aggregates. The anulus and cartilage end plate contain aggregates that closely resemble those found in articular cartilage, but even in disks of infants, nucleus pulposus aggregates are smaller, and their concentration rapidly declines with age[5,12,13] (Fig. 3). In addition, the proportion of nonaggregated proteoglycans progressively increases and the size of the aggrecan molecules decreases dramatically with advanced age, especially in the nucleus pulposus. These extensive alterations in proteoglycan structure begin early in life, years before the occurrence of age-related changes in disk morphology or the development of disk degeneration.

A variety of noncollagenous proteins and small amounts of elastin exist throughout the disk tissues.[4,10,14,15] Although the noncollagenous proteins have not been extensively studied, they appear to contribute significantly to the organization and stability of the matrix.[15] The contribution of elastin to the mechanical properties of the disk remains uncertain, but its low concentration suggests that it does not have a major role.

The unique structure and composition of the intervertebral disk make possible its specialized mechanical behavior. Collagen fibers of the anulus pass into the bone of the vertebral bodies binding together adjacent vertebrae, contributing to the stability of the spine, and joining the anulus to the vertebral bodies. These fibers also contain the nucleus pulposus between the vertebral end plates and the anulus. The dense collagenous circumferential lamellae of the outer anulus fibrosus resist large tensile stresses, minimizing intervertebral disk bulging and anulus fibrosus strains during compression, bending, or torsional loading of the disk. The less dense collagenous matrix of the inner anulus may permit larger deformations in response to loadings, and these larger deformations create fluid flows that dissipate energy. The high water and proteoglycan content of the normal nucleus pulposus enables it to function predominantly as a viscous fluid under static loading conditions. The swelling pressure resulting from the high proteoglycan concentration helps maintain disk height and contributes to support and distribution of loads. The permeability of the cartilage end plates allows water to flow from and into the disk and thereby helps transfer loads uniformly across the inner anulus fibrosus and nucleus pulposus. Thus, the specialized component tissues of the intervertebral disk form a structure that provides spine stability while allowing motion and absorbing and distributing loads. The outer anulus fibrosus resists tensile loads and contains the inner anulus fibrosus and nucleus pulposus, limiting their deformations; the inner anulus fibrosus and nucleus pulposus contribute to the viscoelastic behavior of the disk, including maintaining or restoring disk height and absorbing loads applied to the spine.

Intervertebral Disk Aging

Disk volume and shape change during growth and development and then again when skeletal maturity is achieved.[2,4] The disk rapidly increases in height and diameter after birth to keep pace with the growth of the vertebral column. The changes in volume and shape that occur following skeletal maturity vary among individuals and among disks. Unfortunately, these changes have not been well-defined or correlated with the changes in tissue structure and composition. However, the primary alterations in disk volume and shape that occur with aging include a loss of disk height, or protrusion of the central disk into the vertebral body with a decrease in the height of the anulus, and buckling or bulging of the anulus.

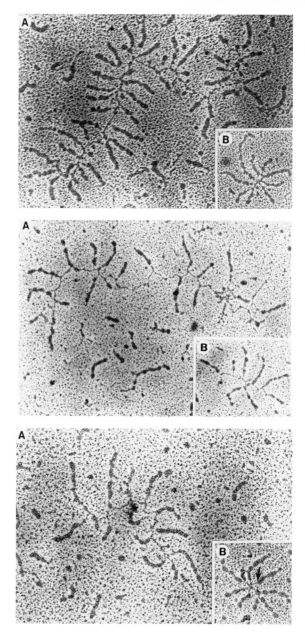

Fig. 3 *Electron micrographs showing aggregating proteoglycans from human infant intervertebral disks. The central filaments consist of hyaluronan and the projecting side arms are aggrecan molecules. The glycosaminoglycan chains are collapsed around the protein cores of the aggrecan molecules in these preparations.* **Top,** *Large (A) and small (B) proteoglycan aggregates from cartilage end plate.* **Center,** *Large (A) and small (B) proteoglycan aggregates from anulus fibrosus.* **Bottom,** *Large (A) and small (B) proteoglycan aggregates from nucleus pulposus. (Reproduced with permission from Buckwalter JA, Pedrini-Mille A, Pedrini V, et al: Proteoglycans of human infant intervertebral disc: Electron microscopic and biochemical studies.* J Bone Joint Surg *1985;67A:284–294.)*

Changes in disk tissue structure and composition precede and accompany the alterations in gross morphology. The changes in disk size, vascular supply, and composition, especially proteoglycan organization and proteoglycan and water concentration, begin during growth and development, well before evidence of disk degeneration appears, but these changes may form the basis for those that occur following skeletal maturity, including degeneration. In this sense the age-related changes of the disk begin soon after birth. Although all disk tissue components and the end plates change from birth through old age,[4,16] the most extensive changes occur in the nucleus pulposus, where a decline in the number of viable cells and the concentrations of proteoglycans and water is accompanied by fragmentation of the aggregating proteoglycans and increases in the concentrations of collagens and noncollagenous proteins.[4,5,10,12,13] All disks eventually develop similar age-related changes, but within the same individual and among individuals these changes vary in rate and extent; thus, specific disks may change more rapidly or more slowly than the time sequence described in the following sections.

Newborn

At birth, hyaline cartilage end plates separate the disk tissues from the vertebral bodies. The outer rim of the anulus consists of dense circumferential layers of collagen fibrils that penetrate the cartilage end plates of the vertebrae. Sparsely distributed elastic fibers lie parallel to the collagen fibrils. Small blood vessels may be found between the lamellae of the outer anulus fibrosus, especially in the posterolateral regions of the disk and adjacent to the cartilage plates, and occasional blood vessels penetrate the inner anulus. Numerous perivascular and free nerve endings lie on and among the most peripheral layers of the anulus. The nucleus fills almost half the disk and consists primarily of notochordal tissue, a soft, gelatinous, clear matrix surrounding syncytial cords and clusters of notochordal cells (Fig. 2, *top left*). The matrix of the nucleus contains few collagen fibrils, and even more rare sheets of elastin embedded in a network of highly hydrated proteoglycans. In the newborn, collagen fibrils have a nearly uniform small diameter. Proteoglycan aggregates from newborn and infant intervertebral disk anulus fibrosus and cartilage end plate have the same structure as aggregates from hyaline cartilages;[3,5,12] only about one third of nucleus pulposus proteoglycan aggregates resemble these large aggregates, and the other two thirds consist of aggrecan clusters that frequently lack a visible central hyaluronan filament (Fig. 3).

Childhood and Adolescence

During skeletal growth there is a several-fold increase in disk volume, increasing distance between the central regions of the disk and the peripheral blood vessels. The blood vessels of the anulus and the vertebral cartilage end plate become smaller and less numerous. The fibrocartilaginous component of the anulus increases in size, but in early adolescence the nucleus pulposus still makes up nearly half the disk and can easily be distinguished from the fibrocartilage of the inner anulus. The number of notochordal cells decreases and chondrocyte-like cells appear in the central regions of the disk (Fig. 2). More collagen fibrils appear in the nucleus, and the collagen fibrils of all disk components increase in mean diameter and variability in diameter. The proportion of proteoglycans that form aggregates and proteoglycan aggrecan size both decrease, and large proteoglycan aggregates similar to those found in articular cartilage disappear.[2,3,5,12,13,16] By adolescence, the proteoglycan population of the nucleus pulposus consists almost entirely of clusters of short aggrecan molecules and nonaggregated proteoglycans (Fig. 3). A decline in the concentration of functional link protein may cause at least some of the change in proteoglycan aggregates.[3,5,12,13,16]

Adult

With skeletal maturity, many of the remaining peripheral blood vessels disappear. The size of the outer anulus fibrosus stays about the same, but the apparent size of the fibrocartilaginous inner anulus expands at the expense of the nucleus as the nucleus becomes progressively more fibrotic. In portions of the anulus, myxomatous degeneration develops with loss of the normal collagen fibril organization. Fissures and cracks appear in the disk and may extend from the periphery to the central regions. The nucleus becomes firm and white rather than soft and translucent. In all regions of the disk inside the outer anulus the concentration of viable cells declines sharply, but especially in the most central regions[4,8,9] (Fig. 4). Few, if any, notochordal cells remain, but the central regions of the nucleus contain scattered viable chondrocyte-like cells (Fig. 2, *bottom*). Proteoglycan and water concentration[6] decrease and collagen and noncollagenous protein concentrations increase[17] as dense granular material accumulates throughout the matrix[4,8,9,18] (Fig. 2, *bottom,* and Fig. 5). Although this material appears throughout the matrix, it appears especially concentrated in the regions immediately surrounding the cells (Fig. 2, *bottom*) and forms thick sheaths around some collagen fibrils.[4,18] Its composition remains unknown, but it may contain degraded matrix molecules or noncollagenous matrix proteins including fibronectin, and its deposition in the matrix may be at least partially responsible for the age-related increase in the concentration of noncollagenous protein. Taken together, the age-related alterations in disk tissue following skeletal maturity appear to decrease the structural integrity of the disk and thereby contribute to the changes in disk volume and shape and the increased probability of mechanical failure of the matrix, leading to disk herniation.[19]

Elderly

Later in adult life, the entire disk inside the outer lamellae of the anulus often becomes a stiff plate of fibrocartilage. It may be difficult if not impossible to distinguish the inner anulus from the nucleus pulposus by gross examination, although the region of the nucleus may still have the smaller diameter, less densely packed collagen fibrils as seen via electron microscopy. Few viable cells remain in the central regions of the disk (Fig. 4). Disk height may continue to decline, and prominent fissures and large clefts may form in the center. The loss of disk height and alterations in disk composition can affect spine mobility and alter the alignment and loads applied to the facet joints, spinal ligaments, and paraspinous muscles.

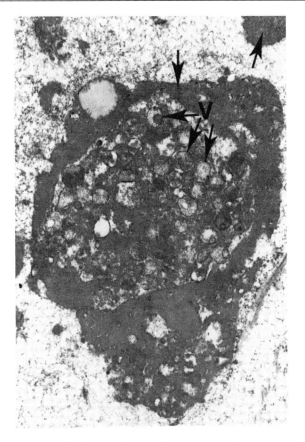

Fig. 4 *Electron micrograph showing the remains of a necrotic nucleus pulposus cell. Arrows show electron dense material. V, vacuoles.*

Intervertebral Disk Degeneration

All disks undergo changes as a result of aging, but not all disks degenerate. Disk degeneration is the age-related deterioration of disk structure and alteration of disk composition that leads to loss of mechanical function, including loss of the ability to maintain disk height, allow normal spine motion, and absorb and distribute loads. Disks that have degenerated to the point where they have almost disappeared, leaving only a thin layer of fibrotic tissue separating adjacent vertebral bodies, represent the end stage of this process (Fig. 6). In many instances advanced disk degeneration is associated with vertebral body osteophytes (Fig. 6), increased bone density or sclerosis of the vertebral bodies adjacent to the disk, and facet joint osteoarthritis.[20,21] Small blood vessels grow into the peripheral regions of degenerated disks[22] and it has been suggested that extensive vascular ingrowth is associated with pain.[23] The loss of disk tissue presumably results from the action of degradative enzymes within the disk and the inability of disk cells to maintain or restore matrix. This last stage of disk degeneration inevitably leads to a loss of spinal mobility and abnormal loading

615

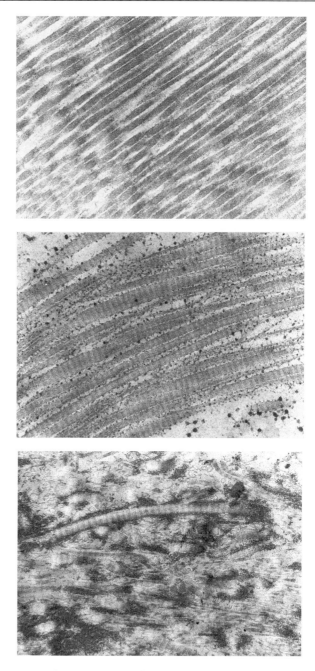

Fig. 5   *Transmission electron micrographs showing collagen fibrils of anulus.* **Top,** *New-born.* **Center,** *Young adult.* **Bottom,** *Older adult. Note the accumulation of granular material between and surrounding the collagen fibrils in the tissue from the older adult. In some areas this material forms elaborate sheaths around collagen fibrils. (Reproduced with permission from Buckwalter JA: The fine structure of human intervertebral disc, in White AA III, Gordon SL (eds): American Academy of Orthopaedic Surgeons Symposium on Idiopathic Low Back Pain. St. Louis, MO, CV Mosby, 1982, pp 108–143.)*

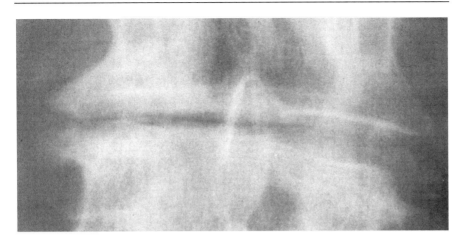

Fig. 6 *Radiograph showing a degenerated L3-4 intervertebral disk. Note the almost complete loss of disk tissue and the formation of vertebral body osteophytes.*

of the facet joints, spinal ligaments, and muscles. In some individuals it is associated with back pain and spinal stenosis.[19]

Although the end stage of intervertebral disk degeneration can be identified by imaging studies and gross examination (Fig. 6), widely accepted criteria have not been established for the diagnosis of disk degeneration and for distinguishing between disk aging and degeneration. Correlation of changes in disk size, shape, composition, and mechanical properties with alterations in spine function may make possible the development of these criteria.[16] Studies may eventually show that disk degeneration differs from the normal aging of the disk much like osteoarthritis or degenerative joint disease differs from normal aging of synovial joints. In both synovial joints and the joints formed by vertebral bodies and intervertebral disks, degenerative changes may or may not be associated with pain. Articular cartilages and intervertebral disks change with age, and degeneration of both these tissues is closely correlated with increasing age,[3] but these tissues continue to function well throughout life in many individuals. Thus, disk degeneration may result from either an acceleration or exacerbation of normal aging or a distinct process that is superimposed on normal aging. At present it is not possible to distinguish between these alternatives.

Mechanisms of Intervertebral Disk Degeneration

A variety of mechanisms that may contribute to age-related disk degeneration have been identified, including declining cell nutrition, decreasing concentration of viable cells, cell senescence, loss of aggregating proteoglycans, modification of matrix proteins, degradative enzyme activity, accumulation of degraded matrix macromolecules, and fatigue failure of the matrix.[2,3] Although each of these mechanisms may alter disk composition and structure, their relative importance and the interactions among them have not been established.[3]

Decline in Cell Nutrition

The most critical event responsible for the changes in central disk cells and their matrices appears to be declining nutrition.[2,7,10] The disk cells rely on diffusion of nutrients through the matrix from blood vessels on the periphery of the anulus fibrous and within the vertebral bodies. The increase in disk volume during growth combined with the progressive age-related decline in the number of arteries supplying the periphery of the disk, and possibly calcification of the cartilage end plates, impair delivery of nutrients and removal of wastes.[7,10] At the same time, the blood supply to the periphery of the disk declines and accumulation of degraded matrix macromolecules and decreasing matrix water concentration within the central disk may interfere with diffusion through the matrix, further compromising cell nutrition. Not only does the supply of nutrients decline, rising lactate concentration caused by increased lactate production, as a result of low oxygen tension and decreased rate of lactate removal, decreases the pH. A decrease in pH compromises cell metabolism and biosynthetic functions, and can cause cell death. Factors that may increase the rate and severity of age-related changes in intervertebral disk by indirectly altering nutrition include increased disk loading caused by demanding physical activities, immobilization, vibration, or spinal deformity.[19] Factors that directly compromise the vascular supply include smoking, vascular disease, and diabetes.[19]

Decline in Concentration of Viable Cells

The age-related decline in nutrition of the central disk region and the accompanying decrease in pH would be expected to adversely affect cell viability, and electron microscopic studies show that the proportion of necrotic cells increases with age[4,8,9] (Fig. 4). In fetal and infant intervertebral disks, no more than 2% of the nucleus pulposus cells showed morphologic signs of necrosis. In disks of adolescents and young adults, more than 50% of the nucleus cells were necrotic, and in samples from elderly people more than 80% of the cells were necrotic.

Cell Senescence

Although age-related changes in disk cell function have not been extensively studied, declining cell function contributes to age-related degeneration in other tissues.[3] Even without an alteration in cell nutrition, many normal differentiated cells become senescent with increasing age. They remain viable, but lose their capacity to replicate DNA and possibly some or all of their synthetic capacity and other specialized functions. Experimental evidence suggests that these alterations in cell capacity result from changes in gene expression, and that transcription factors, proteins that bind to specific sequences of DNA and direct gene expression, control these age-related changes.

Loss of Proteoglycan Aggregates and Decline in Proteoglycan Concentration

Mature intervertebral disks lack large proteoglycan aggregates and aggrecans similar to those found in articular cartilage.[2,5,12,13] The available evidence suggests that a population of articular cartilage-like proteoglycan aggregates exists in the disks of newborns, but that they disappear during maturation and that the aggrecans become shorter.[12,13] Other work shows that a decline in proteogly-can concentration precedes and accompanies disk degeneration.[16,24] The loss of proteoglycan aggregates and large aggrecans and decreased proteoglycan con-centration decrease the ability of the disk to maintain a high water concentra-tion. These changes, combined with the increasing collagen concentration and accumulation of noncollagenous proteins (including fibronectin and others), cause the central disk to become fibrotic and stiff, and limit its ability to main-tain disk height and distribute loads.

Matrix Protein Modification

Connective tissue matrices, including those of the intervertebral disk tissues, tend to lose elasticity and strength with aging. Some of these changes may re-sult from postsynthetic modification of the protein components of elastin, pro-teoglycan, and especially collagens, in the matrix.[3,25] These alterations, includ-ing increased collagen cross-linking and denaturation, may contribute to disk degeneration.[25,26] Increasing collagen cross-links through nonenzymatic glyca-tion or lipid peroxidation may cause an increase in brown pigmentation with age and, more importantly, alter disk mechanical properties. In addition to their potential effects on tissue mechanics, glycation products also can stimulate cells, including chondrocytes, to release cytokines and proteases that contribute to tis-sue degeneration.[25] Examination of adult human intervertebral disks has shown greater denaturation of type II collagen (loss of triple helical configuration) in the anulus fibrosus and nucleus pulposus than in articular cartilage from the same individuals.[26] This difference may result from accumulation of degraded mol-ecules in the intervertebral disk and could alter the mechanical properties of the collagen fibril framework and the interaction of type II collagen fibrils with other matrix molecules.

Degradative Enzyme Activity

Throughout life, newly synthesized molecules replace older ones that are en-zymatically degraded in the matrix. The loss of disk tissue seen in advanced disk degeneration (Fig. 6) must result from excessive degradation relative to syn-thesis. Proteolytic enzymes have been identified within the disk[27,28] and there is evidence of increased proteinase activity in degenerated disks.[29] The cause of the imbalance between synthetic and degradative activity in degenerating disks remains unknown.

Accumulation of Degraded Matrix Macromolecules

With aging, accumulation of partially degraded molecules may alter the prop-erties of the disk, including the mechanical behavior of the tissue and diffusion of nutrients and metabolites through the matrix. Increasing concentrations of de-graded molecules, and possibly noncollagenous proteins, may inhibit or inter-fere with the ability of cells to synthesize new molecules. Accumulation of de-graded molecules may also interfere with assembly of newly synthesized molecules in the matrix. For example, accumulation of hyaluronan binding frag-ments of proteoglycan aggrecan core proteins may interfere with assembly of proteoglycan aggregates.[3,13,30] Accumulation of degraded matrix molecules is most likely to occur in tissues that lack a blood supply and have relatively slow

619

diffusion of molecules through their matrix, such as the central regions of the intervertebral disk.

Fatigue Failure of the Matrix

Normal spine movement requires loading and deformation of disks followed by recovery of disk shape. In addition, maintaining an upright posture decreases disk height by driving water out of the disk matrix. Prolonged recumbency then restores the original disk shape and volume as water returns to the matrix. These repetitive deformations of the disk may lead to fatigue failure of the matrix. This failure may appear as fissures, cracks, or myxoid degeneration, or as more subtle changes in the macromolecular framework of the matrix, including fragmentation of proteoglycans and disruption of collagen fibrils and the relationships between collagen fibrils and other matrix macromolecules. These alterations of the matrix may expose cells to increased loads that compromise their function.

Age-related changes in the disk may render the tissue less able to recover from deformation and more vulnerable to progressive fatigue failure of the matrix. Loss of proteoglycans and water from the central disk regions increase loading of the collagen network. Posttranslational modifications of the collagens, decreased water concentration, and accumulation of degraded matrix molecules may make the collagen framework more vulnerable to failure, and the decline in cell nutrition, decreased concentration of viable cells, and cell senescence, combined with the alterations in the matrix, may compromise the ability of the cells to repair damage to the matrix macromolecules.

Intervertebral Disk Degeneration and Back Pain

The relationships between disk degeneration and pain remain poorly understood. Some individuals with minimal morphologic evidence of disk degeneration have chronic back pain and stiffness, while others with advanced disk degeneration have minimal symptoms. Furthermore, the lack of nerves within disks suggests that disk degeneration may have no relationship to back pain. Yet, the available information suggests that intervertebral disk degeneration may contribute to back pain through two mechanisms: loss of disk structure and mechanical properties, and release of mediators that may sensitize nerve endings. The loss of disk structure and mechanical properties alters loading and alignment of vertebral bodies, facet joints, and spinal ligaments and muscles, and decreases the ability of the disks to absorb and distribute loads applied to the spine. These changes may increase stimulation of nerve endings in bone, spinal ligaments, facet joint capsules, and muscles. By altering the mechanical function of the spine and the alignment of the facet joints, long-standing advanced disk degeneration may initiate or accelerate development of osteoarthritis of the facet joints.[20] In addition to these structural and mechanical changes, the cell and matrix changes associated with disk degeneration, including cell necrosis, may be associated with release of cytokines, free radicals, matrix degradation products, and other molecules. Some of these substances may sensitize nociceptive nerve endings and thereby contribute to the development of back pain.

Summary

Although the causes of age-related degeneration of intervertebral disks and the clinical importance of disk degeneration remain poorly understood, recent advances in understanding of intervertebral disk structure, composition, function, and age-related changes make it possible to develop potential explanations of disk degeneration and of the relationships between this process and back pain. The earliest and most extensive age-related changes occur in the central regions of the disk. These include loss of proteoglycan aggregates followed by decreases in proteoglycan and water concentration, increasing collagen and noncollagenous protein concentrations, and a decline in the density of viable cells. The appearance of myxomatous regions in the anulus, loss of the gelatinous nucleus pulposus matrix, development of cracks and fissures in the disk, and alterations in disk volume and shape precede and accompany the alterations in proteoglycans, water concentration, and loss of viable cells. This sequence of events within the matrix of the central disk suggests that loss of matrix proteoglycan organization, possibly because of a change in cell biosynthetic function, interference with aggregation, or increased degradative enzyme activity, leads to a decline in proteoglycan concentration, accumulation of degraded molecules, and the inability of the matrix to retain water. Once this occurs, the nucleus and inner anulus begin to lose their capacity to maintain disk height and distribute loads. At some point the balance between matrix synthesis and matrix degradation shifts toward degradation, and the cells fail to maintain the matrix. These changes may increase the loads on the collagenous matrix, precipitating failure of the matrix and further loss of disk height and mechanical function.

Demanding physical activities, immobilization, vibration, spinal deformity, smoking, vascular disease, and diabetes may contribute to the initiation and progression of disk degeneration. Disk degeneration may result in back pain by altering the height and mechanical behavior of the disk, resulting in abnormal loading of facet joints, spinal ligaments, and muscles that causes pain. Abnormal loading of the facet joints may eventually cause osteoarthritis, and vertebral and facet joint osteophytes will lead to narrowing of the spinal canal, a change that has been associated with the clinical syndrome of spinal stenosis. It is also possible that disk degeneration releases mediators that sensitize nociceptive nerve endings. Although aging changes of the disk appear to be inevitable, identification of activities and agents that accelerate these changes may help decrease the rate and severity of disk degeneration. Future clinical and epidemiologic investigations should better define the relationships between age-related alterations in disks and loss of spine motion and development of back pain, and more clearly identify the activities and agents that cause or accelerate disk degeneration. Basic scientific work must clarify the mechanisms of age-related changes in human disks and explore the possibilities of slowing the rate of disk degeneration and of regenerating central disk tissue.

References

1. Praemer AP, Furner S, Rice DP (eds): *Musculoskeletal Conditions in the United States*, ed 1. Park Ridge, IL, American Academy of Orthopaedic Surgeons, 1992.
2. Buckwalter JA: Aging and degeneration of the human intervertebral disc. *Spine* 1995;20:1307–1314.
3. Buckwalter JA, Woo SL, Goldberg VM, et al: Soft-tissue aging and musculoskeletal function. *J Bone Joint Surg* 1993;75A:1533–1548.
4. Buckwalter JA: The fine structure of human intervertebral disc, in White AA III, Gordon SL (eds): American Academy of Orthopaedic Surgeons *Symposium on Idiopathic Low Back Pain*. St. Louis, MO, CV Mosby, 1982, pp 108–143.
5. Buckwalter JA, Smith KC, Kazarien LE, et al: Articular cartilage and intervertebral disc proteoglycans differ in structure: An electron microscopic study. *J Orthop Res* 1989;7:146–151.
6. Urban JP, McMullin JF: Swelling pressure of the lumbar intervertebral discs: Influence of age, spinal level, composition, and degeneration. *Spine* 1988;13:179–187.
7. Urban JPG: The effect of physical factors on disk cell metabolism, in Buckwalter JA, Goldberg VM, Woo SL-Y (eds): *Musculoskeletal Soft-Tissue Aging: Impact on Mobility*. Rosemont, IL, American Academy of Orthopaedic Surgeons, 1993, pp 391–412.
8. Trout JJ, Buckwalter JA, Moore KC, et al: Ultrastructure of the human intervertebral disc: I. Changes in notochordal cells with age. *Tissue Cell* 1982;14:359–369.
9. Trout JJ, Buckwalter JA, Moore KC: Ultrastructure of the human intervertebral disc: II. Cells of the nucleus pulposus. *Anat Rec* 1982;204:307–314.
10. Eyre D, Benya P, Buckwalter J, et al: The intervertebral disk: Basic science perspectives, in Frymoyer JW, Gordon SL (eds): *New Perspectives on Low Back Pain*. Park Ridge, IL, American Academy of Orthopaedic Surgeons, 1989, pp 147–207.
11. Buckwalter JA, Maynard JA, Cooper RR: Banded structures in human nucleus pulposus. *Clin Orthop* 1979;139:259–266.
12. Buckwalter JA, Pedrini-Mille A, Pedrini V, et al: Proteoglycans of human infant intervertebral disc: Electron microscopic and biochemical studies. *J Bone Joint Surg* 1985;67A:284–294.
13. Buckwalter JA, Roughley PJ, Rosenberg LC: Age-related changes in cartilage proteoglycans: Quantitative electron microscopic studies. *Microsc Res Tech* 1994;28:398–408.
14. Buckwalter JA, Cooper RR, Maynard JA: Elastic fibers in human intervertebral discs. *J Bone Joint Surg* 1976;58A:73–76.
15. Heinegard D, Lorenzo P, Reinholt FP, et al: Aging and the extracellular matrix, in Buckwalter JA, Goldberg VM, Woo SL-Y (eds): *Musculoskeletal Soft-Tissue Aging: Impact on Mobility*. Rosemont, IL, American Academy of Orthopaedic Surgeons, 1993, pp 349–361.
16. Pearce RH: Morphologic and chemical aspects of intervertebral disc aging, in Buckwalter JA, Goldberg VM, Woo SL-Y (eds): *Musculoskeletal Soft-Tissue Aging: Impact on Mobility*. Rosemont, IL, American Academy of Orthopaedic Surgeons, 1993, pp 363–379.
17. Dickson IR, Happey F, Pearson CH, et al: Variations in the protein components of human intervertebral disk with age. *Nature* 1967;215:52–53.
18. Buckwalter JA, Maynard JA, Cooper RR: Sheathing of collagen fibrils in human intervertebral discs. *J Anat* 1978;125:615–618.
19. Andersson GBJ: Intervertebral disk: Clinical aspects, in Buckwalter JA, Goldberg VM, Woo SL-Y (eds): *Musculoskeletal Soft-Tissue Aging: Impact on Mobility*. Rosemont, IL, American Academy of Orthopaedic Surgeons, 1993, pp 331–347.
20. Butler D, Trafimow JH, Andersson GB, et al: Discs degenerate before facets. *Spine* 1990;15:111–113.
21. Milgram JW: Osteoarthritic changes at the severely degenerative disc in humans. *Spine* 1982;7:498–505.

22. Kauppila LI: Ingrowth of blood vessels in disc degeneration: Angiographic and histological studies of cadaveric spines. *J Bone Joint Surg* 1995;77A:26–31.

23. Stäbler A, Weiss M, Scheidler J, et al: Degenerative disk vascularization on MRI: Correlation with clinical and histopathologic findings. *Skeletal Radiol* 1996;25:119–126.

24. Pearce RH, Grimmer BJ, Adams ME: Degeneration and the chemical composition of the human lumbar intervertebral disc. *J Orthop Res* 1987;5:198–205.

25. Monnier VM, Sell DR, Pokharna HK, et al: Posttranslational protein modification by the Maillard Reaction: Relevance to aging of extracellular matrix molecules, in Buckwalter JA, Goldberg VM, Woo SL-Y (eds): *Musculoskeletal Soft-Tissue Aging: Impact on Mobility*. Rosemont, IL, American Academy of Orthopaedic Surgeons, 1993, pp 49–59.

26. Hollander AP, Heathfield TF, Liu JJ, et al: Enhanced denaturation of the alpha1(II) chains of type-II collagen in normal adult human intervertebral discs compared with femoral articular cartilage. *J Orthop Res* 1996;14:61–66.

27. Melrose J, Ghosh P, Taylor TK: Neutral proteinases of the human intervertebral disc. *Biochim Biophys Acta* 1987;923:483–495.

28. Liu J, Roughley PJ, Mort JS: Identification of human intervertebral disc stromelysin and its involvement in matrix degradation. *J Orthop Res* 1991;9:568–575.

29. Fujita K, Nakagawa T, Hirabayashi K, et al: Neutral proteinases in human intervertebral disc: Role in degeneration and probable origin. *Spine* 1993;18:1766–1773.

30. Roughley PJ, White RJ, Poole AR: Identification of a hyaluronic acid-binding protein that interferes with the preparation of high-buoyant-density proteoglycan aggregates from adult human articular cartilage. *Biochem J* 1985;231:129–138.

Directions for Future Research

Define the factors that affect intervertebral disk nutrition and how alterations in disk nutrition may cause disk degeneration.

Nutrition of the central regions of the intervertebral disk occurs by diffusion of nutrients and metabolites through the disk matrix from blood vessels located within the vertebral body directly adjacent to the cartilage end plate and on the surface of the anulus. A number of studies suggest that a decline in nutrition of the central disk regions may initiate degenerative changes. Further studies are needed to determine how nutrients pass through the disk matrix and, in particular, how matrix changes, including the accumulation of degraded matrix molecules, affect diffusion. Animal experiments in which the blood vessels supplying the disk are interrupted help define the effects of alterations in nutrition on disk cells and matrix and help explain how these alterations affect mechanical properties. Gadolinium-enhanced magnetic resonance studies and possibly other imaging techniques will make it possible to study human intervertebral disk nutrition in vivo and correlate alterations in human disk nutrition with alterations in disk structure and possibly back pain. These methods may also be used to examine the effects of mechanical loading of the spine on disk nutrition.

Develop an animal model to characterize the response of nerve receptors in the disk to mechanical stress and to chemical agents already identified in degenerated or herniated disks.

Neuroanatomic studies demonstrate that the peripheral anulus is innervated by small nerve fibers. Little is known regarding the function of these nerves in the disk, although it is proposed that a subpopulation are nociceptive-specific neurons that can cause low back pain. Other nerves in the disk may include low threshold mechanoreceptors and autonomic fibers. The nociceptive-specific neurons may include high threshold mechanoreceptors and mechanically insensitive chemoreceptors. An animal model should be developed to characterize these receptors.

The pig and sheep are animals with disks large enough that receptive fields can be characterized with sufficient resolution. The pig model has been used extensively in demonstrating nerve root degeneration, so this model can be extended to disk receptors. In addition, the larger animal model would allow visualization of the recurrent sinuvertebral nerve. Studies should include: (1) characterization of receptors in the normal disk, including mechanical threshold and conduction velocity; (2) characterization of nerve receptors in artificially inflamed disks; (3) characterization of the response of anulus nerve receptors to diskogram pressure (applied in normal disks and in those with acute radial tears); and (4) characterization of the response of annular receptors to chemicals identified in degenerated and herniated disks. These chemicals could include phospholipase A_2, nitric oxide, prostaglandin E_2, and normal and degenerate nucleus pulposus.

Determine the cerebral representation of radicular pain and its significance.

Utilizing positron emission tomographic (PET) imaging, functional magnetic resonance imaging (MRI), and other forms of brain mapping, the cortical and thalamic representation of radicular pain should be defined. PET imaging has shed some light on the patterns of acute pain representation. It is likely that radicular pain patterns are different. The significance of these differences should be determined. In addition, the effects of preexisting radicular pain may have implications on the perception of other forms of pain. As a model for examining central patterns of radicular pain, patients studied using PET or functional MRI can be evaluated during a provocative test such as straight leg raising.

Develop and validate an animal model of disk degeneration initiated by changes in the nucleus pulposus.

In the best characterized models of disk degeneration, injury to the anulus fibrosus is the initiating event. However, histologic and MRI studies of human disk degeneration indicate that changes in the nucleus pulposus may occur prior to those in the anulus. In order to investigate the latter possibility, it would be desirable to develop models in which the initiating events occurred in the nucleus pulposus.

Such a model may be created by interrupting the nutritional route through the cartilage end plate, which would compromise the metabolic balance of the nucleus pulposus and may initiate degeneration. An alternative, but more invasive, initiation would involve the introduction of agents into the nucleus pulposus by microinjection.

The use of modern scientific tools, such as MRI, would allow study of the development of degeneration. This knowledge could then be correlated with information about molecular and biochemical changes to provide a comprehensive documentation of the pathway of disk degeneration following nucleus pulposus deterioration.

Delineate the biochemical and biomechanical cascade of events that occur with intervertebral disk degeneration.

The degeneration of the human intervertebral disk is believed to have an important relationship to low back pain. The biochemical and biomechanical sequence of events associated with disk degeneration (either causative or otherwise) is poorly understood, and these two aspects of degeneration are probably closely related.

Because of certain similarities between articular cartilage and intervertebral disk, those biomechanical agents that have been found to be important in cartilage degeneration are probably also important in intervertebral disk degeneration. Examples of these agents are cytokines and growth factors, matrix metalloproteinases, prostaglandins, and nitric oxide.

The mechanical characteristics of whole-disk behavior associated with intervertebral disk degeneration are fairly well understood, but the changes at a finer level of structural components (eg, between anulus fibrosus lamallae or distribution of pore-fluid pressure) have not been extensively studied. However, these changes probably are important, especially in the early phases of intervertebral disk degeneration and also for the interplay between associated biochemical and biomechanical changes.

Examples of useful experimental methods to investigate these issues are human in vitro cell and whole disk cultures, in vitro disk cadaveric specimens, and animal and mathematical models.

Determine the design and physiologic function of the paravertebral musculature.

Because skeletal muscle design is the primary determinant of muscle function, it is critical to determine the design of the major subdivisions of the back musculature, possibly providing insight into the normal function of the different muscle groups and leading to the development of realistic biomechanical models of motion segment function.

The percentage of normal fiber type in paravertebral muscles should also be determined using modern methodology. The literature supports the concept of a type 1 fiber predominance in back muscles, placing these muscles in the category of unusually adaptive and frequently activated muscles. With modern immunohistochemical analysis, we can define those muscles that play the primary stabilizing role and compare them to those that are relatively rarely recruited and may be used only to limit motion in extreme conditions. Similarly, by measuring the changes in back muscles (if any) that occur after various back disorders, it will be possible to infer the muscle activation pattern that accompanies the syndrome.

Finally, although most of the information just described can be obtained from biopsy specimens, it is critical to make noninvasive high quality measurements in patients suffering from well-defined disorders. To this end, it is necessary to develop and refine the noninvasive imaging methods used to measure muscle fiber activation, tissue inflammation, and interstitial fluid shifts. Careful development of the imaging methods in tandem with detailed studies of the imaged tissue will enable the clinician and scientist to refine the definition of various back disorders (at a tissue level) and will permit objective evaluation of the efficacy of interventional studies.

Critically test the hypothesis that cells in the degenerative disk produce clinically significant levels of nociceptive products.

It has been suggested that cells in the degenerative disk can produce nociceptive products and may cause pain when exposed via tears that reach the outer third of the anulus fibrosus. However, this has never been critically tested nor has the presence of these agents correlated with clinically painful disks.

In order to test this hypothesis, a reliable physiologically relevant model of pain will have to be used as a test system. Clinical samples from degenerative disks with known pathology documented by MRI, or histology from painful and nonpainful disks will be needed. It may be possible to obtain the samples via relatively noninvasive methods, such as needle microprobing, and then test their nociceptive effects in neurophysiologic models.

If relevant compounds are identified, studies such as blocking with specific antibodies or antagonists will be needed.

627

Identify the factors that determine when and whether disk structural changes induce low back pain.

Annular fissures and delamination have been noted in intervertebral disks of patients with low back pain, yet it is not clear if these structural abnormalities cause or contribute to back pain. Studies should be undertaken to determine if annular fissures or delamination are associated with changes in cytokines, neural tissues, and inflammatory mediators in the nucleus, anulus, and the end plate or neovascularization and granulation tissue in the disk. The major difficulty will be dissecting the causal relationships between annular abnormalities and pain from secondary effects.

Define the functional roles of the cell populations of the intervertebral disk.

Understanding the cell biology of the disk will provide the groundwork for intervention therapies designed to stimulate tissue reconstruction. With the goal of exploring the repair potential of disk cells, it is important to determine which cell populations are responsible for establishing the nucleus pulposus and anulus fibrosus during development in humans. In the mature individual, do these different cell populations maintain and repair the nucleus and anulus? A developmental study would be necessary, using molecular markers for cell types from early disk/vertebral body differentiation in the embryo to early adulthood. These studies would provide the background for studies that would address the functional capabilities of cells in culture. Cell culture investigations would establish the ability of cells to synthesize a functional extracellular matrix in vitro. Once normal parameters are established, extended investigations using older disks will indicate the changes, such as inappropriate gene expression and cell death, that take place during aging and disk degeneration.

Determine the critical components in disk microstructure that govern mechanical behavior of the disk.

Characterization of mechanical behavior of the components of the nondegenerate disk is essential to the understanding of how the disk supports load and its mechanism of failure. Although some information on anulus fibrosus, nucleus pulposus, and cartilaginous end plate in various loading modes is available, new studies are necessary to fully characterize these material properties.

It is clear that pressurization in the nucleus pulposus and anulus fibrosus provides a crucial role in load support in the nondegenerate disk, and that losses in pressurization with degeneration may result in larger mechanical stresses and strains on the solid matrix.

Future work on modeling and measurement of the swelling pressure is necessary to provide an understanding of load carriage mechanisms and their alterations with degeneration. These studies should include the distinctions between osmotic pressure, hydraulic pressure, and mechanical stresses and strains on the solid matrix.

Further studies aimed at determining accurate material properties should give attention to the anisotrophy and inhomogeneity of the disk tissues, and these studies should be done through noninvasive means that eventually may be used in vivo. A central question remains: Is it possible that with degeneration a shift occurs from isotropic to anisotropic states with subsequent large stress concentrations that initiate local changes? Such questions could be usefully studied with development of a precision finite element model with accurate material properties, geometries true to their anatomic form, and faithful physiologic loading conditions.

Section Five

Epidemiologic and Clinical Issues of Degenerative Stenosis

Section Editor:
Jeffrey N. Katz, MD, MS

Howard An, MD
Gunnar B.J. Andersson, MD,
  PhD
Gordon R. Bell, MD
Steven R. Garfin, MD

Victor M. Haughton, MD
Tae-Hong Lim, PhD
Bruce H. Nowicki, BS
Alexander R. Vaccaro, MD

Overview

This section covers clinical aspects of degenerative lumbar spinal stenosis including epidemiology, evaluation, natural history, and nonsurgical and surgical treatment. Pathophysiologic mechanisms are discussed in the final section of this volume.

Degenerative lumbar spinal stenosis is an increasingly common source of pain and disability in the elderly. The epidemiology of spinal stenosis and spondylolisthesis is discussed in the chapter by Dr. Andersson. Hospital discharge and insurance claims data suggest that rates of surgery for spinal stenosis have increased rapidly over the last decade. It is unclear whether the increase reflects increasing age-adjusted prevalence of spinal stenosis, aging of the population, greater recognition of the syndrome, or a more aggressive approach to treatment. The actual prevalence of symptomatic spinal stenosis is unknown. In asymptomatic persons older than 60 years of age, the prevalence of radiographically defined spinal stenosis on magnetic resonance imaging (MRI) is about 20%. Similarly, population surveys reveal that degenerative spondylolisthesis has a prevalence of 25% in women older than 75 years of age. The lack of data on disease prevalence is due in part to the lack of a standard case definition, which incorporates both radiographic features and clinical characteristics of this syndrome.

Evaluation of Lumbar Spinal Stenosis

The history and physical examination are critical to the diagnosis of spinal stenosis because plain radiographs do not reveal stenosis conclusively and imaging studies are nonspecific, with a high prevalence of cauda equina compression in asymptomatic individuals. Recent studies of their diagnostic utility reveal that several features of the history and physical examination are useful in establishing the diagnosis of this syndrome. The most useful historical feature is a history of pain on standing or walking with absence of pain in the sitting position. Physical examination findings of pain radiating into the buttocks and legs with prolonged lumbar extension; deficits to vibratory, temperature, or pinprick sensibility; lower extremity weakness and a wide based gait; and a positive Romberg sign are all useful in the recognition of spinal stenosis in older patients with back pain.

Imaging studies of the lumbar spine, including MRI, computed tomography (CT), and contrast-enhanced CT, are sensitive but, as noted previously, are extremely nonspecific and, therefore, should be ordered judiciously. As discussed in the chapter by Dr. Haughton, additional features of MRI, including contrast enhancement and dynamic imaging, may further add to its utility in the recognition of spinal stenosis. In general, imaging studies need not be ordered routinely early in the evaluation and management of patients with spinal stenosis. These studies are indicated when the clinical evaluation suggests the possibility of a more ominous source of symptoms, such as tumor or infection. An imaging study is also necessary before surgical treatment in order to assist in preoperative planning.

Natural History

The clinical course of untreated spinal stenosis is essentially unknown because virtually all patients undergo conservative management of one sort or another. However, as reviewed by Drs. Bell and Andersson, observational data suggest that conservative treatment of spinal stenosis, with or without a degenerative spondylolisthesis, is characterized by deterioration in about 10% of patients and improvement in up to one third. Although the literature in this area is limited to small studies, it appears that the majority of patients tend to change little over time.

Nonsurgical Management

There currently are no adequate controlled studies of nonsurgical therapy for lumbar spinal stenosis, except for a negative trial of subcutaneous calcitonin. Limited observational data suggest that lumbar epidural steroid injections may be useful in this syndrome; however, controlled studies of this common therapy specific to patients with spinal stenosis are sorely needed. Patients are often treated with analgesics, lumbar corsets, education regarding the relation between posture and symptoms, activity modification, exercises to stabilize trunk muscles, and aerobic fitness exercises. No definitive statements can be made about the effectiveness of these treatments in lumbar spinal stenosis because there is a lack of adequate studies. Research in this area is a high priority.

Surgical Management

Aspects of surgery in the management of spinal stenosis are covered in detail by Drs. Bell and Garfin. There are no randomized, controlled trials comparing surgery with nonsurgical management for lumbar spinal stenosis. Observational studies indicate that surgery is beneficial in about two thirds of patients.

There are several unresolved questions regarding surgical technique. First, the optimal extent of laminectomy is debated; a wider decompression may ensure greater symptomatic relief, but may also carry the risk of greater postoperative instability. There also is uncertainty about whether to decompress only those intervertebral levels that appear to be responsible for symptoms or to decompress stenotic levels that may not be associated with symptoms at the time of surgery. Although less extensive decompression may lead to greater spinal stability, chronic nerve compression may lead to increased vulnerability to nerve dysfunction.

Several important questions remain about the optimal role of concomitant arthrodesis in the surgical management of spinal stenosis. This issue is addressed by Dr. Bell. In patients with spinal stenosis without degenerative spondylolisthesis, one small, controlled study suggests that laminectomy without concomitant arthrodesis appears to be as beneficial as laminectomy with arthrodesis. In patients with a degenerative spondylolisthesis and attendant spinal stenosis, a noninstrumented arthrodesis appears to produce superior relief of back pain and leg pain as well as improved walking capacity compared with laminectomy without arthrodesis. This conclusion is also based on a study of a relatively small sample and should be confirmed in larger studies.

There is considerable uncertainty regarding the utility of supplementing lumbar arthrodesis with instrumentation. This issue is addressed by Dr. Garfin. Instrumentation improves the rate of bony fusion from approximately 70% to approximately 90%. However, instrumentation also involves higher costs and complication rates. The critical question is whether the higher costs and complications of instrumentation are offset by superior relief of pain and improvement in function. One large, uncontrolled, prospective study of surgery for degenerative lumbar spinal stenosis indicated that noninstrumented arthrodesis resulted in better relief of back pain than instrumented arthrodesis or laminectomy without arthrodesis. At the present time there are no randomized, controlled studies addressing the value of arthrodesis specifically in patients with degenerative spinal stenosis with spondylolisthesis.

Observational studies have yielded information on predictors of outcome in patients undergoing surgery for spinal stenosis, including the role of comorbidity, which is discussed by Dr. Katz. Greater preoperative comorbidity and worse preoperative functional status are associated with worse results. A predominance of leg pain is associated with a better surgical outcome than a predominance of back pain, while age does not appear to be associated with outcome in studies that adjust for comorbidity and functional status. There is little information on predictors of success from nonsurgical therapy. Further studies in this area are needed in order to improve patient selection for surgery.

Chapter 37
Epidemiology of Spinal Stenosis

Gunnar B.J. Andersson, MD, PhD

Introduction

Spinal stenosis has only been a true clinical entity over the last 50 years, even though it reportedly has been found in Egyptian mummies. Variably classified by etiology, pathoanatomy, and symptomatology, it is perhaps not surprising that its epidemiology is largely unknown.[1] Spinal stenosis is more likely to occur in an elderly, nonworking population and, therefore, is not reported to many available disability systems.

However, estimates can be made of the prevalence of symptomatic spinal stenosis based on imaging studies and on hospital and surgical records. These estimates are not ideal, because imaging studies provide an uncertain representation of the population at large or, in the case of radiographs, are suboptimal in the diagnosis of spinal stenosis. Hospital and surgical records reflect only those patients who have severely disabling spinal stenosis.

Hospitalizations and Operations

Deyo and associates[2] reviewed the hospital discharge registry for the state of Washington from 1986 through 1988. There were 18,122 hospitalizations for procedures on the lumbar spine of which 3,380 (18.6%) were for spinal stenosis. This would correspond to 1,126 procedures each year. The mean age of the patients with stenosis was 65 years. The data show that the length of hospitalization and the hospital charges were greater for patients with spinal stenosis than for those with other diagnoses. If 18.6% is representative of the United States, there were almost 52,000 operations for spinal stenosis in 1990. Taylor and associates[3] analyzed the U.S. National Hospital Discharge Survey Data from 1979 through 1990. Operations for spinal stenosis increased dramatically from 4.0 per 100,000 in 1979 to 1981 to 17.7 in 1988 to 1990.

In a meta-analysis of 74 studies involving surgical treatment of 3,381 patients with spinal stenosis, the mean age at surgery was 53.8 years.[4] This age may seem young, but is explained by the fact that some series contain patients with developmental stenosis only, and therefore, the average age of the patients in the included studies ranged from 19 to 67 years. There were more males than females (55.84% versus 44.16%). More than 80% of the subjects had back and leg pain, about 62% had pseudoclaudication, and about 50% some neurologic deficit. How well these data represent the general "stenosis population" is, of course, unknown.

Stenosis on Imaging Studies

Radiographs do not allow determination of spinal stenosis directly because the spinal canal cannot be evaluated. Some aspects of stenosis, such as degenerative spondylolisthesis, which often causes a narrowing of the spine, can be determined. Degenerative spondylolisthesis exceeding 5 mm was found in 5.8% of men and 9.1% of women in a Dutch cross-sectional study.[5] Particularly high prevalence rates (25.3%) were found in women 75 years of age and older (Table 1). The spondylolisthesis occurred at one level in about 90% of cases. The highest relative frequency for men was at L5–S1 (42%), for women at L4–5 (41%).

Computed tomography (CT) allows better determination of stenosis, but cannot be applied to large population groups because of factors such as the availability of the scanner, time and cost, and the required radiation dose, which is quite high. In a CT study of 52 asymptomatic individuals, it was reported that 3.4% of those over the age of 40 years had stenosis.[6] Magnetic resonance imaging (MRI) of asymptomatic individuals results in reports of even higher prevalences. Boden and associates[7] performed radiographic studies on 67 volunteers who were 20 to 80 years old; they reported that 1% of subjects younger than 60 years had at least one level of stenosis, while in those 60 years and older, the prevalence was 21%. For another MRI study, Jensen and associates[8] reported a 7% prevalence of central spinal stenosis among 98 asymptomatic volunteers. Foraminal stenosis was present in 7% of the sample as well.

Measurements of Spinal Canal Dimensions

Early measurements of the spinal canal diameters by Huizinga and associates[9] based on 51 Dutch lumbar skeletons indicated the lowest midsagittal diameter to be at L1 (11-mm average) and the greatest at L5 (14 mm). They further reported that the anteroposterior (AP) and interpedicular diameters were generally not related, and that stenosis mainly occurred in the AP diameter. Eisenstein[10] measured spinal canals in 485 skeletons from South African blacks and whites. His studies confirmed the importance of the AP diameter as a parameter for stenosis, and suggested that the lowest normal limits were 10 mm in blacks and 12 mm in whites. Women and men had similar dimensions. The smallest diameters were at L2 to L4 levels. The interpedicular diameter increased steadily from L1 to L5, confirming earlier reports.[11] Postacchini and as-

Table 1 Age and sex-specific distribution (%) of degenerative spondylolisthesis of at least 5 mm[5]

	Age (Years)				
	35-44	45-54	55-64	65-74	75+
Men	2.2	4.2	8.8	8.5	9.3
Women	2.0	3.1	11.8	14.4	25.3

sociates[12] reported morphologic differences between Italian and Indian skeletons, with the latter having significantly greater dimensions. Hibbert and associates,[13] and Porter and associates,[14,15] in several studies, have addressed the importance of the shape of the vertebral canal to stenosis. In dome-shaped canals there are no true lateral recesses, whereas trefoil-shaped canals have deep recesses, which increase the likelihood for lateral stenosis. In the sagittal plane, the dome-shaped canals are widest at L1, decrease toward L4, and then increase again at L5. In trefoil-shaped canals, L5 width is equal to or smaller than that of L4. Anthropometric measurements have documented only one useful correlation to canal size; the vertebral canal of a tall subject will have a larger transverse diameter.[13] In another skeletal study of spinal stenosis, based on Canadian autopsy specimens, there was a 4.1% prevalence of degenerative spondylolisthesis.[16]

Natural History

The natural history of asymptomatic spinal stenosis is unknown. It is clear from physical findings in patients who have no symptoms of spinal stenosis and imaging studies of patients who only recently became symptomatic that the spinal narrowing can be quite dramatic (causing an almost complete blockage of the spinal canal) without clinical symptoms being present. At the same time, mild narrowing sometimes causes severe symptoms.

Patients with symptoms have been followed by Johnsson[17] over a 3-year period. At 3 years, 32% were improved, 58% remained unchanged, and 10% were worse. Even in the group labeled as having ''severe stenosis,'' 64% improved. Deterioration was more common in this group (36%), but no patient had ''severe deterioration.''

In an attempt to determine the natural history of degenerative spondylolisthesis, a rate of progression was reported of 2 mm per year up to a maximum of 33% of the vertebral body width (which occurred rarely).[18] Symptoms correlated poorly to the rate of progression and/or degree of displacement, confirming conclusions by Valkenburg and Haanen.[5]

Spinal stenosis appears to increase the risk that a bulging or herniated disk becomes symptomatic.[19-21] In adolescents, the importance of canal size in disk herniations requiring surgery has been reported by several investigators.[22-25] Patients with congenital (developmental) spinal stenosis tolerate this narrowing well until the canal is further compromised by a secondary process, such as a disk protrusion or degenerative change.[26] In children with achondroplasia, progressive deformity contributes to the development of symptoms.

Risk Factors

Age is the main risk factor for spinal stenosis because the prevalence of degenerative spinal stenosis is greater in older subjects. Gender appears to be a risk factor as well, with higher prevalence rates among women.[5]

Vanharanta and associates[27] report that the dimensions at several levels of the spinal canal vary depending on occupation. Individuals in physically demanding jobs have smaller canals, probably because of more severe degenerative changes. There is no clinical evidence that spinal stenosis is more common in certain occupations, but more research is needed in this area.

Rosenberg[28] used anatomic specimens and patients to identify risk factors associated with degenerative spondylolisthesis. The level most commonly affected was L4–5. Women developed degenerative spondylolisthesis four times more often than men, sacralization of L5 caused a fourfold increase in risk, and diabetics had a fourfold increase in prevalence.

Summary and Recommendations

Little is known about the prevalence of spinal stenosis. A major obstacle is the lack of a valid case definition, which should include imaging evidence of stenosis along with clinical symptoms of spinal stenosis. While clinical criteria are being developed,[29] standardized imaging criteria are still lacking. More important than prevalence is, perhaps, natural history. This is a difficult research and ethical dilemma that needs to be considered carefully. Still, without knowledge of the natural history, the effect of treatment and, in turn, recommendations to the patient will be difficult to determine.

Degenerative spinal stenosis appears to be a part of aging. Can certain aspects, such as degenerative spondylolisthesis, be prevented? Without additional epidemiologic knowledge, such questions will be difficult to answer.

References

1. Andersson GBJ, McNeill TW (eds): *Lumbar Spinal Stenosis*. St. Louis, MO, Mosby-Year Book, 1992.
2. Deyo RA, Cherkin DC, Loeser JD, et al: Morbidity and mortality in association with operations on the lumbar spine: The influence of age, diagnosis, and procedure. *J Bone Joint Surg* 1992;74A:536–543.
3. Taylor VM, Deyo RA, Cherkin DC, et al: Low back pain hospitalization: Recent United States trends and regional variations. *Spine* 1994;19:1207–1213.
4. Turner JA, Ersek M, Herron L, et al: Surgery for lumbar spinal stenosis: Attempted meta-analysis of the literature. *Spine* 1992;17:1–8.
5. Valkenburg HA, Haanen HCM: The epidemiology of low back pain, in White AA III, Gordon SL (eds): American Academy of Orthopaedic Surgeons *Symposium on Idiopathic Low Back Pain*. St. Louis, MO, CV Mosby, 1982, pp 9–22.
6. Wiesel SW, Tsourmas N, Feffer HL, et al: A study of computer-assisted tomography: I. The incidence of positive CAT scans in an asymptomatic group of patients. *Spine* 1984;9:549–551.
7. Boden SD, Davis DO, Dina TS, et al: Abnormal magnetic-resonance scans of the lumbar spine in asymptomatic subjects: A prospective investigation. *J Bone Joint Surg* 1990;72A:403–408.
8. Jensen MC, Brant-Zawadzki MN, Obuchowski N, et al: Magnetic resonance imaging of the lumbar spine in people without back pain. *N Engl J Med* 1994;331:69–73.
9. Huizinga J, Hejden JA, Von den Vinken PJJG: The human vertebral canal: A biomechanic study. *Proc Royal Neth Acad Sci* 1952;55:23–33.
10. Eisenstein S: The morphometry and pathological anatomy of the lumbar spine in South African negroes and caucasoids with special reference to spinal stenosis. *J Bone Joint Surg* 1977;59B:173–180.
11. Haworth JB, Keillor GW: Use of transparencies in evaluating the width of the spinal canal in infants, children, and adults. *Radiology* 1962;79:109–114.

12. Postacchini F, Ripani M, Carpano S: Morphometry of the lumbar vertebrae: An anatomic study in two caucasoid ethnic groups. *Clin Orthop* 1983;172:296–303.
13. Hibbert CS, Porter RW, Delaygue C: Abstract: Relationship between the spinal canal and other skeletal measurements in a Romano–British population. *Ann R Coll Surg Engl* 1981;63:437.
14. Porter RW, Hibbert C, Wellman P: Backache and the lumbar spinal canal. *Spine* 1980;5:99–105.
15. Porter RW, Pavitt D: The vertebral canal: I. Nutrition and development, an archaeological study. *Spine* 1987;12:901–906.
16. Farfan HF: The pathological anatomy of degenerative spondylolisthesis: A cadaver study. *Spine* 1980;5:412–418.
17. Johnsson KE: *Lumbar Spinal Stenosis: A Clinical, Radiological and Neurophysiological Investigation.* Malmo, Sweden, University of Lund, 1987, pp 7–39. Thesis.
18. Feffer HL, Wiesel SW, Cuckler JM, et al: Degenerative spondylolisthesis: To fuse or not to fuse. *Spine* 1985;10:287–289.
19. Heliövaara M, Vanharanta H, Korpi J, et al: Herniated lumbar disk syndrome and vertebral canals. *Spine* 1986;11:433–435.
20. Ramani PS: Variations in size of the bony lumbar canal in patients with prolapse of lumbar intervertebral discs. *Clin Radiol* 1976;27:301–307.
21. Winston K, Rumbaugh C, Colucci V: The vertebral canals in lumbar disk disease. *Spine* 1984;9:414–417.
22. Gurdjian ES, Webster JE, Ostrowski AZ, et al: Herniated lumbar intervertebral discs: An analysis of 1,176 operated cases. *J Trauma* 1961;1:158–176.
23. Bradford DS, Garcia A: Herniations of the lumbar intervertebral disk in children and adolescents: A review of 30 surgically treated cases. *JAMA* 1969;210:2045–2051.
24. Kurihara A, Kataoka O: Lumbar disk herniation in children and adolescents: A review of 70 operated cases and their minimum 5-year follow-up studies. *Spine* 1980;5:443–451.
25. Epstein JA, Epstein NE, Marc J, et al: Lumbar intervertebral disk herniation in teenage children: Recognition and management of associated anomalies. *Spine* 1984;9:427–432.
26. Hammerberg KW: Spinal stenosis in children, achondroplasia, and spinal deformity, in Andersson GBJ, McNeill TW (eds): *Lumbar Spinal Stenosis.* St. Louis, MO, Mosby-Year Book, 1992, pp 153–167.
27. Vanharanta H, Heliovaara M, Korpi J, et al: Occupation, workload and the size and shape of lumbar vertebral canals. *Scand J Work Environ Health* 1987;13:146–149.
28. Rosenberg NJ: Degenerative spondylolisthesis: Predisposing factors. *J Bone Joint Surg* 1975;57A:467–474.
29. Katz JN, Dalgas M, Stucki G, et al: Degenerative lumbar spinal stenosis: Diagnostic value of the history and physical examination. *Arthritis Rheum* 1995;38:1236–1241.

641

Chapter 38

New Horizons in Imaging

Victor M. Haughton, MD
Howard An, MD
Tae-Hong Lim, PhD
Bruce H. Nowicki, BS

Introduction

Low back pain is a widespread disorder with an immense social and economic impact. Lumbar degenerative disk disease is often cited as the most common cause of persistent back pain and sciatica. Magnetic resonance imaging (MRI) and computed tomography (CT) are effective means of detecting spinal stenosis and degenerative changes in the intervertebral disks; however, the clinical significance of the morphologic changes in the disk is less well defined.[1] Nerve root impingement in the advanced stage of degenerative stenosis or other disk changes is accurately diagnosed with CT, myelography, or MRI, and its treatment is well defined. For example, the accuracy of CT and MRI in spinal stenosis was similar, while that of myelography was slightly poorer.[2] Sensitivities ranged from 0.81 to 0.97 for MRI, 0.7 to 1.0 for CT, and 0.67 to 0.78 for myelography (Fig. 1). In this review of 116 articles,[2] methodologic problems, including failure to assemble a representative cohort for study, small sample size, and failure to maintain independence of readings, were found. Receiver operating characteristic curves, such as those reported for CT, MRI, and myelography for the diagnosis of herniated disk[3] were estimated, but because of the methodologic problems, not calculated. Because no clear-cut advantage is found for one diagnostic modality over another, the choice between CT, MRI, and myelography depends more on cost, equipment used, and skill of the radiologist than on relative diagnostic accuracy. While the sensitivity of imaging studies is high, the specificity is lower because of the frequency of asymptomatic degenerative changes. As the resolution and throughput of MRI improves, more anatomic detail and biochemical information is revealed. Applications of MRI under development suggest a larger role for it in clinical and experimental studies of spine disorders.

Segmental instability of the lumbar spine is a common cause of low back pain, but the anatomic changes in the intervertebral disk, vertebral body, and facet joints associated with instability are not clearly known. Furthermore, spinal instability is not well defined biomechanically or clinically. The criteria for diagnosis of segmental instability are controversial, and a combination of clinical symptoms and imprecise radiographic findings are used. Therefore, results of treatment are often unpredictable and the efficacy of dif-

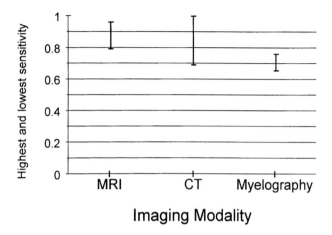

Fig. 1 *Sensitivity of MRI, CT, and myelography. (Reproduced with permission from Kent DL, Haynor DR, Larson EB, et al: Diagnosis of lumbar spinal stenosis in adults: A metaanalysis of the accuracy of CT, MR and myelography.* Am J Roentgenol *1992;158:1135–1144.)*

ferent treatment modalities is difficult to assess. MRI has not been used as extensively to study instability as to study problems such as herniated disks or spinal stenosis. Dynamic MRI studies may improve the diagnosis of instability.

Most patients with segmental instability have some degree of disk degeneration; however, the relationship between instability and degeneration is not clear. Conversely, individuals with apparent disk degeneration may or may not have segmental instability. Patients with a diagnosis of segmental instability and disk degeneration may also have changes in the facet joints. The cause of pain in these patients is often obscure. Because of the widespread nature of both disk disease and segmental instability, it is essential to develop methods to diagnose and treat these disorders more effectively.

Detection of root compression and its causes is considered to be the major role of imaging in patients with back pain or sciatica. However, with a tendency toward more conservative treatment of conditions with nerve root compression, the indications for imaging are changing. Health providers also dictate a more limited use of imaging in patients with back pain. The role of imaging should now be evaluated in terms of the infrequency of nerve root compression as a cause of symptoms. The fraction of patients with back pain or sciatica in which symptoms can be attributed to nerve root compression may be only 5%, or at most 30%.[4] Therefore, the subject of this review is the application of imaging to the detection of pathologic changes in the disk and vertebra, to studying the cause of back and sciatic pain, and to studying the physiology of the spine. Newer imaging techniques that can be applied to clinical or experimental studies of the spine will also be emphasized.

Imaging of Anatomic Changes in the Spine

MRI shows more anatomic detail in the intervertebral disk and possibly in the facet joint than CT or radiography.[5-8] Therefore, in this section, the MRI appearance of morphologic changes in the intervertebral disk, vertebral body and end plate, facet joint, and neural foramen will be reviewed.

Intervertebral Disk

In the intervertebral disk, the peripheral anulus, which is composed predominantly of collagen, is distinguished from the inner anulus and nucleus pulposus, both of which contain fibrocartilage. The changes in collagen content accompanying the development of the disk in the first two decades of life are reflected in changes in the signal intensity and appearance.

Of the tears or clefts that are found in the adult intervertebral disk, several are recognized by MRI.[9-12] One type of tear, called the concentric tear by some investigators, represents a delamination of the anulus fibrosus, with the accumulation of mucoid material in the space. The small fibers that bind the lamellae in the anulus are torn in cases of concentric tears, but the strong annular fibers in each lamella are intact. The concentric tear appears in MRI as a crescentic region of higher signal intensity in the normally lower signal intensity anulus. The transverse tear is a rupture of the insertion or origin of annular fibers from the ring apophysis. Usually, the transverse tear is short. It is recognized as a region of high signal intensity in the peripheral anulus fibrosus. It may be seen in radiographs or CT scans when it contains gas. The radial tear is a rupture of the fibers in each layer of the anulus fibrosus. The tear may occur in the anterior or the posterior anulus. In T2-weighted MRI scans the tear is recognized as a region of abnormally high signal intensity in the normally low signal intensity of the peripheral anulus (Fig. 2). It may also be recognized on MRI scans enhanced with gadolinium (Gd)-containing contrast media as a thin horizontal band of contrast enhancement related to the anulus. About 70% of the radial tears in the anulus that are shown by anatomic or diskographic techniques are demonstrated by MRI.[13]

The intranuclear cleft was studied by anatomic/MRI correlations, which showed that the area of low signal intensity in the equator of the disk, involving the nucleus pulposus as well as the inner anulus, represented a region where the collagen, elastin, and reticulin fibers are denser than in the adjacent fibrocartilage in the disk.[14] The observation that the dark region of the disk is associated with the accumulation of collagenous fibers was confirmed by Pearce and associates.[15]

Gas and calcification can simulate clefts in the intervertebral disk. Gas can cause a low signal intensity region in T1- or T2-weighted images. Dense calcification may also result in a region of reduced signal intensity because of the paucity of mobile protons. However, diffuse calcification in regions of the disk may result in an increased signal intensity in T1-weighted images because of the paramagnetic effect of minute granules of calcium.

Vertebral Body and End Plate

Visualization of the vertebral osseous end plate in MRI is limited by the thin dimensions of the bone in the end plate and the effects of chemical shift and

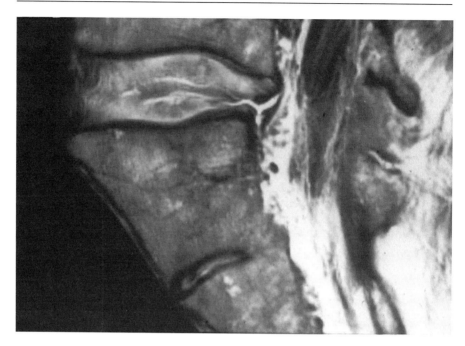

Fig. 2 *Magnetic resonance image showing a region of high signal intensity in the posterior anulus fibrosus of L5-S1 corresponding to a radial tear in the posterior anulus fibrosus.*

truncation artifact, which produce some MRI distortion at all interfaces. In the trabecular bone and marrow adjacent to the end plate, changes can be visualized secondary to disk degeneration. Three characteristic MRI appearances have been described.[16] In the first and probably earliest type, a more vascular tissue replaces the hematopoietic marrow normally adjacent to the vertebral end plate. In MRI this change (Modic type I) appears as a region of increased signal intensity in T2-weighted images and of contrast enhancement in TI-weighted images after the intravenous administration of a paramagnetic contrast medium containing Gd. Another osseous change (Modic type II) is characterized by replacement of the normal red marrow with yellow marrow, which because of the increased fat content appears in T1-weighted images as a region of increased signal intensity. A late stage is characterized by increased density of the trabecular bone adjacent to the end plate because of sclerosis and eburnation of bone. This condition is distinguished by decreased signal intensity in both T1- and T2-weighted images (Modic type III). The pathogenesis of the osseous changes in cases of disk degeneration is not known, but one type is thought to be related to instability.[17]

The microfractures in lumbar vertebrae described by Vernon-Roberts and Pirie[18] have not been identified by MRI. The nodular aggregates of woven bone that were found in trabecular microfractures would decrease signal intensity in the bone marrow. In other joints, bone marrow edema attributed to microfractures has been identified.

Facet Joint

The osseous structures that form the facet joint are effectively shown in CT.[19] Therefore, the later stages of facet joint degeneration such as cartilage thinning, subarticular erosions, and bone hypertrophy as described by Kirkaldy-Willis and associates[20] are demonstrated effectively by CT.[21-23] The cartilage in the facet joint is shown effectively by MRI.[24] The earlier stages of facet joint degeneration involving the cartilage and ligaments may also be shown by MRI.

MRI with small fields of view and special coils shows structure within the cartilage of the facet joints. Three zones are resolved within the articular cartilage on the superior and inferior articular processes. The superficial zone of cartilage, with tangentially oriented bands of collagen, is recognized as a superficial thin band of low signal intensity. Deep to this superficial zone the region of transitional cartilage has higher signal intensity and a pattern of darker radially oriented bands. The deep radiate zone, calcified cartilage zone, and cortical bone have low signal intensity. Pathologic changes in the facet joint cartilage can also be recognized[25] (Fig. 3). The superficial low signal intensity band is absent in eroded cartilage. In regions with degeneration in which the cartilage resembles crabmeat, the surface of the cartilage has an irregular increase

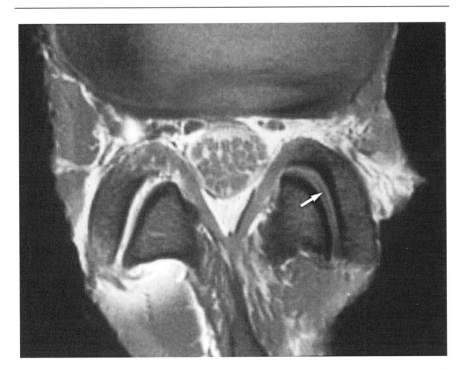

Fig. 3 *Magnetic resonance image with small field of view demonstrating normal and abnormal cartilage in facet joints. In the left facet joint, note the low signal intensity of the normal superficial zones of cartilage (arrow) and the higher signal intensity in the transitional zone. In the right facet joint, where the cartilage is partially destroyed (crabmeat degeneration), the higher signal intensity of fluid replaces the superficial and transitional zones.*

in signal intensity. In regions with disorganized transitional zones, the signal intensity pattern within the cartilage is less homogeneous than normal.

Neural Foramen

The MRI appearance of the nerves and ligaments in the neural foramina has been studied.[26-35] The ligamentum flavum is a significant factor in lateral stenosis. The transforaminal ligament, which has a characteristic MRI appearance, does not appear to be a frequent contributor to lateral stenosis.

Signal Intensity Changes in the Intervertebral Disk

The signal intensity of the intervertebral disk varies significantly with disk degeneration. In the normal disk, the signal intensities of the anulus and nucleus in T2-weighted images are not similar because of the different composition of the two. The outer anulus, which consists primarily of collagen, has a low signal intensity. The inner anulus and the nucleus pulposus, which are composed of fibrocartilage, have a high signal intensity. The high signal intensity of fibrocartilage is caused by the water bound reversibly to the glycosaminoglycans. The diurnal changes in the water content of the disk produce small but measurable changes in signal intensity. The changes in signal intensity with aging and degeneration reflect the changes in biochemical composition. The signal intensity of the lumbar intervertebral disks, exclusive of those with radial tears, normally decreases during seven decades of life by about 10% to 16%, consistent with the normal age-related decrease in proteoglycans and water.[36,37] Most of this change occurs in the first and second decades of life when the disk undergoes rapid maturation. Marked decreases in signal intensity are not observed in normal disks because of aging. Age-related change is appreciated in quantitative studies of signal intensity but not by inspection of MRI scans. By measuring the proton density, T1 and T2 relaxation of the intervertebral disk, Isherwood and associates[37] showed that aging could be distinguished from degeneration. The signal intensity was significantly lower in disks with a radial tear than in normally aging disks (Fig. 4). In the presence of a radial tear, with or without a decrease in height or bulging of the anulus, signal intensity was usually decreased sufficiently that the abnormality was evident on inspection. In degenerated intervertebral disks the signal intensity is conspicuously diminished.

The biochemical correlates of diminished signal intensity were also studied.[15] Disks with a low signal intensity in MRI were characterized by dehydration and decreases in proteoglycan content. On the basis of quantitative studies, it was determined that the low signal intensity probably reflects biochemical changes in the disk rather than changes in water content per se. The concentration of water or of collagen in the nucleus pulposus did not correlate to the signal intensity. Thus, the large differences in disk signal intensity with increasing evidence of degeneration on MRI are probably not caused by water concentration or interactions of water and collagen. In the nucleus, proteoglycan concentration correlated clearly with MRI signal intensity.

Several studies have related the appearance and signal intensity of the disk in MRI to its appearance on CT or radiographs obtained during diskography.

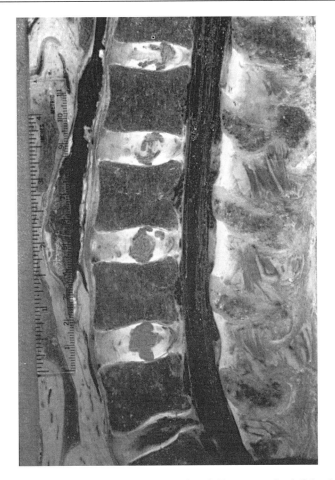

Fig. 4 *Sagittal section showing a radial tear in the L5-S1 intervertebral disk, which has diminished height, and on MRI had diminished signal intensity. The remaining lumbar disks are normal.*

Diskography effectively shows radial tears of the anulus fibrosus.[38] Diminished signal intensity and radial tears of the anulus detected in MRI correlate well with a diskogram that is positive for degeneration. The combination of diminished signal intensity and a defect in the anulus fibrosus correlated in 90% to 100% of patients with an abnormal diskogram in one study.[39] In agreement with Sether and associates,[36] Blumberg and associates[40] found that, regardless of age, a decrease in T2 in the intervertebral disk is virtually always associated with a radial tear.

Magnetic resonance/anatomic correlative studies have shown that in disks with diminished signal intensity, diminished height, and/or bulging of the anulus, a radial tear is likely to be found in the anulus.[41,42] Nordlander and associates[43] observed the same correlation between bulging of the anulus and radial tears in a study of diskography. In a large number of disks with a bulging anulus and no evidence of a herniation at surgery, a radial tear was found at diskography. Diskography in these patients was typically associated with pain resembling or duplicating the clinical symptomatology. Fernstrom[38] demonstrated also that in patients with sciatic pain syndromes, clinical history and physical examination did not distinguish radial tears with or without disk herniations. Disk degeneration has been modeled by creating a tear in the anulus fibrosus.[44-46]

Correlation of Magnetic Resonance Imaging to Provocative Diskography

Although MRI is a good method for demonstrating morphology and pathology in intervertebral disks, it does not differentiate pain-producing intervertebral disks from incidental abnormalities. Several investigators have correlated MRI with the pain produced during diskography to determine if MRI criteria can be developed to identify symptomatic intervertebral disks. It has been reported that there is "a significant relationship of pain and deterioration of disks" as shown by MRI.[47] In one study, the correlation between disk degeneration shown by MRI and diskography positive for pain production was 94%.[48] In another study, the sensitivity and specificity of MRI for identifying painful disks at diskography were calculated to be 81% and 64%, respectively.[49] It was emphasized that despite the relationship between pain and disk deterioration, deterioration is evidently not the only factor required to produce painful disks. Over 20% of the disks classified as normal by the degeneration scale produced some pain. Conversely some severely degenerated disks (6%) were found to be painless. However, only 3% of normal disks had exact reproduction of pain at diskography and 77% of the disks with exact reproduction had severe annular disruption. Others[50] reported 99% correlation of MRI and diskography.

In correlative studies of MRI and diskography it is often noted that exact reproduction of the patient's pain on injection is more common in disks that demonstrate fissures or ruptures diskographically than in disks with less degeneration.[49] In one study, the presence of a defect in the anulus demonstrated by MRI was evaluated as a marker for pain on diskography. In this study, the defect or "high intensity zone" was found only in patients with grade 3 or 4 diskograms. The high intensity zone was 54% sensitive and 89% specific for a grade 4 diskogram. The finding was 82% sensitive and 89% specific for pain production from the disk at diskogram (Table 1).[4] The positive predictive value of the high intensity zone for a disrupted disk at diskography was 86%. Horton and Daftari[39] reported that certain patterns of MRI, such as dark nucleus with annular tears, were highly associated with positive symptoms on diskography. Not in all studies has the correlation been so high. Other studies have indicated that MRI did not accurately reflect the internal architecture of the disk.[51]

Table 1 "Diskogenic pain" on diskography

Radial Tear	Pain	No Pain
Present	31	2
Absent	7	56

Contrast Enhancement in Spine Magnetic Resonance Imaging

After the intravenous administration of a contrast medium, many tissues that have the combination of a vascular supply, a fenestrated capillary endothelium, and an extravascular space show an increase in signal intensity (contrast enhancement) in MRI. Intravenous contrast medium is used in suspected tumors and osteomyelitis to determine the extent of disease. Contrast enhancement in intraspinal nerve roots has recently been studied and will be reviewed in the following paragraphs.

Contrast enhancement is not a normal finding in spinal nerve roots, which have tight capillary endothelial junctions that, like the blood-brain barrier, prevent contrast medium from escaping the capillaries. Enhancement in nerve roots, excluding that caused by neoplasms, is of two types. A faint enhancement of many or all spinal nerve roots probably represents the response of the nerve roots to aseptic inflammation. This type of enhancement is seen, according to Jinkins and associates,[52,53] in 1% to 2% of patients studied with MRI. The other type is the more intense enhancement of a single or a few nerve roots (Fig. 5), which may involve the spinal nerve root from the root sheath to the conus medullaris.

The incidence of enhancing spinal nerve roots depends on the MRI technique and the dose of contrast medium used. Jinkins[54] found the incidence of contrast-enhancement of lumbar nerve roots in MRI performed with gadolinium-diethylenetriaminepentaacetic acid (Gd-DTPA) in unselected patients was 5%. In patients with a herniated disk, it was 20%; in those with spinal stenosis, 74%. Contrast enhancement was more conspicuous in nerve roots if the "double" or "triple" dose of contrast medium was used. Crisi and associates[55] found "selective" enhancement in single nerve roots in 30% of patients with herniated

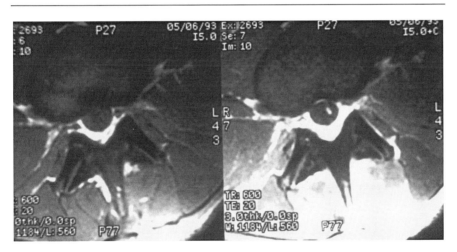

Fig. 5 *Axial MRI scans in a baboon before (**left**) and after (**right**) the administration of contrast medium. Note the enhancement observed in the left S1 nerve root, which had been chronically, mildly compressed. (Reproduced with permission from Nguyen C, Haughton VM, Ho KC, et al: Contrast enhancement in spinal nerve roots: An experimental study.* Am J Neuroradiol *1995;16:265–268.)*

disks and faint, diffuse, nonspecific enhancement in 55%. Overall, Taneichi and associates[56] found it in 39% of those with no history of spinal surgery and in 58% after spinal surgery.

Nerve root enhancement has been suggested by Jinkins[52-54] to be a marker of nerve root pathology. However, it has clinical significance only if nonspecific enhancement is disregarded. The faint enhancement of multiple roots and enhancement of single or multiple nerve roots in the early postoperative period are examples of nonspecific enhancement. Boden and associates[57] found contrast enhancement in nerve roots in all 15 patients studied with contrast-enhanced MRI after successful lumbar laminectomy and resolution of clinical symptoms. However, the enhancement was not detected in the follow-up study at 6 months.

Nerve root enhancement correlates to a degree with clinical symptoms or signs. Taneichi and associates[56] found that the enhancement was correlated with evidence of nerve root edema. They considered the enhancement a means of identifying the affected nerve root because the correlation with clinical symptomatology was good. Jinkins[52-54] found that except in the early postoperative period, enhancement was seen in symptomatic nerve roots only. Twenty-one percent of symptomatic subjects had enhancement in one or more roots, associated with isolated epidural fibrosis in 89%, and with herniated disk in the remaining 11%. Overall, the clinical correlation of single nerve root enhancement with radiculopathy was 96%. However, when there was more than one enhanced nerve root, one of the roots correlated with the clinical symptomatology and others (an additional 21% of nerve roots) did not. There were patients with multiple enhanced nerves postoperatively that were attributed to low grade aseptic inflammation. Jinkins states that the nonspecific enhancement during the first 6 months after laminectomy usually resolves, but enhancement after 6 months is significant. Crisi and associates[55] also studied enhancement in patients with herniated disks. They found enhancement along the entire root in six (30%). The enhancing roots appeared swollen, and all patients were symptomatic at the time. No clinical differences were detected between patients with and without enhancement, except that enhancement tended to be seen in patients with shorter durations of symptoms (40 days or less), which may suggest that the enhancement may be transient. If so, then a decrease in root enhancement and edema is not necessarily followed by resolution of symptoms. There was no correlation with surgical outcome; therefore, contrast enhancement in a nerve root was not a negative prognostic factor.

The pathogenesis of nerve root enhancement has been studied. It was determined that mild or temporary pressure on a nerve root, such as that which may cause paresthesias, is not likely to be a cause of contrast enhancement.[56] Sudden, forceful, mechanical traumatization that produces pathophysiologic changes in the nerve root is likely to cause enhancement. Unlike peripheral nerves, nerve roots have no durable perineurium.[56] Perineurium in peripheral nerves acts as a selective diffusion barrier to macromolecular substances and is part of the blood-nerve barrier, which has considerably more permeability than that of the brain. The minimal enhancement noted in 55% of patients with multiple roots is probably a result of this.[55] The more intense enhancement in single nerves probably reflects the blood-nerve barrier breakdown and centripetal flow of contrast medium through the endoneurium. The endoneurium is connective tissue in which the nerve fiber fascicles are suspended. It extends as far as the Obersteiner-Redlich zone, where the nerve joins the conus medullaris. Histopathologic studies in compressed roots have shown demyelination, hemorrhage, and edema. Nguyen and associates[58] showed that experimental compression of a spinal nerve resulted in contrast enhancement (Fig. 5), which correlated pathologically with degeneration, edema, and changes in the capillary endothelium.[58]

Conventional Applications of Paramagnetic Contrast Media in Spine Imaging

Paramagnetic contrast media are used in spine MRI to improve the detection of tumors, scar tissue, and granulation tissue. Tissues that have a vascularity, a leaky capillary endothelium, and an extravascular space demonstrate contrast enhancement. Bone marrow, dorsal root ganglia, and epidural venous plexus are such tissues; the spinal cord, spinal nerve roots, and intervertebral disks ordinarily are not. The use of paramagnetic contrast media in the diagnosis of neoplasms, osteomyelitis, and epidural fibrosis has been described in detail, but its use in the study of intervertebral disk function has not been widely publicized.

The intervertebral disk is normally characterized as a structure that does not enhance after administration of intravenous contrast medium. A region of enhancement in intervertebral disks is considered a sign of abnormality, such as a radial tear with granulation tissue or diskitis. A series of studies has shown that the normal intervertebral disk may demonstrate contrast enhancement (Fig. 6), which may be used to study the rate of diffusion in cartilage. While the intervertebral disk has no vascular system, it does have a large extravascular space. Nutrients such as oxygen, nitrate, sulfate, and glucose diffuse into the disk in sufficient amounts to sustain the metabolism of the several thousand cells found in each cubic millimeter of disk tissue. Diffusion, not perfusion, through the vertebral end plates and the anulus fibrosus provides the nutrients. Hypothetically, one cause of disk degeneration is diminished diffusion, which restricts the metabolites needed to sustain the biochemical constitution of the disk. Like the small molecular weight metabolites that diffuse in and out of the disk, Gd-chelates with molecular weight around 500 are exchanged between the intervertebral disk and the surrounding tissues. Therefore, contrast enhancement of the disk is detected in MRI if appropriate imaging strategies are used.

Enhancement of Cartilage by Diffusion

After the intravenous injection of Gd-DTPA in normal rabbit intervertebral disks, contrast enhancement is detected by inspection or by measurement of signal intensity.[59] This result may appear to conflict with previous reports that the intervertebral disk does not enhance, except in some pediatric spines. In most of the previous studies, however, contrast enhancement was not studied quantitatively and smaller doses of contrast medium and shorter intervals between injection of contrast medium and imaging were used. With the conventional 0.1 mmol/kg dose of Gd-DTPA, less than a 10% change in signal intensity is measured in rabbit intervertebral disks, and it is not detected by inspection. Enhancement of normal intervertebral disk has been observed in rabbits, dogs, and monkeys (C Nguyen, MD, and VM Haughton, MD, unpublished data, 1994). Rabbits

653

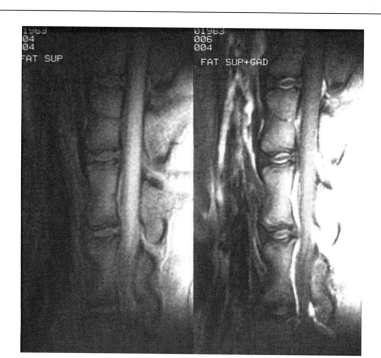

Fig. 6 *Magnetic resonance images obtained before (**left**) and 40 minutes after (**right**) intravenous administration of a nonionic paramagnetic contrast medium. Note the enhancement observed in the intervertebral disk. Contrast medium reaches the disk slowly by diffusion. Enhancement is greater after injection of a nonionic than an ionic contrast medium.*

and dogs have fibrocartilaginous intervertebral disks and porous osseous end plates similar to those of primate and human intervertebral disks. In humans, visible contrast enhancement would not be predicted before 20 to 45 minutes after intravenous injection of a paramagnetic contrast medium or with doses much smaller than 0.3 mmol/kg or with ionic media.

Determinants of Enhancement

Contrast enhancement in intervertebral disks is affected by the structure of the disk and the composition of the contrast medium.[60,61] Factors related to disk structure include the permeability of the end plates, pore size in the collagen structure, and the fixed negative charge density in the cartilage. With respect to the composition of the contrast medium, the charge on the molecule and the molecular weight affect diffusion (Fig. 7).

Contrast enhancement in the intervertebral disk can be described in terms of an enhancement coefficient and a rate constant.[60] After the injection of a bolus of the Gd-complex, enhancement in the intervertebral disk asymptotically approaches a plateau, defined as the enhancement coefficient. The enhancement coefficient is a measure of the maximal enhancement reached after an injection of contrast medium. For different contrast media or disk compositions, the enhancement coefficient may vary. For example, the coefficient is greater for non-

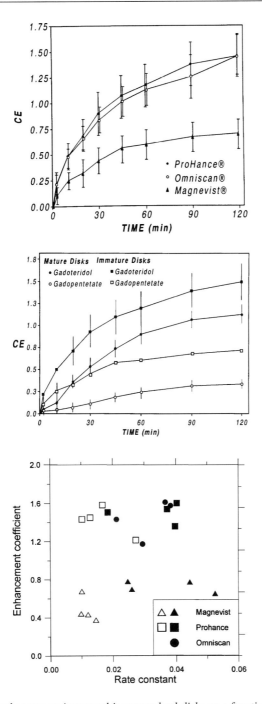

Fig. 7 *Contrast enhancement in normal intervertebral disks as a function of time and dose and type of contrast medium.* **Top**, *The enhancement from ionic (Magnevist) and nonionic media is compared.* **Center**, *The immature and mature disk enhancement is compared.* **Bottom**, *The rate and enhancement coefficients for ionic and nonionic media and mature and immature disks are compared.*

ionic than for ionic media and greater for immature than for mature disks. The greater enhancement coefficient for nonionic media probably represents the greater rate of diffusion of uncharged than of charged molecules in the intervertebral disk. The effect of disk maturation on the coefficient constant probably represents the increasing concentration of fixed negative charges as the disk matures. Intervertebral disk enhancement approaches the plateau at different rates, depending on the composition of the disk and of the molecule. That rate can be described in terms of a rate constant. In a first-order equation the time course of disk enhancement can be described in terms of the rate and the enhancement coefficients: $CE = K(1 - e^{at})$ where K is the enhancement coefficient and a is the rate constant.[60] The rate constants are greater in immature than in mature disks, either because of the effect of greater fixed negative charge density or because of changes in the vertebral end plate with maturation. The ionic contrast medium gadopentetate has smaller constants than do the nonionic media gadoteridol and gadodiamide, presumably because of the fixed negative charges in cartilage that impede the diffusion of charged particles.

Applications of Contrast Enhancement in Imaging Cartilage

With MRI and an intravenous contrast agent, diffusion into the normal intervertebral disk may be measured. While diffusion of isotopically labeled sulfate, glucose, and nitrates into the intervertebral disk has been studied, noninvasive in vivo methods to measure diffusion have not been available. With MRI and a paramagnetic medium, a clinical method of measuring diffusion may be available. Calculations of the enhancement coefficient and the rate constant may provide parameters of enhancement that can be used to identify impairment in diffusion. The effect of drugs, smoking, or surgical procedures on the diffusion of low molecular weight substances into the intervertebral disk may be studied noninvasively in vivo. The hypothesis that diffusion into the intervertebral disk is a marker of early degeneration can be tested by means of MRI and paramagnetic contrast media. The commercially available contrast media are not interchangeable for MRI of the spine. For example, in the differentiation of recurrent herniated disk and scar tissue, ionic and nonionic media may give different results (Fig. 8). The ionic media provide more contrast between recurrent herniated disk fragments and scar tissue than do the nonionic media. The nonionic media are the media of choice if more enhancement of disk or joint cartilage is the objective. Experimental contrast media with greater molecular weights are even more effective than ionic media in differentiating scar and recurrent herniated disk (T Perlowitz, BS, V Haughton, MD, L Riley, MD, unpublished data, 1996).

Application of Dynamic Magnetic Resonance Imaging to Studying Spinal Stiffness and Instability

Most patients with segmental instability have disk degeneration, but the relationship between instability and degeneration is not clear. Toyone and associates[17] reported that MRI of bone marrow adjacent to disks with more than 5° of segmental flexion and more than 3 mm of segmental translation on flexion-extension radiographs had decreased signal intensity on T1-weighted spin-echo images, that is, Modic type I changes. When subjected to an axial load, motion

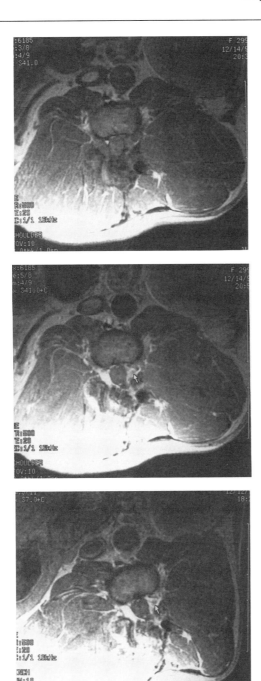

Fig. 8 *Magnetic resonance images in a dog with a disk fragment in the epidural space to model a recurrent herniated disk fragment.* **Top**, *Image obtained prior to contrast medium administration (baseline).* **Center**, *Image obtained after administration of nonionic contrast medium.* **Bottom**, *Image obtained after the administration of the same amount of an ionic medium. The contrast between the fragment and the surrounding scar tissue is greatest after administration of the ionic medium.*

657

segments with a radial tear in the anulus fibrosus have greater changes of the foraminal cross-sectional area than motion segments without such tears.[61,62] In cadaver lumbar spinal motion segments, the application of pure extension, flexion, lateral bending, or rotation moments produced compression of spinal nerves in the neural foramina (occult spinal stenosis) in some specimens (Fig. 9) (BH Nowicki, BS, H An, MD, V Haughton, MD, T-H Lim, PhD, unpublished data,

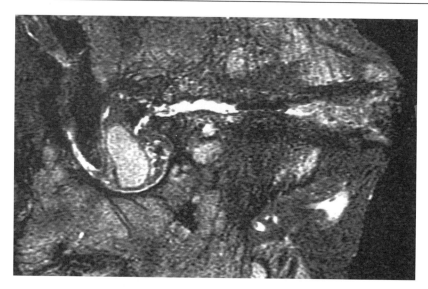

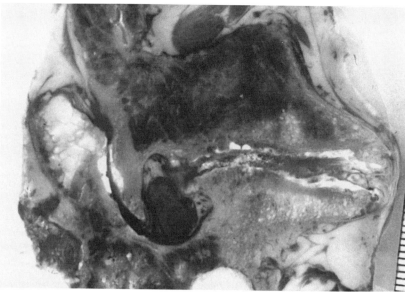

Fig. 9 **Top** *and* **Bottom**, *Parasagittal MRI scans and anatomic sections in a lumbar spinal motion segment subjected to an extension moment. Contact between the spinal nerve and the disk and ligamentum flavum is evident.*

1996). Occult stenosis was common, especially in motion segments with radial tears or advanced degenerative changes in the disk. Extension tended to produce the highest incidence of occult stenosis. Lateral bending produced occult stenosis in a small fraction of cases, usually in association with a radial tear and degeneration in the intervertebral disk. Rotation did not produce occult stenosis in motion segments with degenerating disks.

These studies support the hypothesis that excessive movement or instability in patients with low back pain may be related in some cases to the radial tear of the anulus. Dynamic MRI may be useful to detect occult abnormalities in the central spinal canal or neural foramina in patients with radiculopathy. Dynamic MRI techniques to study stiffness and stability of the spine have been developed. Translation between bones in a joint can be measured by means of three-dimensional reconstructions from CT images[63,64] or MRI.[65] Creep displacements of lumbar disks in flexion and extension postures can be measured. The Department of Orthopedic Surgery at the Medical College of Wisconsin is testing the accuracy and precision of spinal motion analysis systems based on noninvasive imaging. With additional development, MRI may provide both morphologic and kinematic information concerning the intervertebral disk. Such studies may be more accurate than flexion-extension radiographs in determining the degree of spine stiffness and instability. Despite numerous dynamic radiographic studies on spinal instability,[66-74] biplanar stereoradiography, centrode pattern, and invasive techniques requiring the placement of metal beads in the spinous processes,[75-77] methods with sufficient accuracy and acceptance are not available.[78-84] Further studies are needed to correlate types and grades of degenerated disks, biomechanical changes, and eventually patients' symptoms. With technologic improvements, kinematic studies of the spine may be possible noninvasively with three-dimensional CT or MRI. With conventional and dynamic techniques, low back pain and radiculopathy can be investigated more effectively.

References

1. Boden SD, Davis DO, Dina TS, et al: Abnormal magnetic-resonance scans of the lumbar spine in asymptomatic subjects: A prospective investigation. *J Bone Joint Surg* 1990;72A:403–408.
2. Kent DL, Haynor DR, Larson EB, et al: Diagnosis of lumbar spinal stenosis in adults: A metaanalysis of the accuracy of CT, MR and myelography. *Am J Roentgenol* 1992;158:1135–1144.
3. Thornbury JR, Fryback DG, Turski PA, et al: Disk-caused nerve compression in patients with acute low-back pain: Diagnosis with MR, CT myelography, and plain CT. *Radiology* 1993;186:731–738.
4. Aprill C, Bogduk N: High-intensity zone: A diagnostic sign of painful lumbar disc on magnetic resonance imaging. *Br J Radiol* 1992;65:361–369.
5. Pech P, Haughton VM: Lumbar intervertebral disk: Correlative MR and anatomic study. *Radiology* 1985;156:699–701.
6. Ho PS, Yu SW, Sether LA, et al: Progressive and regressive changes in the nucleus pulposus: Part I. The neonate. *Radiology* 1988;169:87–91.
7. An HS, Haughton VM: Non-discogenic lumbar radiculopathy: Imaging considerations. *Semin Ultrasound CT MR* 1993;14:425–436.
8. Yu S, Haughton VM, Rosenbaum AE: Magnetic resonance imaging and anatomy of the spine. *Radiol Clin North Am* 1991;29:691–710.
9. Yu SW, Haughton VM, Ho PS, et al: Progressive and regressive changes in the nucleus pulposus: Part II. The adult. *Radiology* 1988;169:93–97.

659

10. Yu S, Haughton VM, Sether LA, et al: Criteria for classifying normal and degenerated lumbar intervertebral disks. *Radiology* 1989;170:523–526.
11. Wagner M, Sether LA, Yu S, et al: Age changes in the lumbar intervertebral disc studied with magnetic resonance and cryomicrotomy. *Clin Anat* 1988;1:93–103.
12. Sether LA, Yu S, Haughton VM, et al: Ruptures of the anulus fibrosus of cervical intervertebral discs studied by cryomicrotomy and magnetic resonance. *Clin Anat* 1989;2:1–8.
13. Yu SW, Haughton VM, Sether LA, et al: Comparison of MR and diskography in detecting radial tears of the anulus: A postmortem study. *Am J Neuroradiol* 1989;10:1077–1081.
14. Yu SW, Haughton VM, Lynch KL, et al: Fibrous structure in the intervertebral disk: Correlation of MR appearance with anatomic sections. *Am J Neuroradiol* 1989;10:1105–1110.
15. Pearce RH, Thompson JP, Bebault GM, et al: Magnetic resonance imaging reflects the chemical changes of aging degeneration in the human intervertebral disk. *J Rheumatol Suppl* 1991;27:42–43.
16. Modic MT: Degenerative disorders of the spine, in Modic MT, Masaryk TJ, Ross JS (eds): *Magnetic Resonance Imaging of the Spine.* Chicago, IL, Year Book Medical Publishers, 1989, pp 75–119.
17. Toyone T, Takahashi K, Kitahara H, et al: Vertebral bone-marrow changes in degenerative lumbar disc disease: An MRI study of 74 patients with low back pain. *J Bone Joint Surg* 1994;76B:757–764.
18. Vernon-Roberts B, Pirie CJ: Healing trabecular microfractures in the bodies of lumbar vertebrae. *Ann Rheum Dis* 1973;32:406–412.
19. Fletcher G, Haughton VM, Ho KC, et al: Age-related changes in the cervical facet joints: Studies with cryomicrotomy, MR, and CT. *Am J Neuroradiol* 1990;11:27–30.
20. Kirkaldy-Willis WH, Wedge JH, Yong-Hong K, et al: Pathology and pathogenesis of lumbar spondylosis and stenosis. *Spine* 1978;3:319–328.
21. Carrera GF, Haughton VM, Syvertsen A, et al: Computed tomography of the lumbar facet joints. *Radiology* 1980;134:145–148.
22. Xu GL, Haughton VM, Carrera GF: Lumbar facet joint capsule appearance at MR and CT. *Radiology* 1990;177:415–420.
23. Xu GL, Haughton VM, Yu S, et al: Normal variations of the lumbar facet joint capsules. *Clin Anat* 1991;4:117–122.
24. Modl JM, Sether LA, Haughton VM, et al: Articular cartilage: Correlation of histologic zones with signal intensity at MR imaging. *Radiology* 1991;181:853–855.
25. Monson NL, Haughton VM, Modl JM, et al: Normal and degenerating articular cartilage: In vitro correlation of MR imaging and histologic findings. *J Magn Reson Imaging* 1992;2:41–45.
26. Kostelic JK, Haughton VM, Sether LA: Anatomy of the lumbar spinal nerves in the intervertebral foramen. *Clin Anat* 1991;4:366–372.
27. Kostelic JK, Haughton VM, Sether LA: Lumbar spinal nerves in the neural foramen: MR appearance. *Radiology* 1991;178:837–839.
28. Kostelic J, Haughton VM, Sether L: Proximal lumbar spinal nerves in axial MR imaging, CT, and anatomic sections. *Radiology* 1992;183:239–241.
29. Ho PS, Yu SW, Sether LA, et al: Ligamentum flavum: Appearance on sagittal and coronal MR images. *Radiology* 1988;168:469–472.
30. Hasegawa T, An HS, Haughton VM, et al: Lumbar foraminal stenosis: Critical heights of the intervertebral discs and foramina. A cryomicrotome study in cadavera. *J Bone Joint Surg* 1995;77A:32–38.
31. Nowicki BH, Haughton VM: Ligaments of the lumbar neural foramina: A sectional anatomic study. *Clin Anat* 1992;5:126–135.
32. Nowicki BH, Haughton VM: Neural foraminal ligaments of the lumbar spine: Appearance at CT and MR imaging. *Radiology* 1992;183:257–264.
33. Yu S, Haughton VM: Anatomic-radiographic correlations in the spine. *Curr Imag* 1990;2:105–116.

34. Yug DP, Haughton VM, Sether LA, et al: MR appearance of the proximal cerebral spinal nerve: MR appearance. *Radiology* 1992;184:405.
35. Yug DP, Sether LA, Komorowski RA, et al: A multiplanar anatomic study of the cervical proximal nerve roots and spinal nerves. *Clin Anat* 1992;5:433–440.
36. Sether LA, Yu S, Haughton VM, et al: Intervertebral disk: Normal age-related changes in MR signal intensity. *Radiology* 1990;177:385–388.
37. Isherwood I, Prendergast DJ, Hickey DS, et al: Quantitative analysis of intervertebral disc structure. *Acta Radiologica* 1987;369(suppl):492–495.
38. Fernstrom U: A discographical study of ruptured lumbar intervertebral discs. *Acta Chir Scand* 1960;258(suppl):1–60.
39. Horton WC, Daftari TK: Which disc as visualized by magnetic resonance imaging is actually a source of pain? A correlation between magnetic resonance imaging and discography. *Spine* 1992;17(suppl 6):S164–S171.
40. Blumberg ML, Ostrum BJ, Ostrum DM: Letter: Changes in MR signal intensity of the intervertebral disc. *Radiology* 1991;179:584–585.
41. Yu SW, Haughton VM, Sether LA, et al: Anulus fibrosus in bulging intervertebral disks. *Radiology* 1988;169:761–763.
42. Yu SW, Sether LA, Ho PS, et al: Tears of the anulus fibrosus: Correlation between MR and pathologic findings in cadavers. *Am J Neuroradiol* 1988;9:367–370.
43. Nordlander S, Salén EF, Unander-Scharin L: Discography in low back pain and sciatica: Analysis of 73 operated cases. *Acta Orthop Scand* 1958;28:90–102.
44. Nguyen C, Haughton VM, Ho KC, et al: A model for studying intervertebral disc degeneration with magnetic resonance and a nucleotome. *Invest Radiol* 1989;24:407–409.
45. Nguyen C, Ho KC, Yu S, et al: An experimental model to study contrast enhancement in MR imaging of the intervertebral disk. *Am J Neuroradiol* 1989;10:811–814.
46. Osti OL, Vernon-Roberts B, Fraser RD: Anulus tears and intervertebral disc degeneration: An experimental study using an animal model. *Spine* 1990;15:762–767.
47. Vanharanta H, Sachs BL, Spivey MA, et al: The relationship of pain provocation to lumbar disc deterioration as seen by CT/discography. *Spine* 1987;12:295–298.
48. Linson MA, Crowe CH: Comparison of magnetic resonance imaging and lumbar discography in the diagnosis of disc degeneration. *Clin Orthop* 1990;250:160–163.
49. Antti-Poika I, Soini J, Tallroth K, et al: Clinical relevance of discography combined with CT scanning: A study of 100 patients. *J Bone Joint Surg* 1990;72B:480–485.
50. Schneiderman G, Flannigan B, Kingston S, et al: Magnetic resonance imaging in the diagnosis of disc degeneration: Correlation with discography. *Spine* 1987;12:276–281.
51. Zucherman J, Derby R, Hsu K, et al: Normal magnetic resonance imaging with abnormal discography. *Spine* 1988;13:1355–1359.
52. Jinkins JR, Osborn AG, Garrett D Jr, et al: Spinal nerve enhancement with gd-DTPA: MR correlation with the postoperative lumbosacral spine. *Am J Neuroradiol* 1993;14:383–394.
53. Jinkins JR: The pathoanatomic basis of somatic and autonomic syndromes originating in the lumbosacral spine. *Neuroimaging Clin N Am* 1993;3:443–463.
54. Jinkins JR: Magnetic resonance imaging of benign nerve root enhancement in the unoperated and postoperative lumbosacral spine. *Neuroimaging Clin N Am* 1993;3:525–541.
55. Crisi G, Carpeggiani P, Trevisan C: Gadolinium-enhanced nerve roots in lumbar disk herniation. *Am J Neuroradiol* 1993;14:1379–1392.
56. Taneichi H, Abumi K, Kaneda K, et al: Significance of Gd-DTPA-enhanced magnetic resonance imaging for lumbar disc herniation: The relationship between nerve root enhancement and clinical manifestations. *J Spinal Disord* 1994;7:153–160.
57. Boden SD, Davis DO, Dina TS, et al: Contrast-enhanced MR imaging performed after successful lumbar disk surgery: Prospective study. *Radiology* 1992;182:59–64.
58. Nguyen C, Haughton VM, Ho KC, et al: Contrast enhancement in spinal nerve roots: An experimental study. *Am J Neuroradiol* 1995;16:265–268.
59. Ibrahim MA, Jesmanowicz A, Hyde JS, et al: Contrast enhancement of normal intervertebral discs: Time and dose dependence. *Am J Neuroradiol* 1994;15:419–423.

661

60. Ibrahim MA, Haughton VM, Hyde JS: Effect of disk maturation on diffusion of low-molecular-weight gadolinium complexes: An experimental study in rabbits. *Am J Neuroradiol* 1995;16:1307–1311.

61. Ibrahim MA, Haughton VM, Hyde JS: Enhancement of intervertebral disks with gadolinium complexes: Comparison of an ionic and a nonionic medium in an animal model. *Am J Neuroradiol* 1994;15:1907–1910.

62. Nowicki BH, Yu S, Reinartz J, et al: Effect of axial loading on neural foramina and nerve roots in the lumbar spine. *Radiology* 1990;176:433–437.

63. Belsole RJ, Hilbelink DR, Llewellyn JA, et al: Mathematical analysis of computed carpal models. *J Orthop Res* 1988;6:116–122.

64. Wynarsky GT, Harris GF, Orloff S, et al: A non-invasive technique for the description of three-dimensional bone and joint kinematics. *Trans Orthop Res Soc* 1992;17:471.

65. Hedman TP, Fernie GR: In vivo measurement of lumbar spinal creep in two seated postures using magnetic resonance imaging. *Spine* 1995;20:178–183.

66. Boden SD, Wiesel SW: Lumbosacral segmental motion in normal individuals: Have we been measuring instability properly? *Spine* 1990;15:571–576.

67. Dillard J, Trafimow J, Andersson GB, et al: Motion of the lumbar spine: Reliability of two measurement techniques. *Spine* 1991;16:321–324.

68. Dvorak J, Panjabi MM, Novotny JE, et al: Clinical validation of functional flexion-extension roentgenograms of the lumbar spine. *Spine* 1991;16:943–950.

69. Hayes MA, Howard TC, Gruel CR: Roentgenographic evaluation of lumbar spine flexion-extension in asymptomatic individuals. *Spine* 1989;14:327–331.

70. Keesen W, During J, Beeker TW, et al: Recordings of the movement at the intervertebral segment L5-S1: A technique for the determination of the movement in the L5-S1 spinal segment by using three specified postural positions. *Spine* 1984;9:83–90.

71. Knutsson F: The instability associated with disk degeneration in the lumbar spine. *Acta Radiol* 1944;25:593–609.

72. Putto E, Tallroth K: Extension-flexion radiographs for motion studies of the lumbar spine: A comparison of two methods. *Spine* 1990;15:107–110.

73. Shaffer WO, Spratt KF, Weinstein J, et al: The consistency and accuracy of roentgenograms for measuring sagittal translation in the lumbar vertebral motion segment: An experimental model. *Spine* 1990;15:741–750.

74. Tillotson KM, Burton AK: Noninvasive measurement of lumbar sagittal mobility: An assessment of the flexicurve technique. *Spine* 1991;16:29–33.

75. Pope MH, Frymoyer JW, Krag MH: Diagnosing instability. *Clin Orthop* 1992;279:60–67.

76. Pope MH, Panjabi M: Biomechanical definitions of spinal instability. *Spine* 1985;10:255–256.

77. Pope MH, Svensson M, Broman H, et al: Mounting of the transducers in measurement of segmental motion of the spine. *J Biomech* 1986;19:675–677.

78. Brown RH, Burstein AH, Nash CL, et al: Spinal analysis using a three-dimensional radiographic technique. *J Biomech* 1976;9:355–365.

79. Friberg O: Lumbar instability: A dynamic approach by traction-compression radiography. *Spine* 1987;12:119–129.

80. Gertzbein SD, Seligman J, Holtby R, et al: Centrode patterns and segmental instability in degenerative disc disease. *Spine* 1985;10:257–261.

81. Gertzbein SD, Holtby R, Tile M, et al: Determination of a locus of instantaneous centers of rotation of the lumbar disc by moire fringes: A new technique. *Spine* 1984;9:409–413.

82. Kalebo P, Kadziolka R, Sward L: Compression-traction radiography of lumbar segmental instability. *Spine* 1990;15:351–355.

83. Pearcy M, Portek I, Shepherd J: The effect of low-back pain on lumbar spinal movements measured by three-dimensional X-ray analysis. *Spine* 1985;10:150–153.

84. Seligman JV, Getzbein SD, Tile M, et al: Computer analysis of spinal segment motion in degenerative disc disease with and without axial loading. *Spine* 1984;9:566–573.

Chapter 39

Degenerative Lumbar Spinal Stenosis: Natural History and Results of Simple Decompression and Decompression and Fusion for Degenerative Spondylolisthesis

Gordon R. Bell, MD

Introduction

Spinal stenosis is a clinical descriptive condition in which the term ''spinal'' refers to neural and the term ''stenosis'' denotes a narrowing or constriction of a tubular structure. Sachs and Fraenkel[1] were among the first to relate symptoms of sciatica to neural compression within the spinal canal. This condition was subsequently described by Bailey and Casamajor,[2] who described acquired (degenerative) bony compression, and Sarpyener,[3] who described congenital narrowing of the spinal canal. van Gelderen[4] proposed hypertrophied ligamentum as a potential cause of spinal stenosis and reported on a small series of two patients with this condition. The clinical features of the spinal stenosis syndrome and its relationship to congenital narrowing were described in detail by the Dutch surgeon Verbiest[5] who also demonstrated mechanical compression of neural structures by myelography. Kirkaldy-Willis and associates[6] further defined the pathoanatomy of spinal stenosis and helped correlate pathologic changes with symptoms. Since those early mechanical descriptions of spinal stenosis, the importance of vascular, neural, and pain physiology contributions to this condition have been recognized.

The etiology of spinal stenosis may be either congenital (developmental) or acquired (degenerative), or a combination of both (Outline 1).[7] Most cases of spinal stenosis are acquired, caused by degenerative changes in the three-joint complex that consists of the intervertebral disk and facet joints. In some cases, these degenerative changes may be superimposed on a preexisting congenital stenosis. Variations in the shape and size of the spinal canal may predispose the patient to spinal stenosis, with a trefoil canal being associated with lateral recess stenosis more commonly than a round or oval canal.

Natural History of Spinal Stenosis

Large, long-term, prospective studies describing the natural history of spinal stenosis do not exist, partly because many patients with this condition ulti-

Outline 1 Classification of spinal stenosis[7]

Congenital/developmental stenosis
   Idiopathic (hereditary)
   Achondroplastic

Acquired stenosis
   Degenerative
   Combined congenital and degenerative stenosis
   Spondylolytic/spondylolisthetic
   Iatrogenic (eg, postlaminectomy, postfusion)
   Posttraumatic
   Metabolic (eg, Paget's disease, fluorosis)

mately undergo surgery.[8] Several studies describing clinical features of spinal stenosis or its surgical treatment include sporadic cases of patients who had not received treatment.[9-11] In these cases, symptoms progressed in approximately 20% of patients. Blau and Logue,[8] for example, reported on a series of 22 patients, only two of whom were not operated on. One of the two patients showed gradual progression over a 10-year period and the other exhibited no progression over 7 years. Jones and Thomson[11] reported on 13 patients with spinal stenosis, three of whom were treated without surgery. Two of the three patients were followed; one improved and one was unchanged. These studies, however, were neither randomized nor prospective, thereby making conclusions impossible regarding either the natural history of spinal stenosis or comparisons of results of surgical and nonsurgical treatment.

Perhaps the best natural history study to date is that of Johnsson and associates,[10] who compared outcomes of a group of 19 patients treated conservatively with 44 patients treated with surgical decompression (Table 1). The authors found that half of the nonsurgical patients still had neurogenic claudication at an average follow-up of 31 months. In the nonsurgical group, 32% reported subjective improvement (by visual analog scale), 58% were unchanged, and 10% deteriorated. In the surgical group, one third of the patients reported neurogenic claudication at an average of 53 months following surgery. Improvement was reported in 59% of these patients, 16% were unchanged, and 25% deteriorated. Results of surgery did not appear to be related to the degree of stenosis as documented by myelography. Neurophysiologic changes showed progression in almost all cases, and were not prevented by the surgery. Results of this study led to the conclusion that nonsurgical treatment produced reasonably good results

Table 1 Prospective, randomized study comparing surgical versus nonsurgical treatment of lumbar spinal stenosis[10]

	Surgical	Nonsurgical
Stenosis present	37%	53%
Improved	59%	32%
Unchanged	16%	58%
Worse	25%	10%

in one third to one half of patients, with only a 10% chance of deterioration during the 2- to 3-year follow-up period. The study results also suggested that the "decision for surgical decompression in spinal stenosis is not a neurological imperative."[10] This study, however, was neither prospective nor randomized, which made comparisons between the two groups difficult. In the absence of randomization, it is not known whether the conservatively treated patients were comparable to the surgical group.

A recent report evaluating the outcome of patients with lumbar spinal stenosis treated with aggressive nonsurgical measures suggested that such treatment could be very effective.[12] Fifty-two patients were followed for 2 to 8 years. A tolerable pain level without major restriction in daily activities and pain that was controlled with nonnarcotic analgesics was reported in 33 patients (63%); 36 patients (69%) reported "no or minimal restriction in walking tolerance,"[12] although 25 patients (48%) reported "difficulty in standing for long periods."[12] None of the patients experienced any neurologic loss. Transfer to a surgical group for presumed failure of nonsurgical measures was required by four of the 52 patients (8%). The exclusion criteria for this study, however, may have produced some element of bias because patients with preexisting disease (comorbid conditions) or with a "compliance issue that prevented participation in a therapeutic exercise program"[12] were excluded. Furthermore, because this study only included patients receiving some form of therapeutic intervention (therapeutic exercises and epidural steroids, if necessary), it was not a true natural history study. In addition, the study did not include comparison of such treatment with surgery and did not, therefore, offer any comparative data regarding optimal treatment of lumbar spinal stenosis.

Surgical Results

Surgical treatment of lumbar spinal stenosis may be broadly divided into decompressive procedures without concomitant fusion and decompression with fusion. Surgical decompression may vary from limited procedures, such as single level unilateral laminotomy for focal neural compression, to global procedures, such as multilevel bilateral laminectomy with bilateral facetectomies. Types of fusion procedures include anterior lumbar interbody fusion (ALIF), posterior lumbar interbody fusion (PLIF), posterior fusion, posterolateral (intertransverse/bilateral lateral) fusion, or combinations of these procedures. Indirect neural decompression may occur following anterior fusion if disk space distraction occurs, thereby enlarging the central or foraminal canal. Fusion may be augmented by the use of spinal instrumentation, either anterior fixation devices or posterior devices, such as those that use pedicle screw fixation.

Results of Laminectomy

Evaluation of results of an intervention, such as surgery, demands a comparison with either the results of another treatment modality or with the natural history of the untreated condition. As mentioned previously, the natural history of spinal stenosis is poorly characterized, which makes evaluation of even traditional surgical treatments such as laminectomy difficult.[10] Furthermore, a recent review of the literature on spinal stenosis surgery failed to identify even a single randomized trial comparing surgery and conservative treatment.[13] Turner and associates,[13] noting that there had been no comprehensive review of published data, reported an attempted meta-analysis of the literature on surgical outcomes of spinal stenosis. The most definitive finding of their study was the apparent poor scientific quality of the literature, which precluded the authors from conducting the intended meta-analysis. Only 74 of the 625 studies identified as potentially relevant met the inclusion criteria adopted for this study. None of the 74 studies was randomized, only three were prospectively designed, and only seven had independent ratings of outcomes. Based on data supplied in these articles, only 64% (range 26% to 100%) of patients achieved good-to-excellent outcomes at long-term follow-up. Even using the authors' own ratings, the average amount of good-to-excellent outcomes was only 72%. Turner and associates[13] found no statistically significant relationship between outcome and patient age, gender, prior back surgery, or number of levels operated on. In other reviewed articles that reported only on patients with degenerative spondylolisthesis, the reported outcome was better. An interesting finding of the study by Turner and associates[13] was that there was no statistically significant difference in outcome between decompression with or without associated fusion. This finding had also been noted in other literature surveys that reported outcome following lumbar spinal fusion that was performed for a variety of diagnoses.[14] This observation is particularly significant in light of the reported increased morbidity associated with lumbar fusion.[14]

In a large retrospective series in which the results of decompressive laminectomy for spinal stenosis were reported, Katz and associates[15] followed 88 patients for 2.8 to 6.8 years (Table 2). Outcome assessment included a questionnaire in which the patient rated outcome in terms of pain and function. The authors reported a relatively high failure rate with 11% reporting a poor outcome at 1 year and 43% reporting a poor outcome at final follow-up. Repeat lumbar surgery was performed within the first year in 6% and 17% had additional surgery by the time of the last follow-up. Risk factors for poor outcome included presurgical comorbidity and limited (single level) decompression. The authors concluded that the long-term outlook for patients who undergo decompressive laminectomy for spinal stenosis is guarded because of progressive deterioration of results over time. Because spinal stenosis is a global condition, often with diffuse degenerative changes occurring at multiple levels, the authors suggested that more extensive bone removal may be indicated at the time of surgery.

In a recent prospective and randomized study that compared outcomes of decompression with and without fusion for patients who had spinal stenosis with-

Table 2 Long-term results of laminectomy for spinal stenosis[15]

	One Year Follow-up	Final Follow-up
Poor outcome	8/74 (11%)	31/72 (43%)
Severe pain	5/74 (7%)	21/70 (30%)
Repeated surgery	5/88 (6%)	15/88 (17%)
Limited physical function	6/74 (8%)	26/74 (35%)
Walk < 15 meters	6/74 (8%)	15/70 (21%)

out associated instability, Grob and associates[16] reported no significant differences in outcome between the fused and unfused groups. Patients were randomized to one of three treatment groups: group I, decompression without arthrodesis; group II, decompression with arthrodesis of only the most stenotic segment; and group III, decompression and arthrodesis of all decompressed segments (Table 3). Overall, 78% of patients reported very good or good results and 80% of examiner-rated results were very good or good. When the results were broken down by type of procedure performed, no significant differences in outcome with regard to pain relief were indicated between the three groups. The authors concluded that surgical decompression changed the natural history of spinal stenosis, resulting in generally favorable results and improved quality of life in most patients. They further concluded that arthrodesis was not justified in the absence of radiographically proven segmental instability because there was no statistically significant difference in outcome between the three treatment groups. The authors defined such an instability as the presence of either an anterior slip that was greater than 5 mm, a rotational deformity greater than 5 mm of lateral offset, degenerative scoliosis, a spondylolysis, or whether prior lumbar spine surgery had been performed. The technique of radiography was not described, and it is therefore not known whether radiographs were taken in the standing position. It may be presumed that some patients were included who had radiographs taken in a supine position showing as much as 5 mm of anterolisthesis. If these radiographs had been taken in the standing position, the anterolisthesis may have been even more significant, suggesting that some patients may have been included who had a degree of slip that many surgeons would otherwise have elected to fuse at the time of surgery. Despite this, surgical results with decompression alone produced satisfactory results in 87% of patients.

Spinal Stenosis With Degenerative Spondylolisthesis

Introduction and Natural History

Degenerative spondylolisthesis is a condition that was first described by Junghanns in 1930 when he used the term pseudospondylolisthesis to describe the presence of forward slippage of a vertebral body in the presence of an intact neural arch.[17] The clinical and pathologic features of this entity were further defined by Macnab,[18] who described the condition as ''spondylolisthesis with an intact neural arch.'' The term degenerative spondylolisthesis was originally

Table 3 Prospective, randomized study comparing decompression with and without fusion for treatment of spinal stenosis [16]

Evaluator	Group I*	Group II*	Group III*
Patient	13/15 (87%)	12/15 (80%)	10/15 (67%)
Examiner	13/15 (87%)	12/15 (80%)	11/15 (73%)

*Number of very good and good results/total patients (%); group I = decompression without arthrodesis, group II = decompression with arthrodesis of the most stenotic segment, and group III = decompression and arthrodesis of all decompressed segments

used by Newman and Stone[19] and is the terminology most commonly used to describe the anterior slippage of one vertebral body on another in the presence of an intact neural arch.

Degenerative spondylolisthesis may be a source of both low back pain and leg pain and may contribute to radicular or referred leg pain in a characteristic pattern of neurogenic claudication. The diagnosis is typically made from examination of lateral radiographs, but there may be a dynamic component if the slip reduces in the supine position and is therefore readily apparent only on stress radiographs. These radiographs may include supine, sitting, or standing flexion–extension views; standing lateral views; or distraction-compression radiography.[20-23]

As with spinal stenosis, little is generally known about the natural history of degenerative spondylolisthesis. Until recently, the optimal surgical treatment of spinal stenosis associated with degenerative spondylolisthesis had not been known, because prospective and randomized studies comparing the various surgical options had not been done. This problem was noted by Mardjetko and associates,[24] who attempted a meta-analysis of the literature published between 1970 and 1993 in an effort to pool similar data taken from many small studies into a large sample with greater statistical power. Because of numerous design flaws in most of the 152 papers reviewed, they found that their meta-analysis of the literature was unsatisfactory. Only 25 papers, representing 889 patients, were found that satisfied their inclusion criteria. Three papers that delineated the natural history of degenerative spondylolisthesis, encompassing 278 patients, were judged to fulfill their inclusion criteria.[25-27] They found that 90 of 278 patients (32%) achieved satisfactory results without treatment, whereas 188 (68%) had unsatisfactory results, and 12 (reported in only one of the three studies) had progressive slip. The study by Matsunaga and associates[26] represents the best of the three studies and is the only true natural history study. In this study, 40 patients who received no treatment were followed for at least 5 years (range: 5 to 14 years; mean: 8.25 years). Progressive slip was noted in 12 patients (30%), although no correlation was noted between slip progression and deterioration of symptoms. Only four of 40 patients (10%) showed clinical deterioration over the course of the study; all were in the group of 28 patients showing no slip progression over the follow-up period. None of the 12 patients experiencing a progressive slip deteriorated clinically. The majority of the patients in this study, therefore, showed a slight improvement in their clinical symptoms over time.

In summary, the natural history of spinal stenosis, with or without associated degenerative spondylolisthesis, is generally favorable, with only approximately 10% of patients with either condition showing clinical deterioration.[10,26] Clinical improvement seems to occur in approximately one third to one half of patients with either of these two conditions.[10,26]

Results of Decompression Without Fusion

Surgical treatment of spinal stenosis associated with degenerative spondylolisthesis has involved either some form of decompression only or decompression with arthrodesis. In their attempted meta-analysis of the literature published between 1970 and 1993, Mardjetko and associates[24] found only 11 papers, encompassing 216 patients, that met their inclusion criteria and reported the results of decompression without fusion (Table 4). One study was retrospective and nonrandomized,[28] two were prospective and randomized,[29,30] and the remaining eight were retrospective, nonrandomized, and uncontrolled.

The paper by Feffer and associates[28] was a nonrandomized attempt to compare decompression only with decompression and fusion, using two groups of surgeons from two different institutions. A subgroup of 11 patients underwent decompression only; five patients (45%) were rated as good (satisfactory) and six patients (55%) were rated as fair/poor (unsatisfactory).

Similar results were reported in the prospective randomized study by Herkowitz and Kurz[30] that compared decompression only with combined decompression and noninstrumented fusion (Table 5). In the decompression only group, 11 of 25 patients (44%) had satisfactory results. This group of patients was found to have significantly more low back pain and leg pain than their counterparts who had undergone decompression and fusion. Furthermore, the mean slip increased from an average of 5.3 mm presurgically to 7.9 mm postsurgically.

One portion of the study conducted by Bridwell and associates[29] contained a group of nine patients who underwent decompression without fusion. Only three of the nine patients (33%) reported functional improvement and four of the nine patients (44%) were noted to have an increase in their presurgical slip at an average of 3.2 years follow-up. This was one of the few studies that reported an association between progression of slip and recurrence of symptoms with unsatisfactory outcome.

Overall, only 69% of the patients reported on in the meta-analysis by Mardjetko and associates[24] were found to have satisfactory results; 31% of patients in the nine studies in which slip progression actually was recorded showed an increase in the degree of slip. There was generally no correlation between clinical outcome and amount of slip progression except for the study by Bridwell and associates,[29] which showed a positive correlation between the two.

Results of Decompression With Noninstrumented Fusion

In their attempted meta-analysis of the literature, Mardjetko and associates[24] found only six studies meeting their inclusion criteria that reported results of decompression with fusion (Table 6). One study was retrospective and nonrandomized,[28] three were prospective and randomized,[29-31] and the remaining two were retrospective, nonrandomized, and uncontrolled. The portion of the retrospective, nonrandomized study reported by Feffer and associates[28] concerning fusion included eight patients who underwent decompression with in situ posterolateral fusion; five patients achieved satisfactory results (63%).

Table 4 Results of decompression without fusion for degenerative lumbar spondylolisthesis: Meta-analysis of literature 1970 to 1993 (11 articles)[24]

Total No. of Patients	Satisfactory	Unsatisfactory	Progressive Slip
216	140 (69%)*	75 (31%)*	67 (31%)†

*Weighted pooled proportion

†Reported in only nine of 11 articles

Table 5 Prospective, randomized comparison of decompression versus decompression and noninstrumented spinal fusion for degenerative spondylolisthesis[30]

Result	Arthrodesis (No. = 25)	No Arthrodesis (No. = 25)
Excellent	11 (44%)	2 (8%)
Good	13 (52%)	9 (36%)
Fair	1 (4%)	12 (48%)
Poor	0 (0%)	2 (8%)
Mean increase in slip (presurgical to postsurgical)	0.5 mm	2.6 mm ($p = 0.002$)

Table 6 Results of decompression with noninstrumented fusion: Meta-analysis of literature 1970 to 1993 (six articles)[24]

Total No. of Patients	Satisfactory	Unsatisfactory	Fusion
84	59 (79%)*†	16 (21%)*†	62 (86%)

*Weighted pooled proportion
†Data from five of six articles reported

Herkowitz and Kurz[30] reported superior results in their prospective and randomized study that compared decompression only to decompression and noninstrumented spinal fusion in the treatment of L3-4 and L4-5 degenerative spondylolisthesis with spinal stenosis, when concomitant fusion was performed with the decompression (Table 5). This study reported 44% excellent and 52% good results (96% excellent/good total) in the arthrodesis group and only 8% excellent and 36% good (44% excellent/good total) in the nonarthrodesis group ($p = 0.0001$). Outcome was not influenced by either the age or sex of the patient or the presurgical height of the disk space. There was a significant increase in the presurgical slip in patients who did not receive an arthrodesis compared to those who underwent fusion ($p = 0.002$). Of those who underwent arthrodesis, 36% were noted to have a pseudarthrosis; all had either an excellent or good result. The authors concluded that the results of surgical decompression with in situ arthrodesis are superior to those of decompression only in the treatment of spinal stenosis associated with L3-4 or L4-5 degenerative spondylolisthesis. The authors further concluded that the decision for concomitant arthrodesis should be based solely on the presence or absence of a presurgical slip rather than on other presurgical factors. These other factors may include the age or sex of the patient, the disk height, or intraoperative factors, such as the amount of bone resected during the decompression.

The prospective randomized study by Bridwell and associates[29] included a subgroup of 11 patients who underwent decompression and noninstrumented fusion. Of the ten patients available for follow-up, only three (30%) reported improved functional outcome and seven (70%) reported an increase in their presurgical spondylolisthesis.

In a prospective and randomized study of 124 patients who underwent either instrumented or noninstrumented fusion, for a variety of diagnoses, Zdeblick[31] reported radiographic fusion in 65% of the noninstrumented group, and 77% of the semirigid fixation group and 95% of the rigid fixation group fused. When only patients with degenerative spondylolisthesis were considered, 65% of the noninstrumented patients fused, compared with 50% of the semirigid fixation group and 86% of the rigid fixation group.

Subsequent studies have confirmed the superior results obtained when arthrodesis accompanies decompression for spinal stenosis associated with degenerative spondylolisthesis.[15,32,33] Postacchini and Cinotti[33] reported on the relationship between bone regrowth that occurred an average of 8.6 years after surgical decompression for spinal stenosis and long-term outcome. In general, results were satisfactory in patients with mild or no bone regrowth and were less satisfactory in patients with moderate or marked bone regrowth. Sixteen of 40 patients had degenerative spondylolisthesis, and ten of the 16 had concomitant arthrodesis. Although all 16 patients with degenerative spondylolisthesis showed some bone regrowth, there was a greater degree of bone regrowth in the six patients who did not undergo arthrodesis than in the ten patients who were fused (Table 7). Furthermore, there was a significantly higher proportion of good results in the patients who had spinal fusion. Although this study was nonrandomized and retrospective, it suggested that arthrodesis stabilizes the spine, resulting in less bone regrowth and superior long-term results.

Caputy and Luessenhop[32] reported on a retrospective review of 96 patients who underwent decompressive surgery for spinal stenosis and who were followed for at least 5 years. Although the study was retrospective, nonrandomized, and uncontrolled, and the results in the subset of patients with associated degenerative spondylolisthesis were not fully analyzed separately, the authors noted some important trends. Surgery was considered a failure in 16 patients because of recurrent neural involvement and in an additional ten patients because of low back pain (total number of failures, 26). Degenerative spondylolisthesis occurred in 12 of the 26 patients (46%) in whom the surgery failed, a higher incidence than in the 16 of 64 patients (25%) in whom surgery was considered a success. The authors concluded that because of the higher incidence of recurrent symptoms in patients with preexisting degenerative spondylolisthesis, all patients with associated slip should be fused.

Results of Anterior Spinal Fusion

Mardjetko and associates[24] identified three papers that reported the results of anterior spinal fusion in their meta-analysis.[34-36] All three reports were retrospective and nonrandomized. In the report by Satomi and associates,[36] 27 patients treated with ALIF were compared with 14 patients treated by posterior

Table 7   Relationship between outcome and fusion in patients with degenerative spondylolisthesis[33]

	No. of Patients	Excellent	Good	Fair	Poor
Fusion	10	3	5	2	0
No fusion	6	0	2	1	3

decompression, with or without fusion. Follow-up was 3 years. The authors used the Japanese Orthopaedic Association clinical evaluation as a guide to measure the degree of recovery, and found the ALIF group averaged 77% success, and the posterior surgery group averaged only 56%. Those patients treated with ALIF had 93% satisfactory results in self-reported symptoms compared to only 72% of patients in the posterior surgery group. Conclusions regarding optimum treatment were not possible from this nonrandomized study because results of the various types of posterior surgery were not described. Nevertheless, this study did suggest excellent results with anterior surgical stabilization.

The study by Takahashi and associates[35] reported an average 12.5-year follow-up of 39 patients who underwent anterior decompression and interbody fusion for degenerative spondylolisthesis. Clinical evaluation revealed that 76% of patients had satisfactory results for 10 years, 60% for 20 years, and 52% for 30 years. When the results were broken down by the age at which surgery was performed, they revealed that all patients who underwent surgery in their 30s maintained excellent results for 25 years; 80% of those who had surgery in their 40s maintained satisfactory results for up to 16 years; and 73% of those who underwent surgery in their 50s maintained good results for up to 10 years. Only 57% of patients who underwent surgery beyond 60 years of age, however, showed satisfactory results.

Results from the study by Kim and associates[36] are included in the results of the pooled data from the three papers reported in the meta-analysis, which revealed an overall satisfaction rate of 86%, with a fusion rate of 94%.[24] Because randomized studies are not available, no meaningful comparative data can be derived regarding the optimal role of anterior fusion in the treatment of degenerative spondylolisthesis.

Conclusion

A knowledge of the natural history of the untreated condition is required in order to evaluate the results of a treatment. In addition, the evaluation should involve comparison with other treatments in order to make meaningful recommendations regarding the optimal treatment of the condition. In the case of spinal stenosis, either with or without degenerative spondylolisthesis, the natural history of the untreated condition is not completely understood because of the lack of long-term studies.[10,24,26] Furthermore, there are few controlled prospective randomized studies that compare different treatments for these conditions.[29-31] The generally poor quality of the literature that deals with the treatment of both spinal stenosis and degenerative spondylolisthesis and the role of fusion in the treatment of spinal conditions has been summarized and reviewed.[13,14,24]

The available data suggest that the natural history of both spinal stenosis, as well as spinal stenosis associated with degenerative spondylolisthesis, is characterized by improvement in approximately 32% of patients and deterioration in approximately 10%. Approximately 50% to 70% of patients have a generally static clinical course over time with little, if any, improvement.[10,26]

There seems to be little data to support the routine use of arthrodesis in the surgical treatment of spinal stenosis that is not associated with degenerative spondylolisthesis. It is not known which, if any, subgroup of patients might benefit from concomitant fusion. Some surgeons would consider the addition of arthrodesis when decompression has been excessive or extensive, either by excessive bone removal or by the extensive number of levels decompressed. Unfortunately, no prospective randomized studies addressing this issue have been performed.

There seems to be support for the concept that the treatment of spinal stenosis with associated degenerative spondylolisthesis should involve decompression with concomitant arthrodesis.[28-30] Unfortunately, there is not a widespread consensus regarding what exactly constitutes enough radiographic "instability" to warrant the addition of spinal fusion.[20-23] Furthermore, the proper role for augmentation of fusion with spinal instrumentation is unknown because there are few prospective randomized studies.[29,31] Finally, the role of bone graft substitutes in the future is only now evolving. Virtually all of the studies cited above have used autogenous bone graft for arthrodesis.

At the time of this writing, bone screws placed posteriorly into vertebral elements have not been cleared for use in this specific manner by the Food and Drug Administration (FDA). These are Class III devices. This category includes screws placed transfacetally, within pedicles, or in articular, lateral masses. Some bone screws for use within the sacrum have been approved as Class II devices. Some companies have received Class II clearance for use of screws in lumbar pedicles specifically to supplement fusions in the treatment of grade III and IV spondylolisthesis with the proviso that these devices are removed after the arthrodesis has healed. Anterior vertebral body screws (cervical, thoracic, and lumbar) are Class II devices and can be used as labeled in vertebral bodies. Many of the posterior screw-based devices have been shown in laboratory and clinical testing to be useful and may be used in an off-label manner if the physician feels this is appropriate and important for the treatment of the patient. As with all surgeries, informed consent should explain the procedure and why a particular technique has been chosen, as well as its risks and benefits. The question of whether informed consent regarding pedicle screws must include a discussion of the device's FDA clearance status is currently being litigated in several jurisdictions. In cases that have been included in the multidistrict litigation in the Eastern District of Pennsylvania, this additional requirement has not been imposed.

References

1. Sachs B, Fraenkel J: Progressive ankylotic rigidity of the spine (spondylose rhizomelique). *J Nerve Ment Dis* 1900;27:1–15.
2. Bailey P, Casamajor L: Osteo-arthritis of the spine as a cause of compression of the spinal cord and its roots, with reports of five cases. *J Nerv Ment Dis* 1911;38:588–609.
3. Sarpyener MA: Congenital stricture of the spinal canal. *J Bone Joint Surg* 1945;27:70–79.
4. van Gelderen C: Ein orthotisches (lordotisches) Kaudasyndrom. *Acta Psychiatr Neurol* 1948;23:57–68.
5. Verbiest H: A radicular syndrome from developmental narrowing of the lumbar vertebral canal. *J Bone Joint Surg* 1954;36B:230–237.
6. Kirkaldy-Willis WH, Paine KW, Cauchoix J, et al: Lumbar spinal stenosis. *Clin Orthop* 1974;99:30–50.
7. Arnoldi CC, Brodsky AE, Cauchoix J, et al: Lumbar spinal stenosis and nerve root entrapment syndromes: Definition and classification. *Clin Orthop* 1976;115:4–5.
8. Blau JN, Logue V: Intermittent claudication of the cauda equina: An unusual syndrome resulting from central protrusion of a lumbar intervertebral disc. *Lancet* 1961;1:1081–1086.

9. Hawkes CH, Roberts GM: Lumbar canal stenosis. *Br J Hosp Med* 1980;23:498,500,502–503.

10. Johnsson KE, Uden A, Rosen I: The effect of decompression on the natural course of spinal stenosis: A comparison of surgically treated and untreated patients. *Spine* 1991;16:615–619.

11. Jones RA, Thomson JL: The narrow lumbar canal: A clinical and radiological review. *J Bone Joint Surg* 1968;50B:595–605.

12. Tile M, McNeil SR, Zarins RK, et al: Spinal stenosis: Results of treatment. *Clin Orthop* 1976;115:104–108.

13. Turner JA, Ersek M, Herron L, et al: Surgery for lumbar spinal stenosis: Attempted meta-analysis of the literature. *Spine* 1992;17:1–8.

14. Turner JA, Ersek M, Herron L, et al: Patient outcomes after lumbar spinal fusions. *JAMA* 1992;268:907–911.

15. Katz JN, Lipson SJ, Larson MG, et al: The outcome of decompressive laminectomy for degenerative lumbar stenosis. *J Bone Joint Surg* 1991;73A:809–816.

16. Grob D, Humke T, Dvorak J: Degenerative lumbar spinal stenosis: Decompression with and without arthrodesis. *J Bone Joint Surg* 1995;77A:1036–1041.

17. Junghanns H: Spondylolisthesen ohne Spalt im Zwischengelenkstück ('Pseudospondylolisthesen'). *Arch Fuer Orthop* 1930;29:118–127.

18. Macnab I: Spondylolisthesis with an intact neural arch: The so-called pseudo-spondylolisthesis. *J Bone Joint Surg* 1950;32B:325–333.

19. Newman PH, Stone KH: The etiology of spondylolisthesis. *J Bone Joint Surg* 1963;45B:39–59.

20. Boden SD, Wiesel SW: Lumbosacral segmental motion in normal individuals: Have we been measuring instability properly? *Spine* 1990;15:571–576.

21. Friberg O: Lumbar instability: A dynamic approach by traction-compression radiography. *Spine* 1987;12:119–129.

22. Hayes MA, Howard TC, Gruel CR, et al: Roentgenographic evaluation of lumbar spine flexion-extension in asymptomatic individuals. *Spine* 1989;14:327–331.

23. Nachemson AL: Instability of the lumbar spine: Pathology, treatment, and clinical evaluation. *Neurosurg Clin N Am* 1991;2:785–790.

24. Mardjetko SM, Connolly PJ, Shott S: Degenerative lumbar spondylolisthesis: A meta-analysis of literature, 1970–1993. *Spine* 1994;19(suppl 20):2256S–2265S.

25. Fitzgerald JA, Newman PH: Degenerative spondylolisthesis. *J Bone Joint Surg* 1976;58B:184–192.

26. Matsunaga S, Sakou T, Morizono Y, et al: Natural history of degenerative spondylolisthesis: Pathogenesis and natural course of the slippage. *Spine* 1990;15:1204–1210.

27. Rosenberg NJ: Degenerative spondylolisthesis: Surgical treatment. *Clin Orthop* 1976;117:112–120.

28. Feffer HL, Wiesel SW, Cuckler JM, et al: Degenerative spondylolisthesis: To fuse or not to fuse. *Spine* 1985;10:287–289.

29. Bridwell KH, Sedgewick TA, O'Brien MF, et al: The role of fusion and instrumentation in the treatment of degenerative spondylolisthesis with spinal stenosis. *J Spinal Disord* 1993;6:461–472.

30. Herkowitz HN, Kurz LT: Degenerative lumbar spondylolisthesis with spinal stenosis: A prospective study comparing decompression with decompression and intertransverse process arthrodesis. *J Bone Joint Surg* 1991;73A:802–808.

31. Zdeblick TA: A prospective, randomized study of lumbar fusion: Preliminary results. *Spine* 1993;18:983–991.

32. Caputy AJ, Luessenhop AJ: Long-term evaluation of decompressive surgery for degenerative lumbar stenosis. *J Neurosurg* 1992;77:669–676.

33. Postacchini F, Cinotti G: Bone regrowth after surgical decompression for lumbar spinal stenosis. *J Bone Joint Surg* 1992;74B:862–869.

34. Satomi K, Hirabayashi K, Toyama Y, et al: A clinical study of degenerative spondylolisthesis: Radiographic analysis and choice of treatment. *Spine* 1992;17:1329–1336.

35. Takahashi K, Kitahara H, Yamagata M, et al: Long-term results of anterior interbody fusion for treatment of degenerative spondylolisthesis. *Spine* 1990;15:1211–1215. *J Bone Joint Surg* 1968;50B:595–605.
36. Kim NH, Kim HK, Suh JS: A computed tomographic analysis of changes in the spinal canal after anterior lumbar interbody fusion. *Clin Orthop* 1993;286:180–191.

Chapter 40

Degenerative Spondylolisthesis: Fusion With and Without Instrumentation

Steven R. Garfin, MD
Alexander R. Vaccaro, MD

Degenerative spondylolisthesis is a common finding in individuals who present with symptoms of spinal stenosis. If all appropriate forms of nonsurgical care do not help relieve leg pain symptoms, and the patient's quality of life is limited, surgery for the diminution of the leg pain related to the spinal stenosis/degenerative spondylolisthesis is frequently recommended and useful. The primary surgical treatment for the leg pain includes decompressive laminectomies and foraminotomies. A number of authors have demonstrated good results related to decompressive laminectomy in relieving associated leg pain.[1-16] However, when there is concurrent degenerative spondylolisthesis, laminectomies without fusion do not relieve leg pain as reliably for prolonged periods of time.[1,6,8,12,13,17-25]

In a review of 21 patients who had degenerative spondylolisthesis and underwent laminectomy for their associated sciatica, Reynolds and Wiltse[13] reported a 78% good to excellent result rate in those who had careful preservation of their facet joints and pars interarticularis. However, of the patients who underwent wide decompression with complete removal of either the facet or pars, only 33% reported good to excellent results. This difference presumably was related to a postoperative increase in slippage and motion at the degenerative spondylolisthetic segment. Johnsson and associates[21] reported their results on 45 patients who underwent laminectomy and facetectomy for symptoms of spinal stenosis. The majority of these patients had preoperative degenerative spondylolisthesis, and 40% developed increased slippage in the postoperative period. At follow-up, most of those with increased slippage had not improved, or they described increased pain (back and/or leg) after surgery.

Lombardi and associates[9] reported on a large number of patients who had surgical decompression for spinal stenosis and had degenerative spondylolisthesis. Their patients were divided into three groups according to the surgical approach. One group of patients had a wide decompression without fusion. A second group underwent decompression, as necessary, for the cauda equina nerve roots with the addition of a posterolateral fusion. A third group had a limited decompression, with careful attention to preservation of the pars and facets. In the first group (wide decompression without fusion), only 33% reported good to excellent results. In the second group (similar decompression with fusion),

90% reported good to excellent results in relief of leg pain and diminution in back pain. Fewer patients reported good to excellent results when the operation was more meticulous in terms of preservation of the pars and facets, but in the process, may have been less complete in relieving any lateral nerve root compression. Feffer and associates[18] reviewed a series of patients who underwent surgery for leg pain related to degenerative spondylolisthesis. Some of these patients had fusion, and others did not. The good to excellent results strongly favored the addition of a fusion when there was concurrent degenerative spondylolisthesis (Table 1).

A number of other authors have reported similar results.[1,2,9,18,20,26-36] In patients who specifically had a preoperative degenerative spondylolisthesis or "instability" noted on flexion–extension films, usually at the L4-5 level, the addition of a fusion improved the surgical results, particularly over the long term.[1,2,9,26,30,32] Herkowitz and Kurz[20] performed a prospective, controlled, randomized study in which they evaluated patients who underwent one-level decompression at the level of degenerative spondylolisthesis. One group of patients had concomitant noninstrumented fusion and one group had no fusion. Those with a fusion reported 96% good to excellent results at greater than 2-year follow-up. Only 44% of those patients who had a decompression without fusion described good to excellent results at follow-up. The majority of those patients who had poor results, and did not have a concomitant fusion, were noted to have an increased slippage postoperatively at the level of spondylolisthesis. At 2-year follow-up, 33% of the fused patients radiographically demonstrated nonunions, but this finding did not appear to affect their overall results, at least at this point in time.

In addition to the information described, many of the studies listed above, as well as others, have demonstrated an increased slippage postoperatively after decompression without fusion was performed in patients in whom there was a preexisting degenerative spondylolisthesis (particularly early or low grade).[3,20,21,37-41] In general, these patients were associated with results that were less good than results for patients in whom a fusion was added.

It is important to note that at the time that the bone graft is placed in the posterolateral gutters stability is not created. In fact, if a facet fusion is performed there is short-term increased instability created by denuding the capsules and

Table 1 Results of literature review of surgical cases with degenerative spondylolisthesis

Type of Surgery (References)	Patients	Satisfactory	↑ Slip	Fusion
Decompression without fusion[1,2,7-9,12,14,17,18,20,21,26]	216	60%	31%	
Decompression with fusion[7,9,12,17,18,20,32]	84	70%	16%	73%
Decompression with fusion with segmental fixation[17,26-28,31]	101	74%		91%

(Adapted with permission from Mardjetko SM, Connolly PJ, Shott S: Degenerative spondylolisthesis: A meta analysis of literature 1970–1993. *Spine* 1994;19(suppl 20):2256S–2265S.)

placing bone graft in that position, as reported by Boden and associates[42] for an animal model. This result suggests that if stabilization can be performed while the fusion progresses to the point of arthrodesis, the likelihood of good to excellent long-term results may be improved. Admittedly, it may be difficult to exceed the 96% mark noted by Herkowitz and Kurz[20] and the 90% success rate of others who have reported their clinical results following in situ fusions for degenerative spondylolisthesis. The majority of these were either retrospective or reviewed at 2-year follow-up. It has been reported in long-term follow-up studies of patients surgically treated for spinal stenosis that patients note increased symptoms over time (years).[6,9,14,24,43,44] If increased slippage during the time span during which arthrodesis is developing can be minimized, this step may decrease the risk of recurrence. In addition, if a more anatomic alignment can be obtained/maintained and/or lordosis created in the lumbar spine, the potential exists to retard symptoms developing from levels adjacent to a solid fusion.

Advantages of internal, segmental fixation in achieving a spinal fusion include increased rigidity supplied by instrumentation, and enhanced ability to obtain a solid fusion of the lumbar spine. These advantages are similar to the benefits observed in the treatment of long-bone fractures with rigid fixation.[45-63] A number of retrospective studies in the literature support this. Although all studies do not specifically relate to degenerative spondylolisthesis, rigid spinal instrumentation, similar to increased rigid fixation in the treatment of long-bone fractures, is strongly associated with an increased fusion rate.

Kaneda and associates[35] reported on a series of patients who were surgically treated for symptoms of spinal stenosis with the underlying diagnosis of degenerative spondylolisthesis. They reported on 54 consecutive patients who underwent wide decompressions with medial facetectomies. In addition to the decompression, fusions were performed and supplemented with distraction/ compression instrumentation constructs. Twenty-five patients underwent a two or more level decompression and fusion. There were no reported patients who had an increased slip (angle or degree). Only 4% were found to have radiographic evidence of pseudarthrosis. Kaneda and associates[35] reported that their patients had a 96% good to excellent result in terms of relief of leg pain.

Kostuik and associates[64] reported an 86% incidence of union with the addition of Luque rods with sublaminar wiring for multilevel fusions. This result is similar to that reported by Luque[65] in his original series describing the utility of segmental instrumentation to supplement and obtain a fusion in lumbosacral procedures for pain related to degenerative conditions. A number of authors with other techniques have reported similar results. The results are fairly consistent, whether using simple, nonmechanically rigid fixation techniques, such as spinous process plates and screws, or progressing sequentially through segmental fixation with hooks and rods, to sublaminar wires, to rigidly fixed bone screws placed in the pedicles of the spine.

Zdeblick[32] reported on a prospective study of 124 patients who underwent limited segmental spinal fusions. Three groups were entered into the study. One group had an in situ fusion, one had fusion supplemented with semirigid, pedicle screw-based instrumentation, and a third group underwent a fusion supplemented by rigid, segmental pedicle screw-based fixation. The degree of clinical success in achieving relief of pain as well as radiographic evidence of fusion

679

increased progressively through the three groups. The third group, with rigid fixation, had the highest rate of clinical as well as radiographic success. At an average follow-up of 16 months, 64 patients in the in situ fusion group had a successful fusion, with 71% reporting good to excellent clinical results. Patients treated with semirigid fixation to enhance their fusion achieved successful arthrodesis 77% of the time, with 87% reporting good to excellent results. In the last group, those stabilized with rigid internal fixation, 95% reported good to excellent clinical results and, radiographically, 95% were determined to have a solid fusion.

All of this information, as well as studies using animal models, suggest the importance of rigid internal fixation in assisting the surgeon and patient in obtaining a solid lumbosacral fusion.[46-58,60-66] As with the surgical stabilization of long-bone injuries, in addition to providing rigid fixation, instrumentation provides the ability to (1) better align the lumbar spine, (2) regain or maintain lumbar lordosis, (3) close gaps, and (4) place the spine in compression, which enhances the ability to obtain a fusion. Additionally, vascular ingrowth may be enhanced with rigid stabilization because there is diminution in motion. In terms of comfort for the patient, the need for external support is reduced in many cases because internal stability has been achieved.

McAfee and associates[66] have demonstrated in animal models the increased rate of union in bone grafts supplemented with rigid internal fixation. There is an associated stress shielding effect by the metal, but the radiographic and histologic results in terms of a solid fusion are markedly improved with rigid internal fixation. Similar studies have been reported by a number of authors when comparing groups of patients with instrumentation supplementing bone grafting and helping obtain a solid fusion. Ransom and associates[67] reported a high union rate in patients treated with pedicle screw and plate fixation for multilevel spinal fusions. In a similar group of patients operated on by the same authors, only a 36% fusion rate was obtained for patients treated with Luque rods and sublaminar wires and only a 15% rate for those treated with an in situ fusion.

Grubb and Lipscomb[19] reported a 35% radiographic pseudarthrosis rate in patients who underwent a posterolateral fusion without instrumentation, compared to a 6% pseudarthrosis rate for those treated with rigid internal fixation consisting of sublaminar wires affixed to a U rod. Significantly, the patients with a solid fusion reported higher functional levels and less pain than those with evidence of a nonunion. Lorenz and associates[68] evaluated patients who underwent fusion without instrumentation and those fused with instrumentation for the primary diagnosis of lumbar degenerative disk disease. All patients with a rigid screw plate construct had solid fusion, and 80% had improvement in pain and function. This could be compared to a 20% pseudarthrosis rate reported by the same authors in the patients who underwent fusion without instrumentation. The noninstrumented group reported only a 50% decrease in pain, and only 50% returned to work compared to 87% in the instrumented group.

These studies support the importance of adding rigid fixation to help obtain a solid fusion and, therefore, an improved clinical result. Rigid fixation is also important when considering that the ability to physiologically unite bone in the lumbar spine can take from 3 to 6 months, or longer. In that time frame increased subluxation can occur, because there is a race between further progression of deformity and solidification of the arthrodesis. Rigid fixation helps maintain alignment and control the spine, allowing the fusion to succeed before translation increases.

Despite all this supporting information, it still has not been unequivocally proven that it is helpful to use instrumentation to supplement a fusion for patients undergoing laminectomy with degenerative spondylolisthesis. The results need to be analyzed both clinically and radiographically. Ideally, controlled, prospective, randomized studies should be used to document the efficacy of instrumentation in enhancing fusions and clinical results. These forms of studies are difficult to perform. Patients undergoing surgery, in general, request a surgeon to decide on a surgical path. Additionally, for the surgeon as well as the patient, an in situ fusion is an entirely different procedure than an instrumented procedure in terms of cost, risk, intraoperative time, blood loss, postoperative course, postoperative radiographs, risk of infection, and more. Therefore, a purely unequivocal scientific base has not been created to document the utility of instrumentation in assisting with obtaining a fusion.

However, there are a number of reports in which patients with and without instrumentation have been compared. These reports have been subjected to peer review, as well as meta-analysis. In addition, a recent study by Yuan and associates,[25] which coordinates a retrospective, cohort review of over 3,000 patients, with 314 physicians submitting data related to a one-level fusion for degenerative spondylolisthesis with and without instrumentation is available. It is extremely helpful in developing an opinion, and it provides a sound database and support for physicians and patients faced with this dilemma.

In 1994, Mardjetko and associates[22] performed a meta-analysis of the literature available from 1970 through 1993 on patients treated for degenerative lumbar spondylolisthesis (Table 1). They chose a discrete diagnosis with a clear clinical entity characterized by facet arthropathy associated with disk degeneration and subluxation of one vertebral body anterior to the subjacent one. For their analysis of the data, the null hypothesis was that posterior decompression with posterolateral spinal fusion combined with instrumentation demonstrated radiographic (fusion) and clinical success rates equivalent to those of noninstrumented decompressions and fusions. For the review, the authors analyzed all articles that gave enough description to clearly identify the clinical symptoms as pertaining primarily to leg pain (neurogenic claudication). Patients treated primarily for back pain were not included. Additionally, the authors included articles in which they could determine that the outcome of "fusion" was clearly reported at the level of the degenerative spondylolisthesis. Because of the retrospective nature of the review and the fact that many of the articles were 2 decades old, not all publications reported clinical outcome variables, such as relief of back and leg pain, function, and so forth.

Among hundreds of papers reviewed, only 25 met the authors' criteria for inclusion in the study, in terms of providing data in all areas of interest. Six of the papers were in the category of decompression with fusion without instrumentation. In these six papers, the clinical results were available on 74 patients; the majority (86%) were female. The ages ranged from 42 to 84 years. The fusion rate varied from 30% to 100%, with a mean of 86% achieving a solid fusion. In this group, 90% of the patients reported a satisfactory clinical outcome. Of the 74 patients, 14 had progressive slippage occurring while the fusion was healing. In a report by Bridwell and associates,[17] increased slippage was often

681

associated with symptoms, as occurred in many of the patients in the study by Herkowitz and Kurz.[20]

Five studies met the inclusion criteria for decompression with fusion with pedicle screws. In these papers, as with the decompression and fusion without instrumentation group, the majority were female (76%), ranging in age from 19 to 76 years. A wide variety of pedicle screw-based instrumentation systems was used. In this group, the reported fusion rate was 93%, which was not statistically significantly different from the 86% fusion rate reported in the noninstrumented group. Clinically, 86% had a satisfactory or better rating for outcome. This rating was not statistically significantly different from that of the noninstrumented, fused group.

In the reported literature, complications did occur, but were limited. The more common complications included instrumentation failure, screw breakage, screw backout, neurologic deficit, and wound infection. A total of ten complications occurred in the 101 patients reported. The majority of these were mild, did not necessarily interfere with the clinical results, and did not always lead to repeat surgery, delay in hospitalization, or any other clinical sequelae.

Yuan and associates[25] reported in 1994 on the results of an historic cohort study of pedicle screw fixation for degenerative spondylolisthesis and thoracic, lumbar, and sacral spinal fusions. This study looked at two specific diagnoses: degenerative spondylolisthesis and thoracic and lumbar fractures. These diagnoses were assessed in terms of the efficacy and safety of pedicle screw fixation devices. However, important information related to the clinical outcome of degenerative spondylolisthesis treated with laminectomy and instrumented fusions can be gleaned from this study.

Surgeons throughout the world (although primarily the United States) were asked to review their cases of degenerative spondylolisthesis treated with laminectomy and fusion or laminectomy and instrumented fusion from January 1990 through December 1991. A formalized questionnaire was filled in by the treating physicians and data were analyzed by an independent organization. All surgeons submitted all consecutive cases of patients with degenerative spondylolisthesis operated on for leg symptoms related to this condition over the 2-year period. This procedure allowed comparison of noninstrumented, as well as instrumented, cases. In addition, an independent audit was performed to determine the validity of the study with random assessment of a number of reporting physicians' data, compared to the forms they submitted.

Of the 2,684 patients with degenerative spondylolisthesis reported and included in this study, 2,177 were treated with pedicle screw fixations for this disorder. A majority of the patients in the noninstrumented fusion group were older than 65 years of age, whereas only 35% of the pedicle screw fixation group were older than 65 years. The majority of both groups were older than 45 years of age. In both groups, as is common for this diagnosis, there were more females: 62.5% in the pedicle screw fixation group and 69% in the noninstrumented fusion group. In both groups, more than 60% of the patients were nonsmokers. Individuals whose fusions were supplemented with pedicle screw-based instrumentation had a higher percentage of fusion (89%) radiographically than the noninstrumented group (70.4%). For individuals treated with the pedicle screw-based instrumentation, the median time to fusion was approximately 10.5 ± 0.2 months, whereas the noninstrumented group took 13.1 ± 0.8 months to be considered healed radiographically. Clinical outcomes appeared to be enhanced by rigid spinal instrumentation. More patients in the pedicle screw group than in the noninstrumented fusion group demonstrated improvement in neurologic status. More than 90% in the pedicle screw group reported an improved activity level, while greater than 86% in the noninstrumented fusion group had functional improvement. Back and leg pain improved in both groups, with the pedicle screw-based fusion group having a higher level of success (91.5% compared to 84%). Those in the pedicle screw-based group who noted improvement had a fairly consistent result, independent of time from surgery. Conversely, the percentage of patients improving in their back and/or leg pain following noninstrumented fusions tended to drop off as the time from surgery increased.

There are, however, complications related to instrumentation that are not present in noninstrumented fusions (Table 2). The intraoperative events reported in this historic cohort study included pedicle fracture, screw breakout, loss of purchase, implant breakage, nerve root injury, vascular injury, dural tear from a screw, and a few other isolated events. These total approximately 5% of the 2,177 cases. Postoperative complications included instrumentation failure, screw loosening, infection, new radicular pain, and a few other minor events. The postoperative complication rate is unquestionably higher in terms of metal–bone failure when comparing the pedicle screw results to those of the noninstrumented fusion. However, reported complications in the noninstrumented fusion group of patients in terms of infection, postoperative neurologic pain or dysfunction, vascular injury, and associated other injuries were similar to those in the instrumented group.

The results from this study, combined with the meta-analysis of the reported literature review performed by Mardjetko and associates[22] demonstrate the safety, effectiveness, and utility of using internal fixation to supplement fusions

Table 2 Complications of fusion*

	In Situ	Instrumented
Infection	<	
Dural tear	=	
Nerve root injury	=	
Nonunion	>	
Vascular injury	=	
Long-term symptom deterioration	>	
Reoperation[†]	=	
Instrumentation failure	NA	
Pedicle fracture	NA	
Hardware prominence	NA	
Neurovascular injury for screw	NA	

*<: complication rates are less on the closed end of the arrow; =: complication rates are equal in both treatment groups; >: complication rates are higher on the open end of the arrow; NA = not applicable (these complications do not occur when no instrumentation is used)
[†]The reoperation rate in the in situ complications for pseudarthrosis equals the rate in instrumented fusion to remove the metal.

in the treatment of patients undergoing laminectomies to relieve their leg pain related to degenerative spondylolisthesis. Although most of the above listed studies are not prospective (unlike those of Zdeblick[32] and Bridwell and associates[17]), the trends are clear and reproducible throughout the literature.

Patients who undergo surgery for relief of leg pain related to degenerative spondylolisthesis have a better clinical result when segmental stabilization is performed along with a fusion. The rate of achieving posterolateral spinal fusion is enhanced by the addition of spinal instrumentation. Device-related complications do occur, but for the most part are relatively minimal compared to the enhancement of radiographic and, more significantly, clinical success with the use of these techniques. Rigid internal fixation, particularly as now available through pedicle screw-based systems, advances the ability to achieve three-column spinal control and to restore and maintain spinal alignment. The fusion rate is enhanced, which thereby improves the clinical outcome.

Complications, as with any procedure, can occur. If postoperative infection develops with the instrumentation in place, the recommended treatment is to try to leave the instrumentation and graft in place. In addition to parenteral antibiotics, incision, drainage, and wound closure over tubes can usually salvage the original procedure. In general, 6 weeks of systemic antibiotics, followed by oral antibiotics for a period of time, is useful. If neural intravenous injury occurs postoperatively, particularly hyperalgesia, a computed tomography scan should be performed. If there is evidence that a pedicle screw is not properly placed within the pedicle and the symptoms cannot be tolerated by the patient, the screws should be removed and/or replaced. If late in the course, metal failure occurs through failure or pull out from the bone, pseudarthrosis most likely has developed. In this case, elective scheduling for re-exploration, removal of the metal, refusion, and reinstrumentation, if indicated, should be considered. If the screw fractures within the pedicle and cannot easily be retrieved, the options are to leave the broken portion buried within the vertebrae or to burr down the bone of the pedicle to allow access to the broken screw for removal. The latter, however, usually is not necessary. One common complication associated with segmental fixation is local prominence and discomfort over the metal. Once the fusion is healed, if the metal is prominent deep to the muscle and/or subcutaneous tissues, and it creates localized discomfort, removal of the metal may decrease some of the patient's postoperative pain. Routine removal of metal is not necessary, or indicated.

At the time of this writing, bone screws placed posteriorly into vertebral elements have not been cleared for use in this specific manner by the Food and Drug Administration (FDA). These are Class III devices. This category includes screws placed transfacetally, within pedicles, or in articular, lateral masses. Some bone screws for use within the sacrum have been approved as Class II devices. Some companies have received Class II clearance for use of screws in lumbar pedicles specifically to supplement fusions in the treatment of grade III and IV spondylolisthesis with the proviso that these devices are removed after the arthrodesis has healed. Anterior vertebral body screws (cervical, thoracic, and lumbar) are Class II devices and can be used as labeled in vertebral bodies. Many of the posterior screw-based devices have been shown in laboratory and clinical testing to be useful and may be used in an off-label manner if the physician feels this is appropriate and important for the treatment of the patient. As with all surgeries, informed consent should explain the procedure and why a particular technique has been chosen, as well as its risks and benefits. The question of whether informed consent regarding pedicle screws must include a discussion of the device's FDA clearance status is currently being litigated in several jurisdictions. In cases that have been included in the multidistrict litigation in the Eastern District of Pennsylvania, this additional requirement has not been imposed.

References

1. Caputy AJ, Luessenhop AJ: Long-term evaluation of decompressive surgery for degenerative lumbar stenosis. *J Neurosurg* 1992;77:669–676.
2. Dall BE, Rowe DE: Degenerative spondylolisthesis: Its surgical management. *Spine* 1985;10:668–672.
3. Fitzgerald JA, Newman PH: Degenerative spondylolisthesis. *J Bone Joint Surg* 1976;58B:184–192.
4. Garfin SR, Glover M, Booth RE, et al: Laminectomy: A review of the Pennsylvania hospital experience. *J Spinal Disord* 1988;1:116–133.
5. Herkowitz HN, Garfin SR: Decompressive surgery for spinal stenosis. *Semin Spine Surg* 1989;1:163–167.
6. Herno A, Airaksinen O, Saari T: Long-term results of surgical treatment of lumbar spinal stenosis. *Spine* 1993;18:1471–1474.
7. Herron LD, Trippi AC: L4-5 degenerative spondylolisthesis: The results of treatment by decompressive laminectomy without fusion. *Spine* 1989;14:534–538.
8. Jonsson B, Stromqvist B: Decompression for lateral lumbar stenosis: Results and impact on sick leave and working conditions. *Spine* 1994;19:2381–2386.
9. Lombardi JS, Wiltse LL, Reynolds J, et al: Treatment of degenerative spondylolisthesis. *Spine* 1985;10:821–827.
10. Onel D, Sari H, Donmez C: Lumbar spinal stenosis: Clinical, radiologic, and therapeutic evaluation in 145 patients: Conservative treatment or surgical intervention? *Spine* 1993;18:291–298.
11. Paine KW: Results of decompression for lumbar spinal stenosis. *Clin Orthop* 1976;115:96–100.
12. Postacchini F, Cinotti G, Perugia D, et al: The surgical treatment of central lumbar stenosis: Multiple laminotomy compared with total laminectomy. *J Bone Joint Surg* 1993;75B:386–392.
13. Reynolds JB, Wiltse LL: Abstract: Surgical treatment of degenerative spondylolisthesis. *Spine* 1979;4:148–149.
14. Sanderson PL, Wood PL: Surgery for lumbar spinal stenosis in old people. *J Bone Joint Surg* 1993;75B:393–397.
15. Spengler DM: Degenerative stenosis of the lumbar spine. *J Bone Joint Surg* 1987;69A:305–308.
16. Tile M, McNeil SR, Zarins RK, et al: Spinal stenosis: Results of treatment. *Clin Orthop* 1976;115:104–108.
17. Bridwell KH, Sedgewick TA, O'Brien MF, et al: The role of fusion and instrumentation in the treatment of degenerative spondylolisthesis with spinal stenosis. *J Spinal Disord* 1993;6:461–472.
18. Feffer HL, Wiesel SW, Cuckler JM, et al: Degenerative spondylolisthesis: To fuse or not to fuse. *Spine* 1985;10:287–289.
19. Grubb SA, Lipscomb HJ: Results of lumbosacral fusion for degenerative disc disease with and without instrumentation: Two- to five-year follow-up. *Spine* 1992;17:349–355.
20. Herkowitz HN, Kurz LT: Degenerative lumbar spondylolisthesis with spinal stenosis: A prospective study comparing decompression with decompression and intertransverse process arthrodesis. *J Bone Joint Surg* 1991;73A:802–808.
21. Johnsson KE, Willner S, Johnsson K: Postoperative instability after decompression for lumbar spinal stenosis. *Spine* 1986;11:107–110.
22. Mardjetko SM, Connolly PJ, Shott S: Degenerative lumbar spondylolisthesis: A meta-analysis of literature 1970–1993. *Spine* 1994;19(suppl 20):2256S–2265S.

23. Soini J, Laine T, Pohjolainen T, et al: Spondylodesis augmented by transpedicular fixation in the treatment of olisthetic and degenerative conditions of the lumbar spine. *Clin Orthop* 1993;297:111–116.

24. Turner JA, Ersek M, Herron L, et al: Surgery for lumbar spinal stenosis: Attempted meta-analysis of the literature. *Spine* 1992;17:1–8.

25. Yuan HA, Garfin SR, Dickman CA, et al: A historical cohort study of pedicle screw fixation in thoracic, lumbar, and sacral spinal fusions. *Spine* 1994;19(suppl 20):2279S–2296S.

26. Simmons EH, Capicotto WN: Posterior transpedicular Zielke instrumentation of the lumbar spine. *Clin Orthop* 1988;236:180–191.

27. Cauchoix J, Benoist M, Chassaing V: Degenerative spondylolisthesis. *Clin Orthop* 1976;115:122–129.

28. Chang KW, McAfee PC: Degenerative spondylolisthesis and degenerative scoliosis treated with a combination segmental rod-plate and transpedicular screw instrumentation system: A preliminary report. *J Spinal Disord* 1988;1:247–256.

29. Hirabayashi S, Kumano K, Kuroki T: Cotrel-Dubousset pedicle screw system for various spinal disorders: Merits and problems. *Spine* 1991;16:1298–1304.

30. Postacchini F, Cinotti G: Bone regrowth after surgical decompression for lumbar spinal stenosis. *J Bone Joint Surg* 1992;74B:862–869.

31. Garfin SR, Ozanne S: Spinal pedicle fixation, in Weinstein JN (ed): *Clinical Efficacy and Outcome in the Diagnosis and Treatment of Low Back Pain*. New York, NY, Raven Press, 1992, pp 137–174.

32. Zdeblick TA: A prospective, randomized study of lumbar fusion: Preliminary results. *Spine* 1993;18:983–991.

33. Fujiya M, Saita M, Kaneda K, et al: Clinical study on stability of combined distraction and compression rod instrumentation with posterolateral fusion for unstable degenerative spondylolisthesis. *Spine* 1990;15:1216–1222.

34. Hanley EN Jr: Decompression and distraction-derotation arthrodesis for degenerative spondylolisthesis. *Spine* 1986;11:269–276.

35. Kaneda K, Kazama H, Satoh S, et al: Follow-up study of medial facetectomies and posterolateral fusion with instrumentation in unstable degenerative spondylolisthesis. *Clin Orthop* 1986;203:159–167.

36. Knox BD, Harvell JC Jr, Nelson PB, et al: Decompression and Luque rectangle fusion for degenerative spondylolisthesis. *J Spinal Disord* 1989;2:223–228.

37. Johnsson KE, Redlund-Johnell I, Uden A, et al: Preoperative and postoperative instability in lumbar spinal stenosis. *Spine* 1989;14:591–593.

38. Matsunaga S, Sakou T, Morizono Y, et al: Natural history of degenerative spondylolisthesis: Pathogenesis and natural course of the slippage. *Spine* 1990;15:1204–1210.

39. Grobler LJ, Robertson PA, Novotny JE, et al: Etiology of spondylolisthesis: Assessment of the role played by lumbar facet joint morphology. *Spine* 1993;18:80–91.

40. McCullen GM, Bernini PM, Bernstein SH, et al: Clinical and roentgenographic results of decompression for lumbar spinal stenosis. *J Spinal Disord* 1994;7:380–387.

41. Robertson PA, Grobler LJ, Novotny JE, et al: Postoperative spondylolisthesis at L4-5: The role of facet joint morphology. *Spine* 1993;18:1483–1490.

42. Boden SD, Martin C, Rudolph R, et al: Increase of motion between lumbar vertebrae after excision of the capsule and cartilage of the facets: A cadaver study. *J Bone Joint Surg* 1994;76A:1847–1853.

43. Katz JN, Lipson SJ, Larson MG, et al: The outcome of decompressive laminectomy for degenerative lumbar stenosis. *J Bone Joint Surg* 1991;73A:809–816.

44. Herron LD, Mangelsdorf C: Lumbar spinal stenosis: Results of surgical treatment. *J Spinal Disord* 1991;4:26–33.

45. McKibbin B: The biology of fracture healing in long bones. *J Bone Joint Surg* 1978;60B:150–162.

46. Goodship AE, Kelly DJ, Rigby HS, et al: The effect of different regimes of axial micromovement on the healing of experimental tibial fractures. *Orthop Trans* 1987;11:285.

47. Wolf JW Jr, White AA III, Panjabi MM, et al: Comparison of cyclic loading versus constant compression in the treatment of long-bone fractures in rabbits. *J Bone Joint Surg* 1981;63A:805–810.

48. Akeson WH, Woo SL, Rutherford L, et al: The effects of rigidity of internal fixation plates on long bone remodeling: A biomechanical and quantitative histological study. *Acta Orthop Scand* 1976;47:241–249.

49. Bradley GW, McKenna GB, Dunn HK, et al: Effects of flexural rigidity of plates on bone healing. *J Bone Joint Surg* 1979;61A:866–872.

50. Woo SL, Lothringer KS, Akeson WH, et al: Less rigid internal fixation plates: Historical perspectives and new concepts. *J Orthop Res* 1984;1:431–449.

51. Terjesen T, Apalset K: The influence of different degrees of stiffness of fixation plates on experimental bone healing. *J Orthop Res* 1988;6:293–299.

52. Uhthoff HK, Dubuc FL: Bone structure changes in the dog under rigid internal fixation. *Clin Orthop* 1971;81:165–170.

53. Carter DR, Shimaoka EE, Harris WH, et al: Changes in long-bone structural properties during the first 8 weeks of plate implantation. *J Orthop Res* 1984;2:80–89.

54. Wu JJ, Shyr HS, Chao EY, et al: Comparison of osteotomy healing under external fixation devices with different stiffness characteristics. *J Bone Joint Surg* 1984;66A:1258–1264.

55. Hart MB, Wu JJ, Chao EY, et al: External skeletal fixation of canine tibial osteotomies: Compression compared with no compression. *J Bone Joint Surg* 1985;67A:598–605.

56. Goodship AE, Kenwright J: The influence of induced micromovement upon the healing of experimental tibial fractures. *J Bone Joint Surg* 1985;67B:650–655.

57. Kelly DJ, Rigby HS, Watkins PE, et al: The effect of different regimes of axial micromovement on the healing of experimental tibial fractures. *Eur Soc Biomech* 1986;5:173.

58. Kenwright J, Richardson J, Spriggins AJ, et al: Mechanical healing patterns of tibial fractures treated using different mechanical environments. *Eur Soc Biomech* 1986;5:174.

59. Williams EA, Rand JA, An KN, et al: The early healing of tibial osteotomies stabilized by one-plane or two-plane external fixation. *J Bone Joint Surg* 1987;69A:355–365.

60. Sarmiento A, Mullis DL, Latta LL, et al: A quantitative comparative analysis of fracture healing under the influence of compression plating vs. closed weight-bearing treatment. *Clin Orthop* 1980;149:232–239.

61. Lewallen DG, Chao EY, Kasman RA, et al: Comparison of the effects of compression plates and external fixators on early bone-healing. *J Bone Joint Surg* 1984;66A:1084–1091.

62. Terjesen T, Svenningsen S: The effects of function and fixation stiffness on experimental bone healing. *Acta Orthop Scand* 1988;59:712–715.

63. Perren SM, Huggler A, Russenberger M, et al: The reaction of cortical bone to compression. *Acta Orthop Scand* 1969;125(suppl):19–29.

64. Kostuik JP, Errico TJ, Gleason TF: Luque instrumentation in degenerative conditions of the lumbar spine. *Spine* 1990;15:318–321.

65. Luque ER: Surgical immobilization of the spine in elderly patients. *Clin Orthop* 1978;133:273–274.

66. McAfee PC, Farey IO, Sutterlin CE, et al: Device related osteoporosis with spinal instrumentation. *Spine* 1989;14:919–926.

67. Ransom N, La Rocca SH, Thalgott J: The case for pedicle fixation of the lumbar spine. *Spine* 1994;19:2702–2706.

68. Lorenz M, Zindrick M, Schwaegler P, et al: A comparison of single-level fusions with and without hardware. *Spine* 1991;16(suppl 8):S455–S458.

Chapter 41

Comorbidity and Outcome in Degenerative Lumbar Spinal Stenosis

Jeffrey N. Katz, MD, MS

Introduction

Comorbidity refers to the presence and severity of conditions other than the disorder under study or treatment. Comorbidity is associated with poor outcomes across a wide range of surgical and medical conditions.[1-10] This observation has important implications for research and practice. From a research perspective, studies of treatment outcomes or clinical course must be adjusted for comorbidity to avoid potential confounding. From the standpoint of clinical decision-making, clinicians and patients must understand the relationship between comorbidity and outcome to meaningfully discuss the likely benefits and drawbacks of therapy.

This chapter focuses specifically on the relationship between comorbidity and the clinical course and outcomes of degenerative lumbar spinal stenosis. The goals of the chapter are to define comorbidity, examine strategies for measuring it, assess critically the reported associations between comorbidity and outcome, and discuss the implications of these associations for research and practice.

Definition of Comorbidity

Comorbidity is generally conceptualized as the net burden of illnesses that coexist with and are not causally linked to the problem under study or treatment.[1-10] This definition explicitly distinguishes comorbidity from the index condition and from complications arising from treatment of the index condition. For example, in studies of lumbar spinal stenosis, lower extremity muscle weakness relates to the index condition and is not considered a comorbidity. Similarly, postoperative deep venous thrombosis is directly related to treatment of the spinal stenosis and is not considered a comorbidity. However, heart failure, chronic obstructive lung disease, and diabetes mellitus are typical comorbidities in this population.

Comorbidity typically increases with age and is positively associated with worse functional status and a greater use of medications and other health services. In studies of patients with degenerative lumbar spinal stenosis, an index of comorbidity was associated with age, physical functional status, the total number of medications, and the number of cardiac medications with correlations ranging from 0.24 to 0.35 (Spearman's coefficient; J Katz, MD, unpublished data, 1995). These data suggest that comorbidity is related conceptually and empirically to these other variables, but the strengths of these associations are modest. Hence, comorbidity taps a distinctive domain that must be measured directly.

Measurement of Comorbidity

Sources of Data

Data on comorbidity may be obtained from a variety of sources including the medical record, administrative files, and the patient. The medical record generally serves as the standard source of information to be used for research on medical conditions.[11] In some research settings, however, medical record review is impractical or impossible, and other data sources must be used.

Administrative data, such as Medicare claims or hospital discharge abstracts, are attractive sources of information for studying large populations. Medicare claims data, for example, allow study of over 30 million Americans 65 years of age or older. The claims contain principal diagnosis and procedure codes (using International Classification of Diseases codes [ICD-9-CM] for part A claims and Current Procedural Terminology codes [CPT] for part B claims), as well as secondary diagnosis codes that have been used to represent comorbidity. Medicare claims have been used extensively to study the epidemiology and treatment outcomes of numerous conditions.

However, administrative data have important potential limitations that may result in misclassification and bias. The misclassifications are more common for medical diagnoses than surgical procedures,[12] and for secondary versus primary diagnoses.[1] In one study, in which hospital discharge data were used, patients with adult onset diabetes mellitus, previous myocardial infarction, and angina had lower risk of in-hospital death than patients without these conditions coded on the abstracts.[1] This finding is counterintuitive; the diseases under consideration lead to higher, not lower mortality. Such nonsensical findings suggest coding bias. It has been suggested that there is a stronger financial incentive to add chronic disease diagnoses to the discharge abstracts of patients with less serious illnesses (to increase the likelihood of reimbursement) than to those of patients with serious acute illnesses.[1] This coding bias leads to undercoding of chronic illnesses in more seriously ill patients.

Important clinical policy questions may hinge on the validity of using administrative data to assess comorbidity. For example, a large study using administrative data showed a lower rate of mortality in men undergoing open prostatectomy than in those undergoing transurethral prostatectomy, even after adjusting for comorbidity. These results have led to the suggestion that the open procedure may be safer,[13] and have prompted interest in a randomized controlled trial of open versus transurethral prostatectomy. A more detailed review of medical records, rather than hospital discharge data, showed lower mortality with the open procedure in unadjusted analyses, but no difference in mortality between the two procedures in analyses adjusted for comorbidity.[5] On the other hand, in several studies in which administrative data were used, the expected associations were observed between increasing comorbidity and greater mortality and complications.[3,4] Thus, adjustment for comorbidity in studies of administrative data appears to be valid in many circumstances, but must be performed and interpreted cautiously.

In some research settings, such as population-based surveys, medical records may be difficult to obtain. In others, such as studies of outpatients with surgical conditions, medical records may contain limited data on comorbidity. In these situations, patient questionnaires may provide a reliable and valid alternative for obtaining information on comorbidity. Our group[11] has validated a questionnaire version of the Charlson Comorbidity Index and demonstrated it to be reproducible and valid, and to predict a range of health service utilization indicators as accurately as the chart-based version of the Charlson Index.

Measures of Comorbidity

Most measures of comorbidity share generic structural features. Once the source of data is identified, protocols are established for identifying specific comorbid conditions, using explicit criteria. For example, identification of acute myocardial infarction might require evidence of characteristic electrocardiographic changes and elevations of cardiac enzymes. The severity of each condition is then rated, again using explicit criteria. For example, insulin-dependent diabetes mellitus with end-organ complications would be rated as more severe than adult-onset diabetes without end-organ complications that is treated with an oral agent. Finally, the individual comorbidities are aggregated into a final composite comorbidity score. This process generally involves assigning weights to each individual comorbid condition. The weights are often derived empirically.

A commonly used comorbidity system, the Charlson Comorbidity Index,[14] is summarized in Table 1. Charlson and associates[14] collected detailed clinical data on patients admitted to the general medical service of New York Hospital. The authors analyzed associations between comorbid conditions and 1-year mortality in logistic regression models. They assigned weights to each condition significantly associated with mortality; the weights were roughly proportional to the regression coefficients for each condition. The authors then validated the index by assessing its ability to predict deaths due to comorbid conditions in a cohort of patients with breast cancer. The Charlson comorbidity measure has been adapted for use with administrative data[3] as well as in a self-administered format.[11]

Another comorbidity measure that has been used in several studies of lumbar spinal stenosis is the Cumulative Illness Rating Scale,[15] which is also outlined in Table 1. This scale was originally developed as a measure of conditions leading to physical impairment in the elderly, as well as to death. It assigns severity ratings to each of 13 organ systems; ratings range from 0 = no impairment to 4 = extremely severe impairment. The severity scores are summed across organ systems to yield a composite comorbidity score.

Many other instruments are available, some proprietary, others in the public domain. The full range of comorbidity instruments will not be reviewed here.

Not all comorbidity instruments were developed for the same purpose. The Charlson Index,[14] as explained earlier, was developed and validated as a predictor of mortality. The Cumulative Illness Rating Scale,[15] in contrast, was de-

Table 1 Specific disorders or organ systems included in the Charlson Index and Cumulative Illness Rating Scale (CIRS)

CIRS	Charlson*
Cardiac	Myocardial infarction (1)*
Vascular	Congestive heart failure (1)
Respiratory	Peripheral vascular disease (1)
Eye, ear, nose, throat	Cerebrovascular disease (1)
Upper gastrointestinal	Dementia (1)
Lower gastrointestinal	Chronic pulmonary disease (1)
Hepatic	Connective tissue disease (1)
Renal	Peptic ulcer disease (1)
Other genitourinary	Mild liver disease (1)
Musculoskeletal, integumentary	Diabetes, no complications (1)
Neurologic	Diabetes with complications (2)
Psychiatric	Hemiplegia or paraplegia (2)
Endocrine-metabolic	Moderate or severe renal disease (2)
	Tumor, leukemia, lymphoma (2)
	Severe liver disease (3)
	Metastatic solid tumor (6)

*Weights of Charlson items noted in parentheses; CIRS items weighted 0 (no impairment) to 4 (extremely severe impairment)

veloped to predict physical impairment, as well as death. Certain instruments developed for one purpose may be useful for another. The Cumulative Illness Rating Scale, for example, was a strong predictor of mortality 7 to 10 years following laminectomy for spinal stenosis,[16] and the Charlson Index was a strong predictor of resource consumption.[3] Rochon and associates[10] have shown in spinal cord injured patients that the Cumulative Illness Rating Scale was a better predictor of length of stay, while the Charlson Index was a better predictor of mortality. A comorbidity measure was developed by Cleary and associates[9] to predict a range of health outcomes, and it has been useful in adjusting for length of stay. Thus, while comorbidity measures developed for one purpose may be robust in predicting other outcomes, the physician should attempt, if possible, to use an instrument developed to predict the particular outcome of interest.[2]

Comorbidity and Spinal Stenosis

What is the burden of comorbidity among patients undergoing surgery for degenerative lumbar spinal stenosis? Data on comorbidity from several studies of surgery for spinal stenosis[3,6,17-19] are shown in Table 2. Comorbidity is measured differently from study to study, complicating comparisons. Some investigators included specific conditions, others used comorbidity indices. Criteria for establishing the specific conditions are generally not specified. The prevalence of comorbidity in the Medicare data of Deyo and associates[3] appears surprisingly low, suggesting the possibility of undercoding in the claims data. On the

Table 2 Extent of comorbidity in patients undergoing surgery for spinal stenosis

Author, Reference	Sample	Extent of Comorbidity	
Weir and de Leo[17]	N=81 age 30-80, 64% > 50	Cardiopulmonary disease Severe obesity Cancer	23% 6% 3%
Herno et al[18]	N=108 age 23-67 60% > 50	Coexisting illness Cardiac disease Hip or knee osteoarthritis Diabetes	32% 10% 6% 4%
Jonsson and Stromqvist[19]	N=50 age 71-84	Hip or knee osteoarthritis Coronary artery disease Neurologic disease	20% 14% 10%
Katz et al[6]	N=88 age 55-89 mean age 69	Osteoarthritis Congestive heart failure, angina, or arrhythmia Rheumatoid arthritis Chronic pulmonary disease	32% 22% 10% 7%

		CIRS Comorbidity Score:
		     0-2
		     3-5
		     ≥ 3
			
			32%
			42%
			26%

Deyo et al[3]	N=27,111 age > 65, mean age 72	Diabetes mellitus Chronic pulmonary disease Cerebrovascular disease Myocardial infarction	10% 9% 4% 3%

	Claims data
	all diagnoses
	except cancer
		Charlson Comorbidity Score:
		    0
		    1-2
		    ≥ 3
			
			71%
			26%
			3%

other hand, the other investigators may have recruited patients with unusually high prevalence of comorbidity, because the patients were from referral centers.

These concerns notwithstanding, it appears from Table 2 that up to 70% of patients undergoing surgery for spinal stenosis have coexisting medical illnesses that might influence short- and long-term surgical outcomes. The most common conditions include osteoarthritis of the hip and knee and cardiovascular disease. Most of these studies did not account for mental health disorders, which have been associated with outcomes of diskectomy,[20] and might influence the outcome of surgery for spinal stenosis.

The relatively high prevalence of comorbid conditions in patients undergoing surgery for spinal stenosis points to the importance of collecting comorbidity data in studies of older patients. Studies of younger patients with work-associated carpal tunnel syndrome (J. Katz, MD, unpublished data, 1995) or arthroscopic meniscectomy[21] reveal much lower prevalence of comorbid conditions and no influence of comorbid conditions on clinical outcomes.

Associations Between Comorbidities and Outcomes

Cross-Sectional Analyses

Correlates of physical functional status were assessed cross-sectionally prior to decompressive surgery in patients with degenerative lumbar spinal stenosis.[22] Comorbidity (assessed with the Cumulative Illness Rating Scale) explained 20% of the total explained variance in physical disability in these patients, while pain severity accounted for 50%, and physical examination findings for just 8% of the explained variance. Thus, after pain, comorbidity is the most important determinant of physical functional disability in spinal stenosis.

Studies of Surgical Outcomes

Most studies of the relationship between comorbidity and outcome have focused on surgical outcomes. The individual outcomes will be discussed here in three categories, mortality and complications, cost and length of stay, and quality of life following surgery.

Mortality and Complications Deyo and associates[3] studied outcomes of lumbar spine surgery in Medicare recipients. Data were obtained from 1985 Part A Medicare hospitalization claims. The authors studied correlates of 6-week postoperative mortality and in-hospital complications. Diagnoses specified on the claims data were used to construct an adaptation of the Charlson Comorbidity Index.[3] Statistically significant relationships were observed between increasing Charlson comorbidity scores and the proportion of patients experiencing in-hospital complications, as well as 6-week postoperative mortality (Table 3). Multivariate analyses showed that these relationships persisted after adjustment for age.

Oldridge and associates[4] studied mortality using the 1986 Medicare Part A Claims files. The authors examined the relationship between relatively common comorbid conditions and surgical mortality. These data are also presented in Table 3. A greater number of comorbid conditions were associated with greater mortality during the index hospitalization as well as at 30 days and 1 year following discharge.

Oldridge and associates[4] also investigated the influence of specific comorbid conditions on mortality. As might be expected on clinical grounds, cardiovascular and pulmonary disease were associated with greater mortality, while hypertension, paradoxically, appeared to protect against death, as observed by Iezzoni and associates,[1] suggesting coding bias.

The reports of Deyo and associates[3] and Oldridge and associates[4] used administrative data in large populations. One study[16] of 88 patients who underwent laminectomy for spinal stenosis used medical record-based comorbidity data (the Cumulative Illness Rating Scale). Twenty of the 88 patients (23%) died during the 7- to 10-year follow-up period. In logistic regression analyses, inde-

Table 3 Associations between comoridity and outcome of surgery for degenerative lumbar spinal stenosis

Study	Instrument			
Deyo and associates[3]	Charlson Score			
	0	1	3	?3
6-week mortality (%)	0.5	1.0	1.8	2.7
In-hospital complications (%)	7.9	8.4	9.1	10.5
Mean length of stay	12.9	14.0	15.0	16.1
Total hospital charges ($)	6,597	7,463	8,213	8,968
Discharged to nursing home (%)	2.2	2.9	4.4	3.8
Katz and associates[6,8]	CIRS Score			
	0-2	3-5	≥ 6	
Repeated surgery or persistent severe pain (%)	25%	48%	60%	
Satisfied (%)	82%	— 72% —		
Oldridge and associates[4]	No. of Comorbid Conditions			
	0	1	3	≥ 3
Relative risk of in-hospital death	1.0	4.8	12.5	21.6
Relative risk of 1-year mortality	1.0	2.2	4.0	8.7

*CIRS scores ≥ 3 aggregated in analyses of satisfaction

pendent predictors of death included advanced age ($p = 0.0006$), longer follow-up ($p = 0.01$), and higher comorbidity score ($p = 0.04$).

Cost and Length of Stay Deyo and associates[3] presented associations between Charlson comorbidity scores and mean length of stay, total hospital charges, and percentage of patients discharged to nursing homes. These data are shown in Table 3. Higher levels of comorbidity were associated with impressive, graded increases in each of these usage outcomes. At the extreme, patients with three or more comorbidities had 25% longer lengths of stay, 36% greater total hospital charges, and 73% higher rate of discharge to nursing homes than patients with no comorbidity.

Quality of Life Outcomes Our group[6] examined predictors of outcomes 4 to 7 years following surgery for spinal stenosis. Predictors of poor outcome (defined as either severe pain, reoperation, or both) included the comorbidity score ($p = 0.004$) as well as earlier year of operation ($p = 0.01$). The comorbidity score was also an important predictor of limited physical function (unable to walk 50 feet, or shop, $p = 0.02$).

In a prospective study of laminectomy for lumbar spinal stenosis, we[8] found that the comorbidity score was a significant predictor of satisfaction with the results of surgery 6 months postoperatively ($p = 0.03$). Other predictors included baseline physical function as measured with the Sickness Impact Profile ($p = 0.006$) and a predominance of back versus leg complaints ($p = 0.05$).

Mechanism of Association Between Comorbidity and Outcome

The mechanism whereby comorbidity influences outcome is not entirely understood. For example, a higher comorbidity score is associated with greater mortality following surgery for spinal stenosis.[3,4,16] This relationship is intuitive: Patients with potentially life-threatening illnesses die at a greater rate than patients who do not have these illnesses. However, greater comorbidity was also associated with worse pain and higher risk of repeated surgery (performed for pain) 4 to 7 years following the original surgery. This observation raises the question of whether patients with a greater burden of comorbid illness have a lower threshold for tolerating pain or are unable to successfully perform rehabilitation activities following surgery. The effect of comorbidity on pain relief merits further study.

Another unresolved issue is whether specific comorbidities or the total burden of comorbid conditions is the critical factor influencing outcomes. This question was addressed in two reports on the relationship between diabetes mellitus and results of laminectomy. Simpson and associates[23] reported excellent or good long-term results for just 17 of 49 (39%) patients who had diabetes mellitus as compared with 52 of 55 (95%) nondiabetic patients who had disk problems or lumbar stenosis. The authors concluded that diabetes mellitus was associated with poor results.[23] The authors did not report on whether the patients had associated comorbid conditions.

Cinotti and associates[5] reviewed the outcomes of 25 diabetic and 25 nondiabetic patients who had decompression for lumbar spinal stenosis.[5] The authors selected nondiabetic patients who had a high rate of comorbidity in an attempt to match the two groups on this variable. Considerable improvement was reported by 72% of the diabetics and 80% of the nondiabetics. The difference was not significant. Greater comorbidity was associated with worse outcome in both groups, although this was not significant. These authors[5] concluded that with comorbidity matched between groups, diabetes is not a specific risk factor for worse outcomes. Their data suggest that higher comorbidity might underlie the worse outcomes often seen in diabetics.

Unfortunately, the Simpson study[23] was limited by lack of data on comorbidity, and the Cinotti[5] study was limited by a small sample size. Furthermore, Cinotti and associates[5] did not present the raw data on the relationship between comorbidity and outcomes. Nevertheless, the two papers suggest that diabetes may be related to a poor outcome of surgery because of its association with other comorbid illnesses, and not because of direct effects of diabetes per se.

A final methodologic concern is the paradoxical influence of mortality on the effects of comorbidity. Comorbidity was the most important predictor of pain and reoperation 4 to 7 years following surgery for spinal stenosis.[6] However, comorbidity was not an important predictor of pain or reoperation in the same cohort 7 to 10 years following surgery, but it was the most important predictor of mortality.[16] Because patients with greater comorbidity died, they were unavailable for the long-term quality of life analyses, likely explaining the lack of association between comorbidity and outcome at long-term follow-up.

Implications for Research and Practice

From a research standpoint, comorbidity should be ascertained routinely in studies of outcome. Treatment effects should be adjusted for baseline comorbidity. If hospital discharge reports or claims data are the only information available for assessing comorbidity, the results should be interpreted cautiously because of potential inaccuracies in these data sources. Investigators in the ambulatory setting should give more serious consideration to using self-report comorbidity measures. Finally, investigators should use standardized, validated comorbidity assessment instruments whenever possible, to facilitate comparisons across studies.

From a clinical standpoint, the relationship between comorbidity and outcome is a critical aspect of patient selection and informed consent. Patients with a greater burden of comorbid illness are likely to have worse results. This includes short-term outcomes, such as mortality and complications, as well as long-term quality of life outcomes. The direct and indirect costs are likely to be higher in patients with more comorbidity. These observations should not serve to deny surgery to patients with comorbid disease, but should prompt informed discussions with patients about their increased risk of adverse outcomes.

References

1. Iezzoni LI, Foley SM, Daley J, et al: Comorbidities, complications, and coding bias: Does the number of diagnosis codes matter in predicting in-hospital mortality? *JAMA* 1992;267:2197–2203.
2. Rubin HR, Wu AW: Editorial: The risk of adjustment. *Med Care* 1992;30:973–975.
3. Deyo RA, Cherkin DC, Ciol MA: Adapting a clinical comorbidity index for use with ICD-9-CM administrative databases. *J Clin Epidemiol* 1992;45:613–619.
4. Oldridge NB, Yuan Z, Stoll JE, et al: Lumbar spine surgery and mortality among Medicare beneficiaries, 1986. *Am J Public Health* 1994;84:1292–1298.
5. Cinotti G, Postacchini F, Weinstein JN: Lumbar spinal stenosis and diabetes: Outcome of surgical decompression. *J Bone Joint Surg* 1994;76B:215–219.
6. Katz JN, Lipson SJ, Larson MG, et al: The outcome of decompressive laminectomy for degenerative lumbar stenosis. *J Bone Joint Surg* 1991;73A:809–816.
7. Concato J, Horwitz RI, Feinstein AR, et al: Problems of comorbidity in mortality after prostatectomy. *JAMA* 1992;267:1077–1082.
8. Katz JN, Lipson SJ, Brick GW, et al: Clinical correlates of patient satisfaction after laminectomy for degenerative lumbar spinal stenosis. *Spine* 1995;20:1155–1160.
9. Cleary PD, Greenfield S, Mulley AG, et al: Variations in length of stay and outcomes for six medical and surgical conditions in Massachusetts and California. *JAMA* 1991;266:73–79.
10. Rochon PA, Katz JN, Morrow LA, et al: Comorbid illness is associated with survival and length of stay in patients with chronic disability: A prospective comparison of three comorbidity indices. *Med Care*, in press.
11. Katz JN, Chang LC, Sangha O, et al: Can comorbidity be measured by questionnaire rather than medical record review? *Med Care* 1996;34:73–84.
12. Fisher ES, Whaley FS, Krushat WM, et al: The accuracy of Medicare's hospital claims data: Progress has been made, but problems remain. *Am J Public Health* 1992;82:243–248.
13. Roos NP, Wennberg JE, Malenka DJ, et al: Mortality and reoperation after open and transurethral resection of the prostate for benign prostatic hyperplasia. *N Engl J Med* 1989;320:1120–1124.
14. Charlson ME, Pompei P, Ales KL, et al: A new method of classifying prognostic comorbidity in longitudinal studies: Development and validation. *J Chron Dis* 1987;40:373–383.

697

15. Linn BS, Linn MW, Gurel L: Cumulative illness rating scale. *J Am Geriatr Soc* 1968;16:622–626.
16. Katz JN, Lipson SJ, Chang LC, et al: Seven- to 10-year outcome of decompressive surgery for degenerative lumbar spinal stenosis. *Spine* 1996;21:92–98.
17. Weir B, de Leo R: Lumbar stenosis: Analysis of factors affecting outcome in 81 surgical cases. *Can J Neurol Sci* 1981:8:295–298.
18. Herno A, Airaksinen O, Saari T: Long-term results of surgical treatment of lumbar spinal stenosis. *Spine* 1993;18:1471–1474.
19. Jonsson B, Stromqvist B: Lumbar spine surgery in the elderly: Complications and surgical results. *Spine* 1994;19:1431–1435.
20. Spengler DM, Ouellette EA, Battie M, et al: Elective discectomy for herniation of a lumbar disc: Additional experience with an objective method. *J Bone Joint Surg* 1990;72A:230–237.
21. Katz JN, Harris TM, Larson MG, et al: Predictors of functional outcomes after arthroscopic partial meniscectomy. *J Rheumatol* 1992;19:1938–1942.
22. Stucki G, Liang MH, Lipson SJ, et al: Contribution of neuromuscular impairment to physical functional status in patients with lumbar spinal stenosis. *J Rheumatol* 1994;21:1338–1343.
23. Simpson JM, Silveri CP, Balderston RA, et al: The results of operations on the lumbar spine in patients who have diabetes mellitus. *J Bone Joint Surg* 1993;75A:1823–1829.

Directions for Future Research

Perform studies regarding the epidemiology and disease impact of spinal stenosis.

Although there are estimates of the prevalence of low back pain and of radiographic stenosis, the prevalence of the clinical syndrome of spinal stenosis is unknown. Hence, it is not possible to estimate the cost of this syndrome in terms of disability or utilization of resources. Furthermore, the understanding of its natural history is limited. The major obstacle to epidemiologic study of spinal stenosis is the lack of a valid case definition.

Two major research directions are to develop and validate a case definition of the clinical syndrome of spinal stenosis suitable for epidemiologic studies, and to perform population-based studies of disease prevalence, natural history, and disease impact in terms of functional disability and health resource utilization.

Improve the specificity of magnetic resonance imaging and other tests for the diagnosis of the spinal stenosis syndrome.

Magnetic resonance imaging (MRI) is currently the primary imaging study for degenerative spinal stenosis. Its accuracy in clinical studies has been high, up to 97% in some studies. The problem with the MRI diagnosis of spinal stenosis is specificity; there is a high incidence (up to 25%) of asymptomatic narrowing (morphologic narrowing without the clinical syndrome). Measuring the area of the central or lateral canal is not predictive of symptoms. Other factors that affect the pathogenesis of symptoms are not demonstrated by morphologic imaging.

In view of new knowledge about the pathophysiology of pain from stenosis, better tests can be developed. No single test completely predicts the treatment outcomes, but by combining tests that address different aspects of the pathophysiology, a better prediction of outcome may be obtained.

The objective is to develop diagnostic tests that identify physiologically relevant abnormalities. MRI, functional electrical physiologic tests, and intracanal mechanical pressure tests are promising areas for selecting patients for whom treatment will be successful. Specific examples include: (1) Compare the anatomic appearances of the spinal tissues before and after treatment in patients with successful and poor outcomes. (2) Study the morphologic, structural, anatomic, physiologic, and clinical features of stenotic foramina and canals and correlate them with the character of symptoms. (3) Develop diagnostic tests using positron emission tomography and other functional imaging; electrophysiologic measurements; pressure measurements (eg, epidural pressures); and biomechanical, kinematics, and stiffness measures (eg, for the issue of arthrodesis in conjunction with decompression).

In addition, tools for intraoperatively monitoring the adequacy of decompression would be useful. No major obstacles are anticipated in accomplishing the above because most of the relevant technologies exist. One of the challenges will be to relate the developed measures to patient outcome parameters.

Establish methods and studies to assess the role of surgical intervention.

Although surgery is thought to be, in general, efficacious for the management of degenerative lumbar spondylolisthesis and lumbar stenosis, there are few natural history studies. Therefore, it is not known to what extent the results of surgical management exceed the natural history of untreated stenosis. Most studies suggest that concomitant fusion has little role in the surgical treatment of spinal stenosis without spondylolisthesis. However, existing studies have not adequately separated those patients with predominant leg pain from those that have significant back pain as well. Therefore, it is not known whether there is a subgroup of patients that would benefit from concomitant fusion. Furthermore, the role of instrumentation has not been characterized. These variables should be studied.

The exact role of various posterior decompressive procedures is not known, because posterior decompression procedures vary in the amount of bone and extent of decompression performed. Some data suggest that too limited a decompression leads to deterioration over time. Therefore, it would be useful to develop a comparative study to assess the proper role of various decompressive procedures (laminotomy, laminectomy, anterior procedures, and minimally invasive surgical techniques). Furthermore, consideration should be given to the study of selective decompression (only the decompression of the symptomatic levels) versus global decompression of all radiographically stenotic areas.

Conduct randomized, controlled trials and cost analyses of nonsurgical treatment interventions for spinal stenosis.

Many nonsurgical treatment approaches currently exist for patients with spinal stenosis. There is a dearth of data indicating that any of these treatments alter the natural history of the disease. Documentation of efficacy of specific techniques may help to establish treatment protocols and reduce costs.

Commonly used approaches, such as medications, exercise, injections, and trunk orthotics, need to be studied. Design of trials should include well-defined patient populations, comparison of clearly delineated treatments (including placebo control), and use of outcomes including pain, patient function, and patient satisfaction. Direct and indirect cost implications should be addressed. Investigators studying multiple treatments must consider factorial designs to permit independent evaluation of treatments.

Develop, refine, and validate a matrix of outcome measures for application to spinal stenosis (and related spondylotic disease).

There are no universally accepted measures of outcome for treatment of spinal stenosis. Valid techniques have been developed to measure all of the relevant domains, including (1) pain, (2) functional status, (3) work status and performance, (4) neurologic status, (5) psychological impact, (6) patient expectations and satisfaction, (7) need for further therapy, and (8) cost.

A generally accepted spectrum of outcome reporting is key to designing clinical trials, assessing existing and new therapies, and providing a tool for evaluating clinical reporting. Predictors cannot be established without uniform outcome reporting. There are few potential obstacles to such research, and the cost of validation is small.

Identify positive and negative predictors of outcome following surgical treatment of patients with lumbar spinal stenosis.

Surgical treatments for spinal stenosis that is refractory to nonsurgical management are generally thought to be successful, yet some patients have incomplete functional recovery and residual symptoms. To better establish predictors of good outcomes as well as warning signs for potential bad outcomes, a detailed analysis of the prognostic role of preoperative factors is warranted.

An observational study should be performed to include analysis of the effects of the following factors on outcome: age, gender, extent/severity of disease, length of symptoms, rapidity of symptom progression, psychosocial factors, patient expectations, medical comorbidities, and the presence of significant back pain. Specific attention should be focused on the question of whether the subset of stenosis patients with a significant component of back pain but without spondylolisthesis have a better outcome when fusion is added to decompression. In addition, predictors of success or failure with nonsurgical treatments (exercise, corset, epidural steroids) should also be studied. It would be preferable to measure outcome using a combination of generic and disease-specific instruments.

Section Six

Basic and Applied Science Issues of Degenerative Stenosis

Section Editor:
Steven R. Garfin, MD

Ken-ichi Chatani, MD, PhD   *Björn L. Rydevik, MD, PhD*
Mamoru Kawakami, MD, PhD   *Keisuke Takahashi, MD, PhD*
Kjell Olmarker, MD, PhD   *James N. Weinstein, DO, MS*

Overview

The authors of this section have been asked to assess basic and applied science studies related to the signs and symptoms created by degenerative spinal stenosis. This assessment includes a review of the research to date, including modeling, and suggestions for future research directions. In addition, they have attempted to correlate the basic science studies to the clinical condition, trying to help determine the components of the degenerative process that leads to pain, as well as considering the timing of nonsurgical and/or surgical intervention to help alleviate or diminish that pain. As can be seen from the articles in this section, the studies and the animal models are diverse, but the data obtained tend to be consistent. This consistency contributes to the development of a unified thesis for use in explaining and enhancing the understanding of the symptoms and signs related to spinal stenosis.

Based on the classic article by Mixter and Barr in 1934, much of the treatment of back pain and sciatica has focused on the mechanical effects of disk herniation/degeneration. Imaging studies, including myelography, computed tomography (CT), and magnetic resonance imaging (MRI), have provided anatomic bases for sciatica. These studies show nerve root truncation (myelogram) or nerve root compression (CT and MRI), which, when they correlate with the patient's radicular complaints, provide a pathoanatomic explanation for the pain. If nonsurgical treatment fails, the pain can be treated surgically. The surgery is directed at relieving the compression (diskectomy, laminectomy, foraminotomy). Compression of a normal nerve root, however, does not always cause pain. It may lead to numbness, paresthesia, and weakness. Compressed nerves do occur without pain as demonstrated by myelogram, MRI, and CT studies on asymptomatic people. Inflammation, along with some degree of mechanical compression, is needed to create pain.

The focus of the basic science research described in this section is to try to understand the physiologic components of the symptoms and signs of spinal stenosis and sciatica, as distinct from the isolated mechanical-compression effects. Although neurogenic claudication is different from the pain symptoms associated with sciatica, it is a stage in the continuation of neural injury. The spinal stenosis symptoms often are intermittent, but the factors leading to pain probably are similar (although varying in degree) to the sciatica associated with herniated disks. In this regard, some of the articles in this section could also be placed in the section on herniated nucleus pulposus. As described in this section, these factors include: (1) nutritional components affected by alterations in blood–nerve barriers, cerebrospinal fluid (CSF) flow alteration/restriction, and vascular compromise (ischemia); (2) mechanism and rate of compression: slow versus rapid onset, as well as magnitude, duration, and location of compression; (3) anatomic variations: dorsal root ganglia (DRG), spinal nerve root, peripheral nerve root, intrathecal organization (sensory-dorsolateral, motor-ventral-medial); (4) inflammatory component/reaction and edema leading to decrease in nutritional support (vascular, CSF, and/or increased diffusability/permeability through cells), increased metabolic demands, and possibly further compression by the expanding edema/inflammation fluid; and (5) chemical/enzymatic alterations of the internal milieu (pain-enhancing substances, acid-base shifts, etc).

Static components of the process are relatively easily studied in the human (MRI, CT scans). Developing and expanding the basic physiologic understanding, however, is more dependent on creating appropriate animal models, which reproduce the human situation. This is more difficult and currently less precise.

Modeling

Modeling has varied significantly. Researchers have used animals of different size and shape. Rydevik, Garfin, Olmarker, and their associates have used the cauda equina in the spinal column of pigs. Yoshizawa and associates and others have used the spinal cord and spinal nerves of the dog. A number of studies, which are based on histologic analysis as opposed to pressure measurements, neurologic function, or electrophysiologic monitoring, have been done using small animals including rabbits and rats. When function is the parameter being observed, larger animals are used more often.

In a number of earlier studies, peripheral nerves were used to assess the effects of the nucleus pulposus and compression on nerve tissues, as well as to correlate the biomechanical and functional effects of varying stresses and strains on the peripheral nerve, as an explanation for alterations noted in clinical situations affecting spinal nerves. However, as pointed out in the articles by Kawakami and associates and Rydevik and Olmarker, there are distinct anatomic differences between spinal nerve roots, the intraforaminal components including the DRG, and peripheral nerves. Therefore, studies undertaken to correlate neural changes affecting mechanics, function, and nutritional support of the spinal nerves through evaluation of peripheral nerves may have only limited validity and utility in providing understanding of spinal pain mechanisms related to the nerves.

Unfortunately, surgical/artificial manipulation of neural tissues, whether peripheral nerve, spinal nerve, or central neural elements, is used in almost all of the studies, which, therefore, do not truly replicate the degenerative condition. Spinal stenosis evolves gradually. There is persistent blood flow and nutritional support, although perhaps diminished from normal, with the gradual onset of compression. The associated mechanical, chemical, and nutritional alterations occur slowly. Although global in nature, these changes may not affect every component of the nerve root or the surrounding environment and is not necessarily symmetric; whereas, in the laboratory condition, the scar that is created tends to be circumferential and uniform, as does the compressive effect. To date, in the studies reported, compression has been created with silicon tubing, Plexiglass sheets, balloons, chromic suture, etc. Although these devices do provide controlled restriction, they are concentric rather than eccentric, are applied suddenly rather than gradually, and are artificially induced. In addition to the synthetic device, there is also scar related to the surgical manipulation, which in addition to the chemical and mechanical components, may lead to irreversible, relatively complete vascular alterations and compromise.

There has been, to date, no report of the application of a gradual, physiologic insult, introduced in an animal model that replicates the human condition, particularly in a bipedal animal with associated degenerative changes as opposed to a quadruped that, in general, does not demonstrate the degenerative process as consistently or uniformly as humans.

One of the other difficulties with many of the studies that have been performed to evaluate the neurologic and histologic processes that occur with spinal stenosis is clear identification of the level of the spinal cord, conus medullaris, and/or cauda equina in the animal models used. In many quadruped animals, there are more than five lumbar vertebrae, and the spinal cord or conus medullaris extends to the sacrum. Some of the investigators who report to have isolated the cauda equina and, thereby, simulate the human spinal stenosis condition may, in fact, have incorporated some spinal cord or conus medullaris components in the compression, leading to varying abilities of neurologic recovery as well as degrees of impairment because of nerve cell, as opposed to axon/root, inclusion. The most realistic study would be one that involves minimal manipulation and creates an inflammatory response and edema with a slow increase in the amount of compression related to the local reaction. Models that involve the least amount of surgical manipulation/stimulation should provide the most physiologic, reproducible, clinically significant information.

The chapter by Yoshizawa and associates (in the herniated disk section) attempts a more direct analysis of the human condition using a physiologic, dynamic type of MRI study with gadolinium enhancement. This allows the assessment of inflammatory components around the nerve and, perhaps, may assess fluid/vascular flow and/or shifts in the future. In this section, Takahashi has reported on an exciting new technique to measure epidural pressure and correlate it with function. This is dynamic and has direct clinical applicability.

Clinical Correlation

The studies reported in this section all relate to inflammatory type reactions involving the neural elements of the spine and enzymes, which, in the human, correlate with pain. Rydevik and Olmarker have demonstrated that a rapid onset of compression leads to more edema and a greater degree of electrophysiologic impairment than demonstrated with slower, more gradual compression. The "slow" gradual compression they used, however, is still logarithmically more rapid than that which occurs in the human degenerative process. In their studies, particularly those incorporating a "double crush" with a two-level insult to the cauda equina and spinal nerve roots, the physiologic alterations are significant.

Kawakami and associates describe alterations that are ongoing and physiologic. Enhanced MRI has the ability to depict inflammation. This study related to absorbable suture placed around nerve roots demonstrated relatively convincingly the progressive release of neuropeptides and other substances that have been shown to lead to a pain response. These data, correlated with histologic and inflammatory responses observed by them and others, as well as with the hypersensitive reaction of the animals related to this ongoing process, are convincing.

All the studies in this section suggest the importance of understanding the gradual, progressive, dynamic process that occurs. Compression, when associated with inflammation and edema, leads to a reactive cycle that produces increased inflammation and edema. When this cycle occurs at or near the DRG, there is release of substances that implicates these structures in the pain mechanism. Additionally, when the compression and inflammatory components occur separate from the DRG, alterations occur in the nerve tissues diffusion barrier. These alterations can lead to nutritional variations not just locally, but throughout the length of the dural/meningeal sheaths and attachments, and could, in that manner, lead to hyperexcitability and/or associated responses from the contiguous DRG, cells (centrally), and investing tissues.

Discussion

The above discussion, combined with the three chapters in this section, are just beginnings in our attempt to understand through basic science studies the mechanisms of pain response and neurologic deficits observed in certain patients with symptoms and signs of spinal stenosis. More studies, particularly physiologic ones, using models that are closer to the human condition, are necessary. These should involve neural tissues in animals that have structures similar to the spinal nerves and cauda equina in humans, and compression which is progressive and slow that simulates the human degenerative condition. Hopefully, the modeling can use more anatomic-type tissues, as opposed to synthetic barriers and constricting devices.

In addition, most of the studies reported or reviewed in this section have studied nerve conduction. Impulses, either ectopic or persistent, secondary to chemical and/or mechanical sensitization, are recordable. Perhaps more inclusive neurophysiologic studies should/could have been included.

To develop an animal model that could create pain or weakness, and then monitor it long-term is increasingly difficult due to the approval process, animal use constraints (pain, housing, feeding, analgesics, and so forth), the monitoring restraints, and the associated costs (financial, legal, emotional). Overcoming this may be the biggest limitation in our ability to further develop the understanding of the spinal stenosis–pain response process in models that correlate with the human condition, thereby leading to more time and pathophysiologically directed treatment with or without surgery, including specific medications and physiologic alterations targeted at the local condition and response. The clinical and basic science studies point to a multifactorial basis for neurogenic claudication. These factors include mechanical narrowing, instability, inflammation, chemical sensitization of nerves, direct nerve compression/injury, degenerative disk alterations, neuropeptides, and comorbid processes such as atherosclerosis, pulmonary disease (hypoxia), etc.

All the studies suggest that the degree (amount) of compression, the inflammatory/chemical response, and the nutritional alterations, combined with prolonged compromise of the neural tissues and investing elements, increase the overall magnitude of the response. These data suggest that the earlier the inflammatory response and compression are decreased, the less likely permanent changes and fibrosis are to occur. This finding does have some clinical correlation. Studies have demonstrated that surgical decompression of a spinal nerve compressed by a herniated disk can lead to excellent leg pain relief, if the procedure is performed within 3 to 6 months of the onset of the pain complaint, which presumably coincides with concurrent occurrence of inflammation and compression. Prolonged compression (greater than 1 year in the case of herniated disks, and 2 to 3 years for spinal stenosis) leads to less favorable pain (leg) relief following decompression. This fact suggests a time dependency, which may corroborate Kawakami and associates' suggestion that prolonged inflammation and edema can lead to permanent, intrinsic, fibrotic changes, which can create irreversible alterations in nutrition, diffusion/permeability, electrophysiologic excitability, and mechanical/internal stresses.

Chapter 42

Effects of Mechanical Compression on Nerve Roots

Björn L. Rydevik, MD, PhD
Kjell Olmarker, MD, PhD

Introduction

In central and lateral spinal stenosis of the lumbar spine, there is a gradual narrowing of the spinal canal and nerve root canals, which leads to a reduction in available space for the nerve roots. Thus, lumbar spinal stenosis implies involvement of the spinal nerve roots of the cauda equina and, in the case of lateral spinal stenosis, there also may be mechanical involvement of the extrathecal components of the nerve root complex (Outline 1). If the dimensions of the central spinal canal are reduced below critical values, the nerve roots of the cauda equina will be subjected to mechanical compression, leading to neurogenic claudication. In this chapter, structural and functional characteristics of nerve roots are described, in relation to production of symptoms in neurogenic intermittent claudication.

Macroscopic and Microscopic Anatomy of Spinal Nerve Roots

The nerve roots form the structural link between the central and the peripheral nervous systems. Anatomically, the nerve roots are related to central nervous tissue. Physiologically, they are more similar to the peripheral nerves. The structure of the nerve root starts when it leaves the spinal cord as small rootlets before caudally joining and forming the separate nerve root. These nerve roots course through the spinal canal and exit through one of the intervertebral foramina, which are formed by pedicles, articular processes, and vertebral bodies

Outline 1 Lumbar spinal stenosis: Factors of pathophysiologic importance

Pressure levels on nerve roots
Rate of nerve root compression (slow versus rapid)
Single versus double or multiple level compression
Dynamic (intermittent) versus static compression
Impairment of intraneural blood flow and nutritional supply via cerebrospinal fluid
Structural alterations in nerve roots and meningeal membranes

of two adjacent vertebrae, including the intervertebral disk. By definition, the dorsal nerve roots end at the dorsal root ganglion, and the ventral nerve roots end at a corresponding level. However, both the dorsal and ventral nerve roots from one spinal segment join just dorsal to the dorsal root ganglion to form the spinal nerve, which in terms of both structure and function is a peripheral nerve (Fig. 1).

The axons running in the nerve roots are located in the endoneurial space. Both unmyelinated and myelinated axons are present in the ventral and dorsal nerve roots. The diameters of the myelinated axons of the human nerve roots usually range between 1.5 and 16 μm, and diameters of the unmyelinated axons range between 0.4 and 1.6 μm.[1] Thomsen[2] observed that the organization of the nerve root endoneurium is separated into a central glial segment and a peripheral nonglial segment. The glial segment has a microscopic anatomy similar to that of the brain, with astrocytes, oligodendrocytes, and microglia.[3] The microanatomy of the nonglial segment is more similar to that of the peripheral

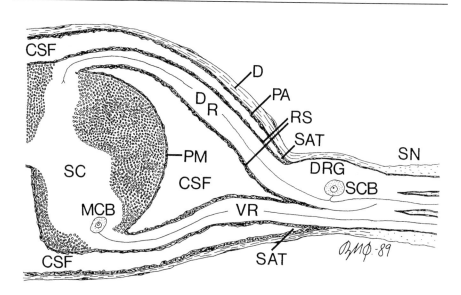

Fig. 1 *Cross-section of a segment of the spinal cord (SC), a ventral (VR) and a dorsal (DR) spinal nerve root. The cell bodies of the motor axons (MCB), which run in the ventral nerve root, are located in the anterior horn of the gray matter of the spinal cord. The cell bodies of the sensory axons (SCB), which run in the dorsal nerve root, are located in the dorsal root ganglion (DRG). The ventral and dorsal nerve roots blend just caudal to the dorsal root ganglion, and form the spinal nerve (SN). The spinal cord is covered with the pia mater (PM). This sheath continues out on the spinal nerve root sheath (RS). The root sheath reflects to the pia-arachnoid (PA) at the subarachnoid triangle (SAT). Together with the dura (D), the pia-arachnoid forms the spinal dura. The spinal cord and nerve roots are floating freely in the cerebrospinal fluid (CSF) in the subarachnoid space. (Reproduced with permission from Olmarker K:* Spinal Nerve Root Compression. *Gothenburg, Sweden, Gothenburg University, 1990. Thesis.)*

nerve, but with small islets of neuroglia. The two segments have a dome- shaped junction 1 to 3 mm after the rootlets leave the spinal cord.[3,4] The endoneurium also contains longitudinally oriented collagen fibrils, fibroblasts, and blood vessels.[1] However, the total amount of protein in nerve roots is only a fifth of that in peripheral nerves, but six times more than that in the spinal cord.[5] In peripheral nerves, the axons run in a wave-form pattern[6,7] that may be seen macroscopically as dark and pale bands across the nerve fascicles when observing the nerve trunk in incident light. These bands are called the spiral bands of Fontana. This anatomic feature, which supposedly compensates for elongation of the nerve, has not been observed in spinal nerve roots.[8]

The endoneural space with its axons is covered by the root sheath, a membrane that separates the axons from the cerebrospinal fluid in the subarachnoid space.[9,10] The root sheath is usually formed by three to four layers of cells.[11,12] However, as many as 12 layers of cells have been observed in some species.[11] The cells of the inner layers are similar to the perineurial cells of peripheral nerves. They are joined by desmosomes and are tightly packed together. There is general agreement that the barrier function of the root sheath is located in these cells and their basal membranes.[11,12]

The spinal cord, cerebrospinal fluid, and spinal nerve roots are enclosed in the spinal dura in a cylinder called the central dural sac or thecal sac.[13,14] Within the central sac each nerve root has a specific location.[15,16] When leaving the spinal cord, the nerve root is centrally located in the sac. However, its location becomes gradually more lateral, and it reaches the spinal dura just prior to leaving the central sac. Upon leaving the central sac, the extrathecal nerve root is covered by a separate extension of the dura called a root sleeve. The extrathecal nerve roots leave the central sac at progressively decreasing angles (Fig. 2).[16] The most prominent difference in takeoff angles between two adjacent nerve roots is at the lumbosacral joint where the angle for the fifth lumbar nerve root usually is about 40°, while that of the first sacral nerve root is about 20°.[16]

The nerve roots of the cauda equina are surrounded by the cerebrospinal fluid, which is likely to provide mechanical protection for the nerve roots and spinal cord. The nerve roots of the cauda equina also seem to derive some of their nutrition via diffusion from the cerebrospinal fluid.[17]

Physiology of Spinal Nerve Roots

Each nerve fiber has two basic functions: propagation of electrical impulses and axonal transport of organelles and various substances such as proteins. Both impulse propagation and axonal transport are energy-dependent processes. The propagation of impulses along the nerve fibers is based on the action potential, which is an all-or-none phenomenon that is elicited in the axon after its resting membrane potential has been altered enough to initiate this process. Because impulse propagation is energy dependent, this process can be blocked, for example, by local ischemia of a nerve or a nerve root.

There is a need for efficient communication systems within the neuron (nerve cell body and its extensions) because of its specific anatomic characteristics, which include long processes (the axons extending from nerve cell bodies). The ratio between length and diameter of an axon is remarkable in that the axonal length may be 10,000 to 15,000 times greater than the diameter of the nerve

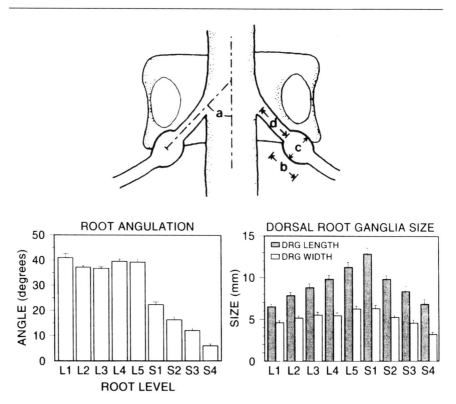

Fig. 2 *Top, Measurement of root takeoff angle (a), DRG length (b), DRG width (c), and distance of proximal ganglia border to root axilla (d). **Bottom left,** Relationship of root take-off angle in the coronal plane to vertebral level (mean ± SE, n = 20). The nerve root angles remain approximately 40° from L1 to L5, decreasing acutely to 22° at S1. The lower sacral nerve root angles decrease progressively thereafter. **Bottom right,** Relationship between DRG length and width and vertebral level (mean ± SE, n = 20). The length and width of the ganglia progressively increase from the L1 to the S1 level. They then decrease progressively in size at the lower sacral levels. (Reproduced with permission from Cohen MS, Wall EJ, Brown RB: Cauda equina anatomy: Part II. Extrathecal nerve roots and dorsal ganglia. Spine 1990;15:1248–1251.)*

cell bodies. Most of the proteins and other substances that are needed for the structural and functional integrity of the neuron are synthesized in the nerve cell body. Such substances are transported from the nerve cell body out to the periphery and also in the opposite direction, through axonal transport systems.

Axonal transport from the nerve cell body to the periphery is called anterograde axonal transport, and the process in the opposite direction is called retrograde axonal transport. Two main components of anterograde axonal transport have been identified.[18-20] Slow anterograde axonal transport takes place at a velocity of about 1 to 6 mm/day and involves transport of cytoskeletal elements, such as microtubuli and microfilaments. Fast anterograde axonal transport takes place at speeds up to about 400 mm/day and involves transport of various enzymes, glycoproteins, lipids, and transmitter substance vesicles.[21-24]

Retrograde axonal transport systems with speeds from about 1 to 300 mm/day have also been identified in several neuronal systems.[25-27]

The exact functions and physiologic significance of axonal transport in both normal and pathologic conditions are not completely understood. Axonal transport systems may be impaired in various pathologic conditions such as ischemia, compression, and axonal degeneration and regeneration.[28-31] The importance of interaction between the nerve cell body and the axon is illustrated by the response of the nerve cell body to nerve injury, including the so-called chromatolytic reaction, which is likely to be based on interruption of the retrograde axonal transport systems.

The axonal transport systems, as well as impulse propagation, require local energy supply along the axon to maintain normal function. Ischemia and anoxia in vitro and in vivo thus may block all types of axonal transport.[32] Although both axonal transport and impulse propagation depend on the supply of energy, these two processes are not based on the same cellular mechanisms. This difference is illustrated by the fact that axonal transport can be maintained over a nerve segment that does not conduct impulses after inhibition of the excitability of the nerve membrane by a blocking substance such as procaine.

The electrophysiologic properties of the nerve root and dorsal root ganglion (DRG) are important in relation to the pathomechanisms of sciatica. The normal DRG can produce spontaneous ectopic discharges and reflected impulses and can also produce mechanically induced discharges; the normal nerve root does not produce discharges.[33-35] Normal variation in the position of the DRG is also important in this regard.

Nociception at the nerve endings and the synapses in the spinal cord is the result of a complicated mechanism that involves several pain-producing substances and neuropeptides. Special attention should be directed to the effector function of antidromically released neuropeptides, which cause neurogenic inflammation. The DRG is an important structure as the site for synthesis of neuropeptides such as substance P and calcitonin gene-related peptide, as well as other substances that are transported both centrally and peripherally by axonal transport.[36-40] In experiments, the synthesis of neuropeptides in the DRG is influenced more by cutting the peripheral nerve than by cutting the nerve root.[41,42]

Vascular Anatomy of Spinal Nerve Roots

The vascular anatomy of the nervous structures of the spinal canal was originally described over 100 years ago.[43-48] Except for some occasional reports,[49,50] there was no particular interest in the blood supply of the spinal cord and roots during the first half of this century. However, an interest in the capability of the spinal cord to recover from vascular lesions and its reaction to vascular surgery initiated a number of investigations on the collateral circulation of the spinal cord arteries.[51-58] There also have been at least two theses on the vascularization of spinal nerve roots.[59,60] The arterial blood supply of the nerve roots is derived mainly from the segmental arteries, which branch from the aorta and the common iliac artery. These vessels divide into three major branches: (1) an anterior branch, which supplies the posterior abdominal wall and the lumbar plexus; (2) a posterior branch, which supplies the paraspinal muscles and facet joints; and (3) an intermediate branch. The intermediate branch, in turn, gener-

713

ally divides into three subdivisions: (1) anterior spinal branches, which supply the posterior aspects of the vertebral bodies and disks; (2) posterior spinal branches, which supply the vertebral arches, the epidural fat, and the spinal dura; and (3) nervous system branches.[57]

The nervous system branches divide into two sets of vessels. The medullary feeder arteries (extrinsic system) supply the arteries of the spinal cord without providing branches to the nerve roots along their course through the subarachnoid space. The other vessels incorporate with either of the two nerve roots (intrinsic system).[61] Thus, the vessels of the extrinsic system do not directly take part in the nutrition of the nerve roots. In the embryo, there are 124 medullary feeder arteries at 31 segmental levels. These arteries are soon reduced in number, and at birth there are only about eight remaining.[61] Thus, the medullary arteries each supply more than one segment of the spinal cord.[56]

The vessels that supply the ventral roots form one to three caudal radicular arteries that are located within the root sheath, run craniad (towards the spinal cord) and are part of the intrinsic system (Fig. 3). In the dorsal root, however, the corresponding vessels form a ganglionic plexus around the DRG before they continue in a cranial direction as caudal radicular arteries. The caudal radicular arteries of both the ventral and the dorsal roots anastomose with the cranial radicular arteries, which are derived from the vascular network of the spinal cord, at the cranial half of the nerve roots. Thus, blood flow is supplied from both cranial and caudal directions. At the location where these two vascular networks anastomose, the vasculature of the nerve roots is less developed. It thus has been suggested that this region of relative hypovascularization may be a particularly vulnerable site of the nerve roots.[61,62]

The arteries of the intrinsic vessels are located mainly in the outer layers of the root sheath. Occasionally they are also found deeper in the nerve root tissue between, or even within the fascicles.[62] The arteries provide each fascicle with a number of parallel interfascicular arterioles via a network of T-shaped branches. There are arterial coils and vascular loops present that will compensate for elongation of the vessels in both the axial direction and between the fascicles.[62,63] Within the fascicles, (ie, in the endoneurial space), the endoneurial capillaries run parallel to the axons.

The venous system has an organization similar to that of the arteries. The largest veins, however, not only course together with the corresponding arteries as in peripheral nerves;[64] they also have a spiraling course deeper in the nerve roots.[62] The veins of the nerve roots also differ from the arteries in that veins occasionally drain through the spinal dura out into the epidural venous plexus.

Permeability of Nerve Root Microvessels and Mechanisms of Edema Formation

In peripheral nerves, there is a diffusion barrier in the wall of the endoneurial capillaries; this barrier is called the blood-nerve barrier, in analogy to the blood-brain barrier of the central nervous system.[65-67] This diffusion barrier seems to be based on the presence of tight junctions between the endothelial cells of the capillaries and/or relative lack of pinocytotic vesicles.[66] However, the microvessels in the epineurium of peripheral nerves are fenestrated and allow a more free

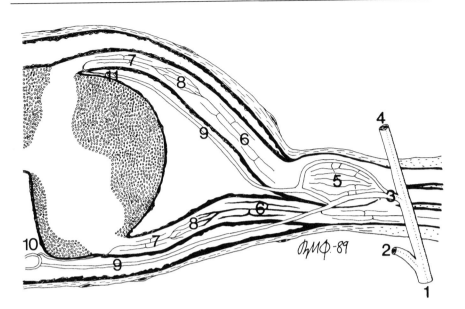

Fig. 3 *Schematic drawing of vascular supply to the spinal cord and nerve roots. When the intermediate branch of the segmental artery (1) enters the spinal canal, it divides into an anterior spinal canal branch (2), a nervous system branch (3), and a posterior spinal canal branch (4). The nervous system branch joins the nerve root and forms a ganglionic plexus (5) and caudal nerve root arteries running in a cranial direction (6). From the vasa corona of the spinal cord, cranial nerve root arteries (7) run in a caudal direction. The caudal and the cranial nerve root arteries anastomose within the cranial half of the nerve root (8). Medullary feeder arteries (9) are also present from the nervous system branch, and run cranially through the subarachnoid space, without any connections to the nerve root arteries, to the vasa corona of the spinal cord, where (10) is the anterior spinal artery and (11) is one of the two dorsolateral spinal arteries. (Reproduced with permission from Olmarker K:* Spinal Nerve Root Compression. *Gothenburg, Sweden, Gothenburg University, 1990. Thesis.)*

passage of various molecules between the intravascular and extravascular compartments.[65] There is experimental evidence that normal transfer of serum albumin from capillaries of nerve root endoneurium is less pronounced than transfer from capillaries in the epineurium of peripheral nerves and the DRG.[65,66] The capillaries of the DRG are fenestrated,[68,69] and there is no blood-nerve barrier in the vessels in the epineurium of peripheral nerves.[67-70] Thus, the permeability of the microvessels of nerve roots indicates a more free passage of fluid and macromolecules than occurs in the endoneurium of peripheral nerves. This difference might imply that edema may form more easily in nerve roots than in peripheral nerves.

The microvessels of peripheral nerves and nerve roots, like all other microvessels in the body, become more permeable when injured. This reaction may lead to formation of edema in the nerve tissue. Such edema may have various effects on nerve fiber structure and function; for example, by altering the ionic balance around the nerve fibers.[70] Furthermore, edema within a confined tissue

715

compartment may result in increased pressure. Such a mechanism has been demonstrated in peripheral nerves following local compression[71] and in DRG following mechanical compression.[72] There is experimental evidence to indicate that formation of endoneurial edema per se may negatively influence the function of axons, without mechanical compression, as indicated by postischemic formation of endoneurial edema.[70]

Effects of Acute Compression on Nerve Roots

The pathophysiology of acute cauda equina nerve root compression has been studied over the last few years.[73-75] In a porcine model, graded compression of the cauda equina is induced by an inflatable balloon, which is fixed to the lower spine after a one- or two-level laminectomy. Using this model, Olmarker and associates[76] have demonstrated that impairment of venular blood flow in terms of congestion in the microcirculation had already been induced at pressures as low as 10 mm Hg. Nutritional impairment of the nerve roots in terms of reduced solute transport was studied using ^{3}H labeled methylglycose; nutrition was reduced by about 55% at 50 mm Hg compression.[77] This nutritional impairment might be related to the formation of intraneural edema.[78]

Nerve root impulse propagation has also been evaluated in the same experimental cauda equina compression model. During a 2-hour compression period, the critical level for impairment of impulse conduction was in the range of 50 to 75 mm Hg. Higher pressure levels (100 to 200 mm Hg) may induce a total conduction block, with varying degrees of recovery following compression release. It has also been shown, in this model, that the sensory fibers seem to be slightly more susceptible to compression than the motor fibers.[74,75]

These functional changes, induced by controlled graded cauda equina compression, also depend on factors such as systemic blood pressure. The threshold for impulse propagation impairment is lowered by experimental hypotension.[79] These observations indicate the pathophysiologic significance of an adequate blood supply to the nerve roots in conjunction with various compression disorders.

Effects of Chronic Compression on Nerve Roots

Recently, a number of models of chronic compresion, ie, experiments in which the animal survives, have been established. Delamarter and associates[80] compressed the dog cauda equina using a plastic band and defined 50% reduction of the dural sac as a critical constriction for inducing slight neurologic deficit and major changes in cortical evoked potentials. A modification of the same model was described by Kim and associates,[81] who obtained the same critical constriction percentage. The dog cauda equina was also subjected to a combination of chronic and acute compression using a system of interconnected inflatable balloons.[82-84] These latter studies showed that chronically compressed nerve roots develop an increased resistance to acute compression and are thus not as susceptible to mechanical deformation as noncompressed nerve roots.[84]

Compression of the single nerve roots has also been assessed.[85,86] Yoshizawa and associates[85] ligated a Silastic tube loosely around the seventh lumbar nerve root in the dog and found that intraneural edema was the most important factor for inducing structural and functional changes. The second sacral nerve root in the pig has been extensively studied.[86] After application of a specially designed constrictor, with a delayed onset of compression during 2 to 3 weeks, fluid is absorbed and the constrictor expands inward because of its rigid outer shell (Fig. 4).[86] The constrictor produced well-controlled changes in structure and nerve conduction velocity when applied for 1 or 4 weeks.[86] Although blood flow was markedly reduced in the compressed segment, the blood flow of the nerve root outside of the segment was not.[87] The constriction, when applied for 1 week, also induced an increase in the synthesis of substance P.[88] After 4 weeks, the amount of substance P was markedly reduced in the nerve root cranial to the constrictor but significantly increased in the DRG. It was suggested that this increase was caused by a compression-induced accumulation of substance P in the DRG, where the synthesis rate was already increased. Based on the assumption that substance P may be involved in pain transmission, it was suggested that this was indirect evidence of painful compression. The constrictor has also been used to compare the effects by mechanical compression to the effects of locally applied autologous nucleus pulposus. It was found that the used constrictor diameter (3.5 mm) induced a similar reduction as compared to the nucleus pulposus, but that the nucleus pulposus also induced changes in the contralateral control nerve root, maybe as the result of diffusion.[89]

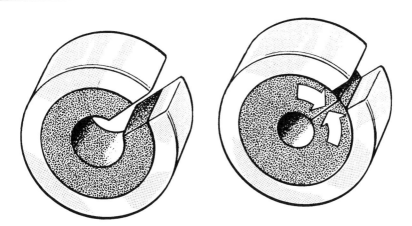

Fig. 4 *Schematic drawing of constrictor used for chronic nerve root compression. The inner surface of the rigid metal cylinder is coated with a thick layer of ameroid. Because of this rigid outer metal shell, the expansion of the ameroid material by absorption of water is directed inward, resulting in compression of the nerve root, which is placed in the center of the constrictor. (Reproduced with permission from Cornefjord M, Olmarker K, Farley DB: Neuropeptide changes in compressed spinal nerve roots.* Spine *1995;20:670–673.)*

Double-Level Nerve Root Compression

It has been shown that central spinal stenosis often is present at more than one spinal level at the same time.[90] A combination of central and lateral spinal stenosis is also commonly seen in patients with symptomatic nerve root compression. The pathophysiologic effects of double-level cauda equina compression have been investigated using a modification of the porcine cauda equina model, in which two balloons were placed at two adjacent disk levels such that there was a 10-mm uncompressed segment between the balloons (Fig. 5). In this experimental setup much more pronounced impairment of nerve impulse conduction was induced by double-level compression than had been found at corresponding compression levels with single-level compression.[91] For instance, a pressure of 50 mm Hg in each of two balloons induced a block of nerve impulse amplitude after 60 minutes of compression, whereas 50 mm Hg in one balloon induced no reduction (Fig. 6). The mechanism behind such changes induced by double-level compression may be based on the particular local vascular anatomy of nerve roots. There are no regional nutritive arteries from surrounding structures to the intraneural vascular system in spinal nerve roots.[62,70,73] Compression at two levels might, therefore, induce a nutritionally impaired re-

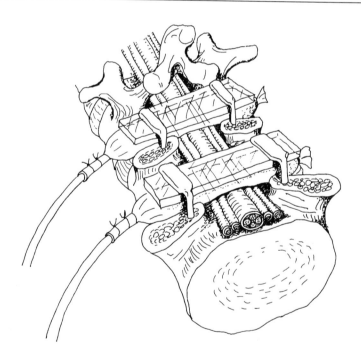

Fig. 5 *Schematic drawing of experimental double-level cauda equina compression. The cauda equina is compressed by two balloons placed across the opened spinal canal and fixed to the vertebrae by L-shaped pins and Plexiglass plates. (Reproduced with permission from Olmarker K, Rydevik B: Single- versus double-level nerve root compression. Clin Orthop 1992;279:35–39.)*

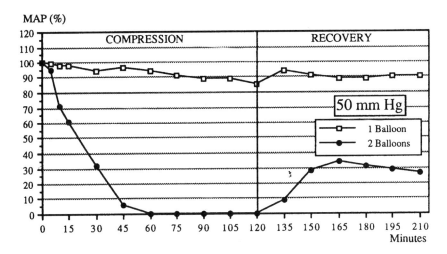

Fig. 6   *Diagram of muscle action potential (MAP) amplitude, comparing the effects of single- and double-level compression. Mean MAP amplitude during compression at 50 mm Hg and recovery. (Reproduced with permission from Olmarker K, Rydevik B: Single- versus double-level nerve root compression.* Clin Orthop *1992;279:35–39.)*

gion between the two compression sites. Experimental evaluation of this hypothesis showed that blood flow in the uncompressed nerve root segment located between two compression balloons was reduced by 64% when both balloons were inflated to 10 mm Hg.[92] The overall conclusion from the experimental studies of double-level nerve root compression, as related to clinical observations in spinal stenosis patients, is that double-level compression induced much more pronounced changes in nerve root nutrition and function than did single-level compression at corresponding pressure levels.

Biomechanics of Nerve Root Compression

Mechanical deformation, such as compression and stretching of nerve roots, affects all the tissue components of the roots (nerve fibers, connective tissue, and blood vessels). Therefore, a discussion of nerve root biomechanics should consider that nerve roots are complex structures in which each tissue component has distinct mechanical properties. Data on peripheral nerve biomechanics cannot be directly applied to spinal nerve root biomechanics owing to the anatomic differences between these two components of the nervous system.[93-95]

Within certain limits, spinal nerve roots may adapt to mechanical deformation without functional changes. However, if the applied force and the resulting deformation exceed those limits, both functional and structural changes may occur. The nerve roots in the subarachnoid space are devoid of epineurium and perineurium, but under tensile loading, they exhibit both elasticity and tensile strength.[96] The limit of elasticity of the nerve roots was found to be 15% of their length, and if nerve roots are stretched more than 20%, complete failure can occur. The ultimate load and stiffness of rat nerve roots are 10% and 20%,

719

respectively, of that of rat peripheral nerves.[97] The ultimate load for human ventral spinal nerve roots from the cauda equina is between 2 and 22 N; for dorsal nerve roots, the corresponding value is between 5 and 33 N.[96]

The mechanical properties of human spinal nerve roots differ depending on whether the root is located in the spinal canal or in the lateral intervertebral foramen region. For example, the ultimate load for the intrathecal portion of the S1 nerve root is 13 N, whereas the ultimate load for the foraminal portion of the S1 nerve root is about 73 N.[98] Corresponding differences between intrathecal and foraminal components have also been verified for the L5 nerve roots. This means that the ultimate load values for the foraminal nerve root sections are about five times higher than those for the intrathecal portion of the same nerve root under tensile loading. However, if the larger cross-sectional area of the nerve root in the intervertebral foramen is compared with the corresponding area in the intrathecal region, the ultimate tensile stress values are more comparable in the two locations.

The biomechanics of nerve root deformation in association with spinal stenosis and disk herniation are different. Spinal stenosis is generally a slowly developing process during which the nerve roots are compressed in a circumferential manner at slow rate. In a dorsolateral lumbar disk herniation, the nerve root deformation is different. There is a local compression, which leads to some flattening of the nerve root, but there also is intraneural tension because the nerve root normally is fixed to the surrounding tissues above and below each intervertebral disk.[99] The contact force between a simulated disk herniation in human cadavers and the deformed nerve root has been evaluated by Spencer and associates.[100] The contact pressure between the disk herniation and the nerve root in these situations was calculated to reach approximately 400 mm Hg. With reduced disk height, the contact pressure between the experimental disk herniation and the nerve root was decreased because of slackening of the nerve root.

Data from human cadaver spine studies, which involve constriction of the dural sac and the enclosed cauda equina with a round clamp, have indicated that the pressure levels among the nerve roots of the cauda equina in spinal stenosis are likely to be considerably lower than the contact pressure associated with disk herniation.[101,102] A pressure level of about 50 mm Hg among the nerve roots of the cauda equina was induced experimentally by constricting the dural sac acutely to a cross-sectional area of 63 ± 24 mm^2 (about 37% of the normal dural sac size at this level). The corresponding degree of acute dural sac constriction needed to elevate pressure to 100 mm Hg is 57 ± 11 mm^2 (which corresponds to 33% of the normal dural sac size at this level).[102] Results from this research also indicated that constricting the cauda equina in the human lumbar spine down to a cross-sectional area less than about 75 mm^2 is likely to induce mechanical compression of the cauda equina nerve roots. Such compression may cause physiologic changes in nerve roots. The values reported here for critical areas of the dural sac correlate with the cross-sectional area of the dural sac in patients with symptoms of central spinal stenosis (90 ± 35 mm^2).[103] However, the dimensions of the spinal canal depend on posture and, for example, flexion and axial unloading can lead to an increase in the available space for cauda equina nerve roots.

The effects of prolonged compression of the cauda equina in dogs has been studied by Delamarter and associates.[80] The cauda equina was acutely constricted circumferentially to 75%, 50%, or 25% of the normal cross-sectional area. The effects of such compression were evaluated at up to 3 months. The result indicated that, with constriction to 75% of the normal value, there were no neurologic deficits. However, with constriction to 50% or 25% of the normal cross-sectional area, there was both motor and sensory impairment, as well as structural damage of the nerve roots. These observations thus correlate with the studies on human cadaver spines by Schönström and associates,[101,102] in which nerve root compression was induced when the cross-sectional area of the dural sac was reduced to about 45% of normal transverse dural sac area.

The effects of compression on spinal nerve roots are related not only to pressure level and duration of compression but also to the onset rate of compression. A rapid onset rate (0.05 to 0.1 second) causes much more pronounced tissue changes and functional deterioration than does a slow onset rate (20 seconds) when compared at corresponding compression pressure levels (Fig. 7). Thus, a rapid onset rate caused more edema formation in the nerve roots, impairment of nutritional transport, and more pronounced changes in impulse conduction than slow onset rate compression.[77,78,104] These rate-dependent physiologic effects are likely to be based on the viscoelastic properties of the nerve tissues.

In cases of local compression, the nerve fibers are displaced from the center of the compressed area toward the noncompressed areas. Such longitudinal displacement as well as intraneural shear stress is maximum at the edges of the compressed segment[67,94,105] and may be called the edge effect. At the edges, where the mechanical deformation is maximum, the damage to both nerve fibers and intraneural microvessels is most pronounced. Thus, in case of local nerve compression, tissue damage does not seem to occur where the hydrostatic pressure in the nerve tissue is the highest (in the center), but where the resulting tissue deformation is most pronounced, namely at the edges of the compressed nerve segment.[94]

Chronic Nerve Root Injury and Experimental–Clinical Correlations

Long-standing compression of spinal nerve roots is likely to induce intraneural edema which may be transferred into fibrotic scar tissue within and around nerve roots.[93] The thin nerve root sheath on the surface of the cauda equina nerve roots may become thickened, leading to impaired passage of nutrients from the cerebrospinal fluid to the nerve root tissue. In case of central spinal stenosis, the free passage of cerebrospinal fluid at the level of stenosis may also be significantly reduced because of the reduction in the dimensions of the dural sac. The nerve fibers can react to long-standing compression by local demyelination and/or axonal degeneration. Such structural nerve fiber injury can, together with the nutritional impairment, lead to ectopic impulse generation,[93] which is likely to be related to pain production in such disorders. Critical dimensions for the dural sac in the lumbar spine as well as pressure levels acting on cauda equina nerve roots have thus been determined by Schönström and associates.[101,103] These data provide a basis for the correlation between experimental data and clinical management regarding diagnosis of central spinal stenosis. Recently, Takahashi and associates[106] have demonstrated variations in epidural pressures in

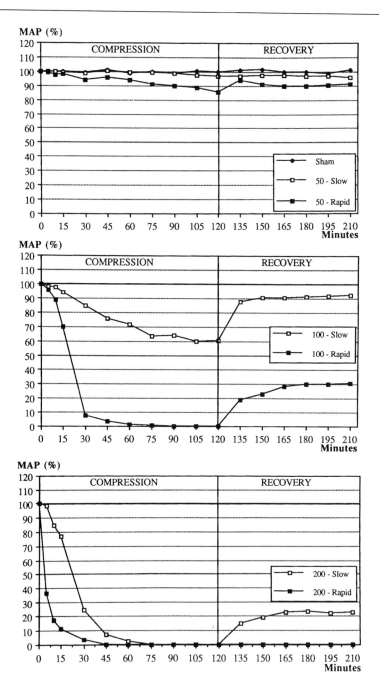

Fig. 7 *Data from experimental graded compression of the pig cauda equina. Average amplitude of muscle action potential (MAP), representing conduction of the fastest conducting motor nerve fibers, expressed a percentage of baseline value. The diagrams show the results of 2 hours of compression and 1.5 hours of recovery for sham compression and for rapid and slow onset compression at 50, 100, and 200 mm Hg. Note that the effects of rapid onset of compression are more pronounced than those of slow onset compression, particularly at 100 mm Hg. (Reproduced with permission from Olmarker K, Holm S, Rydevik B: Importance of compression onset rate for the degree of impairment of impulse propagation in experimental compression injury of the porcine cauda equina. Spine 1990;15:416–419.)*

the lumbar spines of patients with central spinal stenosis. They found that the epidural pressure during standing could reach levels of approximately 110 to 120 mm Hg, which were several times higher than the corresponding pressure measurements while in a lying position. Furthermore, the epidural pressures were found to have a pattern of increase and decrease during walking that provides a basis for description of an intermittent pattern of cauda equina compression in relation to spinal stenosis. Such intermittent compression might be more injurious than constant compression,[107] possibly as a result of tissue injury phenomena caused by reperfusion injury in the spinal nerve root microvasculature. Factors that are likely to be of pathophysiologic importance for nerve root involvement in spinal stenosis are summarized in Outline 1.

Acknowledgments

This chapter is based on research supported by the Swedish Medical Research Council (projects no. 8685 and 9758) and the IngaBritt and Arne Lundberg Research Foundation, Sweden.

References

1. Gamble HJ, Eames RA: Electron microscopy of human spinal-nerve roots. *Arch Neurol* 1966;14:50–53.
2. Thomsen R: Üeber eigenthümliche aus veränderten Ganglienzellen hervorgegangene Gebilde in den Stämmen der Hirnnerven des menschen. *Virchow's Arch Path Anat* 1887;109:459–465.
3. Tarlov IM: Structure of the nerve root: I. Nature of the junction between the central and the peripheral nervous system. *Arch Neurol Psychiat* 1937;37:555–583.
4. Berthold CH, Carlstedt T, Corneliuson O: Anatomy of the nerve root at the central-peripheral transitional region, in Dyck PJ, Thomas PK, Lambert EH, et al (eds): *Peripheral Neuropathy,* ed 2. Philadelphia, PA, WB Saunders, 1984, vol 1, pp 156–170.
5. Stodieck LS, Beel JA, Luttges MW: Structural properties of spinal nerve roots: Protein composition. *Exp Neurol* 1986;91:41–51.
6. Clarke E, Bearn JG: The spiral nerve bands of Fontana. *Brain* 1972;95:1–20.
7. Thomas PK, Olsson Y: Microscopic anatomy and function of the connective tissue components of peripheral nerve, in Dyck PJ, Thomas PK, Lambert EH, et al (eds): *Peripheral Neuropathy,* ed 2. Philadelphia, PA, WB Saunders, 1984, vol 1, pp 97–120.
8. Sunderland S (ed): *Nerves and Nerve Injuries,* ed 2. Edinburgh, Scotland, Churchill Livingstone, 1978.
9. Waggener JD, Beggs J: The membranous coverings of neural tissues: An electron microscopy study. *J Neuropathol Exp Neurol* 1967;26:412–426.
10. McCabe JS, Low FN: The subarachnoid angle: An area of transition in peripheral nerve. *Anat Rec* 1969;164:15–33.
11. Haller FR, Low FN: The fine structure of the peripheral nerve root sheath in the subarachnoid space in the rat and other laboratory animals. *Am J Anat* 1971;131:1–19.
12. Steer JM: Some observations on the fine structure of rat dorsal spinal nerve roots. *J Anat* 1971;109:467–485.
13. Rauschning W: Computed tomography and cryomicrotomy of lumbar spine specimens: A new technique for multiplanar anatomic correlation. *Spine* 1983;8:170–180.
14. Rauschning W: Normal and pathologic anatomy of the lumbar root canals. *Spine* 1987;12:1008–1019.
15. Wall EJ, Cohen MS, Massie JB, et al: Cauda equina anatomy: I. Intrathecal nerve root organization. *Spine* 1990;15:1244–1247.

16. Cohen MS, Wall EJ, Brown RB, et al: Cauda equina anatomy: II. Extrathecal nerve roots and dorsal root ganglia. *Spine* 1990;15:1248–1251.

17. Rydevik B, Holm S, Brown MD, et al: Diffusion from the cerebrospinal fluid as a nutritional pathway for spinal nerve roots. *Acta Physiol Scand* 1990;138:247–248.

18. Black MM, Lasek RJ: Slow components of axonal transport: Two cytoskeletal networks. *J Cell Biol* 1980;86:616–623.

19. Droz B: Synthetic machinery and axoplasmic transport: Maintenance of neuronal connectivity, in Tower DB, Brady RO (eds): *The Nervous System: The Basic Neurosciences.* New York, NY, Raven Press, 1975, vol 1, pp 111–127.

20. Grafstein B, Forman DS: Intracellular transport in neurons. *Physiol Rev* 1980;60:1167–1283.

21. Dahlström A: Axoplasmic transport (with particular respect to adrenergic neurons) *Philos Trans R Soc Lond B Biol Sci* 1971;261:325–358.

22. Lasek RJ: Protein transport in neurons. *Int Rev Neurobiol* 1970;13:289–324.

23. Ochs S: Axoplasmic transport, in Tower DB, Brady RO (eds): *The Nervous System: The Basic Neurosciences.* New York, NY, Raven Press, 1975, pp 137–146.

24. Weiss DG: General properties of axoplasmic transport, in Weiss DG (ed): *Axoplasmic Transport.* Berlin, Germany, Springer-Verlag, 1982, pp 1–14.

25. Bisby MA: Orthograde and retrograde axonal transport of labeled protein in motoneurons. *Exp Neurol* 1976;50:628–640.

26. Kristensson K, Sjöstrand J: Retrograde transport of protein tracer in the rabbit hypoglossal nerve during regeneration. *Brain Res* 1972;45:175–181.

27. Lubinska L: On axoplasmic flow. *Int Rev Neurobiol* 1975;17:241–296.

28. Dahlin LB, Rydevik B, McLean WG, et al: Changes in fast axonal transport during experimental nerve compression at low pressures. *Exp Neurol* 1984;84:29–36.

29. Dahlin LB, McLean WG: Effects of graded experimental compression on slow and fast axonal transport in rabbit vagus nerve. *J Neurol Sci* 1986;72:19–30.

30. Danielsen N, Lundborg G, Frizell M: Nerve repair and axonal transport: Distribution of axonally transported proteins during maturation period in regenerating rabbit hypoglossal nerve. *J Neurol Sci* 1986;73:269–277.

31. Leone J, Ochs S: Anoxic block and recovery of axoplasmic transport and electrical excitability of nerve. *J Neurobiol* 1978;9:229–245.

32. Rydevik B, McLean WG, Sjöstrand J, et al: Blockage of axonal transport induced by acute graded compression of the rabbit vagus nerve. *J Neurol Neurosurg Psychiatry* 1980;43:690–698.

33. Devor M, Obermayer M: Membrane differentiation in rat dorsal root ganglia and possible consequences for back pain. *Neurosci Lett* 1984;51:341–346.

34. Howe JF, Loeser JD, Calvin WH: Mechanosensitivity of dorsal root ganglia and chronically injured axons: A physiological basis for the radicular pain of nerve root compression. *Pain* 1977;3:25–41.

35. Wall PD, Devor M: Sensory afferent impulses originate from dorsal root ganglia as well as from the periphery in normal and nerve injured rats. *Pain* 1983;17:321–339.

36. Carr DB, Lipkowski AW: Neuropeptides and pain. *Agressologie* 1990;31:173–177.

37. Harmar A, Keen P: Synthesis, and central and peripheral axonal transport of substance P in a dorsal root ganglion-nerve preparation in vitro. *Brain Res* 1982;231:379–385.

38. Kashihara Y, Sakaguchi M, Kuno M: Axonal transport and distribution of endogenous calcitonin gene-related peptide in rat peripheral nerve. *J Neurosci* 1989;9:3796–3802.

39. Weinstein J: Mechanisms of spinal pain: The dorsal root ganglion and its role as a mediator of low-back pain. *Spine* 1986;11:999–1001.

40. Weinstein J, Claverie W, Gibson S: The pain of discography. *Spine* 1988;13:1344–1348.

41. Czéh G, Kudo N, Kuno M: Membrane properties and conduction velocity in sensory neurones following central or peripheral axotomy. *J Physiol* 1977;270:165–180.

42. Tohyama M, Senba E, Noguchi K, et al: Different responses in neuropeptide biosynthesis of axotomized dorsal root ganglion cells: An analysis using in situ hybridization histochemistry. *Biomed Res* 1989;3(suppl):349–354.

43. Duret H: Note sur les artères nourricières et sur les vaisseaux capillaires de la moelle épinière. *Progr Méd* 1873:284.

44. Duret H: Conclusion d'un mémoire sur la circulation bulbaire. *Arch Physiol Norm et Path* 1873;50:88–89.

45. Adamkiewicz A: Die Blutgefässe des menschlichen Rückenmarkes: I. Die Gefässe der Rückenmarkssubstanz. *Sitzungsb d k Akad d Wissensch Math Naturw* 1882;84:469–502.

46. Adamkiewicz A: Die Blutgefässe des menschlichen Rückenmarkes: II. Die Gefäse der Rückenmarksoberfläche. *Sitzungsb d k Akad d Wissensch Math Naturw* 1882;85:101–130.

47. Kadyi H: Über die Blutgefässe des menschlichen Rückenmarkes. *Anat Anz* 1886;1:304–314.

48. Tanon L: *Les Artères de la Moelle Dorsolombaire*. Paris, France, University of Paris, 1908. Thesis.

49. Suh TH, Alexander L: Vascular system of the human spinal cord. *Arch Neurol Psychiat* 1939;41:659–677.

50. Herren RY, Alexander L: Sulcal and intrinsic blood vessels of human spinal cord. *Arch Neurol Psychiat* 1939;41:678–687.

51. Adams HD, van Geertruyden HH: Neurologic complications of aortic surgery. *Ann Surg* 1956;144:574–610.

52. Fried LC, Doppman J: The arterial supply to the lumbo-sacral spinal cord in the monkey: A comparison with man. *Anat Rec* 1974;178:41–48.

53. Gillilan LA: The arterial blood supply of the human spinal cord. *J Comp Neurol* 1958;110:75–103.

54. Corbin JL (ed): *Anatomie et Pathologie Arterielles de la Moelle*. Paris, France, Masson et Cie, 1961.

55. Lazorthes G, Gouazé A, Bastide G, et al: Arterial vascularization of the lumbar elevation: Study of variations and substitutions. *Rev Neurol* 1966;114:109–122.

56. Lazorthes G, Gouaze A, Zadeh JO, et al: Arterial vascularization of the spinal cord: Recent studies of the anastomotic substitution pathways. *J Neurosurg* 1971;35:253–262.

57. Crock HV, Yoshizawa H: The blood supply of the lumbar vertebral column. *Clin Orthop* 1976;115:6–21.

58. Dommisse GF, Grobler L: Arteries and veins of the lumbar nerve roots and cauda equina. *Clin Orthop* 1976;115:22–29.

59. Desproges-Gotteron R: *Contribution À L'étude De La Sciatique Paralysante*. Paris, France, University of Paris, 1955, Thesis.

60. Viraswami V: *A Study of the Blood Supply of the Nerve Roots in Man and the Rabbit With an Experimental Analysis of the Collateral Circulation Following Ligature of the Arteries*. London, UK, London University, 1963. Thesis.

61. Parke WW, Gammell K, Rothman RH: Arterial vascularization of the cauda equina. *J Bone Joint Surg* 1981;63A:53–62.

62. Parke WW, Watanabe R: The intrinsic vasculature of the lumbosacral spinal nerve roots. *Spine* 1985;10:508–515.

63. Petterson CÅ, Olsson Y: Blood supply of spinal nerve roots: An experimental study in the rat. *Acta Neuropathol* 1989;78:455–461.

64. Lundborg G: Ischemic nerve injury: Experimental studies on intraneural microvascular pathophysiology and nerve function in a limb subjected to temporary circulatory arrest. *Scand J Plast Reconstr Surg* 1970;6(suppl):3–113.

65. Olsson Y, Reese TS: Abstract: Inaccessibility of the endoneurium of mouse sciatic nerve to exogenous proteins. *Anat Rec* 1969;163:318–319.

66. Olsson Y, Reese TS: Permeability of vasa nervorum and perineurium in mouse sciatic nerve studied by fluorescence and electron microscopy. *J Neuropathol Exp Neurol* 1971;30:105–119.

725

67. Rydevik B, Lundborg G: Permeability of intraneural microvessels and perineurium following acute, graded experimental nerve compression. *Scand J Plast Reconstr Surg* 1977;11:179–187.

68. Arvidson B: A study of the perineurial diffusion barrier of a peripheral ganglion. *Acta Neurpathol* 1979;46:139–144.

69. Jacobs JM, Macfarlane RM, Cavanagh JB: Vascular leakage in the dorsal root ganglia of the rat, studied with horseradish peroxidase. *J Neurol Sci* 1976;29:95–107.

70. Lundborg G: Structure and function of the intraneural microvessels as related to trauma, edema formation, and nerve function. *J Bone Joint Surg* 1975;57A:938–948.

71. Lundborg G, Myers R, Powell H: Nerve compression injury and increased endoneurial fluid pressure: A "miniature compartment syndrome." *J Neurol Neurosurg Psychiatry* 1983;46:1119–1124.

72. Rydevik BL, Myers RR, Powell HC: Pressure increase in the dorsal root ganglion following mechanical compression: Closed compartment syndrome in nerve roots. *Spine* 1989;14:574–576.

73. Olmarker K: Spinal nerve root compression: Nutrition and function of the porcine cauda equina compressed in vivo. *Acta Orthop Scand* 1991;242:1–27.

74. Pedowitz RA, Garfin SR, Massie JB, et al: Effects of magnitude and duration of compression on spinal nerve root conduction. *Spine* 1992;17:194–199.

75. Rydevik BL, Pedowitz RA, Hargens AR, et al: Effects of acute, graded compression on spinal nerve root function and structure: An experimental study of the pig cauda equina. *Spine* 1991;16:487–493.

76. Olmarker K, Rydevik B, Holm S, et al: Effects of experimental graded compression on blood flow in spinal nerve roots: A vital microscopic study on the porcine cauda equina. *J Orthop Res* 1989;7:817–823.

77. Olmarker K, Rydevik B, Hansson T, et al: Compression-induced changes of the nutritional supply to the porcine cauda equina. *J Spinal Disord* 1990;3:25–29.

78. Olmarker K, Rydevik B, Holm S: Edema formation in spinal nerve roots induced by experimental, graded compression: An experimental study on the pig cauda equina with special reference to differences in effects between rapid and slow onset of compression. *Spine* 1989;14:569–573.

79. Garfin SR, Cohen MS, Massie JB, et al: Nerve-roots of the cauda equina: The effect of hypotension and acute graded compression on function. *J Bone Joint Surg* 1990;72A:1185–1192.

80. Delamarter RB, Bohlman HH, Dodge LD, et al: Experimental lumbar spinal stenosis: Analysis of the cortical evoked potentials, microvasculature, and histopathology. *J Bone Joint Surg* 1990;72A:110–120.

81. Kim NH, Yang IH, Song IK: Electrodiagnostic and histologic changes of graded caudal compression on cauda equina in dog. *Spine* 1994;19:1054–1062.

82. Konno S, Yabuki S, Sato K, et al: A model for acute, chronic, and delayed, graded compression of the dog cauda equina: Presentation of the gross, microscopic, and vascular anatomy of the dog cauda equina and accuracy in pressure transmission of the compression model. *Spine* 1995;20:2758–2764.

83. Sato K, Konno S, Yabuki S, et al: A model for acute, chronic, and delayed graded compression of the dog cauda equina: Neurophysiologic and histologic changes induced by acute, graded compression. *Spine* 1995;20:2386–2391.

84. Kikuchi S, Konno S, Kayama S, et al: Increased resistance to acute compression injury in chronically compressed spinal nerve roots. An experimental study. *Spine*, in press.

85. Yoshizawa H, Kobayashi S, Morita T: Chronic nerve root compression: Pathophysiologic mechanism of nerve root dysfunction. *Spine* 1995;20:397–407.

86. Cornefjord M, Sato K, Olmarker K, et al: A model for chronic nerve root compression studies: Presentation of a porcine gradual onset compression model with analyses of nerve root conduction velocity. *Spine*, in press.

87. Sato K, Olmarker K, Cornefjord M, et al: Changes of intraradicular blood flow in chronic nerve root compression: An experimental study on pigs. *Neuroorthopaedics* 1994;16:1–7.
88. Cornefjord M, Olmarker K, Farley DB, et al: Neuropeptide changes in compressed spinal nerve roots. *Spine* 1995;20:670–673.
89. Cornefjord M, Olmarker K, Konno S, et al: Mechanical and biochemical injury in spinal nerve roots. A neurophysiologic study. *Eur Spine J,* in press.
90. Porter RW, Ward D: Cauda equina dysfunction: The significance of two-level pathology. *Spine* 1992;17:9–15.
91. Olmarker K, Rydevik B: Single-versus double-level nerve root compression: An experimental study on the porcine cauda equina with analyses of nerve impulse conduction properties. *Clin Orthop* 1992;279:35–39.
92. Takahashi K, Olmarker K, Holm S, et al: Double-level cauda equina compression: An experimental study with continuous monitoring of intraneural blood flow in the porcine cauda equina. *J Orthop Res* 1993;11:104–109.
93. Rydevik B, Brown MD, Lundborg G: Pathoanatomy and pathophysiology of nerve root compression. *Spine* 1984;9:7–15.
94. Rydevik B, Lundborg G, Skalak R: Biomechanics of peripheral nerves, in Nordin M, Frankel VH (eds): *Basic Biomechanics of the Musculoskeletal System,* ed 2. Philadelphia, PA, Lea & Febiger, 1989, pp 75–87.
95. Rydevik BL, Kwan MK, Myers RR, et al: An in vitro mechanical and histological study of acute stretching on rabbit tibial nerve. *J Orthop Res* 1990;8:694–701.
96. Sunderland S, Bradley KC: Stress-strain phenomena in human spinal nerve roots. *Brain* 1961;84:120–124.
97. Beel JA, Stodieck LS, Luttges MW: Structural properties of spinal nerve roots: Biomechanics. *Exp Neurol* 1986;91:30–40
98. Kwan M, Rydevik B, Brown R, et al: Selected biomechanical assessment of lumbosacral spinal nerve roots. *Orthop Trans* 1988;12:611–612.
99. Spencer DL, Irwin GS, Miller JA: Anatomy and significance of fixation of the lumbosacral nerve roots in sciatica. *Spine* 1983;8:672–679.
100. Spencer DL, Miller JA, Bertolini JE: The effect of intervertebral disc space narrowing on the contact force between the nerve root and a simulated disc protrusion. *Spine* 1984;9:422–426.
101. Schönström N, Bolender NF, Spengler DM, et al: Pressure changes within the cauda equina following constriction of the dural sac: An in vitro experimental study. *Spine* 1984;9:604–607.
102. Schönström N, Hansson T: Pressure changes following constriction of the cauda equina: An experimental study in situ. *Spine* 1988;13:385–388.
103. Schönström NS, Bolender NF, Spengler DM: The pathomorphology of spinal stenosis as seen on CT scans of the lumbar spine. *Spine* 1985;10:806–811.
104. Olmarker K, Holm S, Rydevik B: Importance of compression onset rate for the degree of impairment of impulse propagation in experimental compression injury of the porcine cauda equina. *Spine* 1990;15:416–419.
105. Ochoa J, Fowler TJ, Gilliatt RW: Anatomical changes in peripheral nerves compressed by a pneumatic tourniquet. *J Anat* 1972;113:433–455.
106. Takahashi K, Miyazaki T, Takino T, et al: Epidural pressure measurements: Relationship between epidural pressure and posture in patients with lumbar spinal stenosis. *Spine* 1995;20:650–653.
107. Konno S, Olmarker K, Byröd G, et al: Intermittent cauda equina compression: An experimental study of the porcine cauda equina with analyses of nerve impulse conduction properties. *Spine* 1995;20:1223–1226.

Chapter 43

Distinction Between Nerve Root and Dorsal Root Ganglion Sources of Pain as it Relates to Irritation

Mamoru Kawakami, MD, PhD
James N. Weinstein, DO, MS
Ken-ichi Chatani, MD, PhD

Introduction

Clinical symptoms and signs do not accurately indicate which irritations of either the nerve root or the dorsal root ganglion (DRG) produce "pain." It is important to clarify the differences in responses secondary to irritations of the nerve root and the DRG when elucidating the pathomechanisms of low back pain and radicular pain. In this chapter, we describe the anatomic and neurophysiologic differences between the nerve root and the DRG. In addition, we discuss the disparity in pain-related behaviors, c-*fos* expression, and neurochemistry noted between irritated nerve roots and DRGs. The purpose of this chapter is to define the distinction between nerve root and DRG sources of pain as it relates to chronic irritation. We emphasize that previously developed experimental animal models for radicular pain are reliable and clinically relevant to lumbar radiculopathy with low back pain and sciatica.

Anatomic Distinction Between the Nerve Root and the Dorsal Root Ganglion

The nerve roots in the thecal sac, unlike a peripheral nerve, generally lack epineurium and perineurium; however, under tensile loading they exhibit both elasticity and tensile strength.[1] The mechanical properties of a human spinal nerve root differ according to whether it is located within the central canal and/or the lateral intervertebral foramen. Ultimate loads are approximately five times higher for foraminal segments of spinal nerve roots than for the intrathecal portion of the same nerve roots under tensile loading.[2] The ligaments that connect the anterior dura to the posterior longitudinal ligament and the vertebral periosteum act as a tether to nerve roots. Disk herniation or other types of anterior compression may produce significant nerve root impingement without compressing the nerve root against the posterior elements.[3] Because nerve roots lack a well-developed endoneural blood-nerve barrier, they hypothetically are more susceptible to compression injury than are peripheral nerves, and the nerve roots have increased risk of endoneural edema formation. Anatomic studies focused on compression of the DRG indicate that it plays a significant role as a modulator of low back pain.[4] The epineurally located receptors, such as nervi nervorum, appear to respond similarly to cutaneous nociceptors in the peripheral nervous system.[5] Therefore, the epineurium of the DRG may be directly activated by compression or mechanical stimulation of these receptors.

Neurophysiologic Distinction Between the Nerve Root and the Dorsal Root Ganglion

Compression of nerve roots is thought to be responsible for a number of neurophysiologic changes.[6] However, mechanical compression of the nerve root does not always cause low back pain and radicular pain.[7,8] Although pain may be related to radicular ischemia because the reduction of oxygen intake in patients with neurogenic claudication exacerbates the symptoms,[9] studies on the intrinsic vasculature of the nerve root suggest that the venous side of the system may be the more vulnerable to the spatial restriction of the spinal canal.[10,11] Chronic blockade of axoplasmic transport may lead to wallerian degeneration of a distal axon. Nerve injury may also interfere with transport of neurotrophic factors from the periphery to the cell body and may produce chromatolysis and/or death of the cell body.[12] Thus, interference with axoplasmic transport after mechanical compression or nerve injury may produce degeneration both centrally and peripherally. Increased vascular permeability secondary to mechanical compression of the nerve root results in intraneural edema.

Inflammation of the nerve root tissue must be present for mechanical nerve root deformation to induce radiating pain.[13,14] It seems, therefore, that the nature of inflammation in or around nerve roots is likely to be characterized by edema, inflammatory cell reaction, and local demyelination.[15] Breakdown products from degenerating nucleus pulposus tissue might leak into the epidural space and induce a ''chemical radiculitis'' along the nerve root.[16,17] Furthermore, degenerating disk material may produce an acidic environment that may, in part, promote formation of adhesions around the nerve root.[18] Application of normal, nondegenerated, autologous nucleus pulposus induces a local inflammatory reaction when applied epidurally in the dog.[19] Nucleus pulposus and anulus fibrosus allografted into the lumbar epidural space in the rat produced hyperalgesia, but allografted fat did not.[20] Chemical radiculitis may be significant in the pathophysiology of nerve root pain. Radiculitis may be initiated by directly irritating effects of proteoglycans from the disk[16] and/or by an autoimmune reaction from exposure to disk tissues.[21,22] In an electrophysiologic study using anesthetized cats, it has been reported that there were 14 mechanosensitive units with conduction velocities in the C fiber range whose receptive fields were to sacral dorsal roots and whose afferent projections were to sacral dorsal roots at the same level. These findings demonstrate a pain pathway through excitation of nervi nervorum on ventral roots and suggest this as a possible mechanism of radicular pain.[23]

Compression of roots or ganglia can cause an associated increase in the amount of connective tissue around the Schwann cells. Signs of axon and myelin degeneration are seen in and are associated with a proliferation of Schwann cells. More proximal nerve lesions are associated with more profound degeneration of the cell body, and lesions central to the DRG do not have regenerative potential equivalent to that of lesions peripheral to the ganglion.[24,25] Therefore, an injury proximal to the DRG may produce serious and less reversible neurologic injury than an analogous injury in the periphery.[6]

Neurophysiologic findings suggest that the increased excitability of the DRG is an inherent problem.[26,27] It contributes to reliable afferent impulse propagation past the ganglion but makes the system a likely site of ectopic impulse generation, which can lead to dysesthesias and pain. Spontaneous dorsal root ganglion firing has been reported to increase substantially with tetanic (repetitive) stimulation of neighboring axons, a phenomenon that could contribute to sensory abnormalities, including spatial effects, such as referred pain, and temporal effects, such as after sensation and wind-up.[28] The failure of C fibers to exhibit cross-excitation limits is important in understanding pain states.

The venous and arterial vascular supply of the DRG must play a significant role in its function. The aging and concomitant vascular changes of the DRG are thought to be associated with degeneration and changes in vibratory sensation.[29] It has been suggested that neurogenic claudication appears to begin with venous congestion of the nerve roots and DRG distal to the induced constriction.[29] Cellular degeneration secondary to vascular compression alters the chemical and neurophysiologic response of the nerve root and the DRG.

The DRG contains large cells, which are thought to be responsible for the myelinated fibers, and many small cells, which are thought to be responsible for the unmyelinated C fibers and the finely myelinated A-delta fibers. A large number of primary afferent neurons with small and intermediate diameters produce neuropeptides, such as substance P and somatostatin.[30] Vasoactive intestinal peptide (VIP), cholecystokinin, neurotensin, calcitonin gene-related peptide (CGRP), substance P, somatostatin, dynorphin, enkephalin, angiotensin II, and bombesin-gastric relating peptide have been found in anatomic studies of neuropeptides in DRG cells.[31] Substance P probably acts as a neuromodulator of pain signals at synapses in the region of the substantia gelatinosa where pain perception is first integrated in the spinal cord,[32-34] although neurophysiologic functions of all neuropeptides have not been established.

Experimental Lumbar Radicular Pain Models in the Rat

A major obstacle to a further understanding of the pathophysiologic mechanisms of radicular pain has been the lack of a good experimental animal model. Animal models of painful neuropathy have been described in which hyperalgesia, allodynia, and spontaneous pain are produced by tying loosely constrictive ligatures around the sciatic nerve[35] and the lumbar spinal nerve distal to the DRG[36] in the rat. These models are not clinically relevant to mechanisms of radicular pain in that most spinal problems result from irritation of the nerve root proximal to the DRG or of the DRG itself. We have developed a reliable model for lumbar radicular pain in which behavioral changes resulting from irritations of either the nerve root or the DRG produce quantifiable hyperalgesia.[8,37,38] Different behavioral results were observed between the nerve root and the DRG in these experimental models.

Hyperalgesia

The rats were divided into five groups. The control group had no treatment. Lumbar nerve roots and DRGs were only exposed in the nerve root-exposure (NR-Exp) group and the DRG-exposure (DRG-Exp) group, respectively. Nerve roots and DRGs were ligated with chromic gut in the nerve root-ligation (NR-Lig) group and the DRG-ligation (DRG-Lig) group, respectively. Behavioral measures were evaluated in all five groups preoperatively and postoperatively. Although rats in the NR-Exp group did not show motor paresis, rats in the NR-Lig, DRG-Exp, and DRG-Lig groups showed evidence of motor paresis for up to 2 weeks postoperatively. Changes in withdrawal responses to mechanical and thermal stimuli were measured. Lower scores and shorter latencies were indicative of more sensitivity and a hyperalgesic response. Mechanical hyperalgesia was observed in both the DRG and the DRG-Lig group after surgery, but not in either the NR-Exp or the NR-Lig group (Fig. 1, *top*). Rats in the NR-Lig,

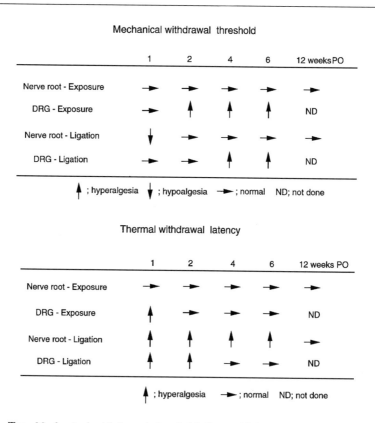

Fig. 1   Top, *Mechanical withdrawal threshold. Rats with irritated dorsal root ganglion (DRG) (the DRG-exposure and the DRG-ligation groups) showed evidence of mechanical hyperalgesia at 2 to 6 weeks postoperatively. Nerve root irritation did not produce hypersensitivity to noxious mechanical stimuli.* **Bottom,** *Thermal withdrawal latency. Time-dependent thermal hyperalgesia was observed in rats with ligated nerve roots and in rats with both only exposed and ligated DRGs. PO = postoperative.*

DRG-Exp, and DRG-Lig groups showed evidence of time-dependent thermal hyperalgesia, but rats in the control and the NR-Exp groups responded normally to thermal stimuli (Fig. 1, *bottom*).

Mechanical irritation secondary to simple exposure of lumbar DRGs produced mechanical and thermal hyperalgesia, while that of lumbar nerve roots did not. Ligatures of both nerve roots and DRGs with chromic gut resulted in thermal hyperalgesia. These results suggest that the pain threshold in DRGs is lower than in nerve roots and that the DRGs were clearly more vulnerable to mechanical irritation than were the nerve roots. Because endoneurial microvessels are more permeable in the DRG than in peripheral nerves,[39] endothelial edema can occur as a result of minor trauma to the DRG.[15] Moreover, because the DRG has a tight capsule acting as a diffusion barrier,[40] edema may lead to an increase in endoneurial fluid pressure within the DRG.[41] This increased endoneurial pressure is likely to result in an impairment of the nutritive blood flow to the nerve cell bodies of the sensory neurons in the DRG,[41] which probably are more sensitive to ischemia and compression than their corresponding nerve fibers.[15] It is hypothesized that these mechanisms may play a role in the development of hyperalgesia associated with the DRG.

Although mechanically irritated normal nerve roots do not produce pain-related behaviors,[37] ligatures of the nerve roots with chromic gut did result in thermal hyperalgesia. The thermal hyperalgesia was maximal in both groups at 7 to 14 days postoperatively and resolved within 3 and 8 weeks postoperatively, respectively, for rats in the DRG-Exp, DRG-Lig, and NR-Lig groups. These results suggest that chemicals contained within chromic gut itself, such as chromium ions or pyrogallol, may be released[42] and produce radiculitis, or a change in pH[43] may be involved in the production of symptoms associated with radicular pain. Compressed and/or inflamed nerve roots in patients undergoing laminectomy and/or disk excision under epidural anesthesia are very sensitive to mechanical manipulation,[13] and stimulation of a stretched, compressed, or swollen nerve root is associated with significant back pain in patients undergoing progressive local anesthesia.[14] These clinical findings are compatible with the results seen in these experimental models.

Expression of c-*fos*

Expression of c-*fos* in the spinal cord increases in response to noxious stimuli.[44-46] Although it has been demonstrated that nonnoxious stimulation also can induce c-*fos* expression,[46,47] accumulating evidence indicates that noxious signals from the periphery induce c-*fos* expression in the nuclei of the spinal cord neurons. Demonstration of continuous c-*fos* expression in the spinal cord suggests a persistent activation of spinal neurons. The total number of cells expressing c-*fos* correlates with thermal hyperalgesia in the NR-Lig, DRG-Exp, and DRG-Lig groups.[37,38] Expression of c-*fos* in the lumbar spinal cord was observed 5 days and 2 weeks postoperatively in the DRG irritated groups (DRG-Exp and DRG-Lig) and the NR-Lig group, respectively (Fig. 2). These results suggest that noxious stimuli are prolonged by chemical irritation due to chromic gut ligatures around the nerve root and DRG, and by mechanical irritation to the DRG.

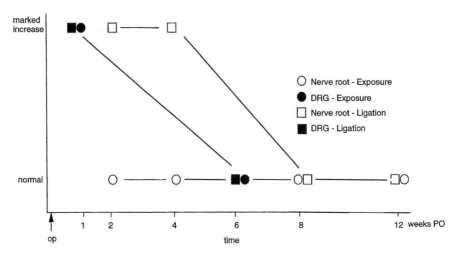

c-Fos expression in the lumbar spinal cord

Fig. 2 *Expression of c-fos in the lumbar spinal cord. Both ligated nerve roots and dorsal root ganglions (DRGs) with chromic gut increased c-fos expression. Only exposure of the DRG also increased c-fos expression in the lumbar spinal cord. The total number of cells expressing c-fos correlates with thermal hyperalgesia.*

Changes in Neuropeptides

CGRP, substance P, and VIP in the DRG and the lumbar spinal cord have been evaluated using immunohistochemistry and radioimmunoassay after irritation of the nerve root and the DRG in each group.[37,38] In each case, there was no apparent change in either CGRP, substance P, or VIP in the spinal cord or the DRG in either the control or NP-Exp groups. However, both substance P and CGRP were increased in the ipsilateral DRGs of rats in the NP-Lig group and both DRG-irritated groups (DRG-Exp and DRG-Lig) at 2 weeks and 5 days postoperatively, respectively. These neuropeptides remained increased in both the DRG-Exp and the DRG-Lig groups at 6 weeks postoperatively, although behavior in these groups returned to normal sensitivity to noxious stimuli (Fig. 3, *top*). The only significant change in CGRP and substance P in the spinal cords of rats in any group at any of the time points measured occurred in the ipsilateral spinal cords of rats in the NR-Lig group at 12 weeks postoperatively.

VIP in the ipsilateral DRG was noted to increase in the NR-Lig, DRG-Exp, and DRG-Lig groups after surgery; however, at 5 days postoperatively, VIP content in the ipsilateral DRG was unchanged in the DRG-Exp and DRG-Lig groups (Fig. 3, *bottom*). VIP content in DRGs in the NR-Exp group was not significantly different from that in the controls. VIP content in the lumbar spinal cord was unchanged for rats in each group except for a significant increase in VIP content in the ipsilateral spinal cord of rats in the NR-Lig group at 12 weeks postoperatively.

CGRP, substance P in the ipsilateral DRGs

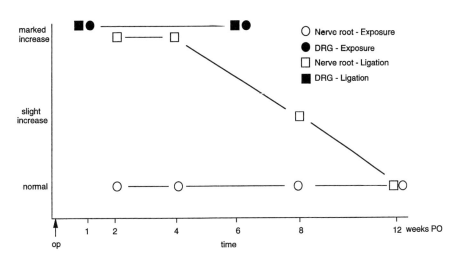

VIP in the ipsilateral DRGs

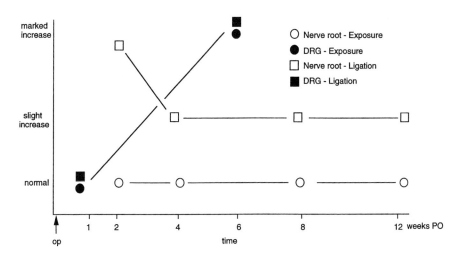

Fig. 3   Top, *Calcitonin gene-related peptide (CGRP) and substance P in the ipsilateral dorsal root ganglions (DRGs). Increases of CGRP and substance P in the ipsilateral DRGs were significantly induced by the nerve root. Changes of these neuropeptides correlate with thermal hyperalgesia in rats with ligated nerve roots. However, these neuropeptides increased in rats with surgically irritated DRGs up to 6 weeks after surgery, when the sensitivity to thermal stimuli returned to normal.* **Bottom,** *Vasoactive intestinal peptide (VIP) in the ipsilateral DRGs. Irritation with chromic gut ligatures to the nerve root enhanced increase of VIP content in the ipsilateral DRG over time. Increase of VIP also was demonstrated in the ipsilateral DRGs 6 weeks after irritation of the DRG. Change of VIP content does not correlate with sensitivity to mechanical and thermal stimuli.*

Although it is thought that the increase in CGRP, substance P, and VIP in DRGs of rats in the NR-Lig group may reflect a disturbance of axonal transport, these peptides remained unchanged in the spinal cord. Therefore, the significant increases in these neuropeptides in the DRGs may not be due to interruption of axonal transport, but may result from an increase in production in response to nerve irritation. Only increases in CGRP and substance P content in the ipsilateral DRGs were correlated with thermal hyperalgesia produced in the NR-Lig group. However, in rats with irritated DRGs, changes in CGRP, substance P, and VIP content were not directly correlated with the maintenance of thermal hyperalgesia, although there were increases after surgical procedures. It has been reported that substance P and CGRP immunoreactivity is decreased in the dorsal horn of the lumbar spinal cord after loosely constrictive ligation of the sciatic nerve,[48] and that substance P immunoreactivity decreases while VIP immunoreactivity increases after sciatic nerve section.[49,50] In our experimental models, there was no consistent relationship between thermal hyperalgesia and alterations in CGRP, substance P, or VIP in the spinal cord. Overall, the noted association between hyperalgesia and changes in c-*fos* expression and neuropeptide content suggests a possible role for c-*fos*, but not the neuropeptides, in the maintenance of hyperalgesia.

Histology

Sections through the nerve root, DRG, and spinal nerve were quantitatively examined for changes in myelinated nerve content. Significant decreases in the number of large diameter myelinated fibers and increases in the number of smaller ones were observed to be similar in both the ipsilateral nerve root, DRG, and spinal nerve in the NR-Lig, DRG-Exp, and DRG-Lig groups, respectively.[8,38] However, thermal hyperalgesia, which was observed in these groups, was not correlated with histologic changes in myelinated fiber content in the ipsilateral nerve root, DRG, or spinal nerve. These results, therefore, suggest that mechanical irritation of the nerve root and DRG, as evidenced by a loss of myelinated fibers, is not sufficient to produce the behavioral effects associated with these models of lumbar radicular pain.

Summary

In summary, mechanical irritation of the nerve root and/or the DRG produces different and distinctive responses to the noxious stimuli. Radicular pain is induced by mechanical irritation of the DRG itself, but not of the nerve root. We consider that endoneural edema seen after mechanical irritation of the DRG may be related to the pathogenesis associated with DRG-related symptoms. The behavioral and neurochemical results suggest that chemical irritation of the nerve root produces hyperalgesia in the animal model and pain in humans.

These experimental models have reliably produced radicular pain resulting from nerve root or DRG irritation and should help to further elucidate our understanding of pain after irritation of a nerve root or the DRG. With further refinements, these models may aid in understanding the mechanisms of lumbar radicular pain and serve as models to study the effects of clinically relevant interventions.

References

1. Sunderland S, Bradley KC: Stress-strain phenomena in human spinal nerve roots. *Brain* 1961;84:120–124.
2. Kwan M, Rydevik B, Brown R, et al: Selected biomechanical assessment of lumbosacral spinal nerve roots. *Orthop Trans* 1988;12:611–612.
3. Spencer DL, Irwin GS, Miller JA: Anatomy and significance of fixation of the lumbosacral nerve roots in sciatica. *Spine* 1983;8:672–679.
4. Lindblom K, Rexed B: Spinal nerve injury in dorso-lateral protrusions of lumbar disks. *J Neurosurg* 1948;5:413–432.
5. Shantha TR, Evans JA: The relationship of epidural anesthesia to neural membranes and arachnoid villi. *Anesthesiology* 1972;37:543–557.
6. Weinstein JN: Anatomy and neurophysiologic mechanisms of spinal pain, in Frymoyer JW, Ducker TB, Hadler NM, et al (eds): *The Adult Spine: Principles and Practice.* New York, NY, Raven Press, 1991, vol 1, pp 593–610.
7. Boden SD, Davis DO, Dina TS, et al: Abnormal magnetic-resonance scans of the lumbar spine in asymptomatic subjects: A prospective investigation. *J Bone Joint Surg* 1990;72A:403–408.
8. Kawakami M, Weinstein JN, Chatani K, et al: Experimental lumbar radiculopathy: Behavioral and histologic changes in a model of radicular pain after spinal nerve root irritation with chromic gut ligatures in the rat. *Spine* 1994;19:1795–1802.
9. Evans JG: Neurogenic intermittent claudication. *Br Med J* 1964;2:985–987.
10. Parke WW, Watanabe R: The intrinsic vasculature of the lumbosacral spinal nerve roots. *Spine* 1985;10:508–515.
11. Watanabe R, Parke WW: Vascular and neural pathology of lumbosacral spinal stenosis. *J Neurosurg* 1986;64:64–70.
12. Grafstein B: The nerve cell body response to axotomy. *Exp Neurol* 1975;48:32–51.
13. Greenbarg PE, Brown MD, Pallares VS, et al: Epidural anesthesia for lumbar spine surgery. *J Spinal Disord* 1988;1:139–143.
14. Kuslich SD, Ulstrom CL, Michael CJ: The tissue origin of low back pain and sciatica: A report of pain response to tissue stimulation during operations on the lumbar spine using local anesthesia. *Orthop Clin North Am* 1991;22:181–187.
15. Rydevik B, Brown MD, Lundborg G: Pathoanatomy and pathophysiology of nerve root compression. *Spine* 1984;9:7–15.
16. Marshall LL, Trethewie ER: Chemical irritation of nerve-root in disc prolapse. *Lancet* 1973;2:320.
17. Marshall LL, Trethewie ER, Curtain CC: Chemical radiculitis: A clinical, physiological and immunological study. *Clin Orthop* 1977;129:61–67.
18. Nachemson A: Intradiscal measurements of pH in patients with lumbar rhizopathies. *Acta Orthop Scand* 1969;40:23–42.
19. McCarron RF, Wimpee MW, Hudkins PG, et al: The inflammatory effect of nucleus pulposus: A possible element in the pathogenesis of low-back pain. *Spine* 1987;12:760–764.
20. Kawakami M, Tamaki T, Weinstein JN, et al: Pathomechanism of pain-related behavior produced by allografts of intervertebral disc in the rat. *Spine*, in press.
21. Bobechko WP, Hirsch C: Auto-immune response to nucleus pulposus in the rabbit. *J Bone Joint Surg* 1965;47B:574–580.
22. Gertzbein SD, Tile M, Gross A, et al: Autoimmunity in degenerative disc disease of the lumbar spine. *Orthop Clin North Am* 1975;6:67–73.
23. Janig W, Koltzenburg M: Receptive properties of pial afferents. *Pain* 1991;45:77–85.
24. Sunderland S: Avulsion of nerve roots, in Vinken PJ, Bruyn GW (eds): *Injuries of the Spine and Spinal Cord: Part I.* Amsterdam, The Netherlands, North Holland, 1975, pp 393–435.
25. Sunderland S, Bradley KC: Stress-strain phenomena in human peripheral nerve trunks. *Brain* 1961;84:102–119.
26. Devor M, Obermayer M: Membrane differentiation in rat dorsal root ganglia and possible consequences for back pain. *Neurosci Lett* 1984;51:341–346.

27. Howe JF, Loeser JD, Calvin WH: Mechanosensitivity of dorsal root ganglia and chronically injured axons: A physiological basis for the radicular pain of nerve root compression. *Pain* 1977;3:25–41.
28. Devor M, Wall PD: Cross-excitation in dorsal root ganglia of nerve-injured and intact rats. *J Neurophysiol* 1990;64:1733–1746.
29. Bergmann L, Alexander L: Vascular supply of spinal ganglia. *Arch Neurol Psychiat* 1941;46:761–782.
30. Delamarter RB, Bohlman HH, Dodge LD, et al: Experimental lumbar spinal stenosis: Analysis of the cortical evoked potentials, microvasculature, and histopathology. *J Bone Joint Surg* 1990;72A:110–120.
31. Hökfelt T, Elde R, Johansson O, et al: Immunohistochemical evidence for separate populations of somatostatin-containing and substance P-containing primary afferent neurons in the rat. *Neuroscience* 1976;1:131–136.
32. Salt TE, Hill RG: Neurotransmitter candidates of somatosensory primary afferent fibres. *Neuroscience* 1983;10:1083–1103.
33. Marx JL: Brain peptides: Is substance P a transmitter of pain signals? *Science* 1979;205:886–889.
34. Naftchi NE, Abrahams SJ, St. Paul HM, et al: Localization and changes of substance P in spinal cord of paraplegic cats. *Brain Res* 1978;153:507–513.
35. Naftchi NE, Abrahams SJ, St. Paul HM, et al: Substance P and leucine enkephalin changes in spinal cord of paraplegic rats and cats, in Naftchi NE (ed): *Spinal Cord Injury*. Jamaica, NY, Spectrum, 1982, pp 85–101.
36. Bennett GJ, Xie YK: A peripheral mononeuropathy in rat that produces disorders of pain sensation like those seen in man. *Pain* 1988;33:87–107.
37. Kim SH, Chung JM: An experimental model for peripheral neuropathy produced by segmental spinal nerve ligation in the rat. *Pain* 1992;50:355–363.
38. Kawakami M, Weinstein JN, Spratt KF, et al: Experimental lumbar radiculopathy: Immunohistochemical and quantitative demonstrations of pain induced by lumbar nerve root irritation of the rat. *Spine* 1994;19:1780–1794.
39. Chatani K, Kawakami M, Weinstein JN, et al: Characterization of thermal hyperalgesia, c-fos expression, and alterations in neuropeptides after mechanical irritation of the dorsal root ganglion. *Spine* 1995;20:277–290.
40. Arvidson B: Distribution of intravenously injected protein tracers in peripheral ganglia of adult mice. *Exp Neurol* 1979;63:388–410.
41. Arvidson B: A study of the perineurial diffusion barrier of a peripheral ganglion. *Acta Neuropathol* 1979;46:139–144.
42. Rydevik BL, Myers RR, Powell HC: Pressure increase in the dorsal root ganglion following mechanical compression: Closed compartment syndrome in nerve roots. *Spine* 1989;14:574–576.
43. Maves TJ, Pechman PS, Gebhart GF, et al: Possible chemical contribution from chromic gut sutures produce disorders of pain sensation like those seen in man. *Pain* 1993;54:57–70.
44. Maves TJ, Pechman PS, Gebhart GF, Meller ST: An acidic milieu around the rat sciatic nerve produces a reversible thermal hyperalgesia. *Soc Neurosci Abstr* 1993;19:518.
45. Bullitt E: Expression of c-fos-like protein as a marker for neuronal activity following noxious stimulation in the rat. *J Comp Neurol* 1990;296:517–530.
46. Hunt SP, Pini A, Evan G: Induction of c-fos-like protein in spinal cord neurons following sensory stimulation. *Nature* 1987;328:632–634.
47. Menetrey D, Gannon A, Levine JD, et al: Expression of c-fos protein in interneurons and projection neurons of the rat spinal cord in response to noxious somatic, articular, and visceral stimulation. *J Comp Neurol* 1989;285:177–195.
48. Kuraishi Y, Nanayama T, Ohno H, et al: Antinociception induced in rats by intrathecal administration of antiserum against calcitonin gene-related peptide. *Neurosci Lett* 1988;92:325–329.
49. Bennett GJ, Kajander KC, Sahara Y, et al: Neurochemical and anatomical changes in the dorsal horn of rats with an experimental painful peripheral neuropathy, in Cervero F, Bennett GJ, Headley PM (eds): *Processing of Sensory Information in*

the Superficial Dorsal Horn of the Spinal Cord. New York, NY, Plenum Press, 1989, pp 463–471.

50. McGregor GP, Gibson SJ, Sabate IM, et al: Effect of peripheral nerve section and nerve crush on spinal cord neuropeptides in the rat: Increased VIP and PHI in the dorsal horn. *Neuroscience* 1984;13:207–216.

Chapter 44

Dynamic Influences of Posture and Walking on the Stenotic Spinal Canal

Keisuke Takahashi, MD, PhD

The clinical history of lumbar spinal stenosis is characteristic. Cauda equina and radicular symptoms often are related to posture. Pain and numbness in the buttock, thigh, and leg are provoked either by walking or by prolonged standing with an upright posture. Symptomatic relief can be obtained by lying, sitting, or standing with lumbar flexion. Neurogenic intermittent claudication, referred to as pseudoclaudication, is the most common symptom. Patients with neurogenic intermittent claudication also complain of posture-related pain and feel more comfortable when walking in a stooped posture.[1,2] These patients can ride a bicycle without symptoms.[3] Walking behind a shopping cart or lawn mower or walking up an incline or stairs generally is better tolerated than simple walking or walking down an incline or stairs.[4]

The phenomena described above suggest that dynamic factors probably are important in the pathogenesis of the clinical presentation of radiculopathy in spinal stenosis. However, the exact mechanisms by which symptoms develop or are relieved by lumbar postures are uncertain, and the pathogenesis of neurogenic intermittent claudication remains obscure.

Pathology of Nerve Root Compression

Clinical Studies

The symptoms of spinal stenosis may be caused by mechanical factors directly interfering with the nerve roots in the spinal canal. The findings of functional myelograms generally indicate that, in lumbar spinal stenosis, the dural sac is more compressed by lumbar extension at the intervertebral disk level than by lumbar flexion (Fig. 1). The shape of the spinal canal varies in different positions.[5] Dynamic variations in flexion and extension are caused mainly by changes in the degree of bulging of the intervertebral disk and in the thickness and buckling of the ligamentum flavum.[6] These size variations might explain the postural dependency of symptoms in patients with lumbar spinal stenosis.

In cadaveric experiments, Schönström and associates[7] found that the first sign of a pressure increase occurred when the cross-sectional area of the cauda equina was 77 ± 13 mm^2, which correlated with corresponding measurement on computed tomography (CT) scans of spinal stenosis patients. To achieve a pressure

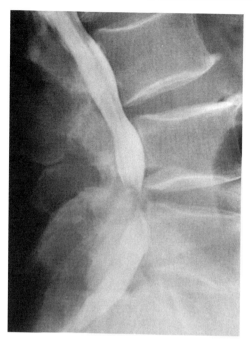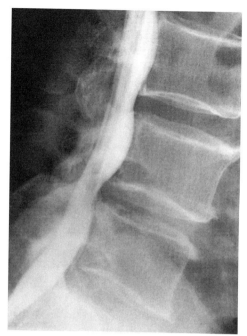

Fig. 1 *Myelograms of spinal stenosis.* **Left,** *Lateral view in lumbar extension demonstrates a complete block of the dye column at the L4-5 level.* **Right,** *Lateral view in lumbar flexion demonstrates mild compression at the L4-5 level. The degree of compression to the dural sac changes by extension and flexion in lumbar spinal stenosis.*

increase of 50 mm Hg, the cross-sectional area of the cauda equina had to be further constricted by an average of 19% ± 8%.[8]

Animal Studies of Nerve Roots Compression

In animal experiments, Olmarker and associates[9-11] and Takahashi and associates[12] demonstrated that mechanical pressure could cause disturbances in the blood supply and nutrition of the nerve roots, and they determined pressure levels critical to impairment of basic physiologic events in the nerve roots. Pressure as low as 10 mm Hg was sufficient to induce occlusion in some venules, a 64% reduction of total blood flow, and a 20% to 30% reduction in nutrition. The pressure required to stop blood flow was slightly less than and directly related to the systolic blood pressure. Nerve roots are thus very sensitive to compression. These data suggest that compression-induced disturbances in the blood supply to the nerve roots play an important role in the production of symptoms in spinal stenosis.

Pressure Measurements in the Stenotic Human Spinal Canal

The cerebrospinal fluid (CSF) pressure changes with posture and walking. Magnaes[13] recorded a high CSF pressure in claudicating patients caudal to a stenosed segment and related to posture, with block pressure relieved by flexion. Lindahl[14] measured the pressure in the epidural space of patients during surgery for sciatica; he used a fine lumbar-puncture needle connected with a doubly-bent glass tube. He demonstrated that normal negative pressure disappeared completely or largely in association with sciatica. This pressure was measured in the prone position only. He also stated in a later report that the nerve roots of a patient with sciatica were hypersensitive to the increased epidural pressure produced by injection of physiologic saline solution.[15]

I have developed a method of measuring epidural space pressure.[16] I used a flexible pressure transducer for continuous measurement of epidural pressure during a variety of movements. A Mikro-tip catheter transducer was used as a pressure transducer. This transducer is flexible and has a diameter of 1.2 mm. A Tuohy needle was inserted into the epidural space using the loss of resistance method through the L5-S1 interlaminar space. The catheter transducer was inserted into the epidural space, and the tip of the transducer was placed at the L4-5 disk level. The course was monitored by fluoroscopy. This transducer was connected with a pressure amplifier and a thermal recorder. Epidural pressure was then measured continuously. The following postures were studied: supine, supine with knee flexion, prone, prone with lumbar extension, sitting in a chair, cross-legged sitting, square sitting, upright standing, standing with lumbar extension, and standing with lumbar flexion. In another study, the epidural pressure was continuously measured as patients walked on a treadmill at a velocity of 2 km/h.[17] The pressure was measured during both simple walking (without lumbar flexion) and walking with lumbar flexion.

Postural Influences on the Stenotic Spinal Canal

Reason for Posture-Dependent Symptoms

Mechanical compressions, which cause symptoms of spinal stenosis, directly influence the nerve roots. The size of the spinal canal changes significantly when the spine is extended or loaded.[18-20] This variation in canal size might explain the postural dependency of the stenotic symptoms in some patients. It has been postulated that pressure to the cauda equina will change with changes in posture. Epidural pressure measurements revealed the amount of pressure in patients with spinal stenosis as they assumed different postures.

Epidural pressure was 18.0 ± 6.9 mm Hg in supine patients and 17.0 ± 8.1 mm Hg in supine patients with flexed knees. This pressure difference was not statistically significant. In prone patients, the epidural pressure was 13.1 ± 6.0 mm Hg, and it was increased to 85.0 ± 39.2 mm Hg by maximum extension (Fig. 2). This difference in pressure was statistically significant ($p < 0.001$). Three sitting positions were investigated. The epidural pressure was 36.4 ± 15.1 mm Hg in patients sitting in a chair, 41.6 ± 19.4 mm Hg in patients during square sitting, and 34.9 ± 19.3 mm Hg in cross-legged sitting (Fig. 3). These pressure differences were not statistically significant. In standing patients, the epidural pressure was 66.9 ± 27.5 mm Hg in the upright position, during maximum extension it was markedly increased to 116.5 ± 38.4 mm Hg, and during 30° forward flexion it decreased to 27.3 ± 19.7 mm Hg (Fig. 4). The epidural pressures during standing with extension and standing with flexion were significantly different ($p < 0.001$), as were pressures during upright standing and standing with

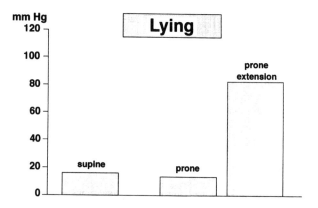

Fig. 2 *Epidural pressures were low in supine and prone positions. Epidural pressure was surprisingly increased by lumbar extension.*

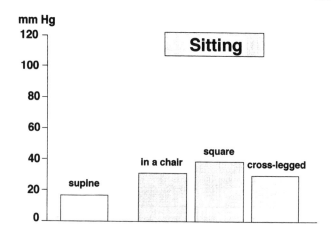

Fig. 3 *Epidural pressure during sitting posture was slightly higher than during lying. There were no differences among types of sitting.*

flexion ($p < 0.01$). The epidural pressure in patients standing with lumbar extension was 116 mm Hg, which was about six times higher than that in supine patients.

The vertebral canal generally has a large reserve space for the nerve structures, and CSF can have a modulating effect on the pressure response of a dural sac subjected to external compression. However, the vertebral canal in spinal stenosis has no reserve space, and the CSF volume at the stenotic level is more or less absent, so that the decrease in size caused by extension may induce compression of the nerve structures. Furthermore, it has been demonstrated using dynamic CT myelography that the subarachnoid space in the

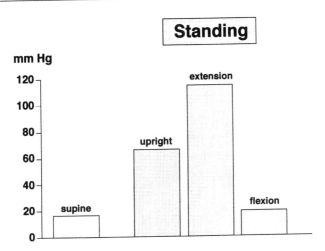

Fig. 4 *Epidural pressure was increased by standing. Pressure was markedly increased by extension to 116 mm Hg, which was about six times higher than the pressure during lying. Pressure was significantly decreased by flexion.*

stenotic region showed bigger changes with motion than that of the normal canal.[21] During standing with extension, the epidural pressure was 116 mm Hg, and cauda equina and radicular symptoms generally were elicited in patients with spinal stenosis. The increase in epidural pressure may induce compression of the nerve roots and impair, for example, the blood supply to the nerve roots, thereby causing these symptoms.

Differences in Spinal Stenosis and Disk Herniation Symptoms

Clinically, symptoms in lumbar spinal stenosis generally are elicited by standing with extension, and are relieved by sitting or standing with flexion. Symptoms in disk herniation usually are elicited by sitting and/or standing with flexion. The relationship between the disk pressure and posture have been carefully evaluated.[22,23] If the patterns of epidural pressure and disk pressure related to posture are compared, it is possible to see that the epidural pressure has different patterns than the disk pressure in each posture (Fig. 5). The disk pressure was increased, and the epidural pressure decreased by sitting as compared with the respective pressures during upright standing. During lumbar flexion, the disk pressure is increased, and the epidural pressure is decreased. These differences in pressure may explain the differences in symptoms at different postures for patients with disk herniation and those with spinal stenosis.

Neurogenic Intermittent Claudication

The Spinal Canal During Walking

Ooi and associates[24] have shown congested cauda equina in claudicating patients using myeloscopic studies. Epidural pressure measurements were used to

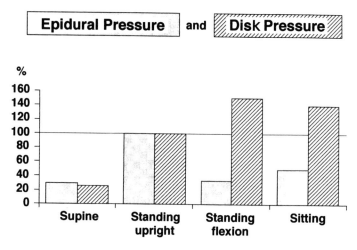

Fig. 5 *Comparison between epidural pressure and disk pressure by posture. Disk pressures were obtained from Nachemson.[22] These pressures were converted to relative values with upright standing posture equal to 100%.*

monitor the changes in extradural pressure during walking. The epidural pressure change had a pattern of increase and decrease, and this pattern was repeated during walking. Intermittent pressure increase was seen at a frequency of about 90 times per minute during walking at a velocity of 2 km/h. The epidural pressure was high during simple walking and low during walking with lumbar flexion (Fig. 6). In simple walking with upright lumbar posture, peak pressure increases were 82.8 ± 14.2 mm Hg in patients with spinal stenosis and 34.2 ± 4.9 mm Hg in individuals with a normal canal (Fig. 7). Peak pressure increases were significantly different ($p < 0.01$) between patients with spinal stenosis and normal individuals. During walking with lumbar flexion, peak pres-

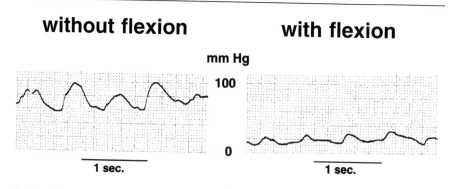

Fig. 6 *Changes in epidural pressure during walking in patients with spinal stenosis. Changes in epidural pressure had a wave pattern of increase and decrease, and this pattern was repeated during walking.*

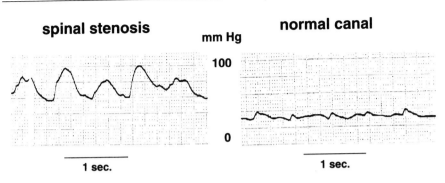

Fig. 7   *Changes in epidural pressure during simple walking in patients with spinal stenosis and in normal individuals. Peak values of pressure increase were significantly different.*

sure increases decreased to 36.8 ± 8.2 mm Hg in patients with spinal stenosis and to 27.4 ± 11 mm Hg in individuals with normal canals. The peak pressure increase was significantly different ($p < 0.01$) for simple walking and walking with lumbar flexion in patients with lumbar spinal stenosis. There was no statistically significant difference between pressure increases during simple walking in normal individuals and during walking with lumbar flexion in patients with lumbar spinal stenosis.

This pattern of changes in pressure might be explained by spinal movement during walking. The response of the pelvis and the spine to the action of the lower limbs produces the characteristic movements during walking. Thurston and Harris[25] showed a spinal movement in a wave pattern in the sagittal plane during walking. The increase of epidural pressure during walking was seen at the double supporting phase in the gait cycle.[17] This result corresponded to the fact that maximum backwards tilt of the pelvis occurred at the double supporting phase.[25] Flexion and extension of the lumbar spine in the sagittal plane were repeated continuously during walking. Because there is a significant difference between epidural pressure in standing with forward flexion (27.3 ± 19.7 mm Hg) and with maximum extension (116.5 ± 38.4 mm Hg),[16] the repeated movements of the lumbar spine during walking induce epidural pressure changes with a pattern of increase and decrease.

Pathogenesis

The mechanism of neurogenic intermittent claudication has been debated by various authors. Some authors have suggested that mechanical compressions induced by standing and walking might directly influence the nerve roots.[26-28] Others have supported an ischemic mechanism at a root level.[29-32] The increase in blood supply to the nerve roots needed during walking may be inhibited by a vascular constriction caused by stenosis. Neurogenic intermittent claudication thus may be caused by compression to the nerve roots and also be a result of nerve root ischemia. These two causes currently are accepted for the pathogenesis of neurogenic intermittent claudication. However, the specific cause of neurogenic intermittent claudication in an individual patient is uncertain, because both of these causes are dynamic in nature.[33] To find a specific cause, it was necessary to measure dynamic changes within the spinal canal.

I have been able to monitor the dynamic changes within the spinal canal during walking. Continuous monitoring of epidural pressure before, during, and after walking is demonstrated in Figure 8. When a patient was standing in a stooped posture, epidural pressure was low. Epidural pressure was quickly increased at the start of simple walking, and there was a repeated pattern of increase and decrease during walking. The pattern of increase and decrease and the magnitude of increase were not changed after symptoms appeared with walking. The patient had to stop walking as a result of the pain. Epidural pressure immediately was decreased to the same level as before walking by stopping and then standing with lumbar flexion.

The magnitude of epidural pressure was significantly different during walking with or without lumbar flexion. The magnitude of the pressure and the amount of the pressure increase during walking with lumbar flexion were lower than during walking without lumbar flexion. The pattern of epidural pressure during walking with lumbar flexion in patients with spinal stenosis was similar to the pattern during simple walking in normal individuals. Walking with lumbar flexion might be associated with few or no symptoms because of the low pressure and low amount of increase. However, neurogenic intermittent claudication occurs during simple walking. This problem may be caused by the frequently repeated increase in epidural pressure. An intermittent increase in the epidural pressure at the stenotic level may induce intermittent compression of the nerve roots. It was recently reported that intermittent compression to the cauda equina also reduced nerve conduction properties.[34] These results indicate that intermittent compression of the nerve roots during walking in patients with spinal stenosis might induce physiologic changes in the nerve roots, such as nerve root ischemia. Thus, intermittent increases in the epidural pressure dur-

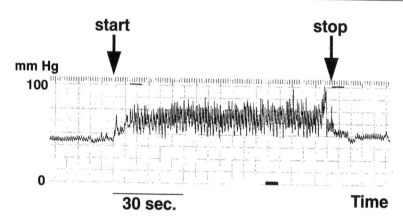

Fig. 8 *Changes in epidural pressure before, during, and after walking. When simple walking was started, epidural pressure was increased, and there was a repeated pattern of increase and decrease during walking. The patient stopped walking because of leg pain. By stopping, the epidural pressure immediately decreased and the leg pain subsided.*

ing walking may have an important role in the pathogenesis of neurogenic intermittent claudication.

Summary

The study of epidural pressure measurements clearly demonstrated that the local extradural pressure at the stenotic level was changed by motion in patients with spinal stenosis. The pressure was low during lying and sitting and high during standing. The pressure was increased by lumbar extension, but decreased by forward flexion. Changes in the epidural pressure correlated with the occurrence of clinical symptoms of nerve root compression. These pressure changes may explain the postural dependency of symptoms in spinal stenosis. The epidural pressure also changed during walking in patients with neurogenic intermittent claudication. The epidural pressure change had a pattern of increase and decrease, and this pattern was repeated during walking. The epidural pressure was high during simple walking and low during walking with lumbar flexion. Intermittent compression to the nerve roots during walking might have an important role in the pathogenesis of neurogenic intermittent claudication.

References

1. Dyck P: The stoop-test in lumbar entrapment radiculopathy. *Spine* 1979;4:89–92.
2. Dong G, Porter RW: Walking and cycling tests in neurogenic and intermittent claudication. *Spine* 1989;14:965–969.
3. Dyck P, Doyle JB Jr: "Bicycle test" of van Gelderen in diagnosis of intermittent cauda equina compression syndrome: Case report. *J Neurosurg* 1977;46:667–670.
4. Porter RW: Spinal stenosis. *Semin Orthop* 1986;1:97–111.
5. Sortland O, Magnaes B, Hauge T: Functional myelography with metrizamide in the diagnosis of lumbar spinal stenosis. *Acta Radiol Suppl* 1977;355:42–54.
6. Rauschning W: Pathoanatomy of lumbar spinal stenosis: A pictorial outline, in Andersson GBJ, McNeill TW (eds): *Lumbar Spinal Stenosis*. St Louis, MO, Mosby-Year Book, 1992, pp 19–29.
7. Schönström N, Bolender NF, Spengler DM, et al: Pressure changes within the cauda equina following constriction of the dural sac: An in vitro experimental study. *Spine* 1984;9:604–607.
8. Schönström N, Hansson T: Pressure changes following constriction of the cauda equina: An experimental study in situ. *Spine* 1988;13:385–388.
9. Olmarker K, Rydevik B, Hansson T, et al: Compression-induced changes of the nutritional supply to the porcine cauda equina. *J Spinal Disord* 1990;3:25–29.
10. Olmarker K, Rydevik B, Holm S: Edema formation in spinal nerve roots induced by experimental, graded compression: An experimental study on the pig cauda equina with special reference to differences in effects between rapid and slow onset of compression. *Spine* 1989;14:569–573.
11. Olmarker K, Rydevik B, Holm S, et al: Effects of experimental graded compression on blood flow in spinal nerve roots: A vital microscopic study on the porcine cauda equina. *J Orthop Res* 1989;7:817–823.
12. Takahashi K, Olmarker K, Holm S, et al: Double-level cauda equina compression: An experimental study with continuous monitoring of intraneural blood flow in the porcine cauda equina. *J Orthop Res* 1993;11:104–109.
13. Magnaes B: Clinical recording of pressure on the spinal cord and cauda equina: Part 2. Position changes in pressure on the cauda equina in central lumbar spinal stenosis. *J Neurosurg* 1982;57:57–63.

14. Lindahl O: The pressure in the epidural space in operated cases of sciatica. *Acta Orthop Scand* 1952;22:232–236.
15. Lindahl O: Hyperalgesia of the lumbar nerve roots in sciatica. *Acta Orthop Scand* 1966;37:367–374.
16. Takahashi K, Miyazaki T, Takino T, et al: Epidural pressure measurements: Relationship between epidural pressure and posture in patients with lumbar spinal stenosis. *Spine* 1995;20:650–653.
17. Takahashi K, Kagechika K, Takino T, et al: Changes in epidural pressure during walking in patients with lumbar spinal stenosis. *Spine* 1995;20:2746–2749.
18. Hansson TH, Schönström NR: The three-joint complex, in Andersson GBJ, McNeill TW (eds): *Lumbar Spinal Stenosis.* St Louis, MO, Mosby-Year Book, 1992, pp 121–128.
19. Penning L, Wilmink JT: Biomechanics of lumbosacral dural sac: A study of flexion-extension myelography. *Spine* 1981;6:398–408.
20. Wilmink JT, Penning L: Influence of spinal posture on abnormalities demonstrated by lumbar myelography. *Am J Neuroradiol* 1983;4:656–658.
21. Hanai K, Hibino K, Satoh N, et al: Dynamic CT myelography in patients with spinal stenosis. *Orthop Trans* 1994;18:841–842.
22. Nachemson AL: The lumbar spine: An orthopaedic challenge. *Spine* 1976;1:59–71.
23. Andersson GB, Ortengren R, Nachemson A: Intradiskal pressure, intra-abdominal pressure and myoelectric back muscle activity related to posture and loading. *Clin Orthop* 1977;129:156–164.
24. Ooi Y, Mita F, Satoh Y: Myeloscopic study on lumbar spinal canal stenosis with special reference to intermittent claudication. *Spine* 1990;15:544–549.
25. Thurston AJ, Harris JD: Normal kinematics of the lumbar spine and pelvis. *Spine* 1983;8:199–205.
26. Ehni G: Significance of the small lumbar canal: Cauda equina compression syndromes due to spondylosis. I: Introduction. *J Neurosurg* 1969;31:490–494.
27. Verbiest H: Further experiences on the pathological influence of a developmental narrowness of the bony lumbar vertebral canal. *J Bone Joint Surg* 1955;37B:576–583.
28. Wilson CB: Significance of the small lumbar spinal canal: Cauda equina compression syndromes due to spondylosis: 3. Intermittent claudication. *J Neurosurg* 1969;31:499–506.
29. Blau JN, Logue V: Intermittent claudication of the cauda equina: An unusual syndrome resulting from central protrusion of a lumbar intervertebral disc. *Lancet* 1961;1:1081–1086.
30. Kavanaugh GJ, Svien HJ, Holman CB, et al: "Pseudoclaudication" syndrome produced by compression of the cauda equina. *JAMA* 1968;206:2477–2481.
31. Watanabe R, Parke WW: Vascular and neural pathology of lumbosacral spinal stenosis. *J Neurosurg* 1986;64:64–70.
32. Porter RW, Ward D: Cauda equina dysfunction: The significance of two-level pathology. *Spine* 1992;17:9–15.
33. Andersson GBJ, McNeill TW: Definition and classification of lumbar spinal stenosis, in Andersson GBJ, McNeill TW (eds): *Lumbar Spinal Stenosis.* St Louis, MO, Mosby-Year Book, 1992, pp 9–15.
34. Konno S, Olmarker K, Byrod G, et al: Intermittent cauda equina compression: An experimental study of the porcine cauda equina with analyses of nerve impulse conduction properties. *Spine* 1995;20:1223–1226.

Directions for Future Research

Study the stages and progression of pathoanatomic changes in spinal stenosis.

Spinal stenosis is a progressive developmental disorder resulting in dysfunction, disability, and pain in many elderly patients. The process tends to progress relentlessly with age, producing greater symptoms over time. The signs and symptoms of advanced disease include leg pain, activity-related pain and weakness, and radiologic findings, such as spondylosis and canal encroachment. The processes involved in canal encroachment include facet hypertrophy, ligamentum flavum hypertrophy, disk protrusion, and spondylosis. Histologic changes seen in experimental animals include perineural and intraneural edema and fibrosis.

A longitudinal and pathoanatomic study should be conducted in a spinal stenosis model. A suitable animal model, correlated to histologic findings in human clinical specimens, should be developed and analyzed to identify the sequence of changes in articular and connective tissues, disk, and nerve roots over time. Volumetric analysis of spur formation and ligamentum and disk protrusion should be compared over time to the development of intraneural fibrosis and reactive changes in the nerve roots and the cauda equina. Early histologic changes related to edema and fibrosis should be followed over time to establish their progression to late changes caused by epidural compression and nerve injury.

Analyze the site of cauda equina compression in spinal stenosis to identify neurophysiologic and neuropeptide changes related to pain generation.

Chronic compression of cauda equina tissue has been proposed as the source of pain in patients with symptomatic spinal stenosis. Although patients frequently experience leg numbness, "heaviness," and/or pain with postural changes and activity, they do not typically complain of the lancinating, unilateral pain symptoms suggestive of acute nerve root or dorsal root ganglion (DRG) compression. A different mechanism of pain generation is suspected, although the nerve root or some segment of the nerve root is still considered the likely source of pain generation. Previous studies have demonstrated histologic changes consistent with early nerve root injury when animals are exposed to circumferential or eccentric compression of the cauda equina. These spinal stenosis models have demonstrated changes in nerve conduction velocity, but have not been studied for ectopic pain generation or neuropeptide changes.

Neurophysiologic analysis of the neural elements exposed to low grade, circumferential and eccentric compression, consistent with a stenosis mechanism, should assess the capacity of compressed nerve segments to generate spontaneous discharges, increased sensitivity to pressure stimulation, and increased discharge rates. Neuropeptide levels should be analyzed relative to other segments of the involved nerve root and to a normal nerve root to identify specific foci of injury/irritation capable of producing ectopic impulses resulting in pain. Immunohistochemical studies should help localize neuropeptides and cytokines in compressed tissue. Local histochemical assessment should be used to identify increases in levels of substance P, vasoactive intestinal peptide, calcitonin gene-related peptide, and other cytokine mediators.

Study the role of the dorsal root ganglion in the development of spinal stenosis symptoms.

There is a different quality of pain in patients with spinal stenosis than in patients suffering from herniated nucleus pulposus and acute nerve root compression. The DRG has been implicated in some pain syndromes, but its role in spinal stenosis is unclear. The most likely point of irritation in the nerve root is proximal to the DRG, and antidromic transmission of responses back through the DRG might activate those neurons in a pathologic fashion. Changes in the nerve root near the DRG may directly stimulate it or result in venous stasis around it, thereby making the DRG a primary generator of pain in spinal stenosis.

A study should be carried out to analyze DRG activity in spinal stenosis as either a primary pain generator or a secondary element responding to ectopic pain generation. Functional magnetic resonance imaging or positron emission tomography technology could be used to image symptomatic and asymptomatic individuals and to assess changes in the DRG activity and blood flow. The addition of contrast materials to the blood supply may provide information about increased blood flow to the DRG in individuals who are symptomatic after activity and asymptomatic when at rest.

Study epidural pressure monitoring and/or other functional evaluations as potential diagnostic tests.

Spinal stenosis is a progressive degenerative disorder resulting in pain and dysfunction in elderly patients. The progressive encroachment of spinal elements on the neural tissues results in the development of leg numbness, tingling, and progressive dysfunction in elderly patients. Studies have demonstrated that pressure in the epidural space correlates with changes in nerve conduction, endoneural edema, and vascular congestion. Epidural pressure changes dramatically with postural changes—a finding that correlates strongly with clinical experience that symptoms are precipitated or increased by standing or extension exercises and are decreased by sitting or flexion activities.

A transducer could be developed to provide epidural pressure measurements from awake, active patients. The mechanism would be percutaneously inserted and capable of providing real time data to a nearby monitoring station. After establishing the validity and reliability of measurements obtained in control subjects, parameters could be developed for patients with elevated epidural pressures secondary to spinal stenosis. These measurements could be used to determine those patients at risk for progressive symptoms or motor dysfunction, and to determine the benefits of postural and medical interventions. Other, yet unexplored functional tests should be developed to help coordinate appropriate timing of treatment interventions.

Validate existing models relating to the clinical situation and design new models that may better mimic spinal stenosis.

To understand the basic pathophysiologic events occurring in the nerve tissue in relation to spinal stenosis, it is valuable to understand how well the existing models reflect the situation in patients.

Investigators should find ways to monitor changes in structure and function that may be assessed in patients. The importance of onset, duration, age of the animal, and number of compression levels must be defined. Models that induce compression due to a narrowing of the spinal canal rather than introduction of foreign material should be developed.

Define the critical time limits for a favorable outcome of surgical intervention.

At present, it is not known when surgery should be performed in relationship to the onset and duration of clinical symptoms. It is currently not possible to know the critical symptom duration that could still have a good or acceptable surgical outcome. In chronic nerve root compression models, surgical decompression should be attempted at various times after onset of symptoms. The results should preferably be assessed by methods that may be used in patients as well.

Clarify the basic events that trigger the onset of symptoms.

To better understand the early pathophysiology of neurogenic claudication, it is necessary to understand what triggers the onset of symptoms. Neurogenic symptoms, as the result of a reduction of the diameter of the spinal canal, usually require years to develop. During this time, the compressed part of the nerve roots adapts to the applied pressure, but may concomitantly be undergoing pathologic changes. These changes may lead the nerve to become a "silent pain generator" that may be symptomatically activated by mechanical or other factors.

Neurophysiologic and histomorphometric studies should be undertaken to define the basic pathophysiologic events in compressed or nutritionally deprived nerve roots. The importance of different factors, such as mechanical deformation, ischemia, or inflammation, as a trigger for neural activity should be assessed.

Measure the endoneurial tissue pressure of the nerve root and the dorsal root ganglion, experimentally and clinically.

In chronic nerve root compression, the perineural sheath (arachnoid and dura) is thickened by scar. There is progressive loss of the subarachnoid space. Edema related to the internal changes leads to nerve root swelling, accentuated by a breakdown of the blood-nerve barrier. The edema fluid remains in the nerve roots as it is encased by a nonporous diffusion barrier in the deeper layer of the arachnoid. At present, the site of nerve ectopic discharge leading to radicular pain is not clear. It may be in the compressed area of the nerve root, the DRG, or both. From experimental studies, it is known that compression leads to cerebrospinal fluid restriction, which produces intraradicular

753

edema and decreases the blood flow by approximately 10% to 20% distally along the root, including the DRG. These factors need further study.

Endoneurial tissue pressure measurement may provide some information to help answer the question as to what is the mechanism of provocation of electrophysiologic discharges leading to radicular pain.

Clinical Questions

On November 1-4, 1995, a workshop was held on the topic of New Horizons in Low Back Pain. This workshop was sponsored by the National Institute of Arthritis and Musculoskeletal and Skin Diseases, the American Academy of Orthopaedic Surgeons, the North American Spine Society, and several corporate contributors. A group of leading basic and clinical scientists gathered to discuss the state of knowledge and directions for future research in this field. These internationally recognized experts were asked to address six practical clinical questions that a layperson might ask a physician regarding low back pain.

The composite answers are summarized below.

Question #1: Doctor, what do the terms slipped disk and spinal degeneration mean?

The term "slipped disk" is often used by patients and journalists as a loose equivalent to the clinical terms disk herniation or herniated nucleus pulposus. Disks are the parts of the spine that separate the bony elements called vertebrae. Each disk looks something like a filled doughnut with an outer fibrous covering called the anulus and an inner gelatin-like substance called the nucleus pulposus. The whole disk does not slip. The words bulging or protruding are more accurate than slipped. In some people, the anulus can crack or tear, thus allowing some of the nucleus pulposus material to escape. The bulging material can cause compression of nearby nerve tissue and lead to pain and, occasionally, some loss of function.

Spinal degeneration means that there is a change in some of the disk and joint components of the spine. As a result of this degeneration, disks lose height and become less flexible, possibly increasing the chance for disk herniation. Each spinal vertebra has a supporting joint (called a facet joint) with the adjacent vertebra. These facet joints may develop degenerative changes and osteoarthritis (referred to by journalists and the general public as arthritis), which is similar to osteoarthritis in other joints (for example, knees and hips) of the body. A moderate degree of spinal degeneration is normal in all of us as we age. For most people, these changes do not lead to pain or other symptoms.

Question #2: Doctor, what can I do to ease the low back pain I got after working in the yard last weekend?

Low back pain like yours typically is caused by injury to muscles or other soft tissues in and around the spine that were overworked, pulled, or stretched. Often the problem was not caused by a single, sudden action, but by a slow accumulation of minor tissue damage. Some symptoms, such as moderate to severe pain, numbness or weakness in the legs, or problems with bladder or bowel control, which are related to pain in the low back region, indicate the need to obtain immediate medical attention. If these symptoms are absent, there is a very strong likelihood that your problem will get better in a few weeks, as long as you are patient and use common sense.

You can try several things to help the recovery process. It is useful to reduce strenuous activity for several days. If your pain is really bad, you may want to spend 1 or 2 days in bed. However, more than 2 days of bed rest may actually slow your recovery. Try to find a comfortable resting position. Many people lie on their side or on their back with a pillow under their legs. Some people get relief from the application of ice or heat to the low back. In either case, you should be careful not to get the skin too cold or too hot, and not to use the treatment continuously. Mild pain medications, either over-the-counter or prescription, may be helpful for a few days. To the best of your ability, continue your normal daily activities as soon as possible. This will not be harmful, even if you experience some mild discomfort. Gradually resume more strenuous activities in about a week. At this time, with your current history, you do not need X-rays or other diagnostic tests.

Once you recover from this low back pain episode, you may wish to learn more about an exercise program to help you gain strength and flexibility of the spine, as well as a general fitness program. You can get further advice from medical-care providers experienced in informing people about these exercises and demonstrating proper methods for doing them. Such a prevention program may make you feel better and help you avoid another severe bout of low back pain.

Question #3: Doctor, what are the best diagnostic tests for my low back pain that has lasted for 1 month?

First, you should have a thorough history and physical examination by a qualified physician. Some conditions may appear similar to low back pain arising from the disks and supporting structures of the spine and, therefore, require special tests if suspected by your physician. An X-ray or other tests may be ordered to rule out these related conditions. The exact nature of your pain (for example, constant versus activity dependent) and the presence of leg pain in addition to back pain will guide the selection of diagnostic tests. It is not necessarily valuable to obtain a magnetic resonance imaging (MRI) test at this time. Scientific studies have shown that many people with no symptoms of any back pain have abnormalities on MRI. Even though your pain has lasted for 1 month, there is a very good chance that you will recover without surgery.

Question #4: Doctor, what can I do about my low back that "goes out" every few months?

Low back pain that periodically recurs is a common problem. It is encouraging that you do not report a continuous level of significant pain. You may have an underlying weakness in the spinal muscles or any of the tissues that make up the spine. If your pain persists beyond 6 weeks you should seek competent medical advice. The severity and distribution of pain will determine whether diagnostic tests are required. For many people no testing will be required.

If the episodes of pain occur after specific activities, it makes sense to avoid or modify the way you perform those activities. For example, carrying heavy objects close to your body, using your legs to assist in lifting objects, avoiding forward bending for long periods of time, and taking breaks every hour or so when driving on a trip are some commonly recommended ways to avoid excessive loading of the spine. Many people have lessened the risk of repeated episodes of low back pain by participating in a well-defined program of stretching, strengthening, and general fitness. Giving up smoking and losing weight are valuable for many individuals.

Question #5: Doctor, should I have a disk operation for the pain in my lower back and right leg that has lasted for the past 3 months?

It is important to know that many people with your condition gradually improve with time and function very well. Some of the medical criteria for consideration of surgery include (1) a specific pattern of pain going down into the leg; (2) confirmation of the anatomic abnormality by specialized radiology tests, such as magnetic resonance imaging (MRI) or computed tomography (CT); and (3) severe and persistent levels of pain. Surgery for your condition is more likely to reduce leg pain than it is to reduce back pain. It is impossible to guarantee that your back will be cured forever. You are at some degree of risk for a return of the original problem or development of a similar condition in another portion of the spine.

You are actually the decision maker. Is the pain impairing your life to the point where you are willing to accept the risks of surgery in order to significantly decrease your pain? Your doctor can explain the likely outcome and risks of surgery.

Question #6: Doctor, should I consider microsurgery for my herniated disk? Does it work? Are there other types of back surgery?

Many people with a herniated disk improve without surgery. Only a minority need any type of surgical procedure. Comprehensive medical examinations should be able to provide a high degree of certainty that a herniated disk is the underlying cause of your pain. Surgery is more likely to relieve leg pain than to relieve back pain. Even with the best of surgical procedures, you will have some risk of recurrence of a disk herniation at or near the site of the original surgery. You should discuss all of the benefits and risks of surgery with your physician and take an active role in the decision whether to have disk surgery or to further pursue nonsurgical treatment.

Microsurgery is similar to traditional surgery for removal of herniated disk material. A smaller incision is made, and the surgeon operates using the aid of a magnifying device to guide the procedure. Not all disk problems can be treated with microsurgery. Both traditional and microsurgery are highly successful when performed on a carefully selected patient. Each procedure has some advantages and disadvantages as compared to the other. Most physicians recommend a post-surgical program to strengthen your back and improve your general fitness.

Several newer procedures that use arthroscopic and other techniques have been under clinical investigation for the past several years. None of these alternative approaches has yet been proven to be equal to traditional surgery or microsurgery.

Index